REGENTS/PRENTICE HALL
TEXTBOOK OF
COSMETOLOGY

THIRD EDITION

MARY HEALY

with a special contribution from
M. Lyal McCaig

REGENTS/PRENTICE HALL
Englewood Cliffs, New Jersey 07632

Library of Congress Cataloging-in-Publication Data

Healy, Mary.
    Regents/Prentice Hall textbook of cosmetology / Mary Healy, --
3rd ed.
      p. cm.
    Rev. ed. of: The Prentice-Hall textbook of cosmetology. 2nd ed.
c1984.
    Includes index.
    ISBN 0-13-690009-7. -- ISBN 0-13-689712-6 (pbk.)
    1. Beauty culture.   I. Prentice-Hall textbook of cosmetology.
II. Title
TT957.H43 1993
646.7'2--dc20   92-46324
                                              CIP

Editorial/production supervision: Kathryn Kasturas
Acquisitions Editor: Elizabeth Sugg
Cover photo/concept: Reginald Wickham/Marianne Frasco
Manufacturing buyer: Ed O'Dougherty
Prepress buyer: Ilene Sanford
Editorial Assistant: Maria Klimek
Page layout: Laura Ierardi
Interior design: Circa 86
Photographer: Michael Gallitelli
Illustrators: Shizuko Horii and Robert Richards
Figures 2.10, 2.11, 2.12, 6.3 courtesy of David Scharf
Figures 2.16, 2.17, 2.18, 2.19, courtesy of Southern Illinois University School
   of Medicine, Division of Plastic Surgery
Figures 6.1, 6.2, 6.7, 6.9, 16.2, 16.3 courtesy of The Wella Corporation, Englewood, NJ
Special thanks to Business Media Resources (New York Office) for their valiant efforts,
   and the administrators and students at the New York International Beauty School, Ltd.

© 1993, 1984, 1976 by REGENTS/PRENTICE HALL
A Division of Simon & Schuster
Englewood Cliffs, New Jersey 07632

Printed in the United States of America

10 9 8 7 6 5 4 3

ISBN 0-13-690009-7 (C)

ISBN 0-13-689712-6 (PBK)

Prentice-Hall International (UK) Limited, *London*
Prentice-Hall of Australia Pty. Limited, *Sydney*
Prentice-Hall Canada Inc., *Toronto*
Prentice-Hall Hispanoamericana, S.A., *Mexico*
Prentice-Hall of India Private Limited, *New Delhi*
Prentice-Hall of Japan, Inc., *Tokyo*
Simon & Schuster Asia Pte. Ltd., *Singapore*
Editora Prentice-Hall do Brasil, Ltda., *Rio de Janeiro*

To past cosmetologists whose mentoring
has created the excitement of today's profession,
and to future stylists who will carry the industry
to even greater heights

CONTENTS

CHAPTER 1

THE LOOK YOU LIKE 1

CHAPTER 2

SKIN, HAIR, AND NAILS 21

CHAPTER 3

ANATOMY AND PHYSIOLOGY 43

CHAPTER 4

BACTERIOLOGY AND INFECTION CONTROL 65

CHAPTER 5

SHAMPOOS AND RINSES 81

CHAPTER 9

PRECISION HAIRCUTTING 163

CHAPTER 10

WET HAIRSTYLING 175

CHAPTER 11

THERMAL HAIRSTYLING 207

CHAPTER 12

WIGS AND HAIRPIECES 227

CHAPTER 13

CHEMISTRY FOR COSMETOLOGISTS 243

CHAPTER 14

HAIR COLORING 267

CHAPTER 15

HAIR LIGHTENING 301

CHAPTER 16

CHEMICAL WAVING 329

CHAPTER 17

CHEMICAL RELAXING 359

CHAPTER 18

SKIN CARE 375

CHAPTER 19

MAKEUP 395

CHAPTER 22

ELECTRICITY 449

CHAPTER 23

HEAT AND LIGHT 463

CHAPTER 24

BUILDING YOUR SALON SUCCESS 475

PREFACE

TO THE INSTRUCTOR

The third edition of the **Regents/Prentice Hall Textbook of Cosmetology** provides you with the optimal instructional tool for teaching basic concepts and services. In preparing this edition, we identified the present state of the industry relating to licensure requirements and job skills salon employers need their entry-level employees to possess. From this analysis, a list of competencies required for a successful career in cosmetology was developed.

Cosmetology is a demanding field, requiring artistic, technical, entrepreneurial, and communication skills. In the technical areas, we considered the changes that have shaped the industry since the second edition and the trends forecast for the future. All of the chemical services areas were completely revised with current procedures and new safety precautions. This edition is the first cosmetology text to approach hair coloring in a comprehensive manner and include the industry's system of level. Chapters for nail technicians and estheticians were completely reworked to include the latest technologies.

As chapters were developed, they were reviewed carefully by instructors, practicing technicians, and trainers for product manufacturers. The content was analyzed against licensing criteria to ensure that requirements were met and exceeded in the United States and Canada. We gave special attention to how easily these materials are used in the classroom.

The approach to artistic development in the **Regents/Prentice Hall Textbook of Cosmetology** is an exciting one. The all-new chapter *Elements and Principles of Design* written by expert Lyal McCaig, demystifies design and instructs budding cosmetologists in how they can creatively enhance their work. The artistic concepts in the chapter are reinforced throughout the text and applied through the chapter projects.

Chapter 24, *Building Your Salon Success*, details the communication skills, the people skills, and the marketing skills vital to a career in today's salon. Real-life job performances assess students' abilities to meet the expectations demanded of today's successful cosmetologist. Client Tips showcase personal and business skills for success in a sales environment.

Performance Goals for skill development are described in the Career Focus beginning each chapter of the new edition. Key Points capture the main idea of each major section, and help you ensure that learning objectives are met. Each competency is reinforced in the Summary and skill level can be assessed by having students complete the chapter's Projects. Safety Precautions are stressed throughout.

The textbook was prepared for the learning tendencies of visually-oriented students. Every procedural step is heavily illustrated. Key terms are introduced in boldface type, spelled phonetically, and defined. Emphasis is placed on problem-solving and thinking skills rather than on rote and recall. Full-color photographs and illustrations detail technique from the perspective of the student in relation to his or her client.

To assist your successful use of the third edition of the **Regents/Prentice Hall Textbook of Cosmetology**, a wide array of supplemental materials are available for you and your students.

TO THE STUDENT

Welcome to the exciting world of cosmetology! You have selected a demanding career field; but one that offers unlimited opportunity to express your creative abilities.

The first step is to become adept at the skills that will serve as the basis for your chosen career. Each chapter in this book will start with a Career Focus. You will receive some background on the history of each area of cosmetology, and more importantly, you will identify the job skills you must master in order to be successful in today's salon. Work with your instructor until you have mastered each Key Point and completed the Projects assigned.

Your instructor is the first link in a network of mentors that will help you find your niche in this stimulating industry. As your network grows you will advance along your career path, prepare for your licensure examination, and begin your salon internship. There you will apply your client skills and demonstrate your proficiency in the art of cosmetology. There you will learn and grow as you choose the services that appeal to you the most; you will establish your career goals.

You have chosen a people-based industry, and you will touch the lives of those with whom you work and upon whom you practice your skills. We at Regents/Prentice Hall congratulate you for selecting cosmetology and wish you the best of luck in your career.

ACKNOWLEDGMENTS

The **Regents/Prentice Hall Textbook of Cosmetology** is the result of a joint effort and an exchange of information from top professional educators and technicians. Recognition is noted for the author team of the first edition, who established the line: Olive P. Scott, Mary G. Callahan, Rose Marie Faulkner, Margaret-Lee Jenkins, Gregory J. Nunz, Sallie Ponce-Hantz, and Wanda Sterner. In the second edition, contributions by Peter Green in the sections on haircutting and styling are noted.

For this third edition, we recognize the special contribution of M. Lyal McCaig for Chapter 7, *Elements and Principles of Design*. Special thanks to Lyal for his additional reviews and input into the quality of the overall text.

We extend our thanks to the following people for their input on the third edition of the **Regents/Prentice Hall Textbook of Cosmetology**:

Morelia Anguiano
   National Career Institute
   Harlingen, TX

Barbara Azan
   K&K International
   New York, NY

Dr. Shirley Ballard
   Ballard Educational Technology Ltd
   Tampa, FL

Marianne Bernotsky
   Englewood Cliffs, NJ

Susan Braddock
   Braddock Dermatology Clinic
   Omaha, NE

Barbara Brant-Williams
   Hair To Die For Salon
   Charleston, SC

Rick Brown
   Academy of Hair Design
   Redding, CA

Johnnie M. Cohen
   NE Texas Community College
   Mt. Pleasant, TX

Leila Cohoon
   Independent College of
   Cosmetology
   Independence, MO

Michael Cole
   Salon Development Corporation
   St. Paul, MN

Brenda Curtis
   National Career Institute
   Independence, MO

Geraldine Dearborn
   Southwest Wisconsin Technical
   Institute
   Fennimore, WI

Michael B. Dick
   Santa Cruz Beauty School
   Santa Cruz, CA

Peggy Dietrick
   Texas State Board of Cosmetology
   Loredo, TX

Gail Donoway
   Potomac Academy of Hair Design
   Falls Church, VA

Don Estes
  Estes Institute of Cosmetology
  Visalia, CA

Aurie Gosnell
  South Carolina State Board of
  Cosmetology
  Aiken, SC

Linda Grant
  Arlington Academy of Beauty
  Culture
  Arlington Heights, IL

Mary Ann Haley
  Solano College
  Suisun, CA

Juanita Harris
  International Beauty Enterprises,
  Inc.
  Lancaster, PA

Carmen Hathaway
  Origi-Nails
  Arlington, TX

Marina de Haydu
  Christine Valmy
  New York, NY

Robert Herlth
  Maryland State Board of
  Cosmetology
  Baltimore, MD

Emmett Hickey
  Origi-Nails
  Arlington, TX

Mary Justman
  Bauder College
  Atlanta, GA

Cher Kelly
  Vogue College of Cosmetology
  Austin, TX

Kenneth Kolle
  Pasadena City College
  Pasadena, CA

Karen Lessler
  National Nail Technicians Group
  Huntington, NY

Evelyn Lockett
  Sheridan VoTech
  Hollywood, FL

Brenda Longhofer
  Roy's of Louisville Beauty Academy
  Louisville, KY

Nelle Lorick
  Southeast College of Beauty Culture
  Charlotte, NC

Charles Lynch
  International Beauty Enterprises,
  Inc.
  Lancaster, PA

Florence March
  Academies of Cosmetology
  Ft. Pierce, FL

Brenda Massey
  JC Penny
  Dallas, TX

M. Lyal McCaig
  Capital School of Hairstyling
  Omaha, NE

Dorothy McKinley-Sorressi
  NY International Beauty School, Ltd
  Queens, NY

Carol McSheffery
  Jhurab Salon
  Hartford, CT

Michael Megna
  Backscratchers
  Sacramento, CA

Ada Menzies
  The Finishing Touch
  Boulder, CO

Loretta Montgomery
  Alaion Products, Inc.
  Chicago,IL

Mary Murphy-Martin
  Birmingham, AL

Carey Nash
  Marinello School of Beauty
  Whittier, CA

Michele Nicoletti
  Flushing, NY

Pat Nix
  Indiana State Board of Cosmetology
  Boonville, IN

Noelle the Day Spa
  Stamford, CT

Pat Oberhausen
  West Columbia, SC

James O'Neall
  Jim's Beauty Studio
  Pochohantas, IA

Penny Parker
  Matrix Essentials, Inc.
  Solon, OH

Ralph Payne
  JC Penny
  Plano, TX

Nancy Phillips
  Lakeland College
  Mattoon, IL

Michael Privette
  Ft. Pierce Beauty Academy
  Ft. Pierce, FL

Cheryl Raty
  Solano Community College
  Suisun, CA

Art Resso
Continental School of Beauty
Culture
Rochester, NY

Richard Rosenburg
RBR Productions, Inc.
Teaneck, NJ

Tom Ross
Ohio State Board of Cosmetology
Columbus, OH

John Saffa
New York International Beauty
School Ltd.
Flushing, NY

Mike Salamone
Westchester School of Beauty
Culture
Mt. Vernon, NY

Sue Sansom
Arizona State Board of Cosmetology
Phoenix, AZ

David Scharf
Los Angeles, CA

George Schaub
International Beauty Enterprises,
Inc.
Lancaster, PA

Christine Schumann
Barcelona Hair Center
Toms River, NJ

Brian Smith
L'Oreal Professional Salon Products
New York, NY

Jo Ann Stowers
National Assessment Institute
Clearwater, FL

Alma Tilghman
National Interstate Council of State
Boards of Cosmetology, Inc.
Beaufort, NC

Veda Traylor
Arkansas State Board of
Cosmetology
Mayflower, AK

Vinny Troiano
Hair Design Institute
Brooklyn, NY

Charlene Van Orden
Arizona State Board of Cosmetology
Phoenix, AZ

Gerald Varkas
North Park College
San Diego, CA

Pat Wake
Ocean County Vo-Tech
Jackson, NJ

Sandra E. Webb
Classic Beauty Colleges
Phoenix, AZ

Wig Discount Center
Flushing, NY

Lois Wiskur
South Dakota State Board of
Cosmetology
Pierre, SD

Elvin G. Zook, M.D.
Southern Illinois University, School
of Medicine
Springfield, IL

THE LOOK YOU LIKE

CHAPTER GOAL

Your appearance and personality will help you establish yourself as a professional and successful cosmetologist. After reading this chapter and completing the projects, you should be able to

1. Outline the importance of self-analysis.
2. Explain the importance of color and demonstrate color analysis.
3. List the guidelines of good grooming for the successful cosmetologist.
4. Demonstrate the posture a cosmetologist should have to avoid muscle aches and back strain.
5. Explain the key elements of wardrobe planning.
6. Describe the personality traits necessary for success in the personal service industry.

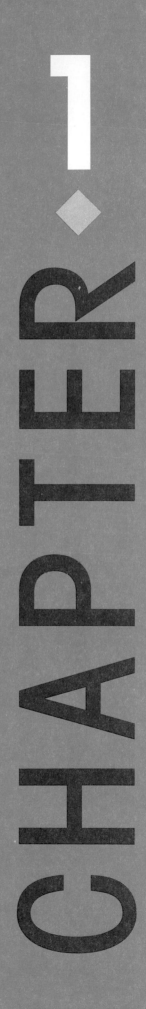

CHAPTER ◆ 1

The industry of cosmetology has developed over many centuries. It started as a duty performed by slaves or servants to the very wealthy. Then, in the Middle Ages, individual artisans began passing along their particular skills. Guilds were formed as a training ground for apprentices and as a source of further information for the practicing artisan. By the time of the Renaissance, independent shops were established. Even though services were still only available to royalty and the very wealthy, the industry of cosmetology had begun.

In this country, cosmetology also began as a household function to the wealthy. The first recorded establishment available to the general public was opened by a freed slave after the Civil War. Once services were available for a fee, hair artisans developed styles that did not require upkeep every day. America became noted for individual styling and avant-garde trends such as the Gibson, and later the Flapper.

To begin your career in the cosmetology industry, first create your own unique look. Improving your own personal appearance will help you develop the skills and techniques to enhance the appearance of others. By analyzing your own wardrobe and color suitability, you will learn the skills to assist your clients. Improving your posture will help you perform your duties without injury or strain. You will soon be on your way to an exciting career in the billion-dollar beauty industry!

SELF-ANALYSIS

Do you see an old or a young woman in Figure 1.1? It depends on how you look at things. Every day we make many observations. Often in our hurry we base decisions on what we think we see.

To carry out self-analysis successfully, you must try to look at yourself as you would look at a stranger. This is difficult to do. It is much easier to be objective when you are evaluating another person. Use a mirror, a tape measure, a scale, and a recent photograph to evaluate yourself as others see you.

The next step is to try to help this "stranger" identify her or his best features and to determine where improvement is desirable. Bone structure and height are two of the physical characteristics that cannot be changed. We learn to live with them and to show them to their best advantage. Many things can be done with color, cosmetics, hairstyling, posture, diet, and wardrobe to correct irregularities and improve your appearance. Your attitude toward your appearance shows (see Figure 1.2)!

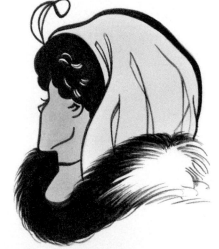

1.1

◆ Key Point ◆

One of the first skills a cosmetologist must develop is that of analysis. Train your eye to notice balance, line, and proportion.

COLOR

Color is a magic word. Surveys have shown that people respond to certain colors in general ways, and that factors in each person's life tend to make that person like or dislike specific colors. Your reasons for liking or disliking certain colors can be traced back to hereditary factors such as your skin tones, your eye color, and your natural hair color. In business and industry, color is used to stimulate efficiency, to quiet the nerves, or to encourage us to buy a product.

Color is organized by a number of systems that are used to explain the physical properties of color. The Newton theory, which is the oldest color theory, dates back to 1660. The color theories devised by Louis Prang (1824–1909), Albert H. Munsell (1858–1918), and Wilhelm Ostwald (1853–1932) are directed primarily at the professional artist and designer. One current-day system of color selection is called *The Color Key Program.**

This uncomplicated color theory was developed in 1950 by Robert Dorr, whose extensive professional background in designing and marketing color began in 1928. *The Color Key Program* is used by designers, artists, manufacturers, retailers, educators, photographers, and the average consumer as a lifetime color guide in selecting and combining color easily and effectively. (The discussion of *The Color Key Program* system of color selection that follows is reprinted with the permission of Color Key Corporation.)

There are many systems of color analysis. Some are based on the seasons of the year; others are divided into a cool series and a warm series. Your instructor can provide references for color analysis.

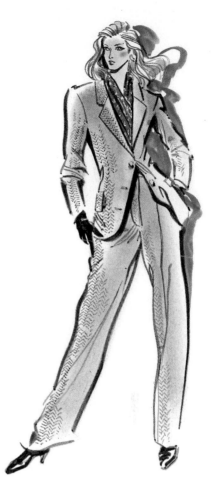

1.2

The Color Key Program

The Color Key Program system of color selection is based upon a scientific way of relating basic pigments of one color with those of another color. *The Color Key Program* system divides all of the colors of the spectrum into only two palettes. All the colors in one of the palettes are visually perfect for use in combination with one another. There are no neutral colors. *The Color Key* theory has been validated by the General Electric spectrophotometer, a device that records the amount of red, blue, yellow, black, and white in any color, whether it be a skin tone or house paint. The color of everything you see is made up of these three colors—red, blue, and yellow—plus black and white. Those colors that harmonize are related to one another in terms of the color pigment in their composition. For example, all red colors do not blend or harmonize, because some reds have yellow pigment in their composition while other reds are blended with blue pigment. All the blue-red colors harmonize regardless of how light

---

* *Color Key*®, and *The Color Key Program*® are registered trademarks of Color Key Corporation, a subsidiary of Grow Group, Inc.

KEY 1

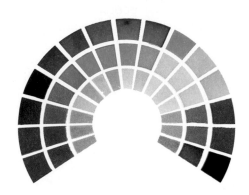

YOUR EYE COLORS

YOUR NATURAL MOST FLATTERING HAIR COLORS

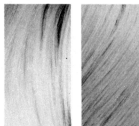 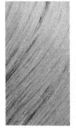 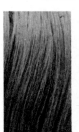 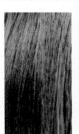 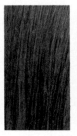 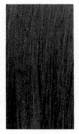  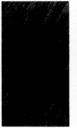 

YOUR BEST SKIN COLORS

KEY 2

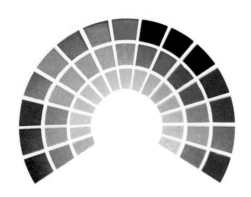

YOUR EYE COLORS

YOUR NATURAL MOST FLATTERING HAIR COLORS

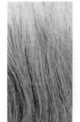 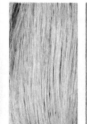 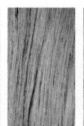 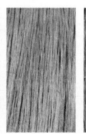 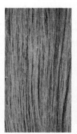  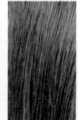  

YOUR BEST SKIN COLORS

 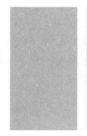      

THE COLOR KEY PROGRAM® SYSTEM

or dark the color is, and the same is true of the yellow-red shades. *The only mistake you can make in color selection is to combine colors from both palettes.*

It has been established, after testing hundreds of thousands of people over many years, that each person during the teenage years forms a choice of color pattern that remains the same throughout his or her lifetime. Professor Robert L. Beardmore, of California State Polytechnic University, Pomona, California, tested the *Color Key* theory scientifically for over a year to determine what made a person naturally choose the proper *Color Key* palette with 100 percent accuracy. He concluded that some people have a more rose-pink (blue) pigmentation, whereas other people have a more peach-pink (yellow) pigmentation. He also concluded that until an instrument is developed to measure and relate one's sight, brain function, and skin pigmentation, we must assume that a sixth sense leads a person to select the right *Color Key* palette. We all prefer, and are more comfortable with, certain groups of colors. Look at the *Color Key* chart on pages 4 and 5. You too will prefer one set of colors.

Colors in the palette you choose will be your most flattering colors because they are made of the same color proportions as your natural coloring. *The Color Key Program* works the same way for people of all skin colors. The correct *Color Key Palette* is determined by the undertone of the skin.

The Color Key Program in Relation to Your Skin, Eyes, and Hair

Any color analysis system can help you determine the best colors for you and your clients. The following guides will start your color education.

Skin Tones

Your skin tone, eye color, and natural hair color will appear in the *Color Key* palette you select. This means the selected palette will complement your skin, eye, and hair coloring. *The Color Key Program* system of colors works for all men and women. A rose-pink complexion indicates a *Key 1* person, whereas a peach-pink skin tone denotes a *Key 2* person. The undertone, not the darkness or lightness of the skin, indicates the appropriate *Color Key* palette. The blue undertone of the *Key 1* person gives the skin a smoky or umber cast, whereas the yellow undertone of a *Key 2* person gives the skin a golden cast. Your skin will darken (tan), lighten, and age in its own *Key*.

Eye Colors

Blue, brown, green, gray, or hazel eyes are found in both palettes. Eye color does not fade or change as do skin and hair colors. It remains the same from infancy or unless it is changed by disease or by the use of contact lenses. Bright blue eyes are found in *Key 1* and yellow-brown in *Key 2*. The different varieties of green, gray, and hazel eyes can be found in your own *Key*.

Hair Colors

Hair may be blonde, red, brown, black, or white in either palette. The undertone of the color determines the palette to which it belongs. The blue or ash undertones of the platinum, silver, and ash blondes are in *Key 1*; so are the smoky or ash undertones of the brunettes, the pink, purple, or wine undertones of the reds and auburns, the blue-blacks and jet-blacks, and the snow-whites and silver-whites. The golden undertones of the honey or golden blondes, the golden or rust undertones of the reds and auburns, the golden or red-gold undertones of the brunettes, the off-blacks, and the cream-whites belong to *Key 2*. When you gray, you will gray in your own *Key*—snow- or silver-white in *Key 1* and cream- or off-white in *Key 2*. When selecting a tint or rinse for a client, remember to select one in the person's own *Key*. Not every gray-haired or white-haired client needs a silver rinse. If the hair is *Color Key 2*, it may have a strong yellow undertone. If so, a rinse may be needed to eliminate the yellow undertone while maintaining a cream-white tone. Remember also to use *The Color Key Program* system of colors when selecting a wig for yourself or for a client.

Selecting Your *Color Key Palette*

Study the *Color Key* illustration on pages 4 and 5 carefully. You will notice pinks, reds, blues, greens, yellows, purples, browns, blacks, and whites in both palettes. Only two colors exist in just one *Key*. Magenta is found only in *Key 1*, and orange is present only in *Key 2*. Both palettes contain warm and cool colors, and both have clear as well as grayed shades. Notice the blue-pink in *Key 1* and the peach-pink in *Key 2*; the snow-white in *Key 1* (left-most hair sample on *Color Key*) and the cream-white in *Key 2* (left-most hair sample on *Color Key*); the jet black in *Key 1* and the charcoal-black in *Key 2*. Note how the models in the pictures harmonize with the colors surrounding them.

As you study *The Color Key Program* system of color selection, do not be influenced by any single color; make your choice instead on the entire group of colors in the *Key*. The choice of one palette does not mean that you dislike the other; it just means you like one group of colors better than the other. Have you decided which *Color Key* palette you prefer? Now look at yourself in a mirror. Can you identify your skin tones and your eye and hair color in the mirror? If you are still having trouble deciding, drape a bright orange towel or scarf (*Key 2*) around your shoulders and look back into the mirror. Now try a bright magenta towel or scarf (*Key 1*) and again look into the mirror. If the towel is in the wrong *Key*, all the wrinkles, shadows, blemishes, freckles, and other pigmentation defects in your skin will be more noticeable.

Now that you have chosen your most flattering colors, avoid using colors from the opposite palette.

Textures and Lighting

Textured materials such as leather, velvet, corduroy, satin, and certain types of paint may cause an article to appear lighter or darker than the *Color Key* sample you have selected. Daylight, at different times, and various types of artificial light will affect each texture differently. Colors may be somewhat grayer or darker in tone than the color sample and yet still be in the same *Key.*

Cosmetics

Selecting makeup of the right color is difficult for the cosmetologist or makeup artist. By using *The Color Key Program* system of color selection, the cosmetologist can determine a client's proper *Color Key* palette and then recommend the correct cosmetics. Foundation colors should match your client's skin tone. Generally, your client needs only two colors of foundation—a lighter one to match your client's skin tone in winter and a darker one for summer. You can mix the two shades for any color in between. (Other shades of foundation may be needed for corrective makeup. See Chapter 19.) Eyeliner, mascara, eyebrow makeup, and eye shadow should harmonize with hair coloring and eye color. Rouge, blushers, lipstick, and nail enamel should be selected according to the *Color Key* palette. The careful selection of lipstick and nail enamel will enhance the beauty of face and hands by complementing skin tones. This will also eliminate the need for changing the color of lipstick and nail enamel constantly as clothing changes, because all the colors in the same palette blend with one another.

Haircoloring

The *Color Key* approach can be a tremendous help to you in haircoloring. Both you and your client will look better, receive more compliments, and be happier with an artificial hair color if it is in the proper *Color Key* palette. The new hair color will also harmonize with makeup and wardrobe. Artificial hair colors in *Key 1* are harder to achieve than the *Key 2* colors because of the lifting (lightening) action of the haircoloring product on the natural pigment of the hair. However, it is possible to achieve *Key 1* colors by adding accent colors to the haircoloring formula. Your extra effort will be rewarded by increased business and client satisfaction.

Wardrobe

Have you ever wondered why some things in your wardrobe do not go together even when they are the same color? You may have a navy blue skirt in a *Key 1 Color* and a deep blue sweater in a *Key 2 Color.* The blues do not blend or harmonize because they are in different *Color Key* palettes. Check the colors in your wardrobe and you will probably find that at least 80 percent of your clothes will be in your *Color Key* palette. By using *The Color Key Program* system of color selection when choosing clothing to add to your wardrobe, you will increase its size considerably. Everything will blend together. Sweaters and jackets will blend with skirts and pants. Shoes will mix and match other articles in the wardrobe. What happens when you select a fabric with a pattern or design of some kind? Will all the colors in the pattern be in the same *Key*? Probably not, in many cases, but keep looking until you do find a fabric all in one *Key*. You will be much happier with your selection. Two wrongs do not make a right—the manufacturer may not have followed *The Color Key Program* system in designing a particular fabric, but this does not mean you have to buy it.

Grooming

Your personal grooming should be suited to your professional life and your leisure activities. Your hairstyle, accessories, and type of clothing will vary according to the formality of your various activities. Neatness and good taste are synonymous with being well groomed. You cannot have one without the other.

Because you are a cosmetologist, your friends, clients, and the public in general will expect you to lead the way in good grooming. Just as you would expect your dentist to keep his or her own teeth in good repair, your clients will expect you to set an example for them.

Some Basics of Good Grooming

Grooming is a habit that you should develop for your professional image.

Care of Yourself

1. Do you take a daily bath or shower? This is a must in order to prevent body odor (see Figure 1.3).
2. Use a **deodorant** or **antiperspirant** that is effective for you. Deodorants mask an odor. An antiperspirant swells the openings of the sweat glands on the surface of the skin. This swelling lasts for a few hours and stops wetness or at least lessens it. Antiperspirants are not harmful. When you stop perspiration in one area, you perspire more freely in another.
3. Perspiration stains should never show on your clothing. If your deodorant or antiperspirant is not effective, try another brand. Some people wear shields in their clothing and tee-shirts to eliminate perspiration stains.
4. Undergarments should be changed daily. Soiled undergarments can cause body odor that is offensive to the people you work with and the clients you serve.
5. Do you eat properly, exercise daily, and get the right amount of sleep? All this has an effect on how you feel and look. You cannot work at top performance unless you practice these three essentials.

Care of Your Mouth and Teeth

1. Brush your teeth twice a day (Figure 1.4), and use dental floss daily.
2. Use a mouthwash to clean the tongue, gums, and roof of the mouth and to sweeten the breath. Remember, "even your best friend won't tell you."
3. Visit your dentist every six months to make sure that your gums and teeth are healthy.

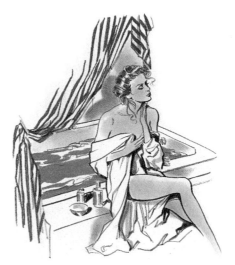

1.3

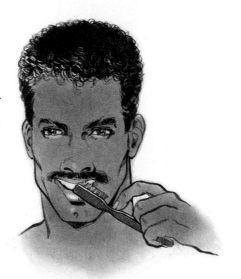

1.4

Care of Your Feet

1. Do your feet look abused and neglected? Shoes that are too small or that do not fit properly can cause calluses, corns, and bunions. You cannot look your best or perform your job well if your feet hurt.
2. Your work shoes are the most important shoes that you buy. Be sure they fit well and give your feet the support they need. Tired feet are usually caused by shoes that do not fit properly. Keep your feet happy by making sure all your shoes fit properly.
3. It is a good idea to have two pairs of work shoes, so you can alternate wearing them. Foot powder sprinkled in your shoes will help to keep them from smelling.
4. Your shoes must be clean and polished, and if laced, the laces should be clean. The heels should not be worn down. Worn heels are hard on your feet and damage your posture.
5. Change your stockings or socks daily. Always wear hose or socks with your work shoes. This will help protect your feet from blisters and calluses.
6. Socks should be free of holes and hose should be free of runs and snags. Have an extra pair of hose or stockings on hand. If you get a bad run, you can switch to your spare.

Removing Body Hair

1. Men should shave daily or twice a day (Figure 1.5) to avoid a "five o'clock shadow." If a beard or mustache is worn, it should be well trimmed.
2. Most women prefer to keep underarms and legs free of hair by shaving or by using a hair remover (Figure 1.6). (See Chapter 20 for a complete discussion of hair removal.) Underarms with hair can collect perspiration that causes an offensive odor.
3. Bleach can be used to lighten dark unwanted hair on the face and on the arms.
4. Eyebrows should be arched or penciled to complement your facial shape (see Figure 1.7 and Chapter 20 for details).

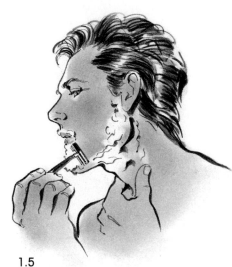

1.5

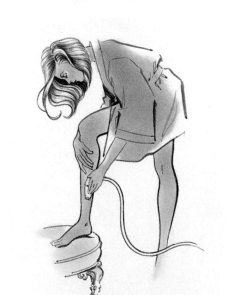

1.6

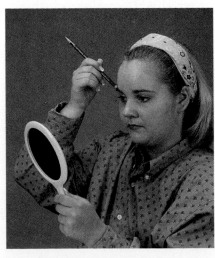

1.7

Skin Care and Cosmetics

1. A daily routine of skin care is a must for everyone. A good complexion is the background for an attractive face. If your skin is in bad condition because of acne, pimples, or blackheads, consult a dermatologist. Cleanliness is the beginning of a clear complexion. Different types of skin require different care (see Figures 1.8 through 1.11 and Chapters 2 and 18).
2. Keep your skin-care program simple, so that you will do it every day. Again, it is the daily care that counts.
3. Wear makeup that is appropriate for you and your job. (See Chapter 19 for a complete discussion of makeup application.)

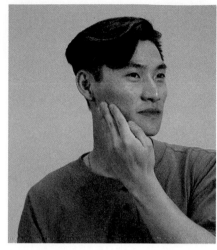

1.8

Care of Your Hair

1. A complimentary hairstyle will enhance your appearance. Select a hairstyle that is flattering to you and appropriate for your job. Be sure your hair will not look messy or unkempt while you are working. If you find you have this problem, select a style that is more suitable (see Chapter 9).
2. A light misting with hair spray or the use of a styling aid holds the style line and keeps hair in place (see Figure 1.12). Experiment with several brands until you find one that satisfies you. It is not necessary to "glue" your hair in place. Avoid using aerosol hair sprays with propellents that damage the environment.
3. Clean, healthy hair is an asset. Many people do not wash their hair often enough to keep it clean. Your hair must be properly cared for as well as shaped and styled for your individual features. (Consult Chapter 6 for hair treatments and conditioners designed to help various hair problems.)
4. If you use color on your hair, retouch it often enough so that the regrowth is not noticeable. (See Chapters 14 and 15 for a discussion of hair coloring.)

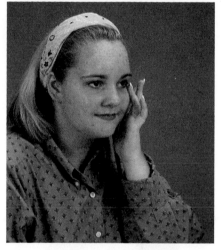

1.9

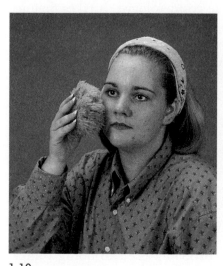

1.10

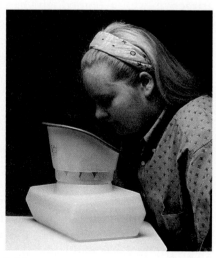

1.11

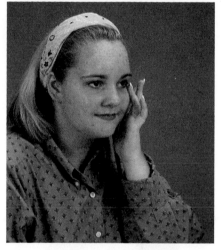

1.12

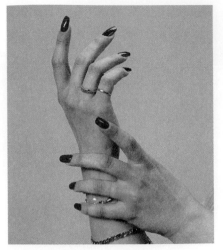

1.13

Nail and Hand Care

1. Be sure your hands look clean, neat, and attractive as in Figure 1.13. A cosmetologist's hands are abused constantly. Wear gloves whenever possible and use protective creams. Use a good hand cream or lotion before going to bed each night.
2. Nail biting is a nervous habit. Applying artificial nails may help you eliminate the habit. Regular manicures will keep your free-edge smooth and cuticles soft.
3. After your bath or shower, take a few moments to care for your cuticles by pushing them back gently with a terry towel.
4. Your nails should be well manicured. If you wear nail enamel or clear gloss, change or repair it whenever it becomes chipped. (See Chapter 21 for a complete discussion of nail care.)
5. Ingrown toenails are usually caused by cutting too deeply into the corners of the nails. Keep the nail slightly rounded or straight across the top.

Care of Your Clothing

1. Your clothes should be clean and pressed and free from perspiration odor. Dark clothes should be brushed and should be free of lint.
2. The clothing you wear should be suitable for your work. Both men and women should avoid low necklines.
3. Hang your clothes up after each wearing. Give them a chance to air out.
4. Your hemline should hang evenly and should not be held in place with safety pins. Mend or sew buttons on as soon as you notice that they are loose.
5. Women should not wear sleeveless dresses that reveal bra straps and slips. Check yourself in a full-length mirror before you leave the house to make sure everything is in order.
6. Keep your clothing free of dandruff flakes and fallen hair.

Self-discipline is required to realize your full potential as an attractive, well-groomed, and capable cosmetologist. It takes time to acquire the skills you will need. Your performance will improve with practice, just as athletes improve through rigorous training. Your approach to personal grooming should be adapted to fit your needs. Start where you are and with what you have and make something out of it.

POSTURE AND PROFESSIONAL BEHAVIOR

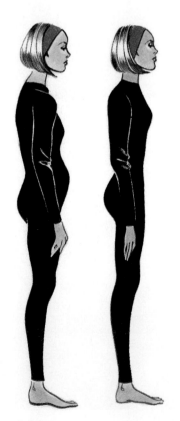

1.14

People judge you by the way you act, as well as by the way you look. The way you carry out simple activities—sitting, walking, and so forth—is important in presenting the best you. The following instructions on how to carry out these activities may seem a bit awkward at first, because you are probably used to doing things differently. A bit of practice will help you to perform them naturally.

Standing

The correct posture creates body alignment and balance (see Figure 1.14). To check your posture, stand with your back to a wall, with your feet slightly apart, and your heels about 3 inches from the wall. Now lean back. If your back, head, and shoulders all touch the wall at the same time, your back is straight, the way it should be. If you find this position uncomfortable, strengthen and straighten your back with exercises.

When standing, turn your body slightly to make the front view look slim and tall. A female cosmetologist should stand with forward foot pointed straight ahead, while the back foot should be at about a 45° angle to the front foot (see Figure 1.15). If you are male, you should stand with your feet spread about 12 inches apart. Your weight should be evenly distributed between the feet. Your knees should be slightly relaxed, never locked.

Walking

Walking should be a smooth, gliding, rhythmic action that conveys an air of ease and confidence. Your feet should move parallel to each other. Do not take too long a step or too short a step, and walk with as little noise as possible. Your shoulders should be relaxed so that the arms will swing easily, the palms of the hands facing inward. Your head should be held up.

You will climb stairs more confidently if your leg muscles are strong and your joints are limber (see Figure 1.16). Keep your back straight and your head up as you go up and down stairs. Place the entire foot on each step with your toes pointing straight ahead and with your legs as close together as possible. Push and lift with your thigh muscles as you go up each step. Glance at the stairs as you start down. Keep your weight on the back leg until the other foot is firmly placed on the step below. Point your toes out slightly, with one foot stepping directly in front of the other. Keep your legs close together.

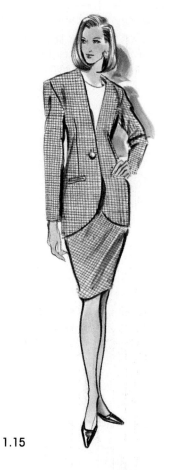

1.15

Sitting

Walk directly to the chair, turn around, and pause in your basic standing position. Touch the chair with the back of one leg, move one foot slightly under the chair, and sit down. Let the foot that is under the chair take most of your weight as you sit down, with your back straight, head up, and knees together. Do not back up to the chair and lead with the buttocks as you sit down.

Foot Positions While Sitting

1. Place your feet flat on the floor, one foot a little in front of the other, with the knees together. This is recommended when you are sitting in front of an audience.
2. Cross your ankles in front of you, one on top of the other. Now turn both feet to the left or right side and rest the weight on the foot that is on the floor (the bottom foot).

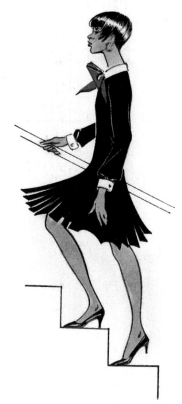

1.16

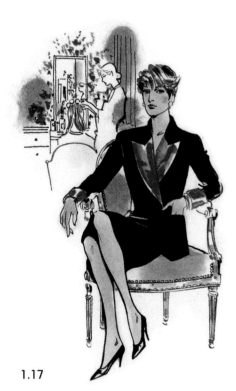

1.17

◆ **Key Point** ◆
Good posture will build your image as a professional cosmetologist and help you avoid strain and injury while working.

3. In order to sit comfortably, you may choose to cross your legs. As a woman, you should keep your legs close together all the way from the knee to the ankle. Point the toes of both feet toward the floor. Turn your body slightly to one side. As a man, you should sit comfortably with legs only slightly apart.

Hand Positions While Sitting

1. Hands may be cupped in your lap, fingertips of one hand in the palm of the other.
2. One elbow or hand may be placed on the armrest, the other resting on your lap or loosely in your pocket. Never place both elbows or both hands on the armrests at the same time (Figure 1.17).

Picking Things Up

If you bend or stoop improperly, you will display some of your most conspicuous features in the least flattering manner. The same technique should be used both for removing something from a drawer and for picking up something from the floor.

Stand directly beside the object you want to pick up or directly in front of a drawer. Place one foot in front of the other for balance. As you stoop to pick up the object, bend deeply at the knees, keeping the buttocks tucked under and the back straight. As you reach for the object, let one hand stop at your knee. Pick up the object (Figure 1.18) and return to a standing position using your thigh muscles to raise yourself. Heavy objects should be lifted with the legs, not the back.

Accessories

If you are right-handed, you probably carry your briefcase, backpack, handbag, umbrella, gloves, and other accessories with your left hand so that your right hand will be free. The points that follow refer to a right-handed person. Switch hands if you are left-handed.

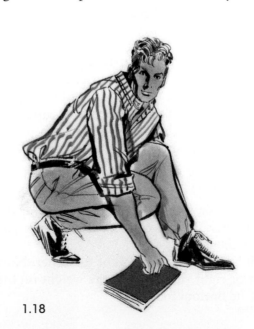

1.18

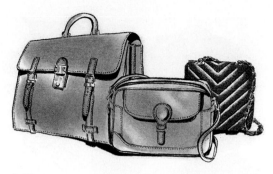

1.19

1. A handbag with a strap is carried on the left arm at waist height.
2. A briefcase or a clutch handbag is carried in the left hand. Do not carry handbags, packages, or magazines under your arm.
3. If you carry gloves, place the gloves together and fold the glove fingers in the palm of the left hand with the cuff (top) placed neatly over the outside of the hand.

WARDROBE PLANNING

Have you ever made the statement, "I haven't a thing to wear?" If you have, something is wrong with your wardrobe planning. A good wardrobe plan is one that fits your individual needs. You can gather ideas from books, magazines, and classes, but you alone can put together a plan that fits your needs. Your present wardrobe, your life style, and the money you have to spend on additional wardrobe items all affect your future wardrobe planning. You need a wardrobe tailored to fit your personal needs, with clothing suitable for all occasions.

Illusion

Your clothes should suit your life style and body type as well as the occasion. Lines can be used to create illusions or impressions. Your eyes tend to follow a line, and repeating the line gives it more emphasis. Vertical lines create height and make you look slimmer. Horizontal lines make you look shorter and heavier. Diagonal lines tend to slenderize, and curved lines suggest grace or movement.

Color is the magic word when planning your wardrobe. Determine your correct *Color Key* palette from *The Color Key Program* system of color selection and then use this to decide on a basic color for your wardrobe. In the past, basic colors have been black, brown, or navy blue. We have more freedom today in selecting a basic color.

The most expensive items, such as a coat, suit, shoes, and handbag should be in the basic color. As you add other items—skirts, pants, shirts, dresses, and accessories—select colors from your palette to harmonize with the basic wardrobe items. It is better to have only a few well-chosen items in your wardrobe than to have a closet filled with things you do not or cannot wear.

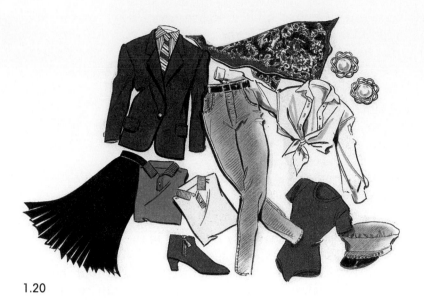

1.20

Clothing Inventory

A planned wardrobe is easier on your bank account. Hit-and-miss buying wastes money and results in a wardrobe that is never quite complete. Make an inventory of your clothes. Lay your garments out on a bed and sort them into three groups:

1. The clothes you will wear.
2. The clothes you will wear if they are altered or repaired.
3. The clothes you know you will not wear.

Start altering and repairing the clothing in group 2. If you are unable to do this yourself, find someone who can. Sell the clothing in group 3 or give it to your favorite charity. Make this inventory with your fall-and-winter, spring-and-summer, and year-round clothes.

Make a list of your wardrobe under various categories. Include what you can wear it with and where you can wear it. The list should include the following categories:

1. Coats and jackets.
2. Suits.
3. Dresses.
4. Skirts, blouses, sweaters, shirts, and slacks.
5. Bags and shoes.
6. Gloves and hats.
7. Scarves and ties.
8. Jewelry and accessories.
9. Lingerie and underwear.
10. Casual and sport clothing.
11. Miscellaneous (bathing suits, ski clothes, and so on).

You will probably find that you have more clothes than you thought you had. There will be some things that do not go with the rest of your wardrobe, probably because they are in the wrong *Color Key* palette. Some outfits need certain things to make them complete. You may find that you have too much of one type of clothing and not enough of another. You now have a shopping list to start with. Do not buy other items until your list has been completed.

Fashion

Clothing fashions change, just as hair fashions change. They change from the simple to the complex and back to the simple again. Skirt lengths and waistlines go up and down. Slacks have cuffs or are straight-legged. Fads come and go.

Read the newspapers and fashion magazines. Look in the better department stores and specialty shops to see what they are displaying. Avoid buying a lot of fad items that will not stay in fashion more than six months or a year.

Newspaper advertisements and magazines will tell you what is in fashion and what the fads are. The fashion magazines will give you an idea of what the fashion trends will be.

PERSONALITY DEVELOPMENT

As a cosmetologist, you will always be working around other people. Some will be your co-workers, the rest your clients. A pleasing personality is essential to success. Consumer surveys reveal that clients will leave a stylist because of a bad personality more often than they will leave for poor technical skills.

In order to be successful, you must develop your personality and your image as well as your technical abilities. Practice these skills now with your fellow students so you will have a pleasant school environment.

Self-Control

One of the first qualities you should develop is that of self-control. Learn to control your emotions so that you don't affect your associates with highs and lows. Try not to reveal your negative emotions such as anger, jealousy, envy, or dislike. Instead, develop methods of expressing what is troubling you without the emotional upheaval. Work to develop an even temper that treats your fellow students and teachers with respect.

Punctuality

A key personality trait of a successful stylist is a good sense of time. You will be working on a schedule and will not want to keep your clients waiting. Practice while in school by being on time and returning as scheduled from breaks and lunch.

Humor

A sense of humor will get you through many trying situations. Develop a pleasant demeanor by always smiling and greeting people pleasantly. Learn to see the lighter side of a difficult situation. This will help cushion disappointments and give you more pleasure out of life. The positive approach will make you a valued employee in any salon. Take yourself less seriously—laugh at those difficult situations and give it another try.

Good Manners

The manners that you have reflect how you think of others. "Please" and "thank you" are always in order. Address your teachers and your clients by *Ms.*, *Miss*, *Mrs.*, or *Mr.* rather than by their first names. Once your clients feel comfortable with you, they will ask that you use their first name, indicating that you have been accepted. Do not interrupt conversations until you have been asked to do so.

Annoying Mannerisms

Nervous habits should be caught as soon as possible and stopped. Do not drum your fingernails or tap your feet. This will annoy your fellow students and will make your future customers nervous. Gum chewing is never acceptable in the cosmetology school or salon. If you smoke, do so only in designated areas and never in front of a client; use mouthwash or breath mints so your breath will not offend others. Cover your mouth if you must cough, and your nose if you sneeze. Always turn away from others and excuse yourself.

Communication Skills

The cosmetology business involves one-on-one contact every day. Develop your ability to communicate so your can meet and greet clients easily. Be able to make conversation with them about their hair and skin-care needs. Convince them that you can perform the services that they desire in a pleasant and competent manner.

Telephone manners will also be important to you, both in the school and later in the salon. Learn to answer the phone more slowly, stating the name of your school. Greet the customer pleasantly and ask how you can be of help. Make a note of the customer's name before answering their question. Repeat back any information you have, such as the appointment just made. Make a note of the telephone number so a return call can be made if necessary. Always thank the customer for calling, no matter what the purpose for the call.

A key part of any good communication is the ability to listen. Start by practicing with other students. See if you can repeat back the main part of the story they just told you. Practice with each other so you can understand client requests. Always say something like, "So, you want to have your hair short in the back, but still full at the top. Did I understand you correctly?" Work with pictures so that you can assure your customer that you do understand and are going to give them what they want.

Keep your conversation in the school and salon professional. Avoid gossip at all times. Learn to study and to work together now so you can enjoy yourself in the close atmosphere of a salon. Practice conversations that center around the beauty business. Talk about current fashion, new products available in the school, a technique you have just mastered. You will find that newspapers and magazines are great sources of information.

Building a professional image begins with building a look you like. Analyze your appearance and learn how to minimize your least attractive features. Personal cleanliness is essential to protecting your image and preventing any offensive odors as you work closely with your clients. A pleasant personality will help you enjoy your school days and help you plan for a successful future in the salon.

Understanding color is necessary to be successful as a cosmetologist. Practice color analysis methods to determine the best colors for you to wear. Work with your fellow students to determine the makeup and hair colors that complement your skin and hair tones. This will help you develop the skills to analyze clients and suggest services as a professional. These same skills will help you develop your wardrobe for both your professional and your personal style.

The posture you develop will enhance your professional image while it helps you avoid fatigue and injury in the salon setting. Practice the basic ways of standing, sitting, and lifting so you can work comfortably through the day.

SUMMARY

QUESTIONS

1. Why is self-analysis important?
2. How is color important to the total look? How can you determine the best color to wear?
3. What effect do texture and lighting have on color?
4. What elements of good grooming are essential to be successful as a cosmetologist? Why is cleanliness important?
5. Describe the correct way to stand. How will good posture help you prevent injury on the job?
6. What are the key elements of wardrobe planning?
7. What personality traits are a successful cosmetologist likely to possess?
8. Which traits enhance your image as a professional?

PROJECTS

1. Make a chart of your five best features. List how you should wear your clothes, hair, and accessories to take advantage of the best features you have.
2. Practice color analysis on three different people. Determine the color tones they have in their skin and the best colors for them to wear.
3. Practice sitting, standing, and bending in cosmetology settings. For example, at the shampoo bowl, behind the styling chair, at the manicure table, and picking up a dropped comb.
4. Arrange your wardrobe by color. Hang each article separately and sort by color. Make up a wardrobe plan for a week with as few pieces as is practical.
5. Do a personality inventory of your best and worst traits. Make a plan to develop and perfect your best traits. List what you need to do to improve your personality.

SKIN, HAIR, AND NAILS

CHAPTER GOAL

A thorough understanding of the structure of the hair, skin, and nails is vital to your success as a cosmetologist. After reading this chapter and completing the projects, you should be able to

1. Explain the structure of the skin.
2. List the six main functions of the skin.
3. Name the divisions of the hair.
4. Describe the structure of the hair.
5. State the function of each structure of the hair.
6. Describe the structure of the nails.
7. List the nail conditions that can be treated in the cosmetology salon.

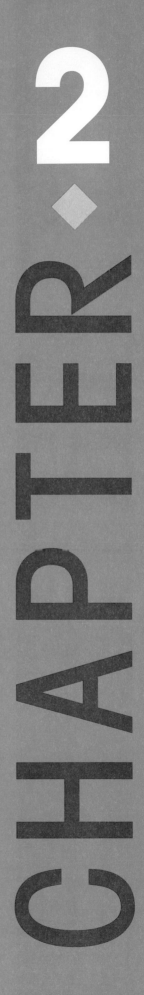

CHAPTER ◆ 2

The scientific study of hair, skin, and nails did not begin until the twentieth century. The discovery of the molecule-by-molecule breakdown of DNA by high-powered microscopes made it possible to study proteins.

Hair, skin, and nails are all made of protein. The closest protein to that of hair is wool. Fortunately, the wool industry has studied fibers in great detail in order to develop fabric that does not wrinkle, holds color better, etc. As a result, cosmetic scientists have been able to build detailed models of the skin, the nails, and the hair. While you do not intend to become a scientist, a thorough knowledge of the underlying structures of hair, skin, and nails will help you protect your client from harm and create the results you want.

Skin

The skin is very elastic, durable, and complex. It is the largest organ of the body. It wraps the adult body in about 20 square feet of tissue that weighs about 6 or 7 pounds. On the eyelids the skin is thinner than a page of this book, but on the soles of the feet it may be 1/4 inch thick.

The skin is frequently called "the mirror of the body." A healthy skin is usually a sign of overall good health. On the other hand, a serious illness often shows its presence first on the surface of the skin. The study of the structure, function, and diseases of the skin is **dermatology**. **Dermatologists** are doctors who specialize in the diagnosis and treatment of skin disorders. In diagnosing, they use **subjective symptoms** (the way the patient feels) and **objective symptoms** (the way the patient's skin looks.)

A cosmetologist's prime task is to help clients acquire and maintain a healthy, attractive skin, not to diagnose skin disorders. However, your training will make you aware of the objective symptoms of various skin disorders. If the condition is not serious, as in the case of dry or oily skin, you can suggest ways to control this condition. If you see evidence of a serious problem, you should recommend that your client see a dermatologist. You may later be able to help the client to follow the dermatologist's instructions or perform a treatment that the doctor has suggested.

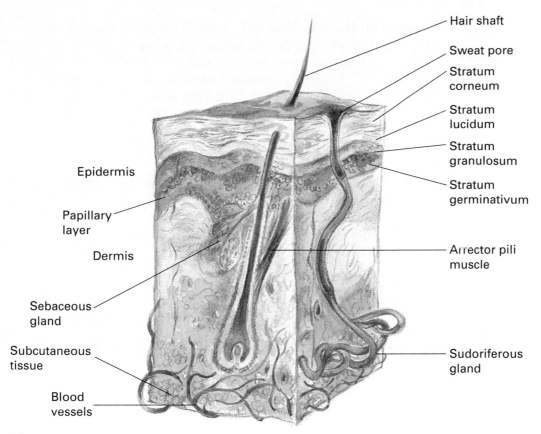

Hair shaft

Sweat pore

Stratum corneum

Stratum lucidum

Stratum granulosum

Stratum germinativum

Arrector pili muscle

Sudoriferous gland

Epidermis

Papillary layer

Dermis

Sebaceous gland

Subcutaneous tissue

Blood vessels

2.1

Structure of the Skin

The skin has two main divisions, an outer one called the **epidermis** (ep ih **DUR** mis) and an inner one called the **dermis** (see Figure 2.1). There is a third layer of **subcutaneous** (sub kyoo **TAY** nee us) fatty tissue. (*Subcutaneous* means "beneath the skin.")

The epidermis itself is divided into four distinct layers. These are, from top to bottom, the **cornified** layer, the **clear** layer, the **granular** layer, and the **germinative** layer.

The cornified layer (**stratum corneum**) (**STRAT** um **KOHR** nee um) is the surface layer of the skin. The cells in this layer contain a hard substance called **keratin**, and the entire surface is covered with a thin film of oil. This layer is very tough and nearly waterproof. The top-most cells are constantly being worn away and shed.

The clear layer (**stratum lucidum**) (**LOO** si dum) consists of a thin layer of small cells through which light can pass.

The granular layer (**stratum granulosum**) (gran yoo **LOH** sum) contains cells that are nearly dead. These cells look like granules and are moving toward the surface of the skin. They replace cells in the cornified layer that have been worn away.

The germinative layer (**stratum germinativum**) (jur mi nah **TIV** um) lies just above the dermis. In this layer, new cells are continually formed. Among these new cells can be found great numbers of special cells called **melanocytes** (**MEL** uh no seytes). These cells contain **melanin**, a brownish pigment that determines skin color.

People with fair skin have only a relatively small number of these cells, but dark skinned people have much greater numbers of them. People with little or no melanin suffer from a condition called albinism, which will be discussed later. Melanin protects the skin from the sun's ultraviolet rays. When the skin is exposed to sunlight, the melanocytes produce a greater amount of pigment for protection. This is what causes tanning.

The epidermis consists almost entirely of dead and dying cells. It has blood supply only in the deepest layer.

The **dermis**, or "true" skin, is made up of many interwoven fibers that form a tough, elastic network. In the dermis are found many nerves, glands, blood vessels, and hairs. This is the thickest part of the skin and is firmly attached to the epidermis. The dermis is divided into two distinct layers—the papillary layer and the reticular layer.

The **papillary** (pa **PIL** ah ry) **layer** gets its name from **papillae**, tiny fingerlike projections that anchor the dermis to the epidermis (see Figure 2.2). The papillae are well supplied with blood vessels and contain **tactile corpuscles**, the **sensory nerve endings** or **receptors** responsible for the sense of touch.

The **reticular** (re **TIK** u lar) **layer** contains a great variety of structures (see Figure 2.3). The sensory nerves that are sensitive to cold, heat, and pain are found in this layer. Oil glands and sweat glands, hair follicles, and blood vessels are also found here. The blood vessels in this layer supply the skin with oxygen and nutrients.

Subcutaneous tissue consists mainly of fat and serves as a cushion between the skin and the muscles. The fats help to keep the skin smooth and can be used for energy if necessary. When this layer shrinks as we grow older, it no longer can support our skin and keep it firm. The surface skin becomes loose, sags, and wrinkles develop.

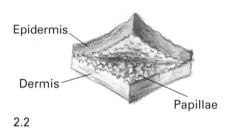

Epidermis

Dermis

Papillae

2.2

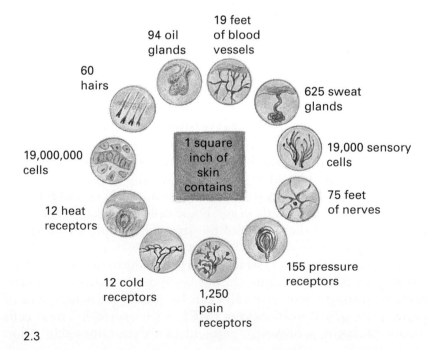

94 oil glands

19 feet of blood vessels

60 hairs

625 sweat glands

19,000,000 cells

1 square inch of skin contains

19,000 sensory cells

12 heat receptors

75 feet of nerves

12 cold receptors

1,250 pain receptors

155 pressure receptors

2.3

Functions of the Skin

The skin has a variety of functions. The most obvious one is to serve as an enclosure for all the other organs of the body. Other functions are temperature regulation, protection, absorption, sensation, secretion, and excretion.

Temperature Regulation

The normal temperature of the human body is 98.6°F. No matter how hot or cold the air is, the skin helps to keep the temperature of the body constant. When the cells of our body break down food, heat is produced. The blood carries this heat to the skin, where evaporation of sweat cools the body. In hot weather, the **sudoriferous** (soo dohr **IF** er us) **glands** (sweat glands) are very active, but in cold weather we sweat very little so that heat can be kept within the body. This function of the skin can affect your work as a cosmetologist. If you allow your client to sit for too long under a very warm hair dryer, that person's sweat glands will become overactive. When you take the set down, the moisture from your client's body will wet the hair, and your hairstyle will be a failure.

Protection

As we pointed out, the skin is very tough and waterproof. This helps the skin to protect the body from harmful bacteria and to prevent the absorption of many chemical substances. Many people are allergic to chemicals in certain cosmetics, and if these substances were able to penetrate the skin, the results could be serious. Because the skin also acts as a cushion, it protects the internal tissues from injuries.

Absorption

Although the skin is a protective covering, some substances can penetrate it in a limited way. Included in this group are such useful substances as topical medicines and some cosmetics, such as emollients and plant extracts.

Sensation

As mentioned in the previous section, the skin is well supplied with **sensory nerve endings** or **receptors** that convey messages to the brain and spinal cord. These nerve endings react to touch, heat, cold, pain, and pressure. The skin is the principal organ of the sense of touch. Sensations such as itching, tickling, and burning result when combinations of nerve endings are stimulated. Other nerves, called **motor nerves**, act on tiny **arrector pili** (a **REK** tohr **PEYE** leye) **muscles** that are attached to the hair **follicles**, the tubelike extensions through which hair reaches the surface of the body. This muscle can make your hair stand on end and can cause gooseflesh when you are chilled or frightened. The arrector pili muscle will be discussed in more detail in the section on the hair. A third type of nerve, the **secretory nerve**, affects the activity of the sweat and oil glands.

Secretion

The skin is well supplied with **sebaceous** (si **BAY** shus) **glands** (oil glands) that secrete oils that are vital to our skin. The function of secretion, then, refers to the oil glands, at least when we are speaking about the skin. (Other glands are also at work in our body, but these will be discussed in Chapter 3.) The oils secreted by the sebaceous glands lubricate the skin and keep it soft and pliable. They also soften our hair. A mixture of sweat and oil makes the surface of the skin slightly acid (see Chapter 13) and helps to keep bacteria from entering the body.

The oil gland itself is a tiny sac that secretes oil (really a fatty substance called **sebum**) through the hair follicles and onto the surface of the skin. All parts of the body are well supplied with oil glands, except for the palms and soles. Diet, hormones, and stress play a large part in determining the amount of sebum produced by the oil glands.

Excretion

Excretion refers to the removal of wastes from the body. As mentioned earlier, the **sudoriferous glands** excrete sweat as a means of keeping the body cool. Sweating also serves another purpose: Waste materials such as salt and other chemicals are removed from the body as sweat is produced.

The sudoriferous glands are composed of little coiled tubes that have their own tunnel, or **duct**, that runs to the surface of the skin and ends in what is called a **sweat pore**. These glands are numerous on the palms and soles, under the arms, and on the forehead, but they are also present on almost all parts of the body. The activity of sweat glands is controlled by the nervous system. These glands are functioning all the time in the elimination process, but they become most active when we are exercising and during warm weather. Certain drugs and emotional stress can also increase sweating.

Common Skin Problems

The following are skin problems that you should be able to recognize. Recommend the proper treatment so the condition is normalized.

Disorders of the Oil Glands

When the oil glands secrete too much or too little sebum, a variety of skin disorders can occur.

Acne occurs when the oil glands secrete too much sebum. During the teenage years, the oil glands become very active. When the pores that allow oil to reach the skin's surface become clogged, pimples can form. Sometimes these pimples go deep into the skin and can leave permanent scars. We usually think of acne as a facial condition, but it can also occur on the chest and back.

In teenagers, acne (acne simplex) is usually a temporary condition that can be helped in a variety of ways—careful cleansing of the skin, and using nongreasy cosmetics. Serious cases of acne (acne vulgaris) should be referred to an esthetician (a licensed skin specialist), or to a dermatologist.

> **◆ Key Point ◆**
>
> The skin serves as a protective barrier from the environment. It protects the body from outside temperature, senses heat, cold, pain, pressure, and touch, and prevents bacteria from entering the body.

Comedones (**KOM** ee donz), or **blackheads**, are clogged pores. Sebum hardens and forms a plug. Steaming the affected area usually helps to clear up this condition.

Milia (**MIL** ee uh), or **whiteheads**, result when sebum accumulates beneath the surface of the skin.

Steatoma (stee ah **TOH** mah), or **wen**, is a sebaceous cyst. This is actually a tumor or abnormal growth of the sebaceous glands that forms under the skin. Steatomas vary in size and look like smooth mounds.

Asteatosis (aye stee ah **TOH** sis) is a disorder that occurs most frequently in older people. The sebaceous glands secrete very little sebum, or sometimes none at all, and so the skin becomes very dry and scaly.

Seborrhea is a condition caused by overactivity of the sebaceous glands. The surface of the skin becomes very oily and shiny, and if the scalp is affected, the hair becomes very oily.

Disorders of the Sweat Glands

There are many disorders of the sweat glands. The most common disorders are discussed here.

Hyperhidrosis (heye per heye **DROH** sis) is a condition that is marked by abnormal sweating. Normally the sweat glands become very active in hot weather in order to keep the body cool. But some people sweat a great deal even in cool weather and when they are at rest. They should consult a physician.

Anidrosis (an heye **DROH** sis) occurs when the sweat glands stop functioning entirely. This may be caused by a fever or some other disorder. A doctor should be consulted if anidrosis occurs, because the body has lost its ability to regulate its temperature.

Bromidrosis or **body odor** refers to foul-smelling perspiration. Actually, perspiration itself has little or no odor. The problem is caused by bacterial action on the skin. Good grooming habits can help to control bromidrosis.

Miliaria rubra (mil ee **AYE** ree ah **ROOB** rah), or **prickly heat**, is caused by the inflammation of the skin around the sweat pores. It usually occurs in hot weather, appears in the form of small red pimples, and is accompanied by intense itching. This condition usually disappears when the weather becomes cooler. Various powders and lotions can provide temporary relief—baking soda works well.

Psoriasis

Psoriasis is one of the most common skin diseases. Its cause is unknown and there is no cure. It generally affects adults but can also appear in children. Most frequently it is confined to the scalp region, but it can affect the elbows, knees, and lower back. Psoriasis usually takes the form of red, slightly elevated lesions, or sores, covered by silver, crusty scales. Do not worry if your client has this problem. Psoriasis is not contagious, and you may work over it. The client needs to keep the lesions clean, and washing the area with shampoo will not harm it. If scales are not present, and the lesions

CLIENT TIP ◆◆◆◆◆◆◆

Always use protective base on sensitive skin areas prior to chemical services.

are not weeping, you may give a chemical treatment to the hair growing from that region. Harsh treatments can make psoriasis worse.

Eczema

The cause of eczema is unknown. It appears as dry or moist patches on the skin that can be mildly annoying or painfully irritating. Eczema should be treated only by a physician.

Allergies

People who have a severe physical reaction to a particular substance that has no effect whatsoever on most people are said to have an **allergy**. They are particularly sensitive to certain substances. The reaction may take the form of sneezing, breathing difficulties, itching, or rashes. **Cosmetic dermatitis** is the term used by dermatologists to describe allergic reactions caused by the application of cosmetics. Some chemicals will harm everyone's skin, but here we are discussing chemical agents that cause skin problems only in certain people. These substances are called **allergens**. **Hypoallergenic** cosmetics are as free of allergens as possible.

Mild cosmetics such as soap, hair spray, perfume, and other products that have an irritating effect on the skin only at the point of contact are called *weak* or **primary irritants**. When they are washed off, these substances cause no further reaction. One exception to this is nail hardeners and polish bases that prevent enamel from peeling for twice the normal time. Since the nail has no nerve supply, there is no sensation recorded when the symptoms of irritation begin. Since the irritation is not felt, the product is not removed and damage occurs. These substances penetrate the nail plate and could cause bleeding under the nail. The nail can also become temporarily deformed.

Strong or **secondary irritants** are chemical agents that cause serious skin eruptions—blisters, oozing sores, burning sensations. These substances are usually fairly alkaline (see Chapter 13). Some of the chemicals that make a permanent change in the structure of the hair—chemical curling and straightening products, hair dyes, lighteners, and depilatories—can be secondary irritants. If a client has sensitive skin, these chemicals may cause serious irritation and can even erode the hair and skin, especially if friction is applied. Other clients will have no reaction.

You should not hesitate to use professional products approved for salon services as long as you read package directions carefully. Always take adequate precautions to protect the client's skin and your own. Either you or your client may be allergic to a product. In the procedure sections of this book you will find lists of precautions to be taken in applying products that could irritate the skin. Study these lists carefully and follow them. You may save your client and yourself a lot of pain and expense.

Hair colors present the greatest danger of irritation. Therefore, the federal Food and Drug Administration requires that you apply a small amount of the haircoloring product to your client's skin (usually behind the ear) at least 24 hours prior to the haircoloring service. This is called a predisposition test, PD test, or patch test (see Chapter 14). Tints are formulated from as many as ten ingredients, and different manufacturers may use different chemicals. Therefore you must make a test application of the brand and color you are going to use for the haircoloring service. The skin test is not always reliable if the product is left on the skin only 24 hours before the general application, and some people may not react until the product is left on for twice as long. The reaction to hair dyes takes the form of blisters, swollen eyes and lips, and inflamed skin, accompanied by itching and redness. A client who reacts to a color application should be referred to a dermatologist.

Occasionally a client who has been using hair tints over a long period suddenly seems to become allergic. The client may experience itching, dryness, or some redness and scaling. Give a skin test behind the ear to determine if the cause is the haircoloring product. It may be that something other than the haircoloring product is causing the problem.

Tanning or Sunburn

Years ago a fair, untanned complexion was a status symbol. Laborers, farmers, and others who had to work long hours outdoors had tanned skin, but those who had well-paid indoor jobs kept their fair skin. Today the opposite is true. A tanned complexion generally indicates a life of leisure and luxury.

Exposure to the sun is not entirely harmful, but with the first warm days of summer we tend to spend too much time in the sun. The ultraviolet rays of the sun penetrate into the deeper layers of the epidermis or dermis, and if you are exposed too long, a severe case of sun poisoning, with chills and nausea, can result. Another result of overexposure to sunlight is dry, leatherlike skin. The cells responsible for the elasticity of the skin break down, and the skin becomes thin and wrinkled. Most importantly, because exposure to the sun increases the risk of skin cancer, it is wise to protect the skin as much as possible.

Until recently, suntanning products other than white zinc oxide offered no real protection. Now, however, more than 20 chemicals have been developed to prevent sunburn. These chemicals act by absorbing only the sun's harmful rays while allowing the sunbather to tan painlessly. The degree of protection is called the "sun protection factor" or SPF. The higher the SPF number, the more effective the product will be in screening out ultraviolet rays. A lotion or cream with an SPF of 15 or more should act as a near-total sun block and prevent all tanning. An SPF of 8 to 14 offers medium protection, while an SPF of 4 or less offers only a small amount of protection.

Pigmentation Defects and Wrinkles

Freckles, vitiligo, and chloasma are common pigmentation problems.

Freckles appear most often on fair skin, especially on the skin of redheads. These blotches of color result from a concentration of pigment in a small area.

Vitiligo (vit ih **LEYE** goh) is white blotches, usually on the arms and neck, which are caused by the absence of pigment. These stand out most clearly after exposure to sunlight, and there is little that can be done, except to avoid the sun and wear clothing that covers the affected area. Dermatolgists can treat this disorder.

Chloasma (kloh **AZ** mah) is dark spots on the face, and it usually makes its first appearance on the forehead around the hairline. The cause of chloasma is unknown, but the condition can be treated by an esthetician or a dermatologist.

Albinism is a hereditary condition that occurs in people with little or no pigment. Albinos have milky complexions, white hair, and pink or blue eyes with deep red pupils.

Wrinkles occur with age as the skin loses its elasticity. If these lines have a negative psychological effect, advise your client to see a dermatologist or plastic surgeon. While a doctor can recommend some medication to help preserve a youthful appearance, it should be pointed out that facial packs, masks, and cosmetic preparations do not remove wrinkles.

Cosmetic Surgery

Cosmetic surgery does not fall within the practice of the cosmetologist, but because your job is to enhance the attractiveness and beauty of your clients, you should be familiar with what the medical profession can do to help your clients.

Dermabrasion (dur mah **BRAYE** shun), or skin planing, is used for removing scars or acne pits from the skin. It does not remove the scars or pits entirely but makes them less noticeable by reducing their depth.

Skin peeling involves applying chemicals to the skin to dissolve or destroy the outer layer.

Facelifting is a surgical procedure performed by a plastic surgeon or dermatologist. It involves making an incision in the skin, pulling up the loose or wrinkled skin to tighten it, removing the excess, and then closing the incision.

Rhinoplasty (**RYE** noh plas tee) is surgery designed to improve the shape of the nose. It is usually carried out by a plastic surgeon or an ear, nose, and throat surgeon.

Hair

Hair is an appendage of the skin. Men and women have been concerned about their hair throughout history. Hair has always had great social significance, and even today some people will judge you by the length and style of your hair. Hair offers protection to your body, helps you to look attractive, and plays a big part in supporting the billion-dollar cosmetic industry of which you have decided to become a part. The scientific study of hair is called **trichology** (treye **KOHL** oh jee).

Think about the hair on your body. You have it on your head, unless you happen to be bald, but you also have it in a lot of other places. In fact, hair covers all parts of your body, except for the lips, palms and soles, and parts of the reproductive organs. You are probably not aware of the amount of hair you have unless it is growing in places where you do not want it.

Hair has a very practical purpose. In your nose and ears, it keeps foreign bodies from invading you. Under the arms and in the pubic area, it protects your body from friction. The hair on your head cushions you from blows and keeps your head warm in winter and cool in summer. Your eyebrows keep sweat from running into your eyes, and eyelashes shade the eyes and help to keep dust out.

Hair is composed mainly of a hard chemical substance called **keratin**. Earlier in this chapter we mentioned that this same substance is present in the topmost layer of the skin. Keratin, which is a protein, is also present in our nails and in the claws, feathers, hooves, and wool in animals. Hair contains varying amounts of **carbon**, **hydrogen**, **oxygen**, **nitrogen**, and **sulfur** (see Chapter 13). Light hair has more oxygen and sulfur, whereas dark hair has more carbon and hydrogen.

Structure and Divisions of Hair

There are two main divisions of the hair, one above the surface of the skin and one below it. The portion of the hair that we are usually most concerned about is called the hair **shaft**. This is the part of the hair that we see sticking out from the skin. The hair **root** is the portion that is below the skin.

The Hair Root

A variety of structures are connected with the hair root.

The hair **follicle** (**FOL** ih kel) is a tiny tubelike pit in the skin. The follicle is like a test tube that holds the hair root. Every hair on your body has its own follicle.

At the base of the follicle is the **papilla** (pah **PIL** ah). The papilla is deep in the dermal layer of the skin and is well supplied with the blood vessels and nerves.

The hair **bulb** lies just above the papilla and fits over it tightly. The bulb is wide at the base but gradually narrows as it approaches the surface of the skin. The hair bulb is nourished by the papilla.

The **arrector pili muscle**, which we mentioned earlier, is attached to the lower portion of the follicle. This muscle causes the hair to stand on end when we are chilled. One or more sebaceous (oil) glands are also attached to each follicle. The hair root and related structures are shown in Figure 2.4.

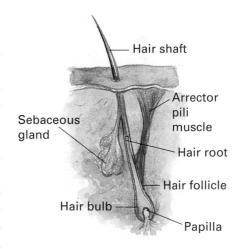

Hair shaft

Arrector pili muscle

Sebaceous gland

Hair root

Hair follicle

Hair bulb

Papilla

2.4

The Hair Shaft

We often think of a hair as something very small. We speak of missing something "by a hair's breadth"; when someone makes a fine distinction, we say he is "splitting hairs." In spite of this, each hair shaft is large enough to have several layers.

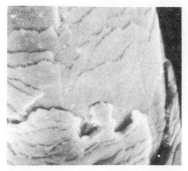

2.5

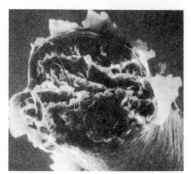

2.6

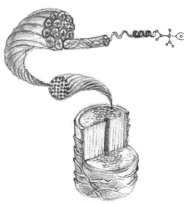

2.7

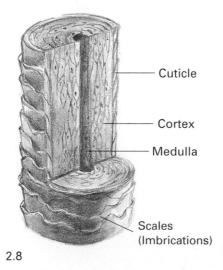

Cuticle

Cortex

Medulla

Scales
(Imbrications)

2.8

The outer layer or covering is called the **cuticle** (**KYOO** ti kul). This layer is composed of tiny, transparent, overlapping cells resembling the scales of a fish or the layers of shingles on the roof of a house. If you stack some paper drinking cups inside one another, the top edges of the cups would represent the cuticle layers as they overlap. This type of overlapping arrangement is called **imbrication** (im brah **KAYE** shun) (see Figure 2.5). The cuticle may or may not completely surround the hair shaft, and normally the imbrications lie flat and close together. They point toward the end of the hair shaft. They cannot be seen by the naked eye, but they can be felt. If you slide your fingers along a dry hair from the end of the shaft to the scalp, the hair will feel sticky or rough. You are sliding your fingers against the cuticle and are lifting the imbrications. Alkali chemicals (see Chapter 13) penetrate the cuticle and damage it to some extent. Thus, hair that has been color treated or chemically waved or relaxed will always feel rough.

Beneath the cuticle lies the **cortex** (**KOR** teks) (see Figure 2.6). The cortex is made up of fibers that coil in a **helix** (**HEE** liks), like the spiral on the back of your notebook. One tiny fiber, a microfibril, will coil around other fibers to make a large or macrofibril. These large fibers then coil around each other to create the cortex. Figure 2.7 shows how the hair develops from a single atom, to a single fiber that then coils until microfibrils, macrofibrils, and finally the cortex is formed. This spiral structure, much like a rope or yarn, makes the hair extremely strong and gives it elasticity. The cortex is the main section of the hair, and it is here that we find the **pigment granules** that give hair its color. When we change the natural color of hair, it is the color granules within the cortex that we change. The cortex also contains the structures that give hair its shape. This is the part of the hair that we affect when we style it. When we have a customer who has hair that is either too straight or too curly, we change the arrangement of elements within the cortex to either add or remove curl. When we apply strong chemicals to the hair shaft, we must use caution. Otherwise we can actually destroy the hair. As you can see, the cortex is the part of hair that the cosmetologist is most concerned about.

The innermost portion of the hair shaft is the **medulla** (mih **DUHL** ah). This is a small core of cells that can run from the hair bulb to the tip of the shaft. Sometimes the medulla is present only in the part of the hair that is below the skin. The medulla is very small in fine hair, and there may be no medulla at all in **lanugo hairs**, the soft, downy hairs that grow on the cheeks, arms, and other parts of the body. The medulla is not involved in cosmetology. Figure 2.8 shows a cross section of the hair shaft.

Forms of Hair

When we speak of the **form** of hair, we mean that it is **straight**, **wavy**, **curly**, or **extra curly**. The shape of the individual hair shaft is generally related to the form of the hair. Straight hairs are usually round, wavy hairs are oval, and curly and extra curly hairs are usually flat. These are only general rules, and there are many exceptions. The shape of the hair is probably due to genetic, or inherited, factors.

Characteristics of Hair

In describing hair, we usually speak of its texture, elasticity, porosity, and density.

The **texture** of hair may be coarse, medium, fine, or very fine. This is usually determined by the diameter of the hairs. Coarse hairs have a large diameter, while very fine hairs have a very small diameter. Another way of saying this is that coarse hairs are thick and fine hairs are thin. All four types of hair can be described as either soft or wiry, depending on how the hair feels. Wiry hair resists treatment, and so it takes longer to wave, tint, or lighten it.

Porosity (po **ROS** i tee) refers to the ability of the hair to absorb moisture. Hair that is very porous takes less time to treat than does less porous hair.

Elasticity refers to the ability of hair to stretch beyond its normal length and then spring back. Normal hair, when wet, can be stretched to about one and a half times its normal length. Dry hair is not so elastic. Dry hair will stretch about 20% of its length and return.

Density refers to the amount of hair per square inch on the scalp. The hair is said to be thin, medium, or thick, depending upon how much hair there is.

Hair Growth and Regeneration

Hair grows, falls out, and is replaced by new hairs. It might surprise you to learn that you normally lose 50–100 hairs a day. You probably have more than 100,000 hairs on your head, though, so you can afford to lose a few. Blondes may not have more fun, but they do have more hair—about 140,000 hairs on the average head. Redheads have the fewest hairs—about 100,000.

Hair growth is influenced by various factors: nourishment, season of the year, time of day, and location of the hair. Hair on the head grows faster than other body hair. It grows fastest in the summer, in daylight, and when properly nourished by the bloodstream. Scalp hair grows at the rate of about 1/2 inch per month. Race, age, and sex also determine the rate of hair growth.

How is the hair replaced? Scalp hair growth follows a cycle. The first stage, that of active hair growth, is called **anagen** (**AN** uh jen) (Figure 2.9a). During this phase, scalp hair continues to grow, anywhere from two to six years. At the end of anagen, hair growth slows during a transitional stage known as **catagen** (**CAT** uh jen). During this phase, the follicle shrinks, and the bulb thickens and slightly lifts from the papilla. The last phase of hair growth is known as **telogen** (**TEE** loh jen). This resting phase lasts about three months and ends when a new hair forming from the papilla pushes the old hair up and out (Figure 2.9b). As long as the papilla is intact and viable, the hair growth cycle is repeated over and over.

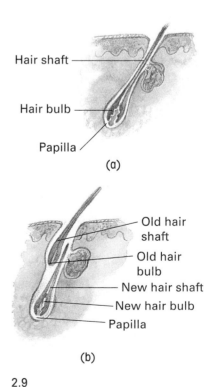

2.9

How Hair Changes as We Grow Older

It is important that cosmetologists understand that age affects the texture and behavior of hair. The hair of an infant is downy soft and differs greatly from the hair of our customers. During the first year of life, a child's hair may change in color, texture, and curl. The hair changes again when the baby teeth begin to fall out and are being replaced by permanent ones. This happens around the age of five or six. The hair changes in texture, and possibly also in color, and becomes very difficult to manage.

Mothers will often consult you about the style and care of the hair of children who are just beginning school because they want them to look their best. The hair may not take a chemical curl successfully unless the curl is very tight. Tight curls can cause problems for the mother and child because combing without pulling the hair is difficult. Stylish haircuts for both young boys and girls are more practical than chemical waving or relaxing.

During the teenage years, when a youngster is maturing sexually, the hair changes again. It frequently loses its resiliency and becomes softer and easier to manage. The texture itself may not change. During this period, teenagers begin to take a greater interest in grooming and in the care of their hair. A chemical wave to give the hair manageability or a chemical relaxer for extra curly hair may be appropriate. The hair will retain the same condition or texture throughout adult life until the graying process begins. At this point, coarse hair may become fine, or fine hair may gradually become coarser.

We do not have any clear explanation as to why these changes take place. We should be aware of them, though, so that we can recommend the proper treatment.

Disorders of the Hair and Scalp

Common disorders of the hair and scalp can be treated in the salon. You should be able to recognize disorders and recommend corrections.

Baldness and Falling Hair

Alopecia (al oh **PEE** shee ah) is the technical term for loss of hair. The four most common forms of hair loss are alopecia areata, pattern baldness, telogen effluvin, and traction baldness.

Alopecia areata (air ee **AH** tah) is a condition in which hair falls out in patches. The patches can vary from the size of a pea to several inches in diameter. There may be a few patches, or the entire scalp may be affected. Other hairy regions of the body can also be affected. There is usually no pain, itching, or inflammation. The hair usually regrows over a period of months, but the condition can recur. You may have a client with this type of baldness who is unaware of the condition if the patches are small. Recommend that the client see a dermatologist, who will probably examine the scalp and take some blood and urine samples. It may be that some physical disorder is causing the condition and that it can be treated with medicines. We should emphasize here that the hair and skin are not nourished by tonics, lights, or electrical stimulators applied by cosmetologists or at home. Do not try to treat this condition; you may worsen it. Other types of alopecia are listed in Table 2.1.

Pattern baldness occurs most frequently in males, but it can occur in females. The hair recedes from the hairline toward the back of the head and also becomes very thin and recedes in the crown area. The blame for this hair loss has been put on diet, drugs, stress, hormones, air pollution, radiation, hats, wigs, cosmetics, and beauty treatments in salons, but no definite cause has been found. Pattern baldness is just as common in tranquil villages where there is no contact with the outer world as it is in big cities; it is common in hot and cold climates and in overpopulated and underpopulated areas. The notion that baldness is inherited seems to be most valid. ("Inherited" here refers to units called genes passed on to us by our parents. These genes determine our hair and eye color, our facial features, and many other characteristics.)

Some women also are affected by pattern baldness. Gradual thinning of the hair can be noted as early as age 20, but usually it does not occur until much later. Women rarely become as bald as men do. The hair becomes thin but is not lost entirely.

Baldness can easily be concealed with a wig or hairpiece (see Chapter 12). In recent years a variety of techniques have been developed to aid in hair replacement. These include hair weaving, hair fusion, and hair transplanting.

Telogen effluvin (**TEL** oh gen ef **FLOO** vihn) is a very common type of hair loss during the resting stage. This type of hair loss is connected with the way hair grows. At any moment, only about 80 percent of the hairs on your head are growing; the other hairs are resting. Each hair grows for two to six years during what is called the **anagen** (**AN** uh jen) **phase**. During the **telogen phase**, which lasts about three months, the hair rests. After this period, the hair falls out. This process goes on all the time, and usually we are not aware of it. Certain conditions, such as childbirth, surgery, serious illness, and emotional stress, can cause a great many hairs to enter the resting stage at the same time. After a few months, all these hairs are shed at the same time, and there seems to be a great increase in hair loss. If an alarmed client comes to you with this problem, explain that this type of hair loss is only temporary and that most of the lost hairs will be replaced.

TABLE 2.1 Types of Alopecia

Technical Name	*Description*
Alopecia adnata	Complete or partial loss of hair shortly after birth
Alopecia follicularis	Loss of hair caused by inflammation of hair follicles, usually in a small area
Alopecia prematura	Loss of hair early in life
Alopecia senilis	Loss of hair in old age
Alopecia totalis	Loss of hair from the entire scalp
Alopecia universalis	Loss of hair from the entire body

Some experts have asserted that reduced circulation in the scalp area contributes to the loss of hair. If this is true, pinning the hair too tightly, as in a ponytail, especially in the case of young children, will tend to reduce circulation and will cause the hair to become thinned. Wigs that are too tight will also reduce circulation. In past years, fashionable hairstyles involved ratting and backcombing the hair, so that the style was protected without combing until the client's next visit to the salon. This type of style minimizes the scalp stimulation that combing and brushing provide.

Hair loss can also be caused by too much stress from pulling and is called **traction baldness**. Very tight braids, especially around the hairline, will cause this type of baldness. Hair that is finer in texture, especially children's hair, is especially prone to this type of baldness. The constant stretching of the hair can pull the hair fiber from the papilla prematurely and result in permanent hair loss.

You can feel whether a client has a tight scalp. If so, brushing and massage, properly performed, will relax the scalp muscles and increase circulation (see Chapter 17).

Superfluous or Excessive Hair

We have concerned ourselves with the loss of hair, but what about persons who have undesirable, superfluous, or excessive hair? **Hypertrichosis** (heye per tri **KOH** sis) refers to abnormal excessive hair growth. This term is not used to describe excessively thick hair on the scalp, which we refer to as density.

Women frequently develop excessive hair on the face, especially on the upper lip. This hair growth has been attributed to a decrease in the amount of the female sex hormone estrogen (see Chapter 3). Certain facial creams and hormones that can be taken orally or injected into the body also tend to produce hair growth on the face. If a client complains about this condition, you should suggest that she see a dermatologist. Certain people seem to be especially prone to the growth of facial hair. This is an inherited characteristic that shows up even in young girls.

There are several services that a cosmetologist can perform to alleviate this condition temporarily. Tweezers, waxes, and chemical depilatories are frequently employed in salons to remove excessive or unwanted hair (see Chapter 20). Shaving is another way of removing hair, perhaps the most common one. This service is usually not provided by cosmetologists but is more often used by the client at home.

The papilla can also be destroyed by electrical means to result in permanent hair removal. This procedure is called **electrology** and should be performed only by a licensed electrologist.

Moles or birthmarks frequently produce some bristly hairs. These hairs can be cut off at the skin surface. Electrolysis can sometimes be used to remove these hairs. Do not try to pull them out with a tweezer and do not use chemical depilatories. The moles themselves can be removed by a doctor.

CLIENT TIP ◆◆◆◆◆◆◆

Make sure that hair pulled away from the hairline is not too tight. Push the hair slightly forward at the hairline before fastening a ponytail. If braids pull the skin at the hairline into bumps, loosen each braid slightly.

◆SAFETY PRECAUTION◆

Never remove hair from a mole without first obtaining a doctor's permission. Some moles are precancerous and the trauma of removing hair could change cell structure.

Gray Hair

The loss of the pigment melanin from the hair is a natural part of the aging process. **Canities** (ka **NIT** eez) is a technical term that is used to describe this loss of color. Like baldness, the tendency to have gray hair is inherited. Some persons who gray early in life would probably find that their ancestors did so also. If the hair turns gray before age 40, it is called premature canities. Because there is a larger amount of pigment in the skin and hair of darker-skinned people, grayness is not as common and does not start as early as in the light-skinned people.

Anyone who finds gray hair unattractive can easily remedy the situation with permanent, semipermanent, or temporary haircoloring (see Chapter 14).

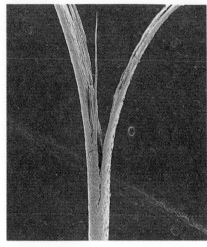

2.10   Split hair (© David Scharf, 1992)

Dandruff

Dandruff is one of the most common scalp disorders. It can be recognized by small white flakes that appear on any hairy region of the body. Medical authorities have listed various causes for dandruff, including poor blood circulation, inadequate nerve stimulation in the scalp, infection, unbalanced diet, and careless grooming habits. Most experts agree that dandruff will spread if it is not treated. The most common cause of dandruff is harsh shampoos and chemicals that dry the scalp. This causes an imbalance in oil production, compounding the problem.

There are two types of dandruff—dry and oily. Dry dandruff is easier to control than oily dandruff. Oily dandruff can be itchy. The scales mix with sebum and are difficult to brush out. Medical treatment is usually the only way to control oily dandruff. Dry dandruff often causes more social problems, however, because small, dry flakes often fall from the hair and adhere to clothing. Dandruff treatments are discussed in Chapter 6.

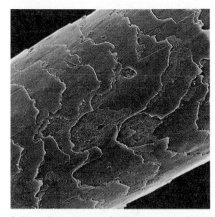

2.11   Coated hair (© David Scharf, 1991)

Other Common Problems

Certain disorders are related to the hair shaft only. Among them are knotted hair known as **trichorrhexis nodosa** (**TRIK** oh rek sis no **DOH** sah), split hair ends known as **trichoptilosis** (TRIK op ti **LOH** sis) (Figure 2.10), and beaded hair known as **monilethrix** (moh **NIL** eh thriks). It is also common to see coated hair (Figure 2.11), and heat-damaged hair (Figure 2.12). Each of these problems can be helped by treatments and conditioners offered in the salon (see Chapter 6).

Contagious Diseases

As a cosmetologist, you should never attempt to diagnose or treat a contagious disease in the salon. If you suspect any disease, refer your client to a physician.

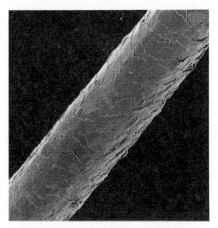

2.12   Heat-damaged hair (© David Scharf, 1986)

Ringworm

Ringworm, or tinea, is not a worm, but a fungus organism present everywhere. When provided with the right environment—warmth, moisture, and food—this fungus can develop on the scalp. The lesion usually takes the form of a red ring. This ring can be as small as a pinhead or up to 3 or 4 inches in diameter. The outer part of the ring is scaly, but the skin within the circle appears normal. As the fungus moves along in its course, it breaks off the hairs and thus causes bald patches. Ringworm of the scalp is called **tinea capitis** (**TIN** ee ah **KAP** ih tis). Do not treat or service anyone who shows signs of ringworm. Recommend that the customer see a doctor.

The disease is passed on by means of scales or hairs containing the fungus. Children often contract the disease by using one another's combs or by trying on another child's hat. Pets and soil may also carry the fungus.

Head Lice

Pediculosis capitis (peh dik yoo **LOH** sis), or head lice, is a disease caused by a tiny louse (see Figure 2.13) that lays eggs, or **nits**, along the hair shaft close to the scalp. You may never see the louse itself, because it may go on to another victim after laying the eggs. The nits resemble tiny flakes of dandruff, but they adhere tightly and cannot be easily lifted off. They hatch in two or three days, and if the conditions are favorable the new family will reside on the scalp and continue to multiply. This condition is extremely contagious. Although some states allow those with head lice to be treated in the salon, it is best never to service anyone who you suspect has the disease. Refer the client to a physician.

NAILS

Nails, like hair, are an appendage of the skin. Neatly trimmed nails of uniform color, whether natural or applied, have always been considered a mark of good grooming. The hair on your head and nails on your fingers and toes seem very different, but in fact they are very much alike. Both originate in the epidermal layer of the skin, and their condition is dependent on the body's overall health. Both can be cut without pain, and both provide protection for the areas that they cover. Both contain the chemical substance keratin, but nails are harder and stronger than hair. Nails also grow somewhat more slowly than hair—about 1/4 inch per month. Nothing you can apply to the nails will cause them to grow, but a good diet can help produce healthy nails. The technical term for nail is **onyx**, and the study of nails is called **onychology** (on ih **KOH** loh jee).

Structure of the Nail

Nails start their growth just under the fold of skin at the point where you see the nail emerging from the flesh. This part of the nail is called the **matrix** and is enriched with blood vessels and nerves. It is

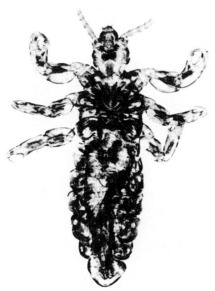

2.13

similar to the papilla of the hair. The nail **root** is attached to the matrix just under the flesh at the back of the nail. The visible part of the nail is referred to as the nail **plate**, and the entire plate is attached to the underlying flesh (the nail **bed**). There is no color in the nail plate; the pink color comes from the blood vessels in the nail bed. The part of the nail plate that is not attached to the nail bed and extends beyond the fingertips is called the **free edge**.

The **lunula** (lu **NOO** lah) is a light-colored, crescent-shaped area at the base of the nail. The light color results from the fact that there are air pockets between the nail plate and the nail bed at this point. The **cuticle** is the tough fold of skin that forms at the base and sides of the nail plate and under the free edge. The cuticle at the base of the nail is called the **eponychium** (ep oh **NIK** ee um). The **hyponychium** (heye poh **NIK** ee um) is the portion of the cuticle beneath the free edge. Figures 2.14 and 2.15 show the structure of a nail.

The nails need to be manicured to keep the free edge smooth and well shaped and the cuticle soft and pliable. Torn, neglected cuticles and frayed edges of nails frequently cause nail biting. **Onychophagy** (on ih **KOH** fah jee) is the technical name for nail biting. Some of your clients may insist that they do not need a manicure because they have no nails. They still need a manicure to remove rough edges and thus stop nail biting and picking (see Chapter 21).

The cuticle protects the nail, but if it is not cared for, it frequently grows forward and covers a large part of the nail plate, especially on the toes. This excessive growth of cuticle is called **pterygium** (te **RIJ** ee um). The cuticle receives much abuse as we go about our daily routine, and it can dry out and split. This results in a condition called **agnails**, or **hangnails**.

Disorders of the Nail

Many common disorders of the nails, such as the cuticle problems just mentioned, can be corrected by regular manicures. Proper care and manicuring can also help improve **onychorrhexis** (on ih koh **REK** sis) (Figure 2.16) (split nails) and **corrugations** (also called wavy ridges).

Hypertrophy and atrophy of nails are two other common complaints. **Hypertrophy**, or **onychauxis** (on ih **KOH** sis), is a thickening of the nails, especially the toenails (Figure 2.17). This can happen when the toenails are not trimmed properly or when tight-fitting shoes prevent the nails from growing normally. **Onychatrophia** (on ih kah **TROH** fee ah), or **atrophied nails**, are very thin and fragile (Figure 2.18). They probably lack keratin and thus tend to split easily. If your client has atrophied nails, advise him or her to avoid placing the hands in very hot water, to use rubber gloves whenever possible, and to apply lotion or olive oil to the fingertips at bedtime. Cotton gloves will keep the oil in place. Nail polish will help to protect the nails. Both hypertrophy and atrophy of nails may be hereditary.

Ingrown nails (**onychocryptosis**) (on ih koh krip **TOH** sis) occur when the corners of the nail press into the skin and cause inflammation.

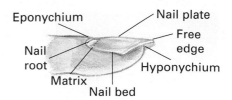

2.14

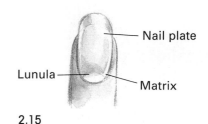

2.15

◆ **Key Point** ◆
Bail irregularities and disorders can be treated with manicuring services.

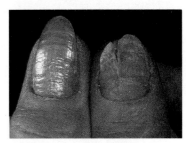

2.16

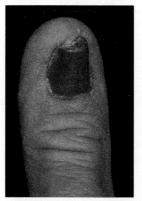

2.17

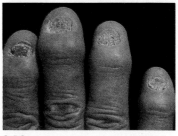

2.18

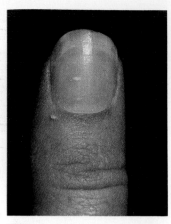

2.19

Improper cutting of the nails and tight shoes can cause this condition, which must be treated by a doctor.

White spots frequently appear on the nail plate, a condition called **leuconychia** (loo koh **NIK** ee ah). This does not necessarily indicate any disease or physical disorder (Figure 2.19); however, some parasites can cause leuconychia. Sometimes **furrows**, or depressions in the nail, can result from an illness or injury.

A blow with an instrument such as a hammer or excessive pressure with manicuring instruments can damage the nail bed and cause the nail to become deformed. In time, however, the deformed nail will be replaced by a new one. More severe damage, such as tearing off the nail completely or dissolving the nail with powerful chemicals, can result in the destruction of the matrix. If this happens, the nail will not grow again.

If the nail is bruised and a blood clot forms under the nail plate, it is called **hematoma nail**. **Eggshell nails**—thin flexible nails that separate from the nail bed—and **blue nail** or **onychocyanosis** are two other disorders you might see.

Diseases of the Nail

Diseases of the nail should be referred to a physician. Do not attempt to treat them in the salon.

Onychosis (on ih **KOH** sis) refers to any disease of the nail. Nail diseases can range from abnormalities in structure to dangerous conditions such as infections and contagious diseases. Examples of structure abnormalities are **onychophosis** (on ih **KOH** foh sis) (accumulation of horny layers of epidermis under the nail) and **onychogryposis** (on ih koh greye **POH** sis) (excessive growth with an inward curvature). Manicures and pedicures should never be given if there is any sign of infection or contagious disease.

Conditions that you should never treat include **paronychia** (pare oh **NIK** ee ah) (an acute infection of the structures around the nail), **onychia** (on **NIK** ee ah) (inflammation of the matrix), and any form of ringworm. **Tinea unguium**, or **onychomycosis** (on ih koh meye **KOH** sis), is fungus of the nails. It attacks the entire nail and can take many forms. Fungus of the hands (**tinea corporis**) and fungus of the feet (**tinea pedis**, commonly called athlete's foot) should also never be treated in the salon. Recommend that anyone with signs of infection or contagious disease see a doctor.

◆SAFETY PRECAUTION◆

Never treat a finger or nail that has signs of infection such as redness, pus, or swelling.

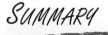

Summary

Study of the hair, the skin, and the nails is essential for the cosmetologist. The proteins that make up these structures build the foundations upon which you will work in the professional salon setting. The structure of each protein is slightly different—giving it unique characteristics. The toughest of the three is the nail, and the softest is the skin.

Hair and nails are an appendage, an outgrowth, of the skin. It is important, then, that we protect these proteins. Both hair and nails are a hard protein, keratin. Cells regenerate from the papilla in the hair, and from the matrix in the nail. As long as these structures are healthy, they will continue to grow.

The skin is made of collagen, a softer protein with a higher moisture content. It is the largest organ of the body; it protects us from the environment, regulates temperature, and provides sensation. The skin can be affected quite easily by salon services. You should know what products can penetrate the skin and what effects they may have on your client. This thorough understanding will help you offer your clients services in a safe and effective manner.

QUESTIONS

1. What is the outermost layer of the skin and what are its functions?
2. What structures are in the inner layer, and what does each contribute to the skin?
3. What are the six main functions of the skin?
4. What are the divisions of the hair?
5. Which division of the hair is most affected by salon services? What are some examples?
6. Describe the structure of each layer of the hair.
7. How is this structure responsible for the characteristics of hair?
8. What is the structure of the nail?
9. How is this structure affected by typical nail services?
10. What nail conditions can you treat in the cosmetology salon?

PROJECTS

1. Make a chart to analyze the structure of the skin. In the first column, describe the structure of each layer. In the second column, detail what quality this structure adds to the skin. In the third column, describe how a salon service could affect it. In the last column, list the products (or specific ingredients) that would affect the skin.
2. Make another chart, this time of the hair. In the first column describe the structure. In the second explain how this structure gives hair its unique properties. In the third column, list the salon services that affect this particular structure. And finally, list the products in the last column that you would use to create that change.
3. Draw a large cross-section of the nail. Label each section and indicate its importance to the overall nail structure.
4. List the portions of the nail that are protective. Beside each item, indicate the best way to preserve its protective function.

ANATOMY AND PHYSIOLOGY

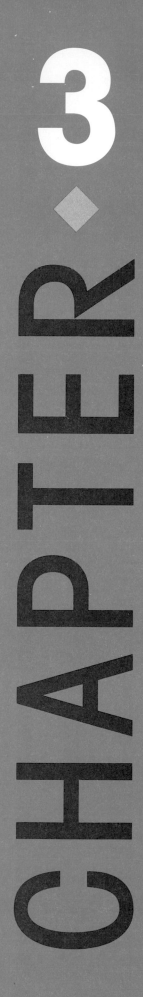

CHAPTER GOAL

Understanding the human body and how it works will help you stay healthy and understand the impact of your services on your clients. After reading this chapter and completing the projects, you should be able to

1. Explain the importance of nutrition and outline the basic food groups.
2. Outline the path of digestion in the body.
3. Explain how circulation works.
4. List the effects an endocrine imbalance can have on hair growth.
5. Describe the function of the excretory system.
6. Outline how oxygen enters the body.
7. Explain the function of the skeletal system.
8. Describe the action of muscles.
9. Explain the importance of nerves to the body.

There are many topics you must study so that you can offer better service in your practice of cosmetology. You will apply the concepts of anatomy and physiology every day.

The art of haircutting, for example, depends upon an understanding of the contours of the bone structure of the head. When you learn the artistry of makeup, you will learn to apply it along certain bones of the face. In skin care, it is necessary for you to understand the muscular system of the body, as well as how nerves are affected by massage movements and techniques. And finally, an understanding of the human body is important to your own health and well-being and that of your clients.

Nutrition

Before discussing the structure and activities of the body, we should study how the body gets the energy to carry on its activities. **Nutrition** refers to the way the food we eat nourishes the cells of our body. The cell is the basic building block of the body. Groups of cells form tissues (for example, the skin), tissues form organs (for example, the liver), and organs become the body systems that keep us functioning. Each one of these systems is dependent on other systems, but each has its own specific function.

Cells have three main parts. There is an outer **membrane** holding the cell together. Within this membrane is a jellylike substance called **cytoplasm** (**SEYE** toh plaz em). Within the cytoplasm is the **nucleus**. All the parts of the cell—the membrane, cytoplasm, and nucleus—are composed of living matter called **protoplasm** (**PROH** toh plaz em). Protoplasm contains water, salt, and particles that have been made from the food that is taken into the body. Cells reproduce themselves by dividing, and these new cells are used to keep tissues, organs, and systems healthy. These processes of growth and repair are fueled by energy from the food we eat. Therefore it is important that we eat the right things.

The foods that are important for adequate daily nutrition can be divided into five groups.

1. THE MILK, YOGURT, AND CHEESE GROUP You should eat two to three servings of dairy foods each day. This group is a good source of calcium, which is needed for strong bones.
2. MEAT, POULTRY, FISH, DRY BEANS, EGGS, AND NUTS GROUP Eat two to three servings from this group each day. Iron and protein are two of the important nutrients in this food group.

3. VEGETABLE GROUP Have three to five servings of vegetables each day. Dark green and yellow vegetables are an especially important source of Vitamin A.
4. FRUIT GROUP Have two to four servings of fruit each day. Citrus fruits are a great source of Vitamin C.
5. BREAD, CEREAL, RICE, AND PASTA GROUP You should have six to eleven servings from this group each day. These foods are high in fiber and low in fat.

There is another group of food that includes fats, oils, and sweets. It is best to eat as little from this group as possible. Eating too much fat, especially saturated fat, is bad for your health. You should also try not to eat too many foods which are high in cholesterol. Finally, when you use oil, try to use olive oil or another oil that is low in cholesterol.

In order to remain healthy—and have healthy skin and hair—a person requires certain kinds of food each day. Each kind of food makes individual contributions to the body. You may not like some of the foods listed in the daily essentials. You may even be allergic to some of them. Unless you are allergic, you should try to eat some of the foods in each group each day.

Proteins

Proteins provide the chemicals that aid growth in childhood and help to repair or replace tissues and blood in people of all ages. Meat, fish, poultry, cheese, milk, and eggs are the animal proteins. Cereals, nuts, dried peas, beans, and lentils are the chief vegetable proteins. Animal proteins more nearly resemble the protein of the human body than vegetable proteins and can be broken down into more of the amino acids needed by our bodies. The **amino acids** are the building blocks of the protoplasm in the cell and are necessary if the body is to function properly. Vegetable proteins cannot supply all of the amino acids required by our bodies.

Carbohydrates

Carbohydrates (sugars and starches) are the energy food. Bread, cereal, pasta, potatoes, and rice are some of the foods that are high in carbohydrates. They are called the energy foods because they supply the body with the fuel it needs to work. Although they are not high in calories, if you eat too many of these foods, you will gain weight, because if the body has more fuel than it needs, it will store the extra fuel away as fat.

Minerals

Certain elements, called "minerals" by dieticians—calcium, phosphorus, potassium, magnesium, iron, copper, and several others—are necessary for the teeth, bones, muscles, internal organs, and body fluids. They control the function of some organs and are needed for normal growth. Milk, whole-grain breads and cereals, fruits, vegetables, eggs, and meat, particularly liver, heart, and kidney, supply minerals.

Vitamins

Vitamins help to protect us from disease and are necessary to maintain good health, an attractive complexion, strong nails, and beautiful hair.

Vitamin A is essential to the health of the skin, hair, and nails. The best sources are fortified margarine, butter, carrots, squash, sweet potatoes, green leafy vegetables, and dried apricots and prunes.

The B vitamins are very important to the nervous system, and their lack can cause skin disorders—roughness, blemishes, inflammation. Whole-grain or enriched bread, cereals, milk, green leafy vegetables, and fresh meat are good sources of B vitamins.

Vitamin C is important for healthy teeth and gums. Citrus fruits, tomatoes, melons, and strawberries are the best sources. Some green leafy vegetables are a good source of vitamin C, but overcooking can destroy this vitamin, so these foods are best eaten raw.

Vitamin D is often called the "sunshine vitamin." Actually this vitamin is not contained in sunlight. Rather the rays of the sun cause vitamin D to form on our skin. If you choose to get your vitamin D from the sun, be sure not to overexpose the skin. You will do more harm than good. Too much sun will cause your skin to have a leather-like texture, and you will hasten the aging process. Ultraviolet light from special lamps can also cause the skin to produce vitamin D, but they should also be used with caution. Milk, egg yolk, and liver are foods that contain a good supply of vitamin D.

> ### ◆ Key Point ◆
> Good nutrition is vital for healthy hair and skin. Good nutrition will help you avoid illness.

Digestion

Digestion is the process of breaking down the food we eat into materials that can be used by our cells in their work of growth and repair. Good digestion is very important for our health and well-being. It is therefore important that we understand how food is digested. Figure 3.1 is a diagram of the **digestive system**.

The Mouth

The process of digestion starts in the mouth, where food is mixed with saliva. **Saliva** is made in three pairs of **salivary glands** located within the mouth. These glands begin to pour out saliva when food is put into the mouth. (Sometimes smelling food, or just thinking about it, can start the salivary glands working.) Saliva contains an enzyme that can change starch to sugar. (An **enzyme** is a protein that can speed up or slow down chemical changes.) As food is chewed, it is mixed with saliva and becomes soft and slippery so that it can be swallowed easily. When we swallow, the food slides down the food pipe, or **esophagus** (ih **SOF** ah gus) into the stomach.

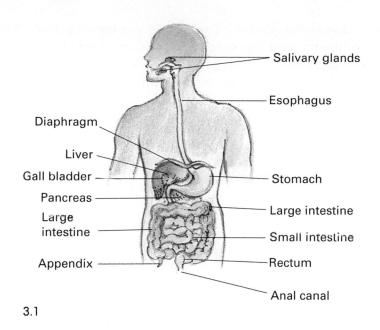

3.1

The Stomach

Once food arrives in the stomach, the walls of the stomach begin to produce a digestive juice containing an acid and the enzyme **pepsin**. The pepsin breaks down proteins in the food we have eaten. The walls of the stomach then press together and gently push the undigested food into the small intestine.

The Small and Large Intestines

The small intestine is where the body absorbs most of the nutrients it needs from the food. **Bile** from the liver and **pancreatic juices** from the pancreas flow into the small intestine and help to digest the food. Bile helps to break down fats and oils into very tiny drops so that they can be digested easily. Bile produced by the liver is stored in the gall bladder. Pancreatic juice contains three different enzymes that help to break down starches, fats, and proteins.

The walls of the small intestine are lined with millions of finger-like projections called **villi**. Nutrients are absorbed into the blood through the villi. Once in the blood, the nutrients can reach the cells of the body.

After the small intestine has taken out all of the important nutrients from the food, whatever remains passes through a valve into the **large intestine**. Here water is absorbed from the digested materials, and the solid waste that remains then passes out of the body through the rectum and the anal canal.

The Abdominal Cavity

The various organs of digestion, starting with the stomach and ending with the large intestine, fill what is called the **abdominal cavity**. This cavity is formed at the top by the diaphragm. The **diaphragm** is a large, dome-shaped, muscular wall in the breast region that has openings for the esophagus, blood vessels, and nerves. The floor of the abdominal cavity is formed by the **pelvic region** and the abdominal walls. The pelvic region contains organs that remove solid and liquid waste from the body as well as the reproductive organs.

THE CIRCULATORY SYSTEM

The blood carries oxygen and nutrients to tissues and organs so that they can function properly. It also carries waste products away so that they can be eliminated from the body. Proper circulation of the blood is essential if we are to remain healthy. If the circulatory system begins to break down, disease and death will follow. In this section we will discuss the role of the heart and blood vessels in the circulatory system. We will also show how the system works and study the composition of the blood that travels through the system. Finally, we will study a second circulatory system, the **lymph system**. The study of the circulation of blood and lymph is called **angiology** (an jee **OHL** oh jee).

The Heart

Your heart is the key to the operation of the circulatory system. Each minute it pumps about five or six quarts of blood on a round trip through your body.

The heart is about the size of a fist and is located in the chest cavity. It is inside the rib cage and behind the breastbone, or **sternum**. It is surrounded by a membrane called the **pericardium** (per ih **KAHR** dee um). The heart is divided into four chambers. The two upper chambers are called **atria** or **auricles**. The auricles receive blood from the veins. The two lower chambers are called **ventricles**. They pump blood out of the heart through arteries.

The Blood Vessels

Blood moves through the body in what is called the **cardiovascular** (kahr dee oh **VAS** kuh lahr) **system**. This system includes the heart and various blood vessels. There are three basic types of blood vessels: arteries, veins, and capillaries. All three types are tubelike structures that can expand or contract as blood moves through them.

The **arteries** carry blood away from the heart. The largest artery is called the **aorta**. Blood leaves the heart through the aorta and travels to all parts of the body. The blood that goes to the lungs is transported by the **pulmonary** (**PUHL** moh ner ee) **artery**.

The **veins** have thinner walls than the arteries and are not so elastic. These vessels carry blood to the heart. Because the blood in the veins flows slowly and is under little pressure, there are valves in the veins to keep the blood from flowing backward. Muscular action

TABLE 3.1 Important Arteries and Veins

Arteries	Description
Internal carotid	Brain, eye sockets, eyelids, and forehead
External carotid	
External maxillary	Skin and muscles of lower region of face—mouth and nose
Occipital	Skin and muscles of scalp, back of head, and neck
Posterior auricular	Scalp behind and above ear
Superficial temporal	Skin and muscles at front, sides, and top of head; also muscles of chewing
Subclavian	Spinal cord, neck, ribs, and upper arm
Transverse scapular	Front and back of shoulder and shoulder joint
Axillary	Armpit, upper arm, and chest
Brachial	Upper arm
Radial	Front of forearm and hand
Ulnar	Back of forearm and hand

Veins*	Draw blood from:
External jugular	Surface of cranium and face
Internal jugular	Internal region of cranium, face, and neck
Cephalic	Front of forearm
Basilic	Back of forearm
Metacarpal palmar	Palm of hand
Metacarpal dorsal	Back of hand
Digital palmar	Surface of fingers

*The veins of the head, neck, and upper arms have the same names and distribution as the arteries, except for the jugular veins.

helps to push blood forward on its journey through the veins. This action is called muscle pumping. Table 3.1 lists some important arteries and veins.

The **capillaries** (**KAP** ih lar eez) are very tiny blood vessels that link the arteries with the veins. Capillaries have very thin walls; oxygen and nutrients in the blood can flow through the walls easily and into the cells of the body. Waste products from the cells enter the capillaries in the same way. These waste products are then carried through the capillaries to the veins, which return the blood to the heart and lungs. Sometimes capillaries can become enlarged and swollen from high blood pressure or from the use of drugs and alcohol. When this happens, you may be able to see capillaries, because some of them are very close to the surface of the skin. This is especially true of capillaries under facial skin.

How Circulation Works

Now that we know something about the structure and function of the heart and blood vessels, we can look more closely at the circulatory system. We have just seen how oxygen in the blood is taken into the cells through the capillaries. Blood without oxygen then flows through the same capillaries and into the veins. The oxygen-poor blood is carried from various parts of the body through the veins to

> ◆ **Key Point** ◆
> Good circulation is essential for healthy hair, skin, and nails. Poor blood supply will cause dull hair, wrinkles, and fragile nails.

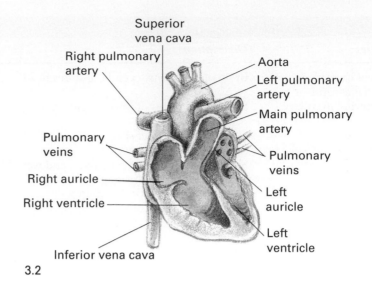

Superior vena cava

Right pulmonary artery

Aorta

Left pulmonary artery

Main pulmonary artery

Pulmonary veins

Pulmonary veins

Right auricle

Left auricle

Right ventricle

Left ventricle

Inferior vena cava

3.2

the heart (see Figure 3.2). The blood enters the right auricle of the heart by one of two large veins, the **inferior vena cava** or the **superior vena cava**. The superior vena cava transports blood from the upper parts of the body (head, chest, and arms). The inferior vena cava carries blood from the lower part of the body (abdomen, legs, and feet). When the right atrium is full of blood, a valve opens and the blood passes into the larger and stronger right ventricle. A contraction of the heart muscle then forces this oxygen-poor blood into the pulmonary artery. The blood travels to the lungs through this artery. While the blood is in the lungs it is purified. It gets rid of carbon dioxide, a waste product that it has collected from the cells, and gets a new supply of oxygen. The blood, now rich in oxygen, returns to the left auricle by way of the pulmonary veins. (We will have more to say about the lungs in the section on respiration.)

When the left auricle is filled with blood, a valve opens, and the blood pours into the left ventricle. The left ventricle is the strongest chamber in the heart. The muscles of this chamber contract and push the oxygen-rich blood into the aorta for its long journey throughout the body. There are two main branches of the aorta. One branch supplies the upper part of the body, the other branch supplies the lower part (see Figure 3.3). The arteries branch over and over again, and the branches get smaller and smaller. The smallest branches supply blood to the capillaries. From the capillaries, the blood travels through very small veins to the large veins (see Figure 3.4).

We should note here that the chambers on both sides of the heart beat in unison. Ordinarily the heart beats from 70 to 80 times a minute. The heart beats faster when we are very active and more slowly when we are resting. All muscles must have rest, and the muscles of the heart rest between beats.

Cosmetologists have to be concerned with the arteries and veins in order to maintain their own good health. Because they are on their feet for many hours at a time, stylists may be bothered by vari-

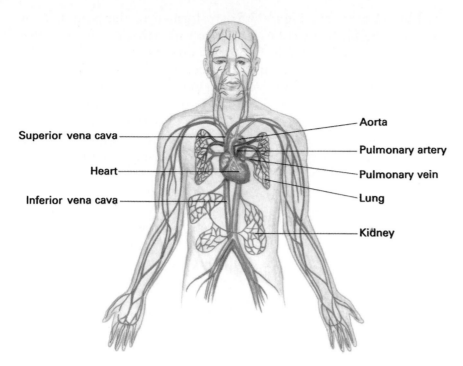

Superior vena cava

Heart

Inferior vena cava

Aorta

Pulmonary artery

Pulmonary vein

Lung

Kidney

3.3

cose veins. Varicose veins are bulges that can form if the veins stretch and lose their elasticity. It is not certain whether people who are on their feet a lot develop varicose veins more easily than others, but preventive measures should be taken. Try not to let yourself become overweight. Early in your career, make sure that you wear well-fitting shoes that will support your weight. Wear elastic hose that are sheer and attractive. Do not wear rolled garters, tight girdles, or undergarments that might impair your circulation.

Another thing to watch for is high blood pressure, or hypertension. This condition can be caused by a variety of factors, but nervous tension is one of the most frequent. As a cosmetologist, you are pressured by a desire to please your customers and by tight schedules. You also have only short and irregular rest periods. Try to teach yourself to remain calm, to eat correctly, and to take a break when you can.

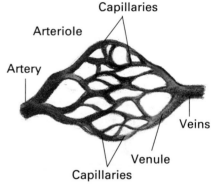

Capillaries

Arteriole

Artery

Veins

Venule

Capillaries

3.4

Blood and Its Cells

So far, we have discussed the "plumbing" of the circulatory system. Now let us look at the fluid that circulates in that system.

Blood is composed of a yellowish fluid (**plasma**) in which red and white blood cells (**corpuscles**) and small objects called **platelets** float.

Plasma is about 90 percent water. The remainder is made up of a variety of minerals, nutrients gathered from the digestive tract, and waste products collected from the cells. Plasma also contains the blood-clotting factor, **fibrinogen**, and antibodies. **Antibodies** are substances that help our bodies resist disease.

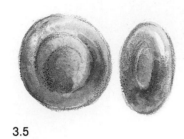

3.5

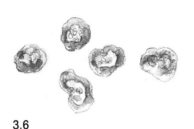

3.6

Red blood cells (see Figure 3.5) are formed in the bone marrow and give the blood its color. They are tiny particles, so small than thousands of them would be found in a drop of blood no bigger that the period at the end of this sentence. The body contains about 25 trillion of these cells and each has a lifespan of about four months. When the life of the red blood cell is over, it is destroyed in the liver or spleen. These cells get their red color from an iron-rich protein called **hemoglobin**. In the lungs, hemoglobin combines with oxygen. The oxygen is carried by the hemoglobin throughout the body to the capillaries, where it is released to individual cells. Hemoglobin also attracts carbon dioxide and carries it to the lungs, where it is exhaled. The blood leaves large quantities of hemoglobin in the muscles, so we have a reserve of oxygen for when we are involved in physical activity that requires a lot of energy.

White blood cells are less numerous than the red blood cells, but they number in the billions. There is one white blood cell for approximately every 700 red corpuscles. The white blood cells (see Figure 3.6) form in the bone marrow, the lymph glands, and the spleen. They differ in shape from the red blood cells.

The white blood cells play the important role of fighting disease and bacteria. When they encounter bacteria, they engulf and digest them. They also attack foreign bodies, such as splinters. During an infection, white blood cells increase rapidly as they try to fight off the invading bacteria. One result of the battle is pus, a thick yellowish fluid composed of dead bacteria and dead and living white blood cells.

Blood platelets are much smaller than the red blood cells. Their primary function is to clot blood. They, too, are manufactured in the bone marrow. When a blood vessel is cut, the platelets collect at the site of the injury. Scientists believe that this begins a complicated chemical process that causes the liquid protein fibrinogen to form threadlike chains that clot and close the wound.

The Lymphatic System

The **lymphatic** (lim **FAT** ic) **system** is a sort of secondary circulatory system that is closely connected with blood circulation. Lymph is a clear fluid that contains white blood cells, some red blood cells, fats, and **lymphocytes**, a type of white blood cell. Lymph removes bacteria from the body. Lymph fills tissue spaces and is continually drained off by the lymph vessels, or **lymphatics**. The fluid is moved along by massaging effects of the muscles as they squeeze together and by action of body movements such as breathing.

The smallest lymph vessels begin in nearly all tissue spaces. These vessels join into larger and larger channels until they form the two major lymph channels—the **right lymphatic duct** and the **thoracic** (tho **RAS** ik) **duct**. The right lymphatic duct drains the head, neck, and right chest, while the thoracic duct drains the rest of the body. These two channels empty into the right and left jugular veins in the neck. Along the course of the lymph channels are **lymph nodes**, also called lymph glands, through which the lymph flows. These nodes are efficient traps for bacteria or foreign particles. They act as collection stations throughout the body, and they are most numerous in the face, neck, and upper torso (see Figure 3.7). The lymph nodes also produce lymphocytes. These cells enter the bloodstream when the lymph enters the jugular veins.

There are more than 100 lymph nodes throughout the body. Each is a potential barrier to the spread of an infection from one part of the body to another. As the glands make an effort to keep infection from spreading to another part of the body, they may swell and cause pain. Those glands most often affected in this way are in the neck and under the arms. There are, however, many other causes of enlarged glands, and a doctor should be consulted at the first sign of swelling.

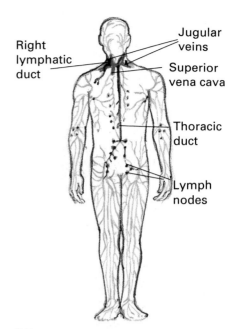

3.7

ENDOCRINE GLANDS

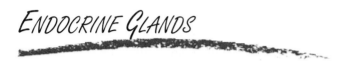

There are two types of glands in the human body—duct glands and ductless glands. **Duct glands (exocrine glands)** produce substances that travel through tubelike ducts. Sweat glands and the glands concerned with digestion are examples of duct glands. Other glands, called the **ductless glands** or **endocrine glands** have no ducts but secrete substances called hormones directly into the blood. **Hormones** are chemicals that are vital to various bodily functions. They can speed up or slow down these activities and can affect growth rate, reproduction, circulation, and nutrition. In this section we shall discuss briefly the most important endocrine glands (see Figure 3.8).

The **pituitary gland** is a pea-sized gland located near the base of the brain. This gland is sometimes called the master gland, because it secretes hormones that affect the activity of other endocrine glands. The pituitary gland also produces a growth hormone. Other pituitary hormones ensure normal sexual development and help to maintain the water balance of the body.

The **thyroid gland** is attached to the windpipe and secretes a hormone called **thyroxine**. This hormone regulates the metabolism of the cells of the body and controls our weight.

The **thymus gland** is located below the thyroid. It is important to the function of the immune system.

The **adrenal glands** are located at the top of each kidney. In times of stress they secrete the hormone **adrenaline** into the bloodstream in greater than normal amounts. It increases the heart rate, causes the body to release stored food, and helps us to take more oxygen into the lungs. In general, the adrenal glands help us to cope with emergencies.

The **pancreas** is both a duct gland and a ductless gland. It is a duct gland because it produces pancreatic juices that help in the process of digestion. But it is also a ductless or endocrine gland because it produces a hormone called **insulin**.

Defects in the endocrine glands can cause many skin disorders. Sometimes a person is given a hormone to correct the defect, but often this only causes more complications.

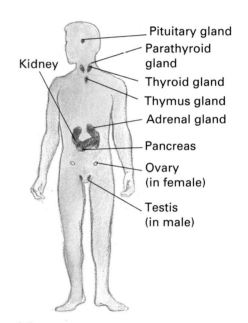

3.8

> ◆ **Key Point** ◆
> Imbalance of the endocrine system can lead to excess hair growth or premature baldness.

EXCRETION OF LIQUIDS

The **excretory** (**EK** skre tohr ee) **system** eliminates solid, liquid, and gaseous wastes from the body. This system consists of the large intestine, the liver, the lungs, the kidneys, and the skin. In the section on digestion we discussed the role of the large intestine and the liver in removing solid waste. Later, we will discuss the work of the lungs, which remove gaseous waste. Here we will be concerned with the kidneys and the skin. These two organs help the body to get rid of liquid waste.

The Kidneys

The **kidneys** (Figure 3.9) are two bean-shaped organs whose job is to filter out waste as the blood passes through them. They are located in the upper part of the abdominal cavity, alongside the spinal column. Liquid wastes are transported through tubes to collection points within the kidneys. They then travel through two large tubes, the **ureters**, to the bladder, where the liquid is stored until it is passed out of the body.

The liquid that passes from the kidneys to the bladder is called **urine**. It is mostly water but also contains various waste materials that the kidneys have filtered from the blood.

The Skin

In Chapter 2 we devoted an entire section to the skin and its functions. Here we will repeat a few key points with regard to the role of the skin as an excretory organ. The sudoriferous, or sweat glands, located in the epidermis, or lower layer of the skin, carry out the removal of waste. They are coiled tubes, similar to the kidney tubes, and are surrounded by capillaries. Like the kidney tubes, the sweat glands filter impurities and water from the blood. This liquid, called sweat, then travels to the surface of the skin and evaporates. Removal of waste is not the only function of the sweat glands. As was mentioned earlier, they also play a key role in keeping body temperature constant.

Artery — Vein
Kidney
Ureter — Bladder

3.9

◆ **Key Point** ◆
The excretory system maintains the health of the body by removing toxins.

THE RESPIRATORY SYSTEM

The body needs a continual supply of oxygen, in addition to food and water. Oxygen is used by the cells to break down food molecules and thus supply us with energy. In doing this, it produces gaseous wastes in the form of carbon dioxide and water. The function of the **respiratory** (**RES** pi rah tohr ee) **system** is to take in the needed oxygen and eliminate carbon dioxide and moisture. The lungs, the windpipe, and the bronchial tubes are the key organs of respiration (see Figure 3.10).

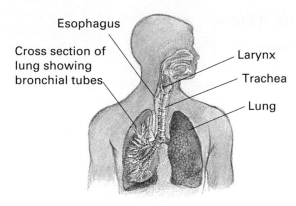

Esophagus

Cross section of
lung showing
bronchial tubes

Larynx

Trachea

Lung

3.10

The Lungs

The lungs are suspended in the chest cavity above the diaphragm. They are spongy masses of tissue containing millions of tiny air cells surrounded by blood-filled capillaries. When we breathe in, air containing oxygen travels through the nose and mouth into the voice box and through the windpipe. The windpipe divides into two branches, each of which enters one of the lungs.

The lung's air sacs are surrounded by capillaries. The capillaries and the air sacs are separated by very thin walls that allow oxygen to pass through them and into the bloodstream. They also permit carbon dioxide to leave the bloodstream and enter the lungs so that it can be exhaled through the windpipe and the nose or mouth.

Inhaling through the nose rather than through the mouth is probably more healthful. Air passing through the nose is warmed, and the fine hairs within the nose act as filters that trap foreign particles and prevent them from entering the system.

> **◆ Key Point ◆**
> Respiration provides oxygen necessary for bodily functioning and removes carbon dioxide.

THE SKELETAL SYSTEM

The bones of our body form a framework called the **skeletal system**. The skeleton supports the body in an upright position and protects vital organs. It is composed of about two-thirds minerals. These minerals are primarily phosphate and carbonate of lime. The skeletal system also helps us to move about efficiently. The study of bones is called **osteology** (os tee **OL** oh jee).

The bones of the human body can be grouped into three classes, based on their shape: long, flat, and irregular (see Figure 3.11). Long bones are found in the arms, legs, hands, and feet. The bones in the hands and feet are sometimes called short bones, but their shape is similar to the long bones. Flat bones are found in the skull, or cranium. They are like plates that protect the brain. Irregular bones come in many different shapes. The bones in the wrists and ankles and the vertebrae in the spinal column are irregular bones.

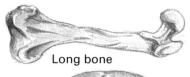

Long bone

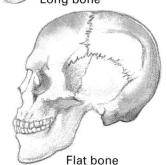

Flat bone

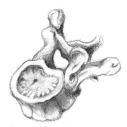

Irregular bone

3.11

The Structure of Bones

Bones are composed of two kinds of tissue. The outer part of the bone is made up of hard, compact tissue. This tough outer shell contains many channels that are penetrated by small blood vessels and nerves. The inner parts and knobby ends of bones are made up of softer, more porous tissue. This tissue is honeycombed with nerves and blood vessels. The large bones have an internal cavity that is filled with bone marrow. Red blood cells, blood platelets, and some white blood cells are formed in the marrow and pass through blood vessels into the bloodstream. The bones in our arms, legs, hips, ribs, and breastbone are most active in blood formation.

Bones have a tough outer covering called the **periosteum** (per ih **OS** tee um). The periosteum is well supplied with nerves and blood vessels, and so it registers pain if there is an injury. It also protects the bone. See Figures 3.12 through 3.15 and Table 3.2.

Cartilage

Cartilage, or gristle, is a tough, elastic tissue that is different from bone in that it lacks minerals to make it hard. It is generally found at the ends of bones, but some of our features, such as the nose and ears, are composed entirely of cartilage. This flexible tissue cushions the bones at the joints and helps to prevent fractures.

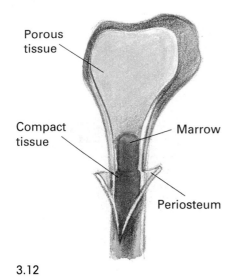

3.12

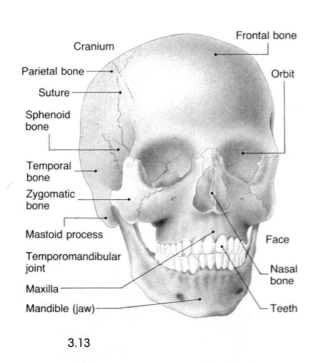

3.13

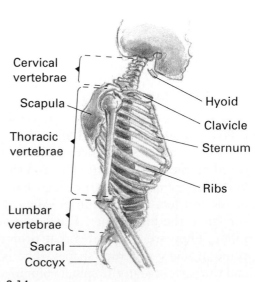

3.14

TABLE 3.2 Some Important Bones

Skull

Name	Number	Location
Frontal	1	Forehead
Parietal	2	Sides and top of skull
Occipital	1	Back of skull
Temporal	2	Sides of skull below parietals
Sphenoid	1	Front base of skull behind eyes and nose
Ethmoid	1	Root of nose between eyes

Face

Name	Number	Location
Zygomatic	2	Upper cheeks and floor of eye cavity
Maxilla	2	Upper jaw
Mandible	1	Lower jaw
Nasal	2	Upper part of bridge of nose
Vomer	1	Back of nasal cavity
Lacrimal	2	Side wall of nasal cavity
Palatine	2	Back of nasal cavity and roof of mouth
Turbinate	2	Side wall of nasal cavity

Neck and Trunk

Name	Number	Location
Hyoid	1	Front of throat between root of tongue and Adam's apple
Cervical	7	Top of spine—top seven vertebrae
Thoracic	12	Next twelve vertebrae to which ribs are attached
Lumbar	5	Next five vertebrae
Sacral	5	Five fused bones beneath lumbar vertebrae
Coccyx	4	Four fused bones forming tail bone
Sternum	1	Breastbone, thorax
Ribs	24	Twelve pairs, thorax

Upper Extremity

Name	Number	Location
Scapula	1 each shoulder	Back of shoulder
Clavicle	1 each shoulder	Top of shoulder
Humerus	1 each arm	Upper arm
Radius	1 each arm	Thumb side of forearm
Ulna	1 each arm	Little-finger side of forearm
Carpals	8 each wrist	Two rows of bones in each wrist
Metacarpals	5 each hand	Palm of hand
Phalanges	2 each thumb 3 each finger	Fingers and thumbs

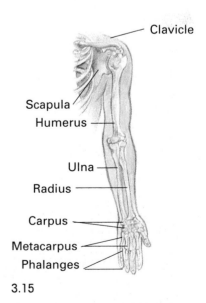

Clavicle

Scapula

Humerus

Ulna

Radius

Carpus

Metacarpus

Phalanges

3.15

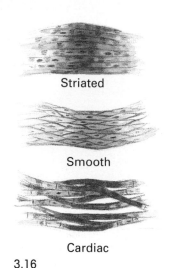

Striated

Smooth

Cardiac

3.16

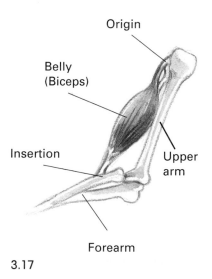

Origin

Belly
(Biceps)

Insertion

Upper arm

Forearm

3.17

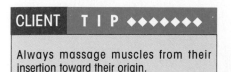
Joints and Ligaments

A **joint** is a point at which bones are connected or joined. Some joints move very easily, such as those in our fingers and arms. Others cannot move at all—for example, the joints between the bones in our skull. Some joints can move only slightly. There are six basic types of joints in the human body:

1. Immovable joints—those in the skull.
2. Gliding joints—the wrist.
3. Hinge joints—the elbow, fingers, and lower jaw.
4. Pivot joints—the neck.
5. Ball-and-socket joints—the shoulder.
6. Slightly movable joints—the spine.

THE MUSCULAR SYSTEM

The muscles of our body, taken as a group, form what is called the muscular system. Muscles make up nearly half our weight; they support our body and give it its shape. Some muscles help us perform actions such as getting out of bed and chewing our breakfast. Others play a key role in the activities of our bodily systems, for example, the digestive and circulatory systems. The study of muscles and their functions is called **myology** (meye **OL** oh jee).

Types of Muscles

There are three types of muscles: voluntary (striated), involuntary (smooth), and cardiac (see Figure 3.16). This last type of muscle is found only in the heart.

The muscles involved in activities such as running and throwing are called **voluntary** or **striated muscles**. Their action is controlled by the will. We can force these muscles to move or not to move. That is why they are called voluntary. When viewed under a microscope, this type of muscle appears to be striated or striped. Voluntary muscles are attached to bones, skin, and other muscles by means of **tendons**.

Involuntary or **smooth muscles** are not controlled by our will and are not striated. They move whether or not we want them to. They are found in the walls of the stomach, intestines, and blood vessels. The cells of the smooth muscles are quite long and are pointed at both ends.

Because cosmetologists deal only with the voluntary muscles, we will look at them more closely. Voluntary muscles are composed of bundles of long, fibrous cylinders.

Each muscle has an origin, belly, and insertion. The **origin** refers to the more fixed, or stationary, attachment of one end of a muscle to a bone or tissue. The **belly** is the thick mid-part of the muscle. The **insertion** is the attachment of the other end of the muscle to a movable bone or another muscle (see Figure 3.17).

Muscles come in many sizes and shapes. Some are very large, such as those in the arms, legs, chest, and back. Some of the muscles of the face and neck are so small that it is difficult to locate their origin and insertion. But, by working along with other muscles, these tiny muscles create many facial expressions and assist in talking, laughing, yawning, and chewing.

Muscles work by expanding and contracting. Muscles are very elastic; they can stretch beyond their normal length or shrink and become thicker than normal. But they always return to their original size and shape. The stimulus for expansion or contraction always comes from outside the muscle. As we shall see in the next section, the nerves are the prime movers of the muscles.

Arteries, veins, capillaries, and lymph vessels arc very abundant in the muscles. The blood supplies oxygen and nourishment to the muscle cells and picks up waste materials. When the muscles are being exercised, the heart rate speeds up, and the flow of blood to the muscles increases.

Muscles are frequently injured when a person falls or receives a hard blow. This causes the muscle fibers and capillaries to rupture, and thus a bruise appears. Muscles can also be pulled or strained. The injury may be painful, but there is usually no permanent damage.

See Table 3.3 for a listing of some important muscles. Some of these muscles are shown in Figures 3.18 and 3.19.

> ◆ **Key Point** ◆
> Muscles provide shape and allow action. The strength of muscles can be increased by exercise and massage.

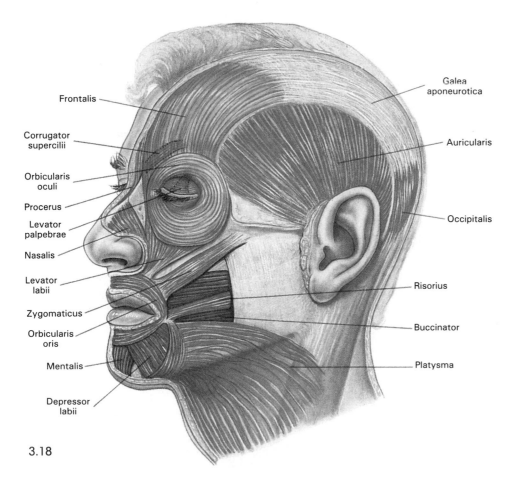

3.18

TABLE 3.3 Some Important Muscles

Head and Face

Name	Location	Function
Frontalis*	Front of scalp, forehead, root of nose	Raises eyebrows, draws scalp back, wrinkles brow
Occipitalis*	Back of scalp	Draws scalp back
Superior auricularis	Above ear	Draws ear upward
Posterior auricularis	Behind ear	Draws ear backward
Temporalis	Beneath superior auricularis	Opens and closes jaw during chewing
Masseter	Back of jaw	Closes jaw
Orbicularis oculi	Encircles eye	Closes eyelid
Corrugator	Eyebrow	Pulls eyebrow down
Procerus	Between eyebrows	Pulls forehead down
Nasalis	Bridge of nose	Opens and closes nostrils
Posterior and anterior dilator naris	Skin in nostrils	Opens nostrils
Depressor septi nasi	Membrane dividing nostrils	Closes nostrils
Quadratus labii superioris	Above upper lip	Lifts upper lip
Quadratus labii inferioris	Below lower lip	Pulls down lower lip
Caninus	Above and at edge of mouth	Draws mouth up and out
Zygomaticus	Corner of mouth to zygomatic bone	Draws mouth up and back
Risorius	Corner of mouth to masseter	Draws mouth out and back
Triangularis	Side of chin from corner of mouth	Draws mouth down
Orbicularis oris	Circles mouth	Contracts and puckers lips
Mentalis	Tip of chin	Raises lower lip, wrinkles chin
Buccinator	Sides of mouth between upper and lower jaws	Compresses cheeks, aids in chewing

Neck, Back, and Chest

Name	Location	Function
Platysma	Runs from chin to shoulders and chest	Draws down lower jaw
Sternocleidomastoid	Runs from collar and chest bones to behind ear	Draws head forward, back, and sideways
Trapezius	Back of neck and upper part of back	Raises and lowers shoulders
Pectoralis major	Runs across chest from breastbone to upper arms	Draws arm across chest, elevates ribs
Pectoralis minor	Underneath and below pectoralis major	Draws shoulders forward and down

*Frontalis and occipitalis are joined by the galea aponeurotica to form the epicranius.

Shoulders, Arm, and Hand

Name	Location	Function
Deltoid	Upper arm and shoulder	Lifts, extends, and rotates arm
Biceps	Front of upper arm	Raise forearm and turn palm outward
Triceps	Back of upper arm	Extend forearm
Pronators	Forearm	Turn hand so palm faces back
Supinators	Forearm	Turn hand so palm faces forward
Extensors	Forearm	Straighten wrist so hand points forward
Flexors	Forearm	Bend wrist and clenched fist backward
Adductors	Base of fingers and thumb	Draw fingers together
Abductors	Base of fingers and thumb	Separate fingers

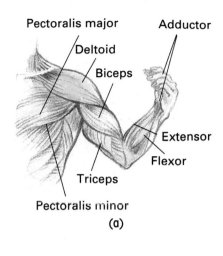

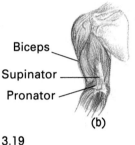

3.19

THE NERVOUS SYSTEM

The nervous system is a complex network of nerve cells and nerve fibers that, together with the brain and spinal cord, coordinate all the activities of our body. The study of the structure and functions of the nervous system is called **neurology** (nuh **ROL** oh jee).

Nerve Cells and Nerves

Nerve cells are different from the other cells in the body. Unlike other cells, nerve cells are not capable of self-repair. Like all human cells, they contain a nucleus, but they also have long and short threadlike fibers called **processes**. The processes carry nerve impulses throughout the body. There are two types of processes: axons and dendrites. The **axons** are long nerve fibers that carry impulses away from the cell body. At the end of the axon are nerve terminals that may be connected to muscles, organs, or dendrites of other nerve cells. The shorter **dendrites** carry impulses toward the cell body. Some of the axons are very long. One of the longest carries signals from the spinal cord to the toes. A **neuron** (see Figure 3.20) is a nerve cell with its axon and dendrites.

A nerve is like a cord that is woven of many thin fibers. These cords or cables carry signals between the brain or spinal cord at one end and muscles, glands, and sensory organs at the other end.

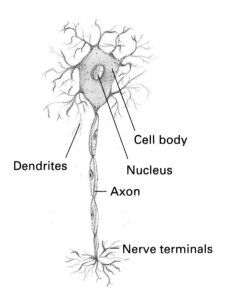

3.20

Types of Nerves

There are two types of nerves: sensory nerves and motor nerves. **Sensory nerves**, called afferent nerves, carry incoming messages from the sense organs to the spinal cord and brain. **Motor nerves**, called efferent nerves, carry outgoing messages from the brain and spinal cord to muscles or other organs.

If we take a look at what is called a reflex action, we can see how the two types of nerves work together. When you touch a hot object, you pull your hand away immediately without thinking. This is a reflex action. As soon as you touch the hot object, the nerve endings of the skin send a signal along a sensory nerve to the spinal cord. Here a connection is made with a motor nerve, and a signal travels along this nerve to the muscles in your hand and arm. The result is that you pull your hand away. Meanwhile, the pain signal continues through the spinal cord to the brain, and you sense pain. All of these actions take place in an instant.

The two types of nerves work together in a reflex action, but they can also work alone. Thus, when you decide to pick up a stone from the ground, the brain sends signals along various motor nerves to many different muscles. These muscles are put into action, and you pick up the stone. The sensory nerves come into play independently. Your eyes tell you where the stone is, and sensory nerves in your hand let you know the texture and feel of the stone.

Divisions of the Nervous System

The nervous system is divided into three main parts: the central nervous system, the autonomic nervous system, and the peripheral nervous system.

The **central nervous system** is composed of the brain and the spinal cord. The brain is made up of billions of nerve cells and their fibers. The spinal cord is made up of a mass of long nerve fibers running to and from the brain. It is enclosed within the spinal column. If we think of the brain as the central switchboard of a telephone system, the spinal cord would be the main lines running to and from the switchboard. Most messages between the brain and all other parts of the body are carried through the spinal cord.

The **autonomic nervous system** controls the activities of our various internal organs—respiration, digestion, circulation, and so on. This system has two divisions, the sympathetic and parasympathetic. These two divisions have opposite effects on our body organs. One may trigger a reaction, while the other may stop it. The autonomic system functions independently of our will. These impulses are carried by the autonomic system.

The **peripheral nervous system** (see Figure 3.21) consists of all the sensory and motor nerves that carry messages to and from the central nervous system. Included in this system are 12 pairs of cranial nerves and 31 pairs of spinal nerves. Some of the cranial nerves that are important to cosmetologists are listed in Table 3.4.

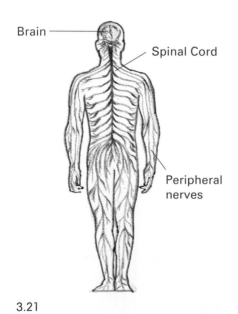

Brain

Spinal Cord

Peripheral nerves

3.21

TABLE 3.4 Important Cranial Nerves

Name and Divisions	Type of Nerve	Function
Trigeminal (5th cranial nerve)		
Ophthalmic	Sensory	Transmits sensations from forehead, eyelids, eyebrows, and nose
Maxillary	Sensory	Transmits sensations from middle of face, lower eyelids, and upper lip
Mandibular	Sensory and motor	Transmits sensations from lower teeth and gums, lower lip and jaw, and sides of head; acts on muscles connected with chewing
Facial (7th cranial nerve)		
Posterior auricular	Motor	Acts on muscles behind ear
Temporal	Motor	Acts on muscles above and in front of ear, eyelid, eyebrow, and upper cheek
Zygomatic	Motor	Acts on muscles of upper cheek, upper lip, and sides of nose
Buccal	Motor	Acts on muscles of upper lip and sides of mouth
Mandibular	Motor	Acts on muscles of chin and lower lip
Cervical	Motor	Acts on platysma muscle on side of neck
Accessory (11th cranial nerve)		
Accessory	Motor	Acts on internal muscles
Spinal	Motor	Acts on the sternocleidomastoid and trapezius muscles

SUMMARY

The study of the anatomy and physiology of the body will help you in practical ways in the salon every day. As you study hair shaping and precision haircutting (Chapters 8 and 9), you will need to understand the bone structure of the head in order to section correctly for accuracy in cutting.

The muscles and nerves are directly affected in esthetic, or skin care services. It is important that you massage from the insertion to the origin of muscles so you strengthen rather than stretch them. Stretching could cause premature aging and sagging. The study of muscles and nerves, especially in combination with nutrition, will also help you through your work day with the least fatigue and strain.

All of the systems of the body work together for good health. Because the hair and nails are appendages of the skin, they often show early signs of illness or disease. Be alert to hair that suddenly goes dull and becomes lifeless, nails that peel, change color, or become thin. As a cosmetologist, you will never diagnose or treat illnesses. But you can do your client a great service by tactfully suggesting an appointment with a physician when you notice changes that could indicate a problem.

QUESTIONS

1. How is nutrition important to you as a cosmetologist?
2. What are the basic food groups and how much should you eat daily from each?
3. What is the process by which food is digested?
4. How does circulation flow from the heart throughout the body?
5. How would the hair, skin, or nails show symptoms of inadequate circulation? What would you do about it?
6. How can endocrine imbalance affect hair growth? What symptoms would you see in the salon?
7. What is the function of the excretory system?
8. How does oxygen enter the body? What is the importance of oxygen to the hair, skin, and nails?
9. What is the function of the skeletal system? What key bones do you need to consider when sectioning the hair for a cut?
10. How do muscles provide for motion?
11. What precautions should you follow when you are massaging muscles?
12. How are nerves important to the body?

PROJECTS

1. Analyze the bone structure of the heads of at least six of your fellow students. Pull the hair straight back from the face, up from the neck, and secure. Working with a headform, draw on paper the outline of each head that you analyze. Note the bone that makes the most prominent feature of the head. List any bone that is within the normal outline of the head-shaped form. Save these analysis sheets for further projects in Chapters 7, 8, and 9.
2. Keep a diary of the food that you eat for one week. Measure it according to servings and compare your normal diet to that recommended for adults. Are all four food groups represented in your daily diet? What foods that you like could provide what you are missing in your daily diet? In what areas do you go beyond the recommended servings? How will the excess affect you? Research the long-range effects of overeating.
3. Research the effect of hormones, especially testosterone and estrogen, on hair and skin growth. Report back to the class on the possible side-effect of too much or too little testosterone. List sources relating estrogen to healthy skin.

BACTERIOLOGY AND INFECTION CONTROL

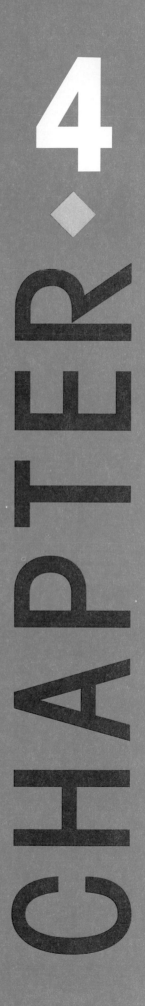

CHAPTER GOAL

Proper infection control practices in the professional salon will protect your health and the health of your clients. After reading this chapter and completing the projects, you should be able to

1. List the two types of bacteria.
2. Explain which bacteria is of concern in the salon.
3. Outline how infection and disease occur.
4. Explain how infection and disease can be prevented.
5. Demonstrate at least three methods of chemical disinfection.

Your career as a cosmetologist, esthetician, or nail technician will bring you into direct contact with the public. Your work will require you to touch the hair, skin, and nails of your clients.

We have learned a great deal in the past century about preventing the spread of disease and infection from person to person through microbiology, the study of minute living things. These studies impact the procedures in the salon. You must take special measures to prevent disease and to protect yourself and your clients in the salon. As a professional, you will determine the best method of infection control for your situation. Next, analyze what chemical will perform best. You must mix the chemical correctly for best efficiency and monitor whether or not it is contaminated. Immerse your implements for the proper amount of time and store to preserve sanitation.

These steps will help ensure your health and safety in the salon and protect your clients from infection. They will recognize you as a professional dedicated to personal service work.

MICROBIOLOGY

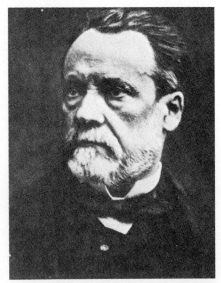

4.1

Germs, or **microbes**, are very small, one-celled plant microorganisms. They are found everywhere in great numbers. They thrive especially well in water, on the skin and hair, in decaying matter, and in the various waste materials produced by man and other animals.

For centuries people knew little or nothing about the nature of diseases and infections that caused the deaths of millions. Some people believed that the fluid that oozed from a wound or infection was caused by evil spirits within the body. Before the twentieth century, many people treated in hospitals died as a result of infection. Doctors did not wash their hands when they moved from one patient to another. Surgical instruments were not kept clean. Whole families died during epidemics because no one guessed that diseases were passed from person to person by means of direct contact. People were not aware that insects or impure food and water could spread disease.

A little over a century ago, Louis Pasteur (1822–1895), a French chemist, discovered that **microorganisms** (very small living things) were the cause of disease and infection (see Figure 4.1). Joseph Lister (1827–1912), an English doctor, accepted Pasteur's theory. In the hospitals where he operated, he attacked the microorganisms responsible for infection by applying an antimicrobial, phenol, over skin wounds and surgical incisions. Because of Lister's work, the occurrence of serious infection in hospitals was greatly reduced. Lister is known as the founder of antiseptic surgery.

The first person to describe bacteria accurately was Anton van Leeuwenhoek (1632–1723), a Dutch businessman and amateur scientist (see Figure 4.2). With a microscope that he had built, he saw little objects moving in water. He called these objects "little animals," but they were microbes.

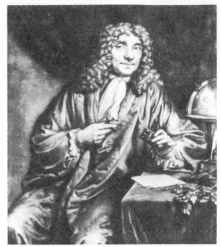

4.2

How Bacteria Grow and Reproduce

Although bacteria are so small that they are invisible to the naked eye, they are complete living things. They carry on all the functions necessary for life. They require food for survival and growth, give off waste material, and reproduce. Some bacteria have hairlike projections called **flagella** (flah **JEL** ah) or **cilia** (**SIL** ee ah), which permit them to move about in a liquid. Bacteria use flagella just as a human being uses arms and legs when swimming. In the environment, bacteria can be found in two forms: active and inactive.

ACTIVE BACTERIA—Bacteria that are growing and reproducing are in what is called the **active stage**. They thrive in a warm, dark, dirty, moist environment. Most bacteria reach full growth in about 20 or 30 minutes. When they have reached full growth, they are ready to reproduce. For bacteria, reproduction is a very simple process. The single bacterial cell merely splits in half, by a process called **direct division**. The two new bacteria are called **daughter cells**. When the daughter cells reach full growth, they too divide in half. This process of growth and reproduction is repeated over and over again. It is during the active stage that bacteria can cause disease.

INACTIVE BACTERIA—Most bacteria cannot grow and reproduce if there is too much light or heat or a lack of food or moisture. Under these conditions, some bacteria die, but others simply become inactive. They form **spores** that have a hard, shell-like outer covering. The spores are resistant to adverse conditions. This permits dormant bacteria to survive for a long time without food and in an environment that is unsuitable for growth. The spores can float in the air, are blown about by the wind, and can come to rest on combs, brushes, or other objects in the salon.

Bacteria in spore form cannot cause disease, but they are still a threat. If conditions change and become suitable for bacterial growth, the spores drop their shells. Then the bacteria start to grow again and reproduce. They become active again and can cause disease. If a bacterial spore enters the body of an animal through a break in the skin, the spore finds a warm, moist haven and begins to grow.

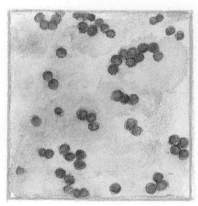

4.3 Cocci

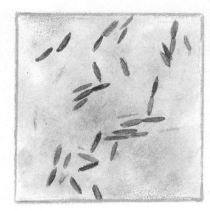

Bacilli

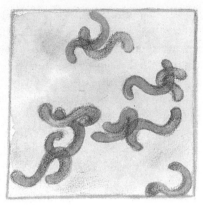

Spirilla

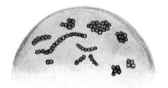

4.4 Cocci grow in groups

Pathogenic and Nonpathogenic Bacteria

There are several thousand different kinds of bacteria, but only about 100 of these can cause disease. These bacteria are said to be **pathogenic** (path o **JEN** ik), "disease-producing." **Nonpathogenic** bacteria are harmless, and some are even useful. In nature nonpathogenic bacteria help decompose dead vegetation and animals and thus fertilize the soil. In the digestive system they help break down the food that we eat. Some are used in the treatment of sewage, and others produce some of the substances that are used by the drug industry in the preparation of **antibiotics** (drugs used to kill bacteria and other disease-producing organisms).

Classes of Pathogenic Bacteria

Pathogenic bacteria can be divided into three classes: **cocci**, **bacilli**, and **spirilla** (see Figure 4.3).

Cocci (**KOK** seye)—These are a group of round or berry-shaped bacteria. They are not able to move in a liquid, but they float in the air and are blown about in dust. Cocci may occur singly, but often they grow in groups (see Figure 4.4). The following are the three main types of cocci:

1. **Streptococci** (strep to **KOK** seye) grow in chains and are commonly found in the respiratory tract and the intestines. Some diseases caused by these bacteria are blood poisoning, sore throat, scarlet fever, and rheumatic fever.
2. **Staphylococci** (staf lo **KOK** seye) grow in bunches or clusters and are among the strongest of non-spore-forming bacteria. Staphylococci are constant inhabitants of the skin and are responsible for many skin disorders. Among the infections they cause are boils, abscesses, carbuncles, pustules, and food poisoning.
3. **Diplococci** (dip lo **KOK** seye) grow in pairs. They can cause pneumonia and other diseases. Often they invade the body following other diseases, such as measles or influenza.

BACILLI (ba **SIL** eye)—These bacteria are shaped like sticks or rods. Some bacilli form spores. Pathogenic bacilli cause some very serious diseases, such as tetanus (lockjaw), typhoid fever, dysentery, and tuberculosis.

SPIRILLA (spi **RIL** ah)—These are the comma- or corkscrew-shaped bacteria. One of the spirilla, *Treponema pallidum*, causes syphilis.

INFECTIONS AND DISEASE

At all times our bodies are inhabited by large numbers of bacteria. As we have said, the nonpathogenic type can be harmless or even beneficial, such as those that aid the digestive process. The pathogenic kind can cause disease. Infection and disease occur when pathogenic bacteria invade the body, overcome the body's defenses, and begin to multiply. As they multiply, they produce complex chemical substances called **toxins.** Toxins are the poisons that cause disease. A **local infection** is one that is confined to one area, for example, a pimple, a boil, or an infected cut. When pathogenic bacteria are carried in the bloodstream to all parts of the body, **general infection** results. Examples are blood poisoning and syphilis.

Pus, the yellowish fluid that oozes from a wound, is a sign of infection. White blood cells attack the bacteria and devour them. The pus contains blood cells, body cells, and dead and living bacteria.

Bacteria may invade the body through cuts, scratches, or punctures in the skin or through any of the body openings (nose, mouth, and so forth). Bacteria are also contained in the food we eat, the water we drink, and the air we breathe. The bite of an insect or animal can also introduce harmful bacteria into the body.

Diseases are said to be **contagious** when they are passed from one person to another by direct or indirect contact. Coughing and sneezing, unclean hands, eating utensils, salon equipment, pets, and insects play a role in spreading disease (see Figure 4.5).

A **communicable** disease is one that can be spread by direct contact when blood or other body fluids are passed from one person to another. Most venereal diseases, and the HIV virus that causes AIDS (Acquired Immune Deficiency Syndrome) are spread in this manner.

4.5

Bodily Defenses

The body has a network of defenses that guard against the invasion of bacteria. Other defense mechanisms control bacteria that are already within the body. The unbroken skin is the body's main defense against invasion. Tears in the eyes, saliva in the mouth, fine hairs in the nose, and mucus help to keep bacteria out of the body.

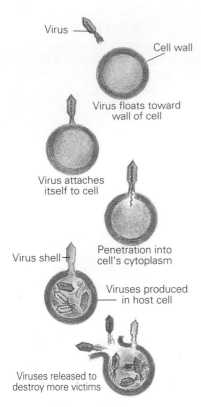

Virus

Cell wall

Virus floats toward wall of cell

Virus attaches itself to cell

Virus shell

Penetration into cell's cytoplasm

Viruses produced in host cell

Viruses released to destroy more victims

4.6   Reproduction of viruses

The acid juices in the stomach kill some germs, as do the white blood cells. Even bleeding helps to wash out bacteria from cuts. Fever is nearly always a sign of trouble. When the body reacts to infection by speeding the defense mechanisms, the temperature of the body rises. Sometimes the fever itself kills some germs.

Viruses

Viruses are infectious (pathogenic) particles that are so small that they cannot be seen through an ordinary microscope. A virus is smaller than the smallest bacteria. It is surrounded by protein and can only multiply inside a living cell. Viruses cause many serious diseases—such as measles, chicken pox, AIDS (HIV-1), Hepatitis B (HBV), and polio—and are responsible even for the common cold.

Viruses cannot reproduce until they enter a living cell of an animal or plant. When the tiny particle enters a cell, something unusual happens—the cell does not fight off the invader. The cell does not recognize the virus as an invader, but instead uses its energy to reproduce viruses until the cell itself is destroyed (see Figure 4.6). It is this characteristic of viral diseases and infections that makes them so dangerous for humans and so difficult to control.

The Acquired Immune Deficiency Syndrome (AIDS), caused by the HIV virus, is incurable. Because there is no cure for the disease, every precaution should be taken to avoid its spread. It destroys the immune system: the white blood cells and antibodies that are produced in the body to fight disease. The HIV virus cannot be spread by casual contact. This means that having a client who is HIV+ or has AIDS does not pose a risk to your health if you follow infection control guidelines. You should take every precaution so the HIV virus is not transmitted in the salon. Always work on a surface cleansed with an approved disinfectant. Use a hospital-grade disinfectant for your implements and completely immerse them as directed. Cleanse your hands and the hands of your clients with an antibacterial cleanser. Wear gloves if the skin is broken or if you know your client is infected.

Immunity

Immunity (ih **MYOO** ni tee) is the ability a person has to fight off or resist disease and infections. There are two kinds of immunity: natural and acquired, as described below.

NATURAL IMMUNITY—Natural immunity seems to be an inborn power to resist certain diseases. This may be due to an inherited characteristic. Many other vague factors may also produce natural immunity—a wholesome diet, frequent exercise, general good health, youthful vitality, and so forth. If one is tired from overwork or lack of sleep and does not eat properly, the bodily defenses against germs are not as strong as they could be, and the body cannot fight off the disease.

ACQUIRED IMMUNITY—This immunity follows after a person has actually had a disease or has been inoculated against it. The actual disease or the inoculation causes the cells in the blood to produce **antibodies**. The antibodies are proteins that fight disease germs. Acquired immunity may be permanent or may last only for a period of time. Immunity can be acquired against polio, some types of influenza, tetanus, typhoid fever, measles, chicken pox, whooping cough, smallpox, and other diseases. Some people who have natural or acquired immunity to certain diseases may still carry the disease germs in their bodies and can infect others. These people are called **human disease carriers**. Typhoid fever and diphtheria are two of the diseases that can be spread in this way.

Fungi

Fungi (fun **JEYE**) are plant organisms that live on dead, decaying, or living matter. **Mold**, **mildew**, and **yeast** are fungi. Some types of fungi consist of one microscopic cell; others are composed of many cells. Certain fungi can cause serious infection, such as ringworm (see Chapter 2). Many other fungi, however, are harmless, and some are even very beneficial. Penicillin, one of the wonder drugs of the twentieth century, can be produced from a type of mold. Yeast is used extensively in the production of alcoholic beverages.

Fungus can cause lifting of the finger or toenails. It usually appears as a discoloration of the free edge of the nail. As the nail grows, the discoloration seems to grow back toward the cuticle. Mold appears as a green spot, and occurs when moisture, air, and heat combine for a perfect breeding ground for germs.

> **CLIENT TIP ◆◆◆◆◆◆◆**
>
> Remove artificial nail or polish from a nail showing signs of mold or fungus. Discard all applicators. Do not treat the affected nail. Refer your client to a physician for further treatment.

Animal Parasites

Certain small organisms and some insects are called **animal parasites**. A parasite lives on or in another living organism. Head and body lice are examples of animal parasites (see Chapter 2). A microscopic parasite carried by a certain kind of mosquito causes malaria. This mosquito bites an infected person and then carries the parasite to another person. Insects like mosquitoes, ticks, and fleas, which carry disease from person to person, are called **disease vectors**.

Avoiding Illness

How can a person avoid getting sick in spite of the fact that disease germs are present everywhere, even within the body? The best defense against disease is a program of personal hygiene. Bacteria thrive in dirt, so you should keep yourself and your surroundings as clean as possible. General good health is also a defense against disease. Eat the proper foods and get plenty of rest. Avoid contact with people who have contagious diseases, and do not work on clients who show signs of infection by plant or animal parasites. Ways to keep the salon and its equipment as free of germs and bacteria as possible are discussed in the following sections.

> **◆ Key Point ◆**
>
> Infection and disease occur when pathogenic bacteria invade the body, overcome its defenses, and begin to multiply.

INFECTION CONTROL

A huge emphasis has been placed on the prevention of disease, especially in light of increasing cases of AIDS (HIV) and hepatitis B (HBV). The term that includes all efforts to prevent the spread of disease is **infection control**. This includes sanitary habits such as general cleanliness, chemical disinfection, and sterilization.

Sterilization is a process by which all germs are destroyed. Sterilization is required whenever the surface of the skin is cut or the body cavity is penetrated. While this is seldom necessary in the professional salon, it does apply to certain skin care, manicuring and pedicuring, and electrology procedures. **Disinfection** is a chemical process identical to sterilization, except it does not kill bacterial spores. State boards of cosmetology and health realize that this is the most practical method for the salon. The guidelines provided in this section are national standards for the industry, approved by the Food and Drug Administration (FDA) and filed with the Center for Disease Control (CDC) in Atlanta. Your instructor will inform you of any guidelines that vary slightly for your state.

Sterilization Methods

The most common method for sterilization is that of heat. Extreme heat under pressure will effectively kill germs. This is a method that is necessary in the medical fields, whenever the protective organ of the body, the skin, is pierced, punctured, or cut. Many professional salons do not have sterilization equipment, such as the **autoclave**, as it is extremely expensive. Instead, they use disposable, presterilized implements for those few instances when the skin is penetrated during a service.

If an autoclave is provided for the sterilization of metal implements, follow the manufacturer's directions for timing. Sterilized implements must also be stored in a sterile environment. Periodic checks must be made to ensure that the autoclave is sterilizing properly.

Chemical Infection Control Methods

Chemical agents used for infection control are called antiseptics and disinfectants (or germicides).

Antiseptics (an ti **SEP** tiks) retard the growth of some microorganisms and kill others. Because antiseptics are used on the skin, they are generally milder than disinfectants. Some of the most frequently used antiseptics are the following:

1. **Tincture of iodine.** A two percent solution (standard purchased strength) is used to cleanse cuts and small wounds.
2. **Merthiolate.** This is a commercial product used to cleanse cuts and wounds.
3. **Boric acid.** A five percent solution is used to cleanse the eyes.

TABLE 4.1 Commonly Used Antiseptics*

Name	Form	Strength	Use
Boric Acid	White crystals	2-5% solution	Cleanse the eyes.
Tincture of Iodine	Liquid	2% solution	Cleanse cuts and wounds.
Hydrogen Peroxide	Liquid	3-5% solution	Cleanse skin and minor cuts.
Isopropyl Alcohol	Liquid, Gel, or Foam	60% solution	Cleanse hands, skin, and minute cuts. Not to be used if irritation is present.
Formalin	Liquid	5% solution	Cleanse shampoo bowl, cabinet, etc.
Antimicrobal Soap	Bar, Cream, or Liquid	2% solution	Cleanse the hands.

*Other approved disinfectants and antiseptics are being used in beauty salons. Consult your state board of cosmetology or your health department.

TABLE 4.2 What Is an Approved Disinfectant?*

Name	Form	Strength	How to Use
Sodium Hypochlorite (household bleach)	Liquid	10% solution	Immerse implements in solution for 10 or more minutes.
Quaternary Ammonium Compounds	Liquid or tablet	1 : 1000 solution	Immerse implements in solution for 20 or more minutes.
Formalin	Liquid	25% solution	Immerse implements in solution for 10 or more minutes.
Formalin	Liquid	10% solution	Immerse implements in solution for 20 or more minutes.
Alcohol	Liquid	70% solution	Immerse implements or sanitize electrodes and sharp cutting edges 20 or more minutes.
Phenol	Liquid	5% solution	Immerse completely for 10 or more minutes.

*Consult with your state board of cosmetology or health department for a list of approved disinfectants to be used in the school. Always follow the manufacturer's directions for mixing and immersion times. For effective disinfection, implements must be completely submersed.

4. **Alcohol.** A 60 to 70 percent solution is used to cleanse hands and skin. Do not use on open cuts. There are two kinds of alcohol in common use: ethyl and isopropyl. Isopropyl alcohol is recommended for salon use because it is noncorrosive, nonstaining, and inexpensive.

5. **Hydrogen peroxide.** A three percent solution is used to cleanse the skin and minor cuts. (A three percent solution of hydrogen peroxide is also called 10-volume peroxide.)

Soap and water can also be used as an antiseptic. Before and after you serve each client, you should cleanse your own hands. An antibacterial soap should be used, and you should pay attention to cleansing thoroughly between fingers and under nails. You may also cleanse your hands by pouring a small amount of 70 percent alcohol into the palm, rubbing the hands together to thoroughly coat the hands and fingers, and letting the alcohol evaporate.

Disinfectants are chemical solutions that destroy most pathogenic and nonpathogenic microorganisms. Disinfectants are used to prepare implements, table tops, and so on, prior to servicing each customer. After use, disinfectants are again used to ensure safety. Some of the disinfectants commonly used in the salon are listed here (check with your state board for a list of approved disinfectants).

1. **Alcohol.** Implements immersed in 70 percent solution of alcohol for 20 or more minutes can be considered sanitized. All traces of oil should be removed from tools before they are immersed in alcohol.

2. **Quaternary ammonium compounds.** These compounds are commonly referred to as **quats** (see Chapter 13). Quats are stable, nonirritating, nonstaining, tasteless, odorless, and inexpensive. They often contain an ingredient that prevents equipment from rusting. Immersion of implements in a 1 : 1,000 quat solution (1 part quat to 1,000 parts water) for 20 or more minutes is sufficient for sanitizing implements (check your state board requirements). The amount of quat to be added to water to make a 1 : 1,000 solution varies, depending on the amount of active ingredient in the quat. Some quat solutions work better in hard water than in soft, and vice versa. Read the label or contact the manufacturer for this information. Quats are seldom used alone but are often a key ingredient of a commercial disinfectant.

3. **Sodium hypochlorite.** Equipment should be immersed in a 10 percent sodium hypochlorite solution (common household bleach) for 10 minutes. This is an excellent, inexpensive disinfectant. **Calcium hypochlorite** has the same characteristics and is used at the same strength and for the same immersion time as sodium hypochlorite.

4. **Formalin.** This is a commercial product composed of about 40 percent **formaldehyde**, a strong germ-killing chemical. Formalin is a good disinfectant, but it has a strong odor and can rust implements. Formalin can be diluted to various strengths, depending on the purpose for which it is intended. A 25 percent solution (two

parts Formalin, five parts water, one part glycerine) is used to sanitize metal implements. A 10 percent solution (one part Formalin, nine parts water) is used for brushes and combs.

5. **Phenol.** Products containing phenol are disinfectants that are reliable and cost-effective for use on implements and salon surfaces. Lysol, Pine-Sol, and CN are among the products that contain these ingredients.

Labels

Always read the label on a product before you use it. Labels contain information about ingredients, about how to get the best results from a product, and about possible dangers connected with the product's use. Follow directions exactly.

Various organizations check the quality of drugs and other medicinal products. **USP** on a label means that the product meets the standards of the *United States Pharmacopoeia*, the official United States book of standard drugs. **NF** on a label means that the product meets the standards of the *National Formulary*, which is published by the American Pharmaceutical Association. An **EPA** (Environmental Protection Agency) number indicates that the product meets the claims on the label. The **NDC** (National Drug Code) number ensures that the product is registered and meets guides established by the Food and Drug Administration (FDA).

Any product that is poisonous must have the word *poison* on the label. Store all poisonous products in a safe place.

Sanitizers

There are three types of sanitizers: wet, dry, and electric.

A **wet sanitizer** is a covered container that is filled with enough germicidal solution to cover tools and implements completely. These sanitizers come in various shapes and sizes, depending on their intended use. (see Figure 4.7).

A **dry sanitizer** is simply an airtight cabinet or drawer in which implements are stored. A small amount of germicide may be poured onto a small blotter and placed into the base of the cabinet. The vapors given off by the germicide keep tools sanitary (see Figure 4.8).

An **electric sanitizer** is a dry sanitizer that contains an ultraviolet lamp (see Figure 4.9). Ultraviolet rays given off by the lamp keep tools sanitary. Before putting tools into either an electric or other dry sanitizer, they should first be immersed in a wet sanitizer containing disinfectant solution.

How to Disinfect Equipment

1. Remove all hair from tools and implements.
2. Wash tools thoroughly with soap and water to remove dirt, grease, and oils.
3. Rinse thoroughly to remove all soap, which may hinder the action of germicides.

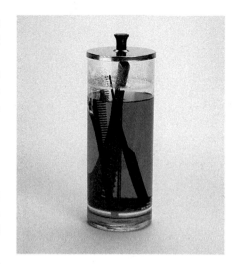
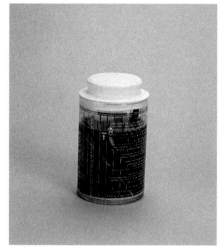

4.7 Wet sanitizers

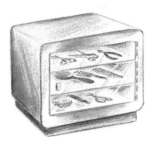

4.8 Dry sanitizer

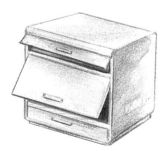

4.9 Electric sanitizer

4. Place tools in a wet sanitizer for the required length of time.
5. Remove tools from sanitizer, rinse with clear water, and dry with a clean towel.
6. Place tools in a dry sanitizer.

Safety Precautions

1. Store all chemicals in a cool, dry area.
2. Keep all containers labeled.
3. Keep all containers tightly covered.
4. Do not taste, smell, or shake any unlabeled liquids.
5. Read the labels on all products carefully.
6. Follow manufacturers' directions when mixing and using chemicals.
7. Wipe up any spilled chemicals immediately.
8. Keep chemicals away from the eyes.
9. Keep a first-aid kit in the salon.
10. Keep emergency telephone numbers (doctor, police, fire department) near the salon telephone.

OSHA and You

The Occupational Safety and Health Administration (OSHA) estimates that at least 32 million workers are exposed to chemical hazards of one degree or another. There are over 575,000 existing chemical products. Many of these are used by the practicing cosmetologist in diluted form. Additionally, there are also risks in the salon due to inhalation of fumes and dust. In 1987, OSHA expanded its ruling to require cosmetic product manufacturers to identify and provide a listing of the potentially harmful ingredients in their products.

Uniform requirements have been established by OSHA to ensure that any hazards from chemicals used in the school or salon are evaluated. OSHA has also established minimum-infection control standards. Information about any risks must then be passed on to employers and employees. This is required for three reasons:

□ To ensure that you know about the hazards related to your work ("Right to Know" Laws).
□ To ensure that you know how to protect yourself from any harm.
□ To reduce injury and illness related to chemicals.

Information about a chemical hazard is detailed on a Material Safety Data Sheet (MSDS) which is provided by the manufacturer for each chemical product that contains potentially harmful ingredients. The MSDS contains important information about toxicity, odor, flammability, and provides safety warnings.

A chemical is listed as a **health hazard** if there is sizable evidence from scientific study that health may be affected by exposure to it. Formalin is an example of such a chemical.

A chemical is listed as a **physical hazard** if there is valid scientific evidence that it is combustible, explosive, or flammable. This category also lists chemicals that are unstable or react with water. Hydrogen peroxide would be an example of such a chemical.

In your school you will find an MSDS manual. You will also notice that the shelves that contain these products are labeled. Familiarize yourself with emergency procedures in the event of an incident at your school.

Used properly, the chemicals employed in the professional salon are very safe. Become familiar with all the chemicals around you to make your work place a safer and healthier place for you and your clients.

General Sanitary Suggestions

1. If you are sick, do not work.
2. Wear clean, neat, washable clothing.
3. Wash your hands carefully after using the bathroom. Remember, many germs are carried on the hands and under the nails.
4. Wash your hands before working on a client.
5. Keep stations and equipment clean and neat.
6. Wash drawers and cabinets regularly with soap, water, and a germicide.
7. Do not keep soiled brushes, combs, and tools in the same drawer or cabinet with clean equipment.
8. Always disinfect equipment after each use.
9. Discard soiled towels and used disposable materials in a covered container.
10. Do not work on a client who has a contagious disease.
11. Do not work directly over any area of the skin or scalp where redness, swelling, or pus is present.
12. Do not allow waste or refuse to collect.
13. Keep garbage cans covered.
14. Cleanse and deodorize garbage cans daily.
15. Provide disposable drinking cups and hand towels.
16. Provide good ventilation and maintain a comfortable temperature in the salon.
17. Clean bathrooms daily with a cleanser and a germicide.
18. Wash walls, floors, windows, and curtains as often as necessary. Use a germicide, in addition to soap and water, on floors.
19. Do not allow animals, except for dogs that assist people with disabilities, in the salon.

Meeting Health Standards

Agencies of the federal, state, and local governments set standards to protect the health and well-being of the public. Various health and safety codes have been set up for salons and schools. Check with your local health department and your state board of cosmetology for rules that apply in your state.

SUMMARY

The theory of bacteriology is important to you as a cosmetologist so that you may protect your own health and that of your clients. It is the applied practice of infection control, however, that you will use every day in the salon. Infection control is critical, and those methods that you learn now in school must be carried with you into the salon.

As a stylist, you will be exposed to a variety of germs and microbes on a daily basis. You will work directly on the skin and nails, two ideal breeding grounds for bacteria. You will, of course, be using your hands and implements—more sources of contagion. As a stylist, esthetician, or nail technician, you should not become overly fearful. You should, however, follow the guidelines outlined by your state board or department of health to protect your safety and the health and welfare of your consuming public.

Avoid cutting of the skin whenever possible. Any implement that pierces the skin or cuts it must be sterilized before and after each use. Implements that cannot be disinfected must be disposed of as directed by your state board. All other implements should be disinfected after each use and stored according to health guidelines to maintain sanitation.

Develop the clean habits now, while you are in school, of keeping hair off the floor, picking up discarded endpapers, disinfecting dropped implements, and so on. These habits will become second nature in the salon. They will impress your clients with your visible sanitation methods and will help reduce any risk of infection in the salon.

QUESTIONS

1. How is microbiology important to the salon professional?
2. What are the two types of bacteria?
3. Which bacteria is of concern in the salon?
4. What procedures should you follow if a client's skin is cut in the salon?
5. How do infection and disease occur?
6. By what means can infection and disease be prevented?
7. What are three methods of chemical disinfection?
8. How will you comply with OSHA requirements for the salon?

PROJECTS

1. Research the disinfectants available in your school. Indicate whether they are phenol, quat, alcohol, or sodium hypochlorite based. Create a master chart that lists the directions for dilution and the immersion time.
2. Check with your local department of health to determine the recommended procedure to follow if you or your client is cut during a salon service.
3. Research the antiseptics or antimicrobals that are available in your school. Make a chart that indicates for each antiseptic the suggested strength for application to the skin. Include any precautions that you should follow.

4. Check with at least two local hair salons, skin care establishments, and nail salons to determine the infection control procedures they use. Analyze how they differ from those you follow in the school and why.

5. Outline the infection control procedures that are followed during a visit to the doctor, the dentist, etc. Explain how the procedures differ in terms of the risk of infection.

6. Properly mix five different infection control products.

SHAMPOOS AND RINSES

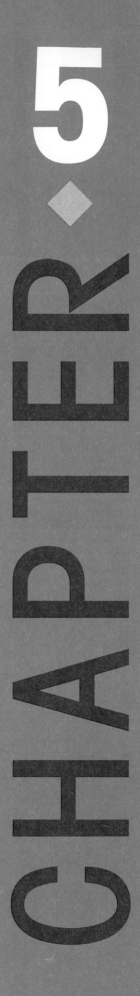

CHAPTER GOAL

Selecting the best shampoo for your client and using correct shampooing techniques prepare your client's hair for a professional salon service. After reading this chapter and completing the projects, you should be able to

1. Explain the importance of the shampoo service.
2. Demonstrate the procedures for preparing a client for a shampoo.
3. Demonstrate the correct procedure for a professional shampoo.
4. Explain the types of shampoos available and the purpose for each.
5. Outline the purposes for which hair rinses are used.

The word *shampoo* comes from the Hindi language and means "to cleanse." Since prehistoric times, man has found ways to cleanse the body in order to prevent disease. Earliest history notes that various herbs such as agave, amole, and soapwort were used to cleanse the hair. Herbs were also used as ingredients in rinses to make the hair shine, and later to add color.

Commercial shampoos became very effective cleansing agents as chemical ingredients replaced natural ones during the 1940s. Later, shampoos were modified in order to preserve and protect the natural pH balance of the hair. The interest in health extended to shampoos; growing concern about harshness led to the addition of conditioning agents. Recently we've seen a return to natural ingredients in the form of herbal additions to shampoos.

You must be able to select the correct shampoo for your client's hair type. You should be able to alter your shampoo techniques, especially before chemical services. Recommend that the client purchase the proper shampoo to use at home. Give instructions to protect your salon work.

SHAMPOOING

Shampooing is very important for the various hair treatments given in the salon. The purpose of a shampoo is to cleanse the hair and scalp and remove dandruff, dirt, and cosmetics. Shampooing also increases the circulation of blood and stimulates the scalp.

Hair should be shampooed as often as necessary, depending on the condition of the hair and how quickly the hair and scalp become soiled. You should know that hair collects more dirt each day than the skin does. Oily hair usually needs to be shampooed more often than dry hair.

There are many kinds of shampoos on the market today, and cosmetologists should know what shampoos are best for each type of hair. They should be familiar with the effects of shampoo and should have some knowledge of the composition and action of the shampoo being used.

When selecting shampoos, you must consider the degree of hardness of the water you use for shampooing. You must also take into account the chemical nature of the shampoo and the condition of the

---

◆ **Key Point** ◆

The ability to give a good shampoo is essential. It establishes a good customer relationship and prepares the hair for your professional services.

client's hair. Hard water contains calcium and magnesium salts and other minerals which curdle some shampoos. This leaves a dulling deposit on the hair shaft and makes the hair difficult to comb. Water can be softened by distillation or by using special cosmetic preparations. Washing soda (sodium carbonate) will soften water. Many salons install water softeners.

Client Draping

After seating your client at the station, ask the client to remove any neck and head jewelry. Turn the client's collar down and inside the neck so that the clothing does not get soiled or wet.

Place a disposable neck strip or towel around the client's neck and hold with the fingers. Fasten a shampoo cape over the neck strip (see Figure 5.1). The neck band of the cape should not touch the client's skin. Fold the neck strip or towel over the cape to form a cuff. Remove all hairpins and ornaments from the client's hair. Examine the scalp and hair so that you can recommend the correct shampoo.

Brush the hair to remove dirt and stimulate the scalp. Follow the procedures for scientific brushing that are explained on page 4. After you have finished brushing the hair, place a towel over the client's shoulders and secure it with a clamp (see Figure 5.2).

Scientific Brushing

Scientific brushing is important to remove any tangles or backcombing before a shampoo. Brushing also relaxes your client and removes dust and hair spray debris.

There are two general types of hairbrushes—those with **natural bristles** and those with **synthetic bristles**. Natural bristle brushes are made from animal hair, usually boar's hair. Boar's hair bristles have a structure that is similar to human hair. The bristles have imbrications, little scalelike cells that overlap one another (see Chapter 2). These scales help clean the hair as it is brushed. The bristles are tapered on the ends and are not sharp. A stiff, natural bristle brush is recommended for regular brushing.

Synthetic bristle brushes are usually nylon. Some synthetic bristle brushes have very sharp bristles that can irritate, scratch, or cut the scalp. This type of brush is not recommended. Some first-quality nylon bristle brushes have beveled bristles. The brushes are very useful for smoothing the hair during comb-outs, because the bristles are very smooth and sleek.

It is important to brush the hair and the scalp prior to a shampoo. Using a natural bristle brush on the scalp and hair helps remove skin debris (skin cells that have been shed), dust, and oil. However, if the hair is fragile, weak, or thinning, avoid brushing and use scalp massage and combing only.

The first step of the procedure is to wash your hands, which you must always do before touching your client. As a rule, wash your hands as the first step of *every* procedure.

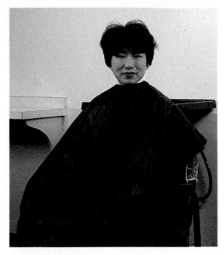

5.1   Fasten cape over neck strip

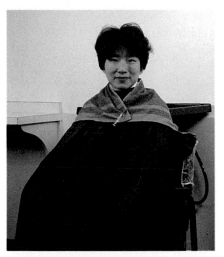

5.2   Secure towel with clamp

Materials

Drape	Brush
Towel or neck strip	Tangle comb
Clips	

Procedure for Scientific Brushing

1. Wash your hands.
2. Drape the client.
3. Examine the scalp for abrasions.
4. Remove tangles from the hair with a comb or brush.
5. Part the hair in four equal sections from center front to center nape and from ear to ear over the crown of the head. Secure three sections with clips.
6. Begin brushing the section that is not clipped.
   a. Divide the section into smaller segments approximately $\frac{1}{2}$ inch in width.
   b. Brush each small segment three times. Roll the brush on the scalp, and brush through the entire length of the hair. Always brush away from the client's face and away from yourself. Otherwise you will get dandruff or skin debris on the client or on yourself.
   c. Part another section and repeat the brushing procedure. Continue through all four sections.
7. Brush the hairline around the entire head and brush all sections together.
8. Place equipment in a container reserved for soiled equipment.

◆SAFETY **PRECAUTION**◆

Always test water temperature on your wrist before wetting client's hair.

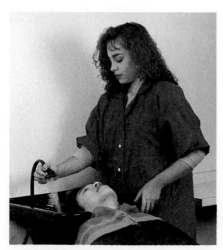

5.3   Check water temperature

Giving a Basic Shampoo

Make sure your client is in a comfortable position. Adjust the shampoo chair to fit under the neck of the shampoo bowl. If the chair has a footrest, check to see that it is in the proper position.

Adjust the water temperature by first turning on the cold water and then the hot water (see Figure 5.3). Test water temperature on your wrist. This is a safety precaution in case the hose should slip and spray the client with hot water.

Assemble all materials before starting the shampoo. It is very annoying to a client to be left with wet hair at the shampoo bowl while you run off to get shampoo and other needed materials.

Materials

Neck strip	Shampoo
Shampoo cape	Hair rinse
Towel	Clamp to secure towel
Comb and hairbrush	

Procedure for Giving a Basic Shampoo

1. Drape client.
2. Brush hair.
3. Pin towel firmly around the neck.
4. Adjust the shampoo chair.
5. Regulate the water temperature and thoroughly wet the hair by holding the spray slightly away from the hair. Protect the client's face and ears from the spray by placing your hand as shown in Figure 5.4. With your hand in this position, the thumb and first finger help to control the flow of water around the hairline, moving the water through the hair and away from the face. Make sure that you do not allow the hand to rest on the forehead. This might remove the client's makeup. Figure 5.5 shows how the hand is curved around the ears, thus allowing the hairline to be wet thoroughly and rinsed without getting water in the ears.

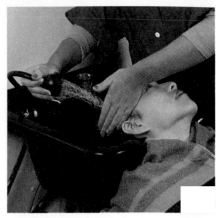

5.4   Protect face and ears

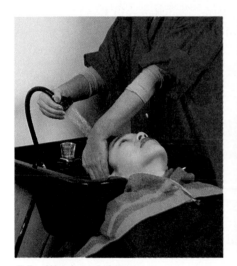

5.5   Wet down hairline

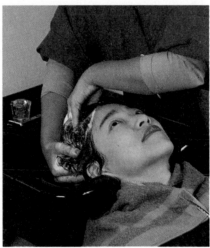

5.6   Start shampoo

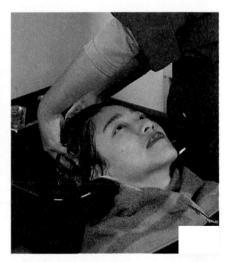

5.7   Shampoo crown

6. Apply shampoo. Lift the hair slightly from the scalp with one hand and pour the liquid shampoo on various areas of the hair.
7. Starting at the center hairline, massage the scalp by using the cushions of the fingers in a back-and-forth movement (see Figure 5.6). Massage this area several times, working back to the crown area.
8. Move to the sides of the head above the ear area and massage from hairline to crown area (see Figure 5.7).
9. With the head still resting on the shampoo bowl, massage the crown area, working the fingers back and forth in this area.
10. Gently raise the client's head, supporting it with one hand (see Figure 5.8). With your fingers spread apart, start massaging from the right ear, working up and down across the nape area to the left ear. Repeat several times. Using the cushions of the fingers, gently massage in a circular pattern along the neck to a one-two-three count. This is very relaxing to the client.

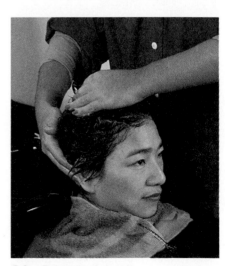

5.8   Raise client's head

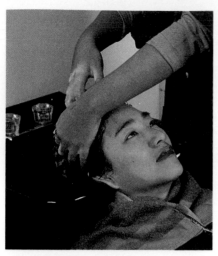

5.9 Massage front hairline

11. Rest the client's head on the shampoo bowl. Keep both hands underneath the head at the nape area and make sure there is no hair between the shampoo bowl and the neck. Repeat the rotating massage described in step 10 along the front hairline (see Figure 5.9).

12. Rinse the hair thoroughly with a strong spray of water, protecting the face and ears.

13. Apply shampoo for a second time and massage the entire scalp, using the various manipulations described in steps 7 through 11.

14. Rinse the hair thoroughly as in step 12.

15. Follow with a cold-water rinse if the client wishes one. A cold rinse stimulates circulation and closes the pores, but you should never give one without first telling the client.

16. Apply a rinse or instant conditioner if necessary.

17. Remove excess moisture from the hair by squeezing it between your hands. This keeps the towel from getting wet and the water from dripping down the client's neck.

18. As you raise your client's head from the shampoo bowl, place the towel over the hair and with the corner of the towel dry the area behind the ears. By doing this, you will make the client more comfortable and will protect the clothing from water stains.

19. Move the client to the styling salon.

TYPES OF SHAMPOOS AND PROCEDURES

Many brand-name shampoos are designed for use with particular types of hair and scalp conditions. It is important that you read the labels carefully so that you know how to use the product properly. Make sure you analyze the hair and scalp before selecting a shampoo.

Plain Shampoo

Plain shampoos contain soap or a detergent base and are usually transparent. If you have hard water, it is better to use a shampoo with a detergent base, rather than a soap base. Detergent shampoos are also better for oily hair.

Plain shampoo can be used on normal hair that is in good condition and has not been chemically treated. But plain shampoos are not recommended for hair that has been lightened, tinted, permed, straightened, or damaged by the sun or improper care. Most plain shampoos should be followed by an acid rinse to counteract the effect of alkalies on the hair.

Cream Shampoo

Cream shampoos have a milky appearance and contain oily compounds that not only cleanse the hair but have a reconditioning effect. They make the hair feel softer. Cream shampoos are manufactured and packaged in liquid and semisolid form. They come in bottles, tubes, and jars.

CLIENT TIP ◆◆◆◆◆◆◆

Work the shampoo into a lather as you pour. This relieves the initial shock of cold shampoo.

CLIENT TIP ◆◆◆◆◆◆◆

When using a cream or concentrated shampoo, squeeze the shampoo into the palm of your hand. Rub your hands together to break down the consistency, then proceed with shampoo manipulations.

Shampoo for Lightened Hair

If hair has been lightened, use a shampoo designed for damaged or chemically treated hair. Use water just warm enough for your client to be comfortable. Keep in mind that lightened hair tangles easily. Apply shampoo slowly and work with your hands underneath the hair to avoid matting. To make the hair easier to comb, use a detangling rinse or an instant conditioner.

Nonstripping Shampoo

Special shampoos for tinted hair are called nonstripping or acid-balanced shampoos. They do not remove color from the hair, as many alkali shampoos do. They are milder and contain conditioners. These shampoos are also recommended for dry, damaged, or chemically treated hair. Many manufacturers make special shampoos for permanent waving. Always be sure to follow the manufacturer's instructions when using these shampoos.

Soapless Oil Shampoo

Soapless oil shampoo has an oil base that is soluble in water. It is a **sulphonated** (**SUL** fuh nay ted) **oil** (an oil mixed with sulfuric acid) and is an excellent cleanser. These shampoos do not attack the structure of the hair like soaps that are strongly alkaline. These shampoos also work well when hard water is used. They are easily rinsed from the hair, and so the scum problem is eliminated.

Dandruff Shampoo

Most dandruff shampoos contain a medicated ingredient that helps resist dirt buildup and unsightly dandruff. They also contain a special conditioner that leaves hair more manageable.

There are many dandruff shampoos on the market, and they must be used according to the manufacturers' instructions. Be guided by your hair and scalp analysis when using a dandruff shampoo. It is important to massage the scalp vigorously and to rinse the hair thoroughly.

Medicated Shampoo

There are special medicated shampoos that are made to treat scalp and hair disorders other than dandruff, such as seborrhea and psoriasis. Some medicated shampoos must be prescribed by a physician, but others can be purchased over the counter. When using any medicated product, always be extremely careful to follow the instructions. Never service a client who appears to have ringworm or head lice (see Chapter 2).

Powder Dry Shampoo

A powder dry shampoo is given when a client's physical condition will not permit giving a wet shampoo. A commercial dry shampoo is commonly used, but almond meal, cornmeal, or orris root also work well.

Materials

Neck strip	Comb and hairbrush	Gauze
Shampoo cape	Powder dry shampoo	Clamp to secure towel
Towels		

Procedure for a Powder Dry Shampoo

1. Drape the client for a shampoo.
2. Divide the hair into four sections.
3. Working with one section at a time, start at the top of the head and stroke the dry shampoo into the hair so that it forms a coating on the hair shaft from the scalp to the hair ends.
4. Continue until all sections are covered and allow the dry shampoo to remain on the hair for 3 to 5 minutes.
5. Taking a small section of hair at a time, brush the hair from scalp to hair ends, carefully going over the entire head in all directions. Keep the brush clean as you work by rubbing it with a clean towel. A piece of gauze may be placed over the brush and changed as it becomes soiled. It is important to work with a clean brush so that the hair is not left looking dusty or powdery.

Peroxide Shampoo

This shampoo is sometimes referred to as a brightening or highlighting shampoo. Hydrogen peroxide and ammonia water are added to a commercial shampoo. The original hair color, the strength of the shampoo, and the length of time it remains on the hair are important to the end results. Too strong a solution or repeated use will result in an obvious color difference between shampooed hair and new growth.

Materials

Neck strip	Shampoo	Measuring cup
Shampoo cape	Hydrogen peroxide	Clamp to secure towel
Towels	Ammonia water	Timer

Procedure for a Peroxide Shampoo

1. Prepare the client as for a plain shampoo.
2. Prepare shampoo by mixing ½ ounce of hydrogen peroxide with 1 ounce of shampoo and 3 drops of ammonia water.
3. Lather shampoo mixture into the dry hair and leave on hair for 5 to 10 minutes. The length of time the shampoo is left on the hair depends on how much lighter you are trying to get the hair.
4. Rinse hair thoroughly.
5. Give a shampoo that is recommended for lightened hair.
6. Style the hair.

Henna Shampoo

The shade achieved from a henna shampoo will depend on the original color of the hair. The lighter the shade of hair, the more auburn-red it will be after the shampoo. Darker shades of hair will acquire a brightness rather than a definite change of color. Do not use a henna shampoo on blond, white, or gray hair. To do so would give the hair an orange shade. (For more information, see Chapter 14.)

Materials

Neck strip	Shampoo	Comb
Shampoo cape	Measuring cup	Hairbrushes
Towels	Henna powder	
Bowl and spoon for mixing	Clamp to secure towel	

Procedure for a Henna Shampoo

1. Prepare the client as for a plain shampoo.
2. Shampoo the hair.
3. Rinse thoroughly.
4. Prepare formula by mixing 1 cup Egyptian henna powder with enough boiling water to make a creamy consistency.
5. Test to make sure the mixture is not too hot for the scalp.
6. Work mixture well into the hair.
7. Leave the mixture on the hair for 5 to 15 minutes, depending on the shade desired.
8. Strand-test by rinsing the mixture off a few strands of hair. A wet towel may be used to wipe the strand for a color check.
9. Rinse thoroughly with warm water.
10. Shampoo hair according to regular procedure and rinse.
11. Complete record card (see Chapter 14).
12. Style the hair.

Safety Precautions for All Shampoos

1. Make sure cape and towel are fastened securely.
2. Check water temperature before wetting the client's head.
3. Avoid scratching the client's scalp with your fingernails when giving a shampoo.
4. See that the client's head is back far enough into the basin.
5. Read and follow instructions for all special shampoos used.
6. Clean and sanitize shampoo bowl after each use.
7. Do not permit water to remain on the floor.

> ◆ **Key Point** ◆
> Shampoos are available for all hair types and conditions. Analyze the hair to select the appropriate shampoo.

HAIR RINSES

Hair rinses are given after a shampoo to remove soap from the hair, to make the hair more manageable, to temporarily highlight or brighten the hair, to give a lustrous appearance, and to temporarily change the color.

Vinegar (Acetic) Rinse

A vinegar (acetic) rinse, often referred to as an acid rinse, is used to remove soap curds from the hair and make it brighter and more manageable. This rinse is used as the last rinse after a shampoo. Pour through the hair and rinse from the hair to remove any odor. To prepare an acetic rinse, mix ¼ cup of vinegar with 1 pint of tepid water. Lemon juice also makes an effective acid rinse.

Finishing Rinses

There are many finishing rinses on the market today. These are recommended for hair that has been tinted, bleached, or permanent waved. It softens the hair and helps to remove tangles.

Color Rinses

Color rinses are used to highlight the color of the hair (including gray hair) without changing the natural shade. If a person desires to change the hair coloring, rinses are easily removed. Color rinses usually last from one shampoo to the next. (See Chapter 14 for more information.)

HAIR CONDITIONERS

Hair that has been damaged or is dry and brittle should be treated with a conditioner. Instant conditioners can be used each time the hair is shampooed. If the hair is severely dry or damaged, a more penetrating treatment should be given. See Chapter 6 for more information on conditioners.

> ◆ Key Point ◆
>
> Almost every shampoo will be finished with a rinse or conditioner for the hair type. Thoroughly rinse the treatment from the hair before proceeding with your service.

SUMMARY

The key to attractive hair is its cleanliness. The hair should be shampooed as often as necessary with a product designed for the hair type and condition. As a stylist, you will determine the best shampoo for the hair type, based upon your analysis. You will then shampoo according to any special instructions for the condition and follow through with the appropriate rinse or conditioner.

The shampoo is a chance for you to put your client at ease about the service to come. A quality shampoo expresses that you are qualified to offer the services the client desires, and gives you an excellent opportunity to analyze the hair for future retail sales.

Not all chemical services require a shampoo, and in the case of relaxers, you should definitely not shampoo prior to the service. A shampoo before a chemical service should be very gentle, especially on the scalp. Avoid tangling the hair; rinse thoroughly so that the shampoo does not interfere with chemicals that you later apply.

Choosing the correct shampoo for the hair type is the first step of a professional service. This builds the foundation for successful services and for continued retail sales.

QUESTIONS

1. What is the importance of the shampoo service?
2. What preparation should be done for the client before shampooing?
3. What is the correct procedure for a professional shampoo?

4. What types of shampoos are available and for what purpose should each be used?
5. How would you alter the shampoo procedure before a chemical service in the salon?
6. What are the purposes for which hair rinses are used?

1. Research the shampoos that are available in your school and at home. Make a chart indicating the ingredients common to all. Categorize the shampoos according to recommended use: dry, damaged, oily, thinning, etc. Note any differences in the directions for proper use.
2. Compare the inventories of shampoos and rinses at three local salons. Note the differences between the products used in the salon and those available for retail.
3. Working with hair swatches, compare the results of available shampoos on normal, permed, color-treated, and relaxed hair. Repeat each shampoo six times on the swatch and then report the effects of each shampoo. Make recommendations for the ideal shampoo for each swatch.
4. Using manufacturer directions as a guide, make a list of services that recommend a shampoo and those that do not. Indicate the correct shampoo, if directed, and any special techniques to be used prior to the service. Outline how the hair is prepared in those instances where a shampoo is not recommended.
5. Properly prepare a client for a chemical service from the moment you greet him/her at the reception area. Demonstrate the correct massage techniques for a shampoo.

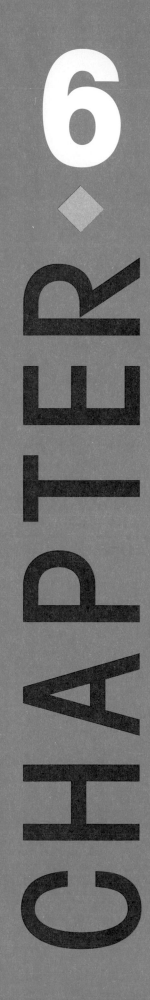

HAIR DAMAGE AND TREATMENT

CHAPTER GOAL

Your goal as a cosmetologist is to help your clients have healthy, beautiful hair. After reading this chapter and completing the projects, you should be able to

1. Define the categories of hair damage and describe the characteristics of each.
2. Outline the corrective measures for each type of hair damage.
3. Demonstrate the procedure for simple and multiple treatment conditioning.
4. Explain the procedure for hair analysis.
5. Demonstrate analysis techniques for each hair characteristic.
6. Demonstrate basic scalp manipulation movements.
7. Prescribe at least seven methods to prevent hair damage.

CHAPTER 6

Beautiful, healthy hair is desired by women and men of all ages. As a future stylist, you will advise your clients on the best care and treatment of their hair outside of your salon and provide the products they need to follow your suggestions. In the salon, the simplest service you will offer is that of conditioning.

Conditioning treatments are a part of nearly all services: shampoos, cuts, styles, and chemical treatments. Determining the right conditioner for the specific hair problem will put you head and shoulders above the competition.

The key to understanding the different types of hair damage and the corrective conditioning treatments is knowledge of the hair itself. Each layer of the hair has particular characteristics and is responsible for specific hair qualities. As a cosmetologist, you must be able to analyze the type of hair damage, prescribe a remedy, and advise your client on the way to avoid hair damage in the future.

CATEGORIES OF HAIR DAMAGE

There are four distinct categories of hair damage. They are

1. Cuticle damage
2. Moisture imbalance
3. Protein loss
4. Chemical or elasticity damage

Cuticle Damage

The cuticle layer, the outer part of the hair, protects the hair. It is the first line of defense against all the other forms of hair damage and should be considered in all hair services in the salon and at home. Figure 6.1 shows a normal, healthy cuticle.

When the cuticle is damaged, the hair appears dull and lacks sheen. It tangles easily, and has a rough texture. Hair with cuticle damage will wet easily which means that it absorbs liquids very fast. This characteristic, porosity, can lead to further damage of the interior layers of the hair.

Cuticle damage, such as that shown in Figure 6.2, can be caused by heat, by mechanical abuse during styling, and by chemical services. It is important that your clients understand how to care for their hair at home to prevent this damage from occurring. Excess heat from blow dryers, curling irons, and hot rollers can weaken the cuticle layers, leading to split ends (see Figure 6.3) and a dry, dull appearance. Mechanical abuse such as brushing the hair while wet

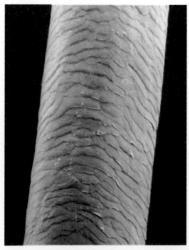

6.1 Healthy cuticle

can cause extreme damage to the hair that is nearly impossible to repair. Chemical services, since they must penetrate the cuticle layer to alter properties of the cortex, always cause some degree of cuticle damage.

Cuticle damage is the first to occur. It can be present with no other hair problems evident. It is important that you treat it right away so that no further harm can happen to the hair shaft. How? The first method is **acidification** (a SID i fi **KAY** shun), the application of a product with a low pH to the hair. In the past, vinegar or lemon rinses were used. Today, magnesium salts or citric acid solutions are used to "superacidify" the hair after chemical services. Spray clean, damp hair with a citric acid or magnesium solution. Work the solution through the hair for a few minutes and apply moisturizing cream directly over acidifier. Time according to manufacturer's directions and rinse. Products with acidifying ingredients in diluted form combined with **emollients** (i **MOL** yents) to make the cuticle surface feel smooth are used to maintain the cuticle.

Occasionally, cuticle damage is so severe that it cannot be effectively treated in this manner. Discuss the situation with your instructor to see if a product that provides a synthetic cuticle must be applied. Follow your instructor's guidelines for use.

Moisture Imbalance

Healthy hair should have a moisture content of nine to eleven percent. This gives it the pliability that it needs to hold a style and lubricates the interior layers of the hair so that it has bounce and body. Moisture imbalance can only happen if the cuticle is damaged, so it is important to consider that as well. There are two types of moisture problems that the hair can have: too much or too little. The first, that of too little moisture, is more common. Dry hair looks and feels brittle. If the atmosphere is also dry, this hair will have static electricity, more commonly known as "fly-away hair." Moisture loss can be caused by exposure to the elements; however, the most common cause of moisture damage is thermal styling. Advise your clients to avoid excess heat when drying, curling, or pressing their hair. Dryness is also a side effect of chemical services. You can correct it in the salon during the process, but your client should maintain the moisture level with quality products at home.

To treat dryness, add moisture to the hair. While this can be done by simply wetting the hair, the correction will not last. The best method is to use a moisturizer, a special conditioner that contains **humectants** (hyoo **MECK** tants) that carry moisture and bind it inside the hair. Most moisturizers also contain ingredients that protect the cuticle to prevent further damage.

The second type of moisture damage, that of too much, is less common but occurs in humid areas and when chemical services such as permanent waves have not been properly finished. This hair is limp and lifeless. It often takes a very long time to dry and does not hold a curl or style. If the hair is wavy or curly, it will have a tendency to frizz when dry, especially around the hairline.

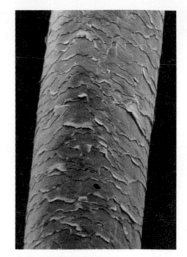

6.2   Cuticle damage

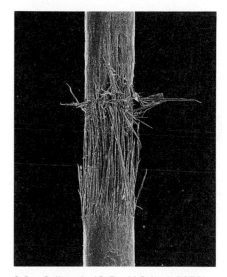

6.3   Split ends (© David Scharf, 1979)

To treat excess moisture, first superacidify the hair. Spray clean, damp hair with a citric or magnesium solution. Work the solution through the hair for a few minutes and apply a moisturizing cream directly over the acidifier. Time according to manufacturer's directions and rinse.

Protein Loss

The primary component of hair is protein, accounting for over 85 percent of its structure. Any chemical service that alters the **cortex**, the second layer of the hair containing its bonds, may cause protein damage. The bonds occur between amino acids, building blocks to protein. So any alteration of those bonds results in protein loss.

Hair that is lacking protein will break easily. Natural color will look dull and lifeless and appear lighter in spots. Haircolor services will fade rapidly and permanent waves will not take or hold curl. The primary culprit in protein loss is chemical services that are not done properly, especially those that are done at home. Excessive exposure to the sun can rob protein from the hair and even fluorescent lighting can cause mild protein loss!

Hair with this damage should be treated with a protein conditioner. Today's professional conditioners contain protein that has a small molecular weight. This means that the size of the ingredient is small enough to be easily and rapidly absorbed into the hair. Common ingredients are plant and herbal extracts, and hydrolyzed animal protein. Liquid protein conditioners are used for fine, thin, or moderately damaged hair. They are also incorporated into chemical services. Cream protein conditioners are used for more seriously damaged hair and often include moisturizers as protein damage almost never occurs without moisture loss.

Chemical or Elasticity Damage

Normal hair will stretch about 20 percent of its length when dry and return to its normal position. When elasticity damage occurs, the hydrogen and the salt bonds in the cortex have been seriously disrupted or even destroyed to such an extent that the elasticity of the hair is gone. The hair is extremely brittle when it is dry, breaking easily. When the hair is wet, it feels soft and spongy and stretches excessively without returning to its normal position. This hair has serious problems! The most common cause is chemical services; either given improperly or too often or both. Elasticity damage can also be caused by brushing the wet hair, stretching the hair beyond its limits. Figure 6.4 shows hair in its virgin, or unstretched position. Figure 6.5 indicates the stress placed on the bonds of the cortex as the hair is stretched. Figure 6.6 shows severely damaged hair that has been stretched beyond its elasticity limit. The bonds have been destroyed.

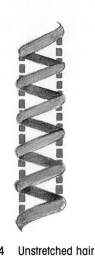
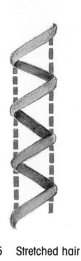
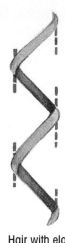

6.4   Unstretched hair   6.5   Stretched hair   6.6   Hair with elasticity damage

Treatment for elasticity damage should be done only in the salon. First, the hair should be gently shampooed. Take care not to tangle the hair by keeping your fingers underneath the hair and using only gentle manipulations. Next, rinse the hair thoroughly with warm water and low pressure. Blot the hair with a towel and then spray the hair with an acidifying solution. Use your fingers to gently work the liquid through the hair and remove tangles. After a few minutes, apply a cream protein conditioner according to manufacturer's directions. Gently work through with a wide-tooth comb. Place a plastic cap over the hair and put your client under a warm dryer. When the suggested time has elapsed, rinse thoroughly and moisturize.

Familiarize your client with quality products which will continue to protect the repair of the hair. Try to determine what originally caused the elasticity damage to the client's hair. Discourage any further chemical services until the damage is corrected. If the damage occurred at home, suggest that future services be performed by a qualified professional. Encourage your client to allow hair to dry naturally or be wet set. Thermal styling should be discouraged until the hair reaches normal elasticity levels.

CORRECTIVE TREATMENTS

Corrective treatments should be as specific as possible to adjust the damage that you determine is present. In the salon, it is very likely that you will be correcting several characteristics of the hair in one treatment. Always apply conditioning products on clean, towel-dried hair and follow the manufacturer's directions. If you are choosing a treatment to correct multiple problems, always correct elasticity damage first, then protein, then moisture, and finally cuticle damage. This is known as the ARM method; acidifying, reconditioning, moisturizing.

Conditioning Techniques

The following procedure is the most common for liquid and for cream conditioners. Always follow manufacturer's directions for best results.

Materials

Drape	Wide-tooth comb	Timer
Towels	pH balanced shampoo	Brush
Neck strip	Conditioner prescribed	Spatula

Procedure for Conditioning Techniques

1. Seat client comfortably at shampoo bowl.
2. Wash your hands with antibacterial soap.
3. Drape your client.
4. Remove tangles from the hair gently.
5. Shampoo the hair with the appropriate shampoo for the type of hair damage, usually one formulated for dry, or chemically treated hair.
6. Rinse thoroughly with warm water and moderate pressure. Re-apply shampoo for second lather only if hair is heavily soiled.
7. Blot gently with a towel to remove excess water.
8. Apply appropriate conditioner. Acidify first if necessary, then recondition, then moisturize and/or treat cuticle damage.
    a. Spray liquids onto the hair with a pump sprayer. Lift crown hair to apply to nape area and ends.
    b. Remove cream conditioners from the container with a spatula. Measure the correct amount into the palm of your hand. Rub your hands together to break down or emulsify the conditioner.
9. Work your fingers through the client's hair, especially on the fragile ends and more damaged areas.
10. Comb through the hair with a wide-tooth comb from forehead to crown, from nape to crown, and from sides up and back to the crown.
11. Time according to manufacturer's directions. For deeper penetration, the manufacturer may direct you to place a plastic cap over the hair and place under a warm dryer.
12. Rinse thoroughly.
13. Blot with towel.
14. Proceed with next salon service.

Hair Analysis

Every contact that you have with a client should begin with a consultation. This is the time when you determine what it is that your client wants, what is working, what is not. Then, as a professional stylist, you make decisions to correct problems and continue successes.

> **◆ Key Point ◆**
>
> Corrective treatments are a major part of your professional services. Always incorporate corrective treatments into all chemical services.

Every consultation that you do should include hair analysis. Depending upon the situation, that analysis may be very detailed or quite brief. Every analysis considers the following characteristics of the hair:

1. Porosity
2. Texture
3. Elasticity
4. Density
5. Condition
6. Scalp condition

Analysis Techniques

Materials

Cape	Clips	Wide-tooth comb
Towel or neck strip	Brush	Record card

Procedure for Analysis

1. Seat your client comfortably at the area designated for analysis or at your styling station.
2. Sanitize your hands.
3. Drape your client.
   a. Place a towel or a disposable neck strip around the client's neck and hold it with your fingers.
   b. Fasten a shampoo cape over the towel or neck strip. Make sure that the band of the cape does not touch the client's neck.
   c. Fold the upper half of the towel over the cape to form a cuff.
4. Remove tangles from the hair gently.
5. Part the hair in four equal sections from the center of the forehead to the nape of the neck and from ear to ear over the crown of the head. Clip hair out of your way for ease of examination.
6. Examine the scalp for abrasions and check for hair qualities in the following descriptions.
7. Record all readings and comments on the client record card along with treatments given.

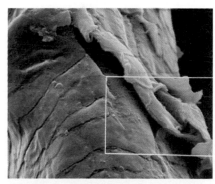

6.7 Hair with extreme porosity

Porosity

This characteristic of the hair is measured by touch. Hair that has low porosity is resistant to penetration by liquids. It has a cuticle layer that is hard and compact and feels smooth. Hair with more porosity will feel rough. Hair with extreme porosity will be raspy (see Figure 6.7).

Another way to check for porosity is to take a small section of hair, lift it from the scalp and move your fingers along the hair shaft toward the scalp (see Figure 6.8). The more the hair ruffles as you slide with your fingers, the more porous the hair is. Hair that is very porous will make a sound and will resist your fingers as you try to slide them down the hair.

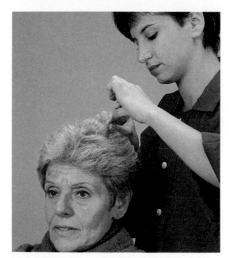

6.8 Check hair porosity

Finally, you can observe the hair as you wet it to gauge porosity. Hair with a lifted cuticle will absorb liquids more rapidly. Hair that is resistant will not; and if the hair is extremely resistant or glassy, it will almost repel moisture.

Texture

Texture refers to the diameter, or the actual size of each hair (see Figure 6.9). It also includes the feel of the hair, whether it is fine, medium, or coarse.

Texture can be measured by touch or by specialized equipment that measures the protein content of the hair (the higher the protein level, the coarser the hair). The texture of the hair is linked to genetic tendencies.

Elasticity

The ability of the hair to stretch and return to its normal length can be measured by hand, although it is difficult to determine the exact level of elasticity. Take a single dry hair and stretch it 20 percent of its length. Release the hair and observe if it springs back to its original position (see Figure 6.10). The speed and the degree of its return will give you a reasonable estimate of its elasticity.

Accurate measurement of elasticity can only be done by analysis machines. An **analysis machine** is a device that tests the strength, elasticity, and moisture content of hair. Hair that stretches 20 percent of its length and then returns to its original state has good elasticity. Any instrumental measure of moisture content will also give you a good estimate of the elasticity level.

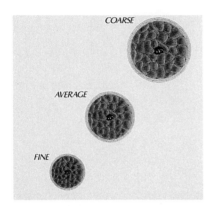

6.9   Hair texture

Density

Density refers to the amount of hairs per square inch of scalp. Usually, blonde hair is thickest and red hair is the thinnest. The reasons for this are unknown, although it is assumed to be a genetic characteristic.

Condition

This complex term considers all of the characteristics of the hair. Hair that is in good condition is also described as resilient, being able to withstand the normal pressures of styling and chemical services. While the term *condition* is quite vague for a professional stylist, it is a good word to use when you begin consultation analysis with your client.

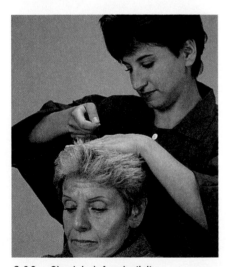

6.10   Check hair for elasticity

Scalp Condition

No analysis of the hair is complete without assessing the scalp. Chemical services should not be performed on a scalp that has abrasions, redness, or sores. To do so could further irritate the scalp and lead to an allergic condition. Excess oiliness or dryness leads to damage of the hair and, in many instances, hair loss. While you cannot return hair that is gone, you can often advise your client on methods to prevent future hair loss. Topical application of several of the B vitamins in conjunction with scalp treatments is thought to reduce hair loss. Additionally, your client may wish to see a physician to ensure that the hormones are in the correct balance.

SCALP MANIPULATIONS

Scalp manipulations are recommended as part of many scalp and hair treatments to relax the client and loosen the scalp. A basic procedure for scalp massage follows.

Materials

Shampoo cape   Brush or comb   Neck strip or towel

Procedure for Scalp Massage

1. Wash your hands.
2. Drape the client using a neck strip or a towel and a shampoo cape.
3. Examine the scalp for lesions or abrasions.
4. Comb tangles from the hair.
5. Perform the seven basic scalp manipulations, as described in the following section (movements should be performed in order, without interruption).

Basic Scalp Manipulations

Movement 1: Rotating the Hairline (Figure 6.11)

1. Place your fingers on the hairline, spreading them from the front top of the ear to the top of the head. The pads of your fingertips should be pressing on the scalp. Avoid scratching your client with fingernails. Curve your hands so that your palms do not rest on the scalp.
2. Pressing firmly, rotate all fingers in upward circles, counting one-two-three.
3. Repeat two more times.

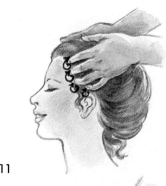

6.11

Movement 2: Rotating the Sides of the Head (Figure 6.12)

1. Lift one hand at a time and place the fingers on the scalp 1 inch behind the hairline, with the little fingers about 1 inch above the ear. One hand should be in the new position before the other hand is lifted.
2. Spread the fingers as in movement 1.
3. Rotate as in movement 1.
4. Repeat two more times.

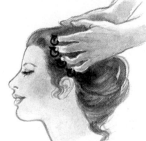

6.12

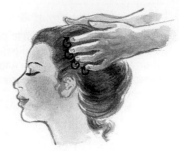

6.13

Movement 3: Rotating Behind the Ears to the Top of the Head (Figure 6.13)

1. Lift one hand at a time and place fingers in the scalp about 1 inch behind the ears. Do not break contact with the scalp as you massage.
2. Spread the fingers as in movement 1.
3. Rotate as in movement 1.
4. Repeat two more times.

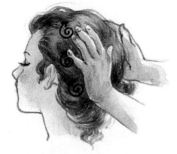

6.14

Movement 4: Massaging the Back of the Head (Figure 6.14)

1. Cup the bones at the top of the head with the hands.
2. Using the heels of the hands, rotate at the crown, counting one-two-three.
3. Lift the hands off the head one at a time and place them at the middle of the back of the head. Rotate, counting one-two-three.
4. Lift the hands off the head again and place them at the nape of the head. Rotate, counting one-two-three.
5. Repeat the entire procedure two more times.

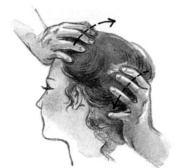

6.15

Movement 5: Twisting the Scalp (Figure 6.15)

1. Move to the side of the client without breaking contact.
2. Place the heels of the hands at the front and back hairlines, spreading the fingers on the scalp.
3. Applying pressure with the hands, twist the scalp by moving your hands in opposite directions, counting one-two-three.
4. Repeat two more times.

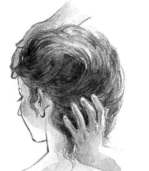

6.16

Movement 6: Rotating the Nape (Figure 6.16)

1. Move to the side of the client, grasping the forehead with one hand.
2. With the other hand, cup the crest of the occipital bone on the side of the client's head at the back. With the heel of the hand in the hollow of the nape, directly under the bone, rotate one-two-three.
3. Go to the middle of the head and rotate as in step 2. Then go to the other side of the head and rotate as in step 2.
4. Repeat the entire procedure two more times.

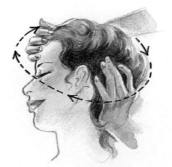

6.17

Movement 7: Rotating the Head (Figure 6.17)

1. Place the hands on the head at the front hairline and nape.
2. Move the client's head in slow, rhythmic circles, counting one-two-three.
3. Make three circles in one direction and then three circles in the other direction.

PREVENTION OF HAIR DAMAGE

Even though the environment, styling methods, chemical services, and just plain wear and tear all contribute to hair damage, it can be prevented. As a qualified professional, you will learn the methods to compensate for side effects of your salon services and how to advise your client to care for the hair and scalp at home. The following guidelines are the ABCs of hair care.

Shampoos

It is very important that you and your client always use a shampoo that is balanced on the pH scale between 4.5 and 5.5. This is the natural pH of the scalp's acid mantle and ideal for the protection of the hair. Additionally, become familiar with the cleansing agents in shampoos, known as **surfactants** (sir **FACT** ants), and choose products with more gentle agents. Shampoos for chemically treated or dry hair contain natural oils and sometimes conditioners to reduce damage and deposit essential fatty acids in the cuticle layer of the hair.

Extremely oily hair should be shampooed gently as well to avoid further stimulation of the glands. If the hair is very soiled, apply the shampoo to dry hair, massage, then rinse and shampoo again.

Conditioners

Manufacturers have provided us with thousands of conditioners, but they fall into four general categories: detanglers, moisturizers, protein conditioners, and styling aids. Do your research and find the best conditioners available and the ones that are right for each of the types of damage outlined.

Detanglers either acidify or coat the cuticle to prevent and remove snarls. They do not usually offer any other benefits to the hair. Detanglers are recommended for hair in good condition, or as a final step in the treatment of hair with more complex problems. Be sure that any coatings left on the hair do not build up and are easily removed with a single shampoo.

Moisturizers contain humectants that carry moisture into the cuticle and sometimes the cortex layers of the hair. The best also regulate the level of moisture in the hair to the normal balance of nine to eleven percent. These conditioners should be the last step in each and every chemical service that you perform and should be used for at-home maintenance for all clients that you determine have dry hair. Moisturizers can also be used to treat the scalp.

Protein Conditioners add amino acids to hair that has been weakened by chemical services or exposure to the environment. Both liquid and protein conditioners may be used in chemical services to prevent damage. Liquid formulas are used on hair that has moderate damage or is fine or thin. Cream conditioners are used to prevent overlapping chemicals on previsously treated hair and for hair types that are more severely damaged, thick, or coarse.

> **CLIENT TIP ◆◆◆◆◆◆◆**
>
> If your client has double-processed hair, is undergoing chemotherapy, or has naturally fragile hair, keep your fingers underneath the hair and use only your fingertips while shampooing. A single lather is enough; follow with a thorough rinsing and conditioning.

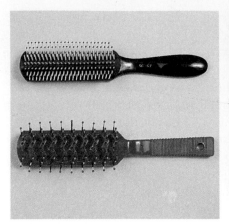

6.18

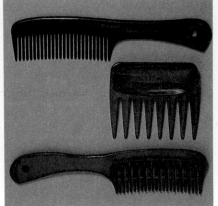

6.19

Styling Aids are not actually conditioners but are very important as preventive products. A styling aid should always be used when wet or thermal styling the hair in order to prevent damage to the hair in its fragile condition. Those designed for thermal styling add **lubricity** (loo **BRI** si tee); they make the hair more slippery and smooth so that thermal styling is easier and less harmful. Styling aids are available in many forms so that you can pick the one best suited for your client's hair type and style.

Equipment

Damage to the hair can be avoided by the proper choice of styling tools. Today's styling equipment is varied and offers many different effects. Keep in touch with new materials and know the features and benefits of each.

Hairbrushes should be considered in the prevention of hair damage. It is best to use natural bristle brushes, or synthetic bristles that have rounded tips. Hairbrushes should not be used on wet hair as they can cause severe damage. Vent type or widely spaced plastic-bristle brushes should be used for blow drying the hair (see Figure 6.18). If the hair is chemically treated or damaged, round brushes should not be used for thermal styling. Damaged hair will tangle around the brush, causing further harm to the cuticle and frayed hair ends.

Combs should always be used on wet hair. Wide-tooth combs or rakes are best for distributing conditioners and removing tangles in dry or wet hair. Combs with narrow teeth should only be used when tangles have been removed from wet hair or for dry hair styling. Metal combs should be avoided because they tear the cuticle layer of the hair (see Figure 6.19).

> ♦ **Key Point** ♦
>
> It is easier to avoid hair damage than it is to treat it. Encourage your client to preserve healthy hair.

Summary

Everyone wants hair in excellent condition. Your client wants to have hair that shows off the best of your design. You want your chemical and styling services to be successful and that can only be possible if the hair is in good condition. The best cut will never look attractive if the hair is dull, lifeless, or frizzy.

As a cosmetologist, you will carefully analyze each client's hair. You will determine if the cuticle is damaged and lifted from the shaft. Hair with protein damage lacks strength and is prone to breakage. Moisture damage, either too much or too little, interferes with styling and can lead to further problems. Check for elasticity damage by noting the hair's resistance to stretching.

As a professional, you will select the correct product to treat each type of hair damage by comparing manufacturer's information. The products you choose should help correct the problem and prevent it from progressing. Advise your client how to care for his or her particular type of hair. Your prescription should include salon treatments and maintenance products to be used at home. When you and your client work together, the result will be healthy hair and successful salon services.

QUESTIONS

1. What are the categories of hair damage? What are the characteristics of each type of damage?
2. What corrective measure would you recommend for each type of damage?
3. What is the correct procedure for conditioning? If multiple treatments are required, in what order are they given?
4. What is the correct procedure for hair analysis? What key indicators help you determine hair condition?
5. When analyzing a client's hair, what do you look for in each hair characteristic and how do you test for it?
6. What are the steps for a basic scalp massage?
7. What would you suggest your client do at home to prevent hair damage?

PROJECTS

1. Conduct a hair analysis on at least three people. Outline the types of damage present and suggest corrective treatments. What improvements will you expect to see?
2. Perform follow-up analysis on the same three people after one, four, and eight weeks. Record improvements in hair condition and/or change your recommendation until hair meets your expectations.
3. Research features of conditioners available in your school and outline the benefits for using each one.

ELEMENTS AND PRINCIPLES OF DESIGN

CHAPTER 7

CHAPTER GOAL

Your challenge as a professional cosmetologist will be to bring the various components of a client's appearance together to create an artistic and pleasing image. After reading this chapter and completing the projects, you should be able to

1. Define *form* and explain its importance.
2. Explain how space functions within the form.
3. List three ways you will use line in the practice of cosmetology.
4. List five effects that color can have on hair design.
5. Outline how texture is used for variety in hair design.
6. Define *proportion* and explain how it is applied to hair design.
7. Give examples of symmetrical and asymmetrical balance.
8. Illustrate three types of rhythm applied to hair design.
9. Explain three methods of creating emphasis in the hairstyle.

Art is a form of communication. Most frequently, we use words to communicate ideas and express feelings; however, people also communicate through appearance. A particular hairstyle, application of makeup, or choice of clothing makes a statement about a person. This chapter offers guidelines for putting together a custom look for each of your clients.

The principles of design are studied by fashion designers, makeup artists, image consultants, and cosmetologists in an effort to create the most attractive and adaptable designs possible. Contemporary standards of design can be traced to the ancient Greek principles of purity of line, proportion, and harmony. Although hairstyles are many and varied, only those that adhere to the early Greek principles are considered classic examples of good design.

As a professional cosmetologist, you must be able to use the elements of form, space, line, color, and texture as tools to create hair designs. You will analyze your client's features to place each element. You will use the principles of proportion, balance, rhythm, emphasis, and harmony to create the desired style with the appropriate elements.

THE ELEMENTS OF DESIGN

The elements of form, space, line, color, and texture could be thought of as the building blocks of art or as pieces of a puzzle. We study each of the elements to establish definitions and guidelines for their use. Thorough understanding of these elements will enable you as a cosmetologist to put them together in a pleasing manner.

Form

We live in a world of shapes and forms. Whether it be a car, an apple, or you, it has shape and form. The shape of a hairstyle is two-dimensional when you look at it from only one angle. In reality, it is three-dimensional and its outline, shadow, or silhouette is referred to as **form** (Figure 7.1).

Form is the most important of the elements. Most people will judge how well they like their hair design by its size and shape. The hair form is pleasing when it is in proportion with the shape of the head and face, the length and width of the neck, and the line of the shoulder. Good form is not difficult to achieve if you keep it

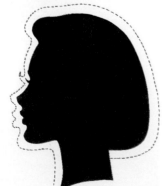

7.1   The outline is the form

simple. Be sure that the proportion is correct, design for the individual's everyday activities, and take into consideration the limitations of the hair.

Simplicity in Form

The size or shape of the form should never overpower the size of the face. The form should not distract. It should serve as a well-planned part of the person's overall proportion. A simple hair form will never overpower the face or the body (Figure 7.2).

Proportion in Form

The form should be in proportion to the face and body. A form that is too large will diminish the importance of the face and be out of balance with the body (Figure 7.3).

Design Form for Lifestyle

Take into consideration the client's day-to-day activities and ability to maintain a style when determining form. The hair is an everyday part of good grooming, and the style must meet both the practical needs and the individual image requirements of the consumer. For example, the client who is active outdoors must have a simple, easy-care style (Figure 7.4). The professional client must have controlled, well-groomed, and practical hair (Figure 7.5). A well-designed form (Figure 7.6) can be adapted easily to suit any occasion.

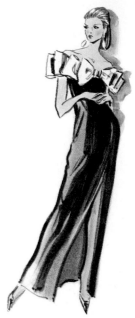

7.2   Simple hair form

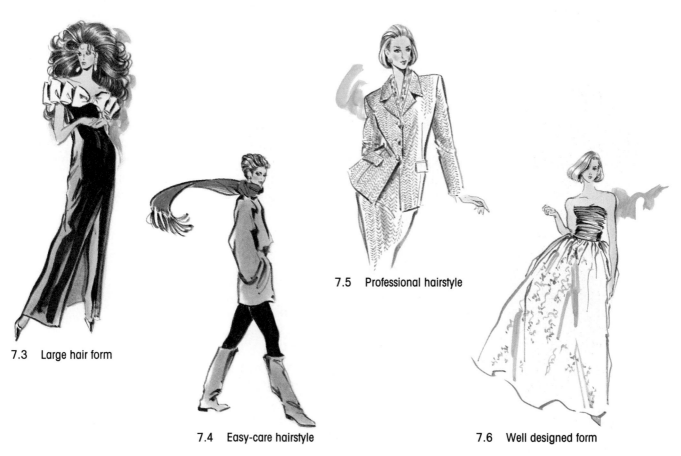

7.3   Large hair form

7.4   Easy-care hairstyle

7.5   Professional hairstyle

7.6   Well designed form

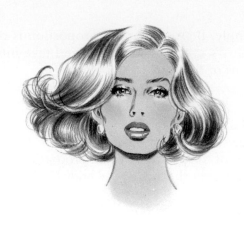

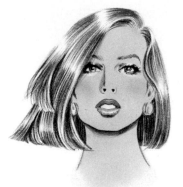

7.7   Quality of hair must support the form

Form and Hair Type

The quality of the hair will determine whether it can support the desired form. Density, texture, and elasticity will be guides to the correct length and proper procedures to use (Figure 7.7).

Space

The movements, directions, and shapes inside the form are referred to as **space** (Figure 7.8). The design may contain curls, curves, waves, straight hair, or a combination of these shapes. Good design uses the elements of space to enhance the shape of the head and facial features.

The term *adaptability* is used when describing space as well as form. **Adaptability** is the quality that makes the hair design suitable to the client. Shapes within the space must support the form and complement the facial features within the limitations of the hair type. The requirements of good design are moderation, simplicity, and support for the form. In the final analysis, the space and the form seem to become one.

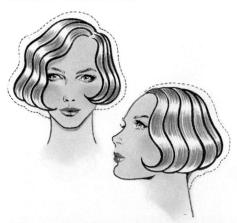

7.8   Movements, directions, and shapes inside form are the space

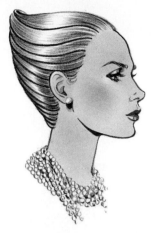

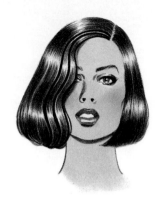

7.9   Keep design simple   7.10   Keep background space simple

Moderation in Space

Keep the design simple by limiting the number of different patterns. When shapes within the space are simple and easy to look at, they are easy to appreciate (Figure 7.9).

Simplify Background Space

Most of the space should enhance the form and provide a background for the most important shapes in the design. The most beautiful hairstyles make one area stand out against a simple background (Figure 7.10).

Space Supports Form

The movement within the form should support and strengthen the shape of the form. Form and space must work together to bring continuity and harmony to the finished hairstyle (Figure 7.11).

Line

Everywhere you look, you see lines! You draw lines on a dot-to-dot puzzle. Trees are planted in lines along a roadway. You write numbers in a line, and you comb curved lines in the hair to make a wave. Some objects look like lines, for example, a wire, or a piece of string. Your eyes will usually follow the movement of lines, making lines very important elements in design.

   Line is the tool we use to produce form and design in the hair. We work with both straight and curved lines. Straight lines are more demanding and aggressive. Curved lines are softer, no matter how they are used in the design. We use straight lines in horizontal, vertical, and diagonal positions. We use curved lines in circles, parts of a circle, or in wave patterns. Any of the curved patterns may be placed in a horizontal, vertical, or diagonal position. Use various types of lines in combination to create interest, versatility, and variety in design. The combinations are endless and will help you produce new and exciting work.

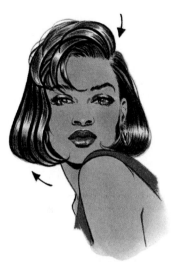

7.11   Space supports the form

> **◆ Key Point ◆**
> Although almost any form can seem modern, the shapes within the form will be the major factor in dating or modernizing the hairstyle.

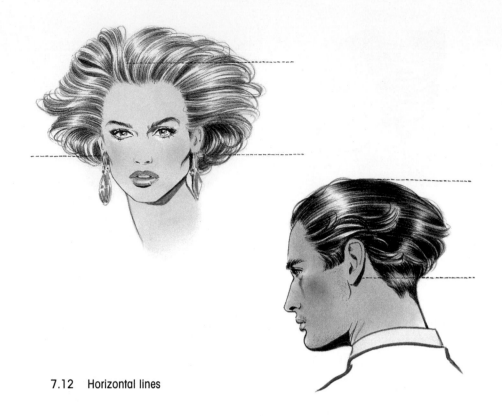

7.12   Horizontal lines

Horizontal Lines

Horizontal lines are straight across, or parallel with the horizon. Horizontal lines add width, whether they are straight or curved (Figure 7.12). The eye will follow the horizontal line out and away from the face. This adds the illusion of width in form or design.

Vertical Lines

Vertical lines are straight up and down; they add length, whether they are straight or curved (Figure 7.13). Because the eye will follow and even continue the vertical line, the form or design appears longer.

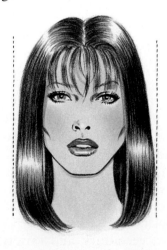

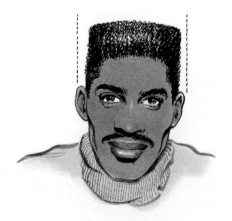

7.13   Vertical lines

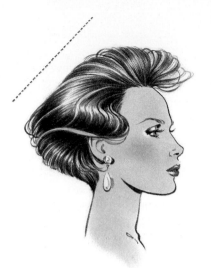

7.14   Diagonal line

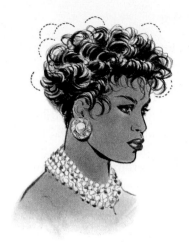

7.15   Curved lines

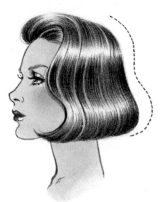

7.16   Repeating line

Diagonal Lines

Diagonal lines are positioned anywhere between vertical and horizontal. Diagonal lines, whether straight or curved, are used to soften, while adding length and width (Figure 7.14).

Curved Lines

Curved lines can be any part of a circle, without completing it. They can be thin or wide; they can curve slowly or rapidly. The curved line softens a direction or an element. Use curved lines to complement angular facial features (Figure 7.15). The curved line can repeat in opposite directions to form a wave. Waves are a classic component in hair design (Figure 7.16).

Repeating Lines

Repeating lines move parallel to each other. They repeat any number of times, creating impact and simplicity (Figure 7.17). Parallel lines can be straight, curved, or in a wave pattern.

Contrasting Lines

Contrasting lines, such as horizontal lines and vertical lines that meet at a 90° angle, create hard edges and an aggressive design. Use angular lines to give form and shape to round facial features (Figure 7.18). Contrasting lines suggest strength of personality.

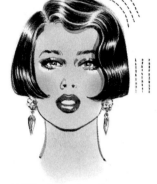

7.17   Repeating lines

> ◆ **Key Point** ◆
>
> Too many lines of one type become boring. A balanced variety is the key to creating interest in a design.

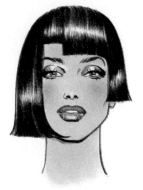

7.18   Contrasting lines

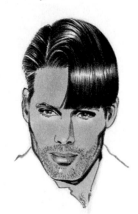

Color

Color is exciting! We respond to color with emotion, and everyone has a favorite color. We see hair color because of the way light shines on a three-dimensional object, causing highlights and shadows on the hair.

Hair color looks different in natural light from the way it looks in artificial light. Artificial light can dramatically change the appearance of the hair color, depending on the intensity of the light and the color content of the incandescent bulb or fluorescent tube.

Hair color plays a significant role in determining design. Color can be used to enhance a design, complement skin tones, or change the shape of the face through the illusion of light and shadow.

Add Emphasis with Color

Color can be used to emphasize a particular area of the hair design by making that area lighter or darker. Lighter colors make an area appear larger and closer; they attract attention. Darker colors make an area appear smaller, recessed, or farther back. Darker colors do not attract attention, but make the form, or silhouette, more obvious. Lighten, brighten, or add complementary shading to clarify and enhance natural hair color (Figure 7.19).

Add Dimension with Color

Add strength to the dimension of a design by adding highlight or shadow to intensify the effect (Figure 7.20). Highlights will bring a movement or part of a movement closer. A darker color will create a shadow, making that part of the movement appear farther away. Dimension will strengthen shapes and forms, and make the design more interesting.

Create Illusions with Color

The face can be enhanced by illusions that seem to change its shape through the use of color. Lighter areas can make the face seem longer or wider. Darker areas can make the face seem shorter or more narrow (Figure 7.21). Light colors will emphasize; dark colors will decrease size and importance.

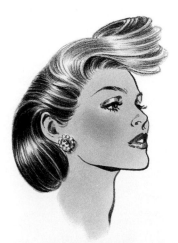

7.19   Emphasis with color

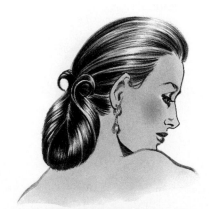

7.20   Dimension with color

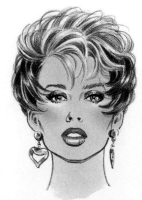

7.21   Illusion with color

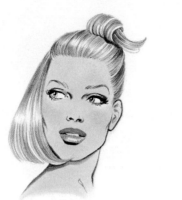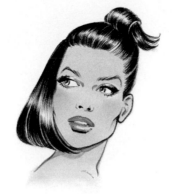

7.22   Different colors create different moods

Create Moods with Color

Color can be used to create a mood and to add a distinct personality to the hairstyle. Figure 7.22 shows how the same style in a different color will result in a different mood or feeling. Lighter colors will seem larger and softer; red colors will seem warmer and dark colors will appear smaller.

Assure Unity with Color

Color can provide unity and harmony to the style by blending complementary shades to tie the design components together (Figure 7.23). Color blending can add a finished touch to the design.

Color Characteristics

Each color has particular characteristics that you should consider when designing a hairstyle. Blue adds coolness and depth to a form. Red adds warmth and vibrancy. Yellow adds brightness and lightness. For a more in-depth study of the effects of color, refer to Chapter 14, Hair Coloring.

Darker colors emphasize lines around the features and make a person look older. A dark color will make the hairstyle look smaller, heavier, and thicker (Figure 7.24).

Lighter colors will soften the lines of the skin and add a more youthful look. Light colors will make a style look larger and seem lighter (Figure 7.24).

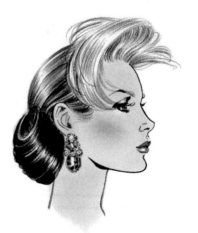

7.23   Blend shades to tie the design together

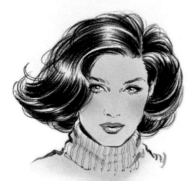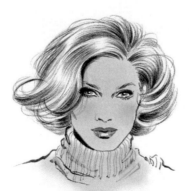

7.24   Darker and lighter colors have different characteristics

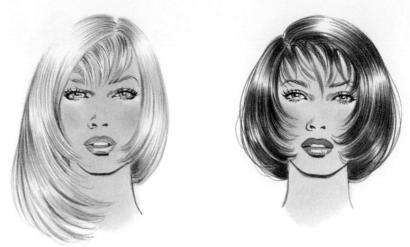

7.25 Warm and cool tones should complement personality

Warm colors appear to come forward, and personalities seem more friendly and extroverted and even a little aggressive. Cool colors recede, seem calm, and the personality more soothing, even aloof. Warm and cool tones should complement the personality of your client (Figure 7.25). If the personality is quiet and introverted, a warm tone would be a good choice. A cool blond with a quiet, introverted personality may seem shy. If the personality is outgoing, a cool tone will add balance. Warm colors with an extroverted personality could make the individual seem aggressive.

Guide for Good Hair Color Choices

□ To shade a design with an equal amount of two or more colors, use colors that are reasonably close in value (the depth or darkness of a color). This will make the finished effect more natural (Figure 7.26).

□ When placing multiple colors in the hair, use a variety of levels of the same hue, or color, creating a design that is easy to look at. Using colors with very different base pigments will produce dis-

◆ Key Point ◆

The color or colors you choose for your client must appear natural, or even improve upon the natural color.

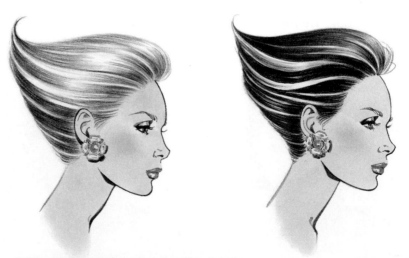

7.26 Shade a design with colors close in value

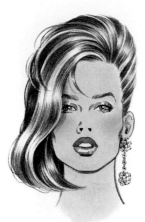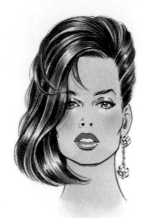

7.27 Compatible colors are soothing, contrasting colors cause discord

cord, and an unnatural feeling about the design (Figure 7.27). Compatible colors are soothing. Contrasting colors cause discord.

□ High-contrast combinations such as dark brown and light blond should use a small percentage of one of the colors for interest only (Figure 7.28). The contrasting color should accent the primary design element.

□ Midrange colors, neither too light nor too dark, are the most flattering to the skin and are the most youthful. All colors used must be in harmony with the skin tone.

Texture

Texture refers to how things feel, or perhaps how they look like they would feel. Sometimes you have to touch an object just to see if it is smooth or rough! You can feel the texture of the hair if you touch it, but you can also sense the texture just by looking at it. Texture is an element that gives variety to a design.

Natural Textures

All hair has a natural texture that should be considered when designing a cut or style for your client. Hair may have a straight, wavy, curly, or extra curly texture. If more than one texture is present, try a unique style that takes advantage of the natural condition Create a sleek line, for example, with straight hair. Provide a larger and more open form for curly hair (Figure 7.29).

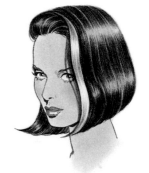

7.28 Contrasting color to accent the primary design element

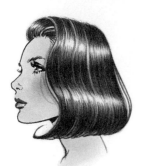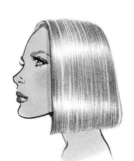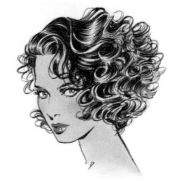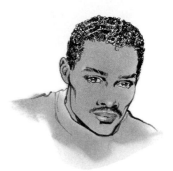

7.29 Texture can be used as a design element

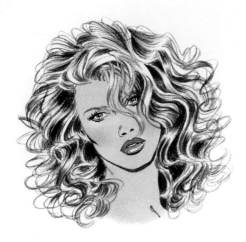
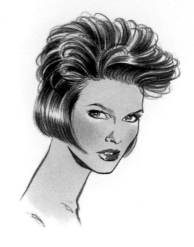
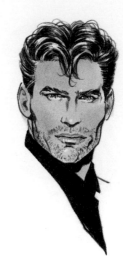

7.30 Create interest in a design with chemically altered textures

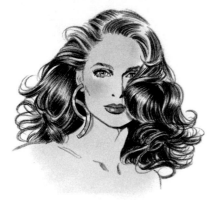

7.31 Hairstyling techniques can alter textures temporarily

Chemically Altered Textures

All natural textures can be altered chemically to a new texture that is more appealing to the client or perhaps more fashionable. Curly hair can be relaxed and straight hair curled through permanent waves, relaxers, or reconstructors. These techniques will be discussed in Chapter 16, Chemical Waving, and in Chapter 17, Chemical Relaxing. In some cases, only part of the natural hair texture is changed to create interest in the design (Figure 7.30).

Temporary Textures

Rollers, pin curls, and thermal iron techniques will produce smooth textures that give curl or wave movement. Combinations of these movements will offer you many ways to accent your overall design (Figure 7.31).

There are a variety of tools that will give spiral, square, zig-zag, and crimped textures to the hair. These tools are used as temporary styling aids to use in design. Many types of braids can be used to supplement a style or give texture variety (Figure 7.32).

Shapings and finger waves display unique texture and give a slightly different look from the conventional pin curl wave. Very small curls give another unique and interesting texture (Figure 7.33).

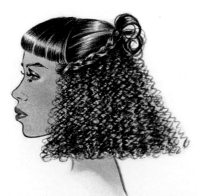

7.32 Create temporary texture with braids and other tools

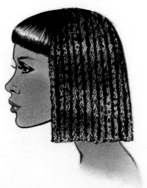

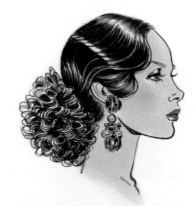

7.33 Waves and shaping change texture

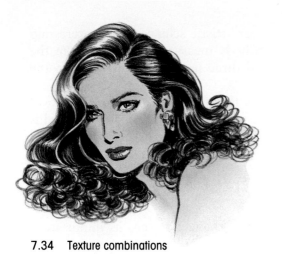

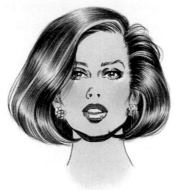

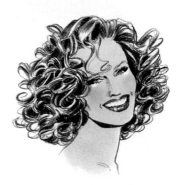

7.34　Texture combinations

7.35　Smooth texture

7.36　Curly texture

Guide for Good Texture Choices

- ☐ Texture combinations make hair styles interesting (Figure 7.34).
- ☐ Smooth textures accent the face, while curly textures draw attention away from the face (Figures 7.35 and 7.36).
- ☐ Smooth textures give more structure and strength. They make round features seem less round (Figure 7.35).
- ☐ Curly textures soften angular features (Figure 7.36).

> **◆ Key Point ◆**
>
> Curly textures can appear dry due to the refraction or absorption of light, while smooth textures appear lustrous due to the reflection of light.

THE PRINCIPLES

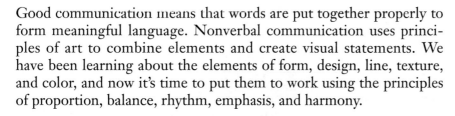

Good communication means that words are put together properly to form meaningful language. Nonverbal communication uses principles of art to combine elements and create visual statements. We have been learning about the elements of form, design, line, texture, and color, and now it's time to put them to work using the principles of proportion, balance, rhythm, emphasis, and harmony.

Proportion

"My ears are too big!" "This chair is too small for me!"

These comments are about problems with proportion. Proportion is the principle that deals with the comparative relationship of one part to another with respect to size. A hairstyle that is too large for the face or one that is too small on the body are examples of problems of proportion. When the proportion is correct, we find the object pleasing; when proportion is lacking, we are uneasy. An understanding of the correct proportion of hair to face, head, and body size will help you design adaptable hairstyles for your clients.

Universal Proportion

Through the ages, people have sought an ideal proportion that would apply to all things. The ancient Greeks found that a ratio of 2 to 3 was a proportion that would control the relationship of parts in

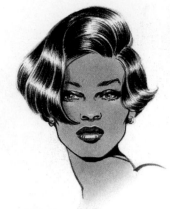

architecture, art objects, and other artistic sciences. It is interesting to note that the average human body measures two parts from the top of the head to the navel, and three parts from the navel to the feet.

Three parts hair to two parts face provides a formula that will adapt hair proportionately to the face. A variation of this standard is normal to accommodate personalities, style preferences, body and face sizes. Following are several examples of the standard and its variations.

3 Parts Hair; 2 Parts Face

A volume of hair slightly larger than the face lessens its importance, but gives a pleasing harmony (Figure 7.37). Irregular features, poor skin, or a lack of facial makeup are less noticeable with the use of more hair volume. More hair volume reduces the emphasis to the face for both men and women.

2 Parts Hair; 3 Parts Face

When smaller volumes of hair are used, the face becomes more important and catches the eye before the hairstyle (Figure 7.38). Regular features; clear, smooth skin; and well-applied facial makeup are emphasized by the use of less hair volume. This smaller hair volume emphasizes the man's or the woman's face.

Profile Proportion

The standard proportion of three parts hair to two parts face remains the same from a profile view (Figure 7.39). The area of hair growth is larger in profile, however, and in many cases five parts hair to two parts face would be a pleasing proportion.

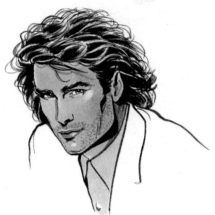

7.37   3 parts hair; 2 parts face

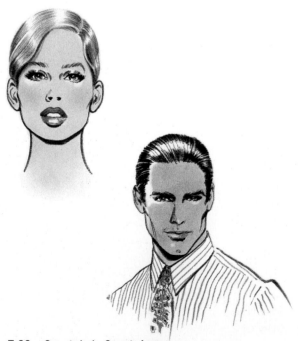

7.38   2 parts hair; 3 parts face

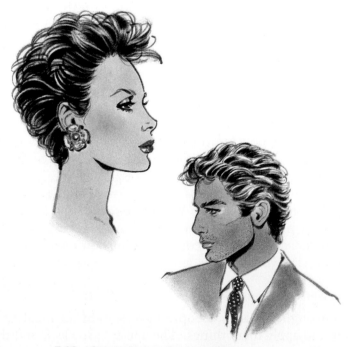

7.39   Standard proportion in profile

Larger than Standard Volumes of Hair

During some periods, a larger amount of hair around the face is considered fashionable. Longer hair has always been popular and creates a larger than standard proportion. Remember, when more hair is around the face, the importance of the face is diminished (Figure 7.40). A larger amount of hair is sometimes used for the theatre or other purposes requiring extreme emphasis.

Head and Face Sizes

Every head and face has an existing size relationship that should guide decisions of hair length and style.

After shampooing the client, comb the hair completely away from the face so you can clearly see the entire face and head (Figure 7.41). Note how low the hairline grows onto the forehead, and how low it grows on the neck. This entire area of hair growth should be considered in decisions of design.

If the total hair area is as large or larger than the face, it will take less length or hair volume to accomplish the proportion you have in mind (Figure 7.41).

If the total hair area is smaller than the face, it will be necessary to have more length or hair volume to meet the correct proportion (Figure 7.42).

Make note of irregularities in head shape. It may be necessary to adjust the shape of the cut or style to fill in areas that are flat or to conceal protruding areas.

Guide to Adjusting Proportion

□ Combing the hair off the face will increase the face size. A larger volume of hair will be required to achieve a proportion of 3 parts hair to 2 parts face (Figure 7.43). As more hair is combed off the face, the form becomes larger.

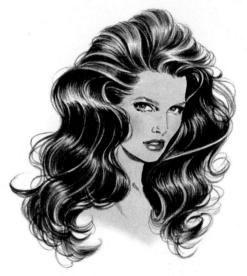

7.40   Large hair volume

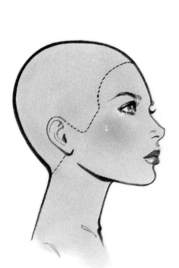

7.41   Large hair area

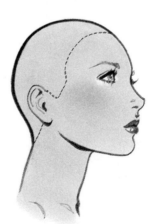

7.42   Small hair area

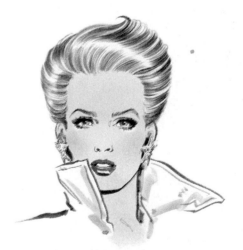

7.43   Comb hair off face

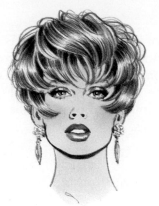

7.44 Comb hair onto face

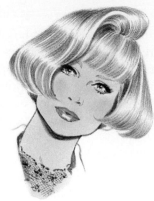

7.45 Combine volume and design on face

- □ Combing the hair onto the face will diminish the face size. In this case, less hair volume will be necessary to achieve a proportion of 3 parts hair to 2 parts face (Figure 7.44). As more hair is placed on the face, the form will become smaller.
- □ Combining volume of hair with design on the face is a good way to achieve proportion. Styles of this type are most easily adapted to individual facial features (Figure 7.45).

Proportion in the Hair Design

Proper proportion within each hair design is equally critical. The manner in which the form is constructed or the design planned can produce correct proportions that are pleasing to see.

Areas of volume in the form should not be equal, but must be in proper proportion. One area should be of primary importance and another of secondary importance. If a third area exists, it should be least important (Figure 7.46). Movements within the design should also display good proportion (Figure 7.47).

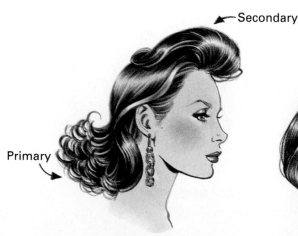

Secondary

Primary

7.46 Areas of volume should not be the same size

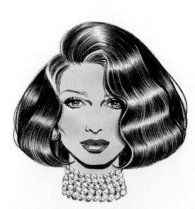

7.47 Movements should show good proportion

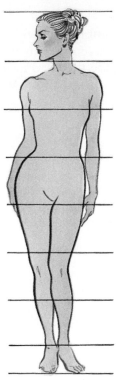

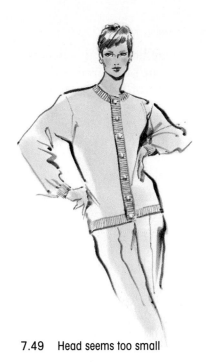

7.49 Head seems too small

7.48 Body proportion

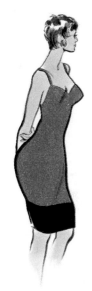

7.50 Hips seem too large

Body Proportion

Although the average human body is said to have universal proportion, there are many exceptions. The hairstyle you chose should be adaptable to the height, weight, and proportion of your client.

The head is used to define the proportions of each individual. The average adult is 7½ heads tall, and the shoulders and hips should be in proportion (Figure 7.48).

Hairstyles too small for the shoulders will make the head look too small. The same hairstyle can make hips that are too large seem even larger (Figure 7.49). The professional cosmetologist should consider the proportion of the head, shoulders, and hips when making hairstyling decisions.

Profiles

From the profile, the bust and buttocks are the areas to note when striving for good proportion. Styles that are too small can emphasize the bustline or the buttocks. Decisions of hair length and style that you make can help balance the proportion of your client's body. Misproportions can seem more visible if the hair form is small (Figure 7.50).

Balance

Balance is a principle of life. Small children are said to have a hard time keeping their balance when they first learn to walk. Later they learn to balance each other's weight on a teeter-totter. In cosmetology, balance is a pleasing harmony of weights or visual attractions. When a style is out of balance, you will be dissatisfied with the results.

> ◆ **Key Point** ◆
> Proportions can dictate what you see first. Just as the eye will go to a bright color, the eye will also look quickly at a misproportion.

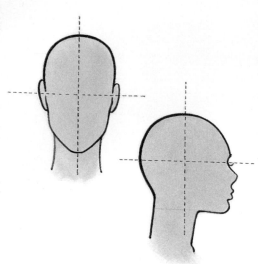

7.51   The central axis

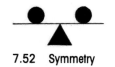

7.52   Symmetry

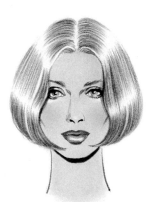

7.53   Mirror image symmetry

The Central Axis

To judge balance, it is necessary to have a point of reference. We call that point of reference the **central axis**. The central axis works like the point of balance on a balance scale. Divide the head in half with an imaginary horizontal and an imaginary vertical line. Where the lines cross, a center point is formed around which we will judge balance (Figure 7.51).

Symmetrical Balance

A style that displays **symmetry** balances at the same distance from the central axis, with equal attractions and weights (Figure 7.52). Symmetry can be achieved by changing the elements of form and space.

In **mirror-image symmetry**, there will be an exact duplication of form and design on either side of the axis. Figure 7.53 shows one side of the style is a mirror image of the other. This style either has no part, or is parted in the center.

A style that displays equal attractions on either side of the central axis is known as **approximate symmetry**. Both sides will equally attract the viewer's eye, but each side will be different and have its own personality (Figure 7.54).

When viewing a hairstyle from the front or the side, your eye will draw an **imaginary balance line** through the fullest two points of the form. These points will be the dominant weights, or largest attractions, in the design and will assist you in determining balance. The most important part of the design should be placed along the balance line. Facial features on the balance line will receive more emphasis than the rest of the face (Figure 7.55).

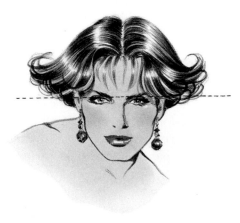

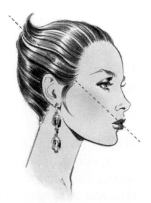

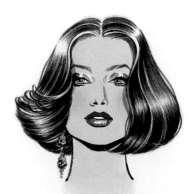

7.54   Approximate symmetry

7.55   Imaginary balance line

Asymmetrical Balance

Asymmetrical balance involves unequal weights or unequal attractions. These weights must be balanced at different distances from the central axis. The larger attraction must be placed closer to the central axis and the smaller one farther away (Figure 7.56).

Imagine a board across a support, like a teeter-totter. The smaller part of your hair design must be far enough from the center to "balance" the heavier part. For example, asymmetry in a hairstyle can be created by balancing the style in a horizontal (Figure 7.57) or a diagonal manner (Figure 7.58).

Lines drawn in asymmetry should create perspective and enhance the best facial features. Read on to see how you can create these effects.

Creating Perspective

By bringing the larger movement of the hairstyle (symmetrical or asymmetrical designs) to the front, and placing the smaller movement in the back, you create depth or perspective depth. Designs that display this type of positioning are both attractive and adaptable to many facial types. Horizontal perspective has an overall effect of increasing width, while diagonal perspective creates length (Figure 7.59).

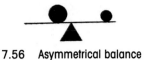

7.56   Asymmetrical balance

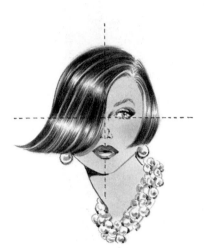

7.57   Horizontal asymmetry

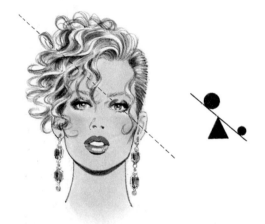

7.58   Diagonal asymmetry

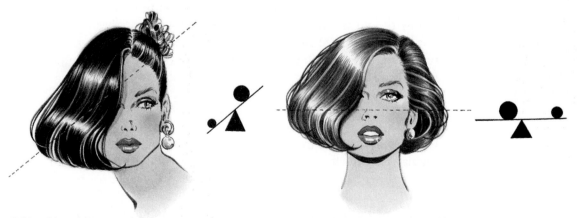

7.59   Diagonal perspective creates length   Horizontal perspective creates width

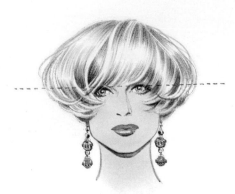

7.60   Emphasize eyes

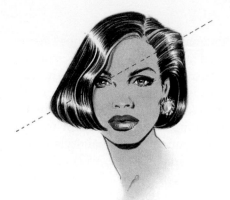

7.61   Diminish round features

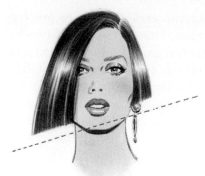

7.62   45° slant is pleasing to eye

┌─────────────────────────────────┐
│   ◆ **Key Point** ◆   │
│ When the balance is correct and the bal- │
│ ance line emphasizes the most attractive │
│ features, the hairstyle will be adaptable to │
│ the individual and pleasing to the eye. │
└─────────────────────────────────┘

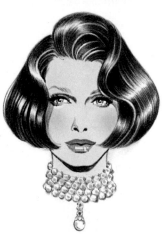

7.63   Rhythm in design

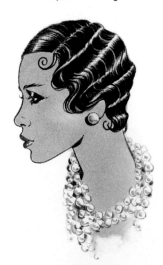

7.64   Regular rhythm

Guide for Using Balance

▫ Use balance to draw attention to the most attractive or interesting features of the face. Use volume at the eye level, for example, and the balance line will emphasize the eyes (Figure 7.60).

▫ Use the diagonal balance line of asymmetry to diminish the effect of round features or a round jaw. Because the eye follows the diagonal line, an illusion of length is created (Figure 7.61).

▫ When cutting the hair in an asymmetric design, the sides should not differ by more than a 45° angle. When the balance line shows a more dramatic slant, the viewer will feel that the style is out of balance and too heavy on one side. Remember, this will give emphasis to whatever feature it passes through (Figure 7.62).

Rhythm

Everyone knows what rhythm is! It's the beat of the music and the marching feet of a band. In hair design, the rhythm is visual. We see it rather than hear it, but what a difference it makes in the way we feel about a hairstyle. If the design has rhythm, it allows our eyes to follow the visual beat as if we could hear it. Though all patterns do not have rhythm, all rhythms do have a pattern. **Rhythm** is a form of repetition intended to create the feeling of movement. When designs have rhythm, your eyes will pick up the beat (Figure 7.63).

Regular Rhythm

Regular rhythm is the repetition of regular motion. Hairstyles with regular rhythm feature an even repetition of design. It has an even, steady flow, and can be beautiful because of its precise, regular pattern. It should be noted, however, that regular rhythm without a break can be boring and even uninteresting. Figure 7.64 shows a classic wave design. Without the interest at the forehead and the nape, this style would be quite boring.

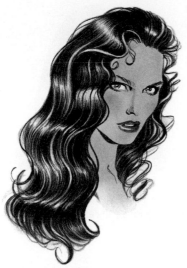

7.65 Progressive rhythm

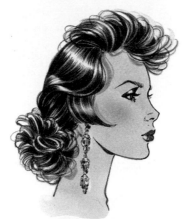

7.66 Alternating rhythms

Progressive Rhythm

In **progressive rhythm**, patterns repeat and become gradually larger or smaller. Figure 7.65 has small waves and curls that gradually enlarge in a line down the length of the hair. Progressive rhythms can be irregular and the sizes can alternate from one size to a larger size and back again. Figure 7.66 shows the option of creating an interesting design that uses alternating rhythms.

Continued Line Rhythm

Rhythm expressed through continued line movement will most likely be made up of curves moving in the same direction (curl) or curves moving in first one direction and then the opposite direction (wave) (Figure 7.67).

Radial Rhythm

Radial rhythm features regular and even patterns emerging from a center point (Figure 7.68). Radial rhythms can resemble progressive rhythm when the hair flows from an off-center point in a pattern that progressively becomes larger or smaller. Figure 7.69 is an example of radial rhythm. The hair flows larger on one side of the design, and smaller on the other.

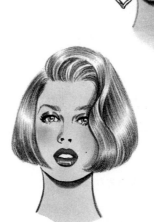

7.67 Continued line rhythm

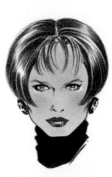

7.68 Radial rhythm

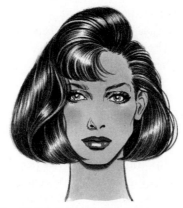

7.69 Radial rhythm that flows larger on one side

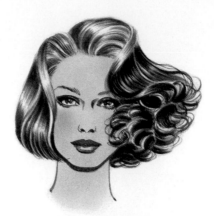

7.70   Interest in design diminishes face

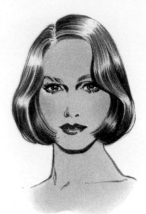

7.71   Regular rhythms emphasize face

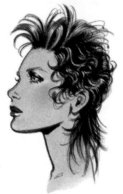

7.72   Progressive rhythm allows spontaneity

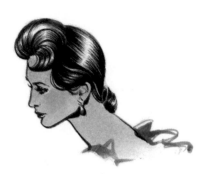

7.73   Radial rhythms can look formal

Guide for Using Rhythm

□ A combination of rhythms can make a hairstyle interesting and pull attention away from facial features which are plain or out of proportion. Creating interest in the hair design will decrease attention to the face (Figure 7.70).

□ A regular rhythm gives a classic look to any hairstyle, and is complimentary to symmetric designs. Regular rhythms are simple, and therefore attract attention to the face (Figure 7.71).

□ Progressive rhythms provide interest, and give you more freedom for spontaneous design (Figure 7.72).

□ Though radial rhythms are simple, they look complex, and sometimes give a formal feeling to the hairstyle (Figure 7.73).

□ Radial motion appears to have a rhythm like a seashell, growing outward from a point of origin.

Emphasis

If you have ever underlined a word or raised your voice to make a point, then you have created emphasis. In hairstyling terms, emphasis means creating a focal point. A **focal point** exists when it differs in some way from the rest of the design or when something about it draws the eye. Focal points control what people see first, second, and so on. The focal point in Figure 7.74, for example, is the full design above the eyes.

Some designs have a secondary focal point that is a smaller, less important part of the hair design. Figure 7.75 shows a hair ornament

---

◆ **Key Point** ◆

Rhythms are used in a hairstyle to create the pattern of the space and form. Rhythms also can be used to emphasize the facial features.

7.74   Focal point above eyes

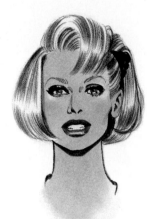

7.75   Ornament as second focal point

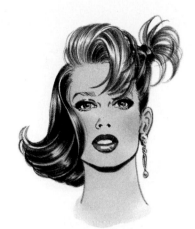

7.76   Multiple focal points can be confusing

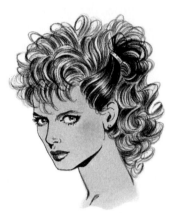

7.77   Color can emphasize an area

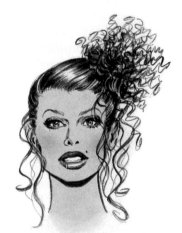

7.78   Focal point of contrasting texture

used as a secondary focal point. The fullness of the forehead is still seen first, the comb pulling back the side is seen second, and the straight side is seen last.

Designs that have several focal points of equal emphasis confuse the viewer. It is not clear what is important, or where you should look first (Figure 7.76).

Emphasis Through Color

Color can be used for emphasis by highlighting within the design. Add lighter, brighter, or darker color and you will create emphasis. Color should be placed so that it draws attention to the primary design feature of the finished style (Figure 7.77).

Emphasis Through Texture

A focal point can be created by using a contrasting texture. In Figure 7.78, the eye is first drawn to the top of the head because of the primary areas of contrasting texture.

Emphasis Through Simplicity

A simple design set against a plain background of hair becomes a focal point (Figure 7.79). Hair ornaments should be small and serve a purpose in the design.

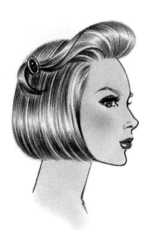

7.79   A simple design against plain background

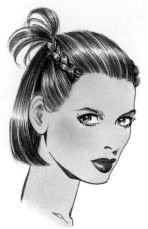

7.80   Braid directs eye to focal point

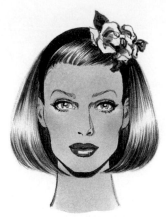

7.81   Focal point creates interest

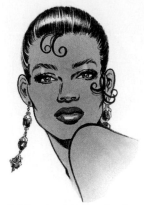

7.82   Accents stand out from simple background

Using design to lead the eye to a focal point is also an example of emphasis through simplicity. In Figure 7.80 the braid is a secondary focal point and leads the eye upward to the explosion of hair—the primary design emphasis.

Guide for Using Emphasis

- Use a focal point to draw attention to a part of the head or face you would like to accentuate.
- The focal point adds interest to a symmetric style (Figure 7.81).
- The simpler the hairstyle, the more emphasis is placed on the focal point or accents (Figure 7.82).
- A general rule in the use of ornamentation in the hair is that the ornament must have a purpose, or at least appear to have a purpose (Figure 7.83). The ornament will usually become a focal point because of the difference in material and texture.
- An ornament can become the focal point of the entire design much like a hat that dominates the hair (Figure 7.84).

Harmony

When you look at an object, a room, or a person, and think, "I wouldn't change a thing," you experience the pleasing effects of harmony. Harmony is the bringing together of different parts in such a way that we see the result as beautiful or suitable.

In terms of hairstyling, **harmony** (or unity) simply means that all of the elements of the hairstyle complement the facial features.

In creating total harmony of face, hair, and clothing, you must see the total person without special emphasis on any one part. This section will concentrate on facial features and types to give you the information needed to properly adapt hairstyles to the face.

Facial Features and Types

The bone structure and the features are made up of lines and shapes that give the face its personality. Harmony is maintained when angular features are complemented with lines and shapes in the hair that are curved or rounded (Figure 7.85). Rounded features can be offset

---

◆ **Key Point** ◆

Use emphasis to direct the eye to important features of the face or hairstyle.

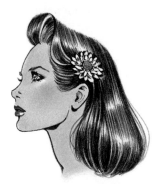

7.83   Ornament is holding the hair

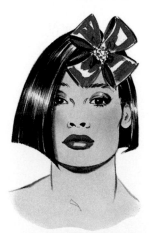

7.84   Dominant ornament

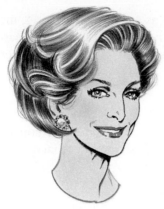

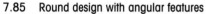

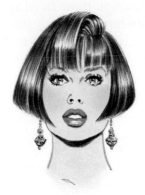

7.85 Round design with angular features   **7.86** Round features need angular design

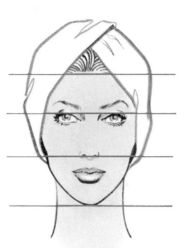

by using angular lines in the hair design (Figure 7.86). This gives you, the hair designer, full freedom to adjust the shape of facial features through the design of the hairstyle.

The face is divided into three areas:
- ☐ Hairline to eyebrow (the upper face)
- ☐ Eyebrow to the end of the nose (the middle face)
- ☐ End of the nose to the bottom of the chin (the lower face)

If the face is correctly proportioned, each area will represent a third of the face length (Figure 7.87). The eyes will be located in the center of the face, and the distance between the eyes will be the length of one eye. This proportion varies from person to person. In this section, we will learn to change the appearance of some facial features to make the face look its best.

When each third of the face is equal, it is said to be ideal, and we term that facial type **oval** (Figure 7.87). The six other facial types are square, round, heart, oblong, pear, and diamond (see Figures 7.88-7.93).

7.87 Three areas of the face

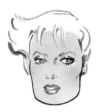

7.88 Square

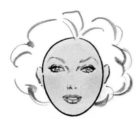

7.89 Round

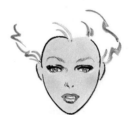

7.90 Heart

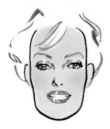

7.91 Oblong

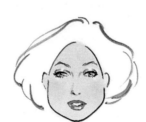

7.92 Pear

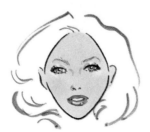

7.93 Diamond

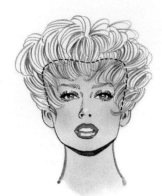

7.94   Cover wide forehead

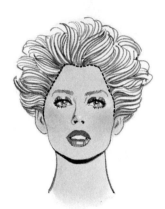

7.95   Brush hair off narrow forehead

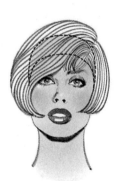

7.96   Cover hairline to disguise high or low forehead

Although these facial types can serve as a guide to learning, most faces do not fall exactly into any one of the types. It is for this reason that each third of the face should be analyzed separately to alter a face that is too long or too wide.

Adapting to the Face on View

By moving a design in a variety of ways over that area, you may change the way in which people perceive the shape of the face.

Guide to Forehead Correction

- □ To correct a forehead that is too wide, select a design that will cover a portion of the forehead with hair (Figure 7.94).
- □ To correct a forehead that is too narrow, either cover it with hair (Figure 7.95) or brush the hair back as in Figure 7.96.
- □ Brushing hair off the forehead adds width to the form and offers a narrow forehead better proportion (Figure 7.95).
- □ To correct a forehead that is too short or too high, cover the hairline. This makes it impossible to tell how low or high the hairline really is (Figure 7.96).

Adapting to the Middle Face

Middle face correction can:

- □ Make eyes seem closer.
- □ Make eyes seem farther apart.
- □ Correct protruding ears.
- □ Emphasize eyes.
- □ Take away from eyes.

Guide to Middle Face Correction

- □ If the ears are higher than the eyebrows, they should not be fully exposed unless the hairstyle has enough height. In that case, they will appear lower (Figure 7.97).
- □ If the ears are no higher than the corner of the eye, exposing the ear is not a problem unless they protrude from the head (Figure 7.98).
- □ If the eyes are close-set, correct by widening the hairstyle slightly.

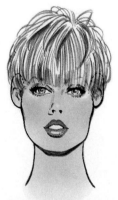

7.97   Cover high ears

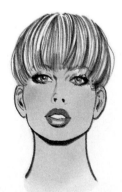

7.98   Exposed low ears

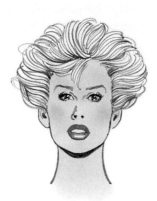

7.99   Eyes seem close with wide hair

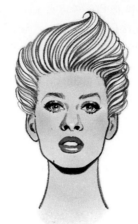

7.100   Full hair demphasizes wide nose

Hair too wide or too close would make the eyes look closer together (Figure 7.99).

□ Most nose correction from the front facial view is best done with makeup (see Chapter 19). However, creating the major fullness in the hairstyle away from the nose area will direct attention away from the nose (Figure 7.100).

Guide to Lower-jaw Correction

□ This area of the face is the most crucial in adapting properly. Unlike the forehead, which can be covered with hair, the lower face must have hair that frames it, or a form that balances it.

□ When the jaw is square, shorter hair looks terrific. Place the major width of the hair in the middle third of the face to soften the squareness (Figure 7.101).

□ When the jaw is pointed, longer hair is the key to filling in the lower jaw area (Figure 7.102).

□ When the jaw is long, either rounded or rectangular, the fullness of the hairstyle should fall in the lower third. This creates an optical illusion of a shorter jaw (Figure 7.103).

□ When the jaw is round, use angularity of form to offset the roundness. Angular fullness in the upper two-thirds of the face will help the round jaw appear more structured (Figure 7.104).

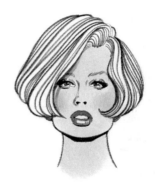

7.101   Square jaw with short hair

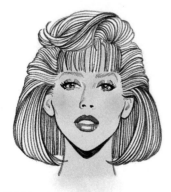

7.102   Long hair with pointed jaw

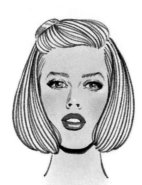

7.103   Long jaw with lower fullness

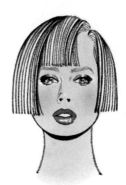

7.104   Use angular form with round jaw

The Face in Profile

The profile is divided into three parts, exactly the same way as the face on view. Divide the profile from hairline to eyebrow, from eyebrow to tip of the nose, and from the tip of the nose to the chin. Ideally, each area would represent an equal third (Figure 7.105).

The ideal overall facial angle is about 10° from an imaginary vertical line in the upper two-thirds of the face. In Figure 7.106, the dotted line indicates the ideal angle, drawn from the forehead to the tip of the nose.

The lower third of the face, from the tip of the nose to the chin, should ideally form the same 10° angle from an imaginary vertical line (Figure 7.107).

Guide to Forehead Correction

- To correct a large forehead, allow enough hair to be placed or to fall around part or all of that area. Covering a large forehead will bring it into proportion (Figure 7.108).
- A receding forehead can easily be adapted by bringing hair over it to fill in the space that seems empty (Figure 7.109).
- Foreheads with a gentle curve look best from profile when uncovered altogether or with only a slight amount of hair for fashion purposes (Figure 7.110).

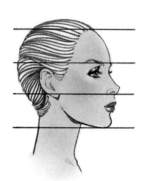

7.105   Three areas of the profile

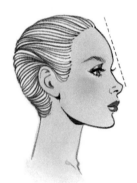

7.106   Ideal angle of upper face

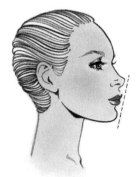

7.107   Ideal angle of lower face

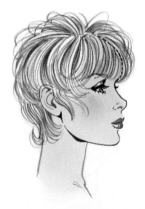

7.108   Cover large forehead

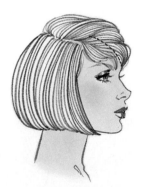

7.109   Bring hair over receding hairline

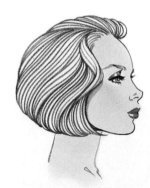

7.110   Leave well proportioned forehead uncovered

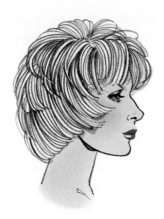

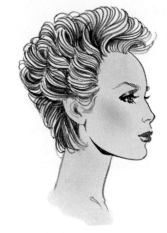

7.111   Move hair forward with large nose   7.112   Leave face open with small nose

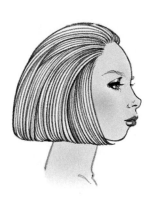

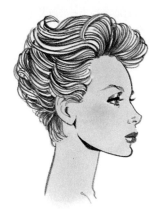

7.113   Move hair forward in chin area   7.114   Move hair up and away with short chin

Guide to Center Profile Correction

- From an adaptation point of view, the nose will affect the total appearance more than the other features.
- When the nose is too large (making the profile convex), balance the nose with hair falling over the forehead (Figure 7.111), and/or hair moving slightly forward.
- A small nose is best handled with an open face. Too much hair around the face will make the nose appear even smaller (Figure 7.112).

Guide to Lower Face Correction

- When the chin recedes and the nose appears large, the hair shape should move forward in the chin area. This creates an optical illusion that moves the chin into balance with the nose (Figure 7.113).
- When the distance from the chin to the neck is short, hair moving backward and upward takes the eye away from the chin area (Figure 7.114). This movement would also take the eye away from a double chin.

The neck-and-shoulder structure differs greatly with each individual. Hair lengths and styles can be used to show off positive features and disguise problems.

Guide to Neck and Shoulder Correction

☐ Rounded shoulders will be concealed when the hair is left long enough to cover the rounded area (Figure 7.115).

☐ A rounded shoulder can also be corrected with short hair, provided an area of fullness is created behind the head. The line created from hair to back will give the illusion of balance (Figure 7.116).

☐ A very straight neck can be on a vertical plane with the back of the head. When this is the case, some fullness in the hair design will give the head softness and shape (Figure 7.117).

☐ A neck that angles forward from the shoulders should have hair at the nape of the neck to keep the shoulders from looking rounded (Figure 7.118).

◆ **Key Point** ◆

You will know when a hairstyle suits an individual perfectly. To create harmony in hairstyling, carefully analyze your client's features. The cosmetologist who creates adaptable designs is a more marketable professional technician and consultant.

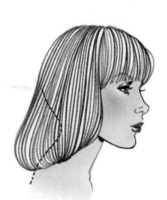

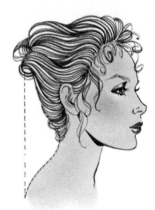

7.115   Concealing round shoulders

7.116   Concealing round shoulders

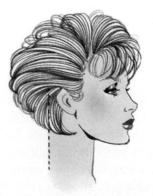

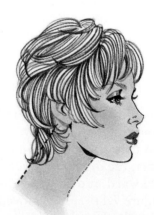

7.117   Fullness softens straight neck

7.118   Hair at nape softens angled neck

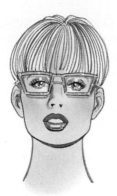
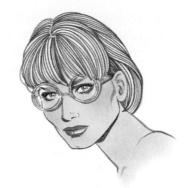

7.119   Angular style for rounded features   7.120   Rounded style for angular features

Eyeglasses and the Hair Design

Frames for eyeglasses should be recommended on the basis of the facial features rather than the hairstyle. A hairstyle is likely to change more often than it is necessary to change the glasses. Though most people selecting eyeglasses will seek the advice of a trained optician, many cosmetologists include glasses in a general consultation. Following are some important points to consider when recommending shapes of glasses.

- People with rounded features should select glasses of an angular style to offset the roundness (Figure 7.119).
- People with angular features should select glasses of a rounded style to offset the angular features (Figure 7.120).
- The size of the frames selected should not overpower small features, nor be too small for stronger or larger features, as in Figure 7.121.
- For an unobtrusive frame, match the skin or hair color. To add authority or drama, make a selection a few shades lighter or darker than the hair color (Figure 7.122). The less ornamentation found on the frames, the more the face is featured.

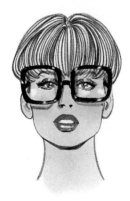
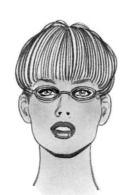
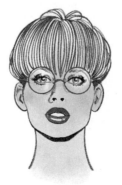
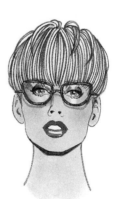

7.121   Glasses should not overpower or be too small   7.122   Color can match skin or be a few shades darker or lighter

SUMMARY

As a cosmetologist, your ability to select, adapt, and execute a hairstyle is vitally important. You will apply the elements and principles of design to add the extra creative dimension to your work.

The elements of form, space, line, color, and texture are the building blocks of art. Form, the most important of the elements, is the shadow or silhouette of the style. Space refers to the movements inside the form. Line is an important element because the eye will follow it, creating a design in the hair. Color adds excitement, warmth, or coolness. Texture, the feel of the design, adds variety naturally, or it can be created chemically.

As a cosmetologist, you will use the elements of form, space, line, color, and texture as tools. You will create hair designs based on your analysis of your client's features, and you will use or place each element to best suit your client.

You will apply the elements by the use of the principles of art and design. The principle of proportion is used to balance facial features. The universal proportion is two to three. You will apply balance in hair design along a central axis to create symmetry, or will use imaginary balance lines for asymmetrical designs. The principle of rhythm is a form of repetition that you will use to create a feeling of movement. You will use emphasis to draw attention to the desired area of the design you create considering your client's best features. Harmony is a principle used to ensure that all of the elements of the hairstyle complement the facial features and the body size.

As a professional cosmetologist, you will use the principles of hair design—proportion, balance, rhythm, emphasis, and harmony—to create the desired style with the appropriate elements. You will adapt hair shapes to the face and body of your clients, thereby creating demand for you as a fashion consultant.

QUESTIONS

1. What is form? How is it important in hair design?
2. How does design function within the form?
3. In what three positions can lines be drawn?
4. What is the importance of lines?
5. What are five effects that color can have on hair design?
6. How is texture used for variety in hair design?
7. What is the definition of *proportion*? How is proportion applied to hair design?
8. What is an example of symmetrical balance?
9. How can asymmetrical balance be used in hairstyling?
10. What three types of rhythm can be applied to hair design?
11. What are three methods of creating emphasis in the hairstyle?
12. How can you obtain harmony when working with the hair and face?
13. How are elements and principles related?

1. Choose several photos of hairstyles you like. Analyze the form and make notes on how it complements the face. Indicate two other forms that would also look good on that face.

2. Choose several photos of hairstyles and decide which of the design elements contributes the most to the overall attractiveness of the style (form/space/line/color/texture).

3. As you create haircuts and hairstyles on your clients, keep a journal and record what art elements and principles you have used to make design decisions, and evaluate your decisions by answering the following questions:
   a. Is each element used properly?
   b. Which element is the most important?
   c. Are all elements in harmony?
   d. Is the design balanced?

4. Create hairstyles and identify the type of rhythm you have used. Observe the purpose that rhythm serves.

5. On a mannequin, place 5 different types and sizes of ornaments in the hairstyle one at a time. Note the alteration of the style by the ornament used.

6. Pull the hair straight back from the face on at least 10 clients and observe the profiles. Using the Guide for profile corrections, make suggestions to the client, and carry through with as many points as your consultation will allow. Evaluate the results.

7. Identify the balance line on at least 10 hairstyles you create on clients. Does the balance line feature the best part of the face?

8. Observe the jaw shape of several people that you know. Does the haircut or style they wear complement and enhance that jaw shape? Analyze why or why not.

HAIR SHAPING

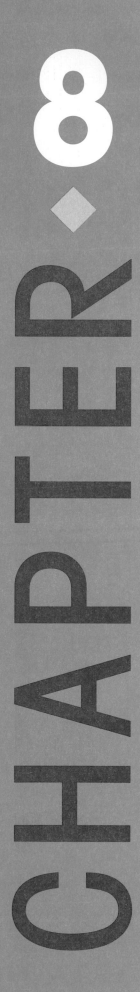

CHAPTER • 8

CHAPTER GOAL

The basis of every hairstyle is a good haircut. After reading this chapter and completing the projects, you should be able to

1. List the basic hair shaping instruments and explain their use.
2. Demonstrate how to hold the shears and the razor with a comb.
3. Explain why sectioning is important in hair shaping.
4. Explain how the texture of the hair will determine the cut that you will give.
5. Define *composition* as it relates to haircutting.
6. Explain the terms *length* and *perimeter*.
7. Demonstrate the three main levels of elevation and explain the purpose of each.
8. Demonstrate a medium-length haircut.
9. Demonstrate a long-length haircut.

Hair shaping has been around since earliest recorded history. While those early methods were quite primitive, we know that ancient peoples removed hair for coolness in the summer and let it grow for protection and warmth in colder months. Later, history tells us that hair length was seen as a sign of strength. Victorious generals would shear the hair of their enemies, often making them adapt the style of the winning nation.

Throughout history, women generally had long hair. Styles for men ranged over time from long to short and back to long again. Hair shaping, as an art, began in the Middle Ages with the very earliest of guilds. As a service, it was available only to royalty, knights, and the very wealthy. By the 1800s, cutting the hair to the shape of the head had become the style among men. It was not until the 1900s that this concept was applied to women as well.

Hair shaping is a term which describes cutting the hair into longer, looser styles. It is to be distinguished from **precision haircutting** which involves cutting the hair into shorter styles with crisp lines (see Chapter 9). Every hairstyle you create should be determined by the individual features of your particular client. The shape of the face and head, the texture and density of the hair, and the height and weight of the person are all important factors to be considered before choosing a style.

In order to become a professional stylist, you must master the basics of hair shaping. You should be able to analyze the shape of the head and section the hair according to that shape. You must be able to establish a guide for the correct length and follow it through the entire cut. You must be able to select the proper elevation as well as the correct shaping implement to achieve the desired cut.

HAIR SHAPING INSTRUMENTS

Each hair shaping instrument produces a particular effect. You should master the correct use of each and know the results it will give you. Each instrument should be chosen according to the texture, density, and condition of the hair.

Shears or Scissors

A pair of **shears**, or **scissors**, is the instrument that is used for most hair shaping or haircutting. It can be used to give a blunt cut—cutting the hair straight across—or for **slithering**. Slithering removes hair at various lengths. To slither the hair, slide the shears up and down the hair shaft. Shears come in various lengths, weights, and qualities of steel. Figure 8.1 shows the various parts of a pair of shears.

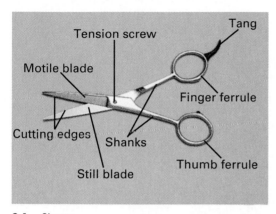

8.1   Shears

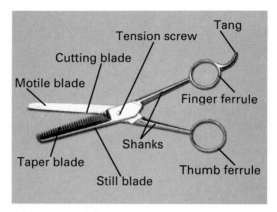

8.2   Tapering Shears

Tapering Shears

Tapering or **thinning shears** are used to thin the hair where there is too much bulk. They may also be used to blend in and shape a haircut that has left the hair with stubby, blunt ends. Tapering shears have notched edges and come in two styles, those with one notched blade and one regular blade and those with two notched blades. Tapering shears with one notched edge remove more hair than shears with two notched edges. This is because the hair that fits into the notches is not removed when the blades are closed. Thinning shears also vary in length from shears with 30 teeth to those with 46 teeth. The more teeth the shears have, the finer the thinning. Figure 8.2 shows the various parts of the tapering shears. Note that one blade is slightly longer than the other. This makes it easier to pick up hair or weave it into the section to be thinned.

Razor

The **razor** is a very useful hair shaping tool for certain textures of hair. It is very versatile. With a razor you can blunt-cut, thin, or taper out the ends of the hair. Parts of the razor are shown in Figure 8.3.

Changing the Razor Blade

Usually the manufacturer provides instruction for changing blades. If not, the procedure is simple. First, remove the guard from the razor. Clasp the guard at the back, opposite the notched edge, and pull it off. Then use the guard to push off the old blade. Next, insert the new blade into the blade slot, making sure to push it in all the way. Finally, remove the paper or plastic covering from the cutting edge of the blade and place the guard over the blade, with the notched edge facing you.

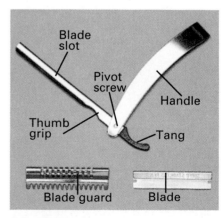

8.3   Razor

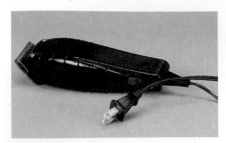

8.4   Electric clippers

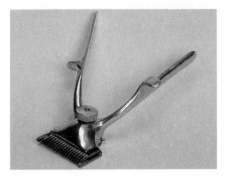

8.5   Hand clippers

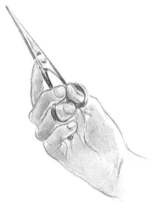

8.7

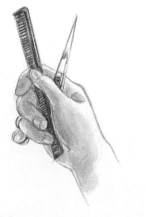

8.8

Clippers

Clippers are sometimes used to cut off undesirable hair at the neckline and to cut the outline for styles such as the Afro. Clippers can also be used as a haircutting implement, especially on thick, coarse hair. Although electric clippers (Figure 8.4) are the most popular kind in use today, hand clippers (Figure 8.5) are still available.

Hair Shaping Combs

Two different combs are used for hair shaping. Figure 8.6 shows the **style comb** and the **barber comb**. The backs of some of these combs have a numbered scale that can be used to measure lengths of hair. These combs have coarse and fine teeth, so they can be used effectively on any texture of hair.

The barber comb is very flexible and is most commonly used to feather out (taper) a short, close, neckline haircut.

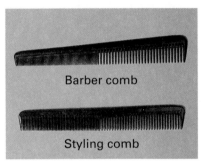

Barber comb

Styling comb

8.6

How to Hold the Shears and the Razor

Learn to hold the shears and razor correctly to avoid fatigue. Proper techniques will produce more accurate results and help you avoid injuring your clients.

Holding the Shears

To hold the shears, place the ring finger in the smaller handle opening, the finger ferrule (refer to Figure 8.1), and the little finger on the tang. Place the middle finger on the shank under the finger ferrule, and the index finger near the middle of the shears to help balance and control them when cutting hair. Place the thumb in the larger handle opening, the thumb ferrule (Figure 8.7). The thumb is used to control the movement of the cutting blade. To prevent the thumb from sliding too far through the opening, tension should be applied between the index finger and the little finger.

In Figure 8.8, note the position of the fingers when the shears are not in use. The same fingers and thumb hold the shears, but the shears slide farther up on the fingers. This leaves the ends of the fingers and the thumb free to hold the comb.

To return the shears to cutting position, place the comb in the left hand and slide the scissors down on the fingers to about the first knuckle or to any other comfortable position.

Another technique for holding the shears when they are not in use is that of "palming" the shears by removing your thumb from the opening and folding the shears into the center of your hand. To return to cutting after combing the next section, move the comb to your other hand, replace your thumb in the ferrule, and proceed to cut.

Holding the Razor

The proper balance of implements is the first step in proper hair shaping. It is particularly important that you feel comfortable when using a razor. In order to ensure proper balance of the razor in your hand, first place the razor on your extended middle, ring, and index fingers (Figure 8.9). Then close your hand partially, placing the thumb on the thumb grip (see Figure 8.10). Next, place your small finger on the tang (see Figure 8.11). Make sure that you keep your wrist very flexible, with the cutting edge directed toward you (see Figure 8.12). For a vertical movement, hold the razor as shown in Figure 8.13. When combing the hair, hold the comb and razor with the same hand (Figure 8.14).

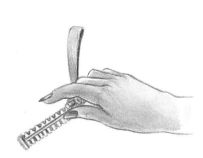

8.9   Balance razor

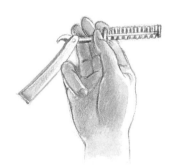

8.10   Grip razor

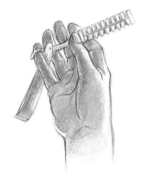

8.11   Little finger on tang

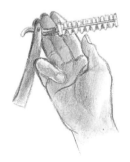

8.12   Cut position

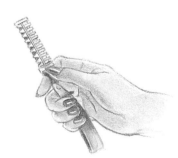

8.13   Optional position

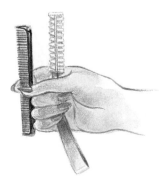

8.14   Palming razor

SECTIONING FOR A HAIRCUT

The purpose of sectioning for a haircut is to determine the bone structure and actual size of the head. This is important because you must know the distribution of hair at the top, the sides, the crown, and the nape in order to shape the haircut. If you consider that sectioning is done for this reason alone, you will understand why all haircuts require similar sectioning. Depending on the style you want to achieve, the angles of the cut will vary in direction within the sections.

Sectioning for the Top

The correct amount of hair to be parted off for the top section corresponds to the area of the head covered by the frontal bone (see Figure 8.15). To determine the width of the frontal bone, place your fingers at the center part of the top of your head. Now run your fingers down the side of your head toward your ears. At about eye level you will feel a slight indentation and then a small bump or protrusion. You have these bumps on both sides of your head. They are caused by the parietal bones. The width of the top section goes from one parietal bone to the other. After determining the width, make two partings going toward the hairline and ending at a point above the natural peak of the eyebrows. Extend the partings back to the highest point of the head. You can determine the highest point by parting the hair down the center and looking at the head from the side.

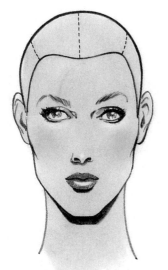

8.15   Sectioning for top

Sectioning for the Crown

Behind the top section and between the parietal protrusion on either side of the head, there is a slight outline of the crown extending down to the base of the skull (the occipital area). You will find another bulge in this section. Although it may not be as pronounced on some heads as on others, there will always be a curve as the back of the head blends into the neck. The bottom of the crown section is parted off just below this curve. Study Figure 8.16 and run your hand over the back of your head to identify the crown section.

Sectioning for the Nape

With the crown section of the hair clipped up out of the way, you can see the hair that belongs in the nape section. You can find the width of the nape section by placing your fingers behind the ears and feeling for the projection of the end of the temporal bones (see Figure 8.16). By using these bones as your guide, you will have the exact amount of hair for the nape, and it will be centered exactly in the middle of the back of the head. (Because the head is covered with hair, it will be almost impossible for you to find the center of the head unless you use these bones as guides.)

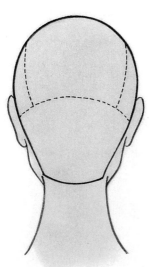

8.16   Sectioning for back

Sectioning for the Sides

The hair remaining after the top, crown, and nape have been sectioned off belongs to the side sections. In Figure 8.17, you can see the division among the top section, the crown section, and the nape section. If you have followed the sectioning accurately, the side sections will be exactly the same size.

Hair Partings Within the Section

For ease in handling and to help you to see the distribution of hair, each section is parted off into smaller divisions. How many partings are made within the section is determined by the haircut to be given, but usually the top and crown sections are divided into thirds (Figure 8.18).

For a layered haircut, vertical partings are used within the sections (Figure 8.19). For a one-length cut, horizontal partings are used (Figure 8.20). The angle used for each of the partings will vary depending upon the style. The sides and the nape section are parted in the same way.

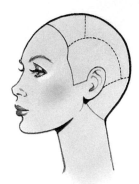

8.17   Sectioning for sides

◆ **Key Point** ◆

Sectioning helps you maintain control of the haircut while determining the bone structure and size of the head.

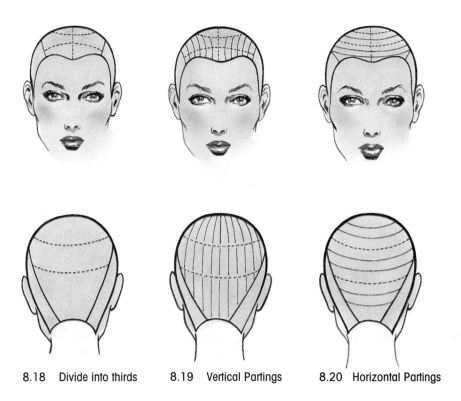

8.18   Divide into thirds   8.19   Vertical Partings   8.20   Horizontal Partings

HAIR TEXTURE AS IT RELATES TO HAIR SHAPING

The **texture** of hair will play a major role in deciding what kind of cut you will give. It will also affect the technique and the type of tool you will use.

Cosmetologists usually use the terms very fine, fine, medium, and coarse to describe hair textures. Hair density is the number of hairs per square inch on the scalp. Density determines whether the hair will be thick or thin. You will find thin and thick hair in all hair textures. Refer to Chapter 16 for further information regarding hair texture.

Based on a client's hair texture, you should follow a few basic rules to achieve the right style for the individual.

Very Fine and Fine Texture

The client with fine or very fine hair will usually complain that the style does not hold well and that it is difficult to manage. Fine-textured hair should be blunt-cut with shears, and it should be one even length. A blunt cut (cutting the hair straight across) with shears does not take away the weight from the ends of hair. The hair will seem thicker if it is cut to the same length. One-length cuts are also the easiest to manage. Fine-textured hair should never be dressed up toward the top of the head unless it is long enough to be pinned.

Medium Texture

People with this type of hair can wear a slightly layered cut (the hair becomes progressively shorter toward the top of the head). It should also be cut with shears. The style can be worn brushed up or down. Generally, styles that are considered good for fine hair are also best for medium-textured hair. However, medium-textured hair will hold more design and curl in the style than will fine hair.

Coarse Texture

A layered cut is better for this type of hair. It can be cut with a razor, especially if it is extremely thick, because the razor gives more taper to the ends of the hair. Usually, coarse hair is styled using a little less curl than medium-textured hair.

It is difficult to make definite rules regarding hair texture. Each head of hair is different. However, very fine hair always presents some problems.

> ### ◆ Key Point ◆
> The texture of hair will determine what kind of cut you can give. Coarser textures can have more layers while very fine textures cannot.

Composition as It Relates to Haircutting

Composition in haircutting refers to the amount of hair to be cut short as compared to the amount to be left long. It also refers to the right distribution of hair as it relates to each section (nape, sides, top, and crown) of the individual head. The head from the profile view is divided into three parts: (1) top and sides, (2) crown, and (3) nape (Figure 8.21). To determine the correct composition (amount of hair), use the client's bone structure as a guide.

Think of the face as being divided into six parts: three vertically and three horizontally. The horizontal sections go from the hairline to the eyebrows, from the eyebrows to the tip of the nose, and from the tip of the nose to the tip of the chin. Vertically the face is divided into thirds from the peak of the eyebrows to the high point of the cheekbone to the hinge of the jawbone (see Figure 8.22). These facial points are important in determining the right composition of hair mass for the individual face shape.

> **◆ Key Point ◆**
>
> Composition refers to the amount of hair and its distribution. You will adjust haircuts according to the composition of the hair. In this way, your haircuts will respond appropriately to your client's facial shape.

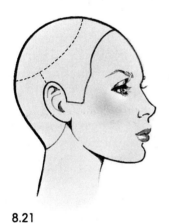

8.21

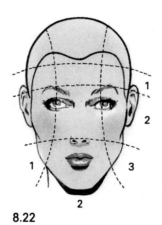

8.22

Length and Perimeter

Length refers to the distance of the hair shaft from the scalp to the end, and **perimeter** refers to the circumference (outer edge) of the cut. Length is determined by the perimeter, while the perimeter is usually determined by the shape of the section or of the head.

For example, the length and perimeter of the hair on the forehead (commonly referred to as the fringe or bangs) are determined

> **◆ Key Point ◆**
>
> Length is the distance from the scalp to the ends of the hair. Perimeter is the outer edge of the haircut.

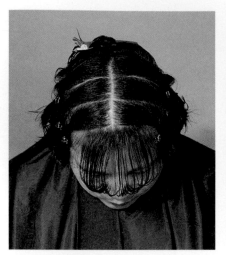

8.23   Section top

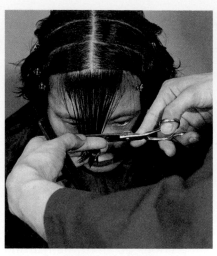

8.24   Cut front third for bangs

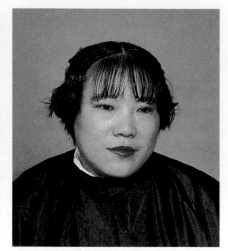

8.25   Finished bangs

by the depth of the section and the width of the forehead. To create bangs, first section the top then divide the section into thirds. Each third should have equal portions of hair (Figure 8.23). The length of the bangs is determined by drawing the first third of hair forward to the brow (Figure 8.24). The finished cut (Figure 8.25) reflects uniform lengths on either side and results in a perfect perimeter outlining the natural shape of the brow. The right amount of hair—one-third—covers the forehead, and two-thirds is left for the top. Also note that one-third of the face is covered, while two-thirds is left open. If you were to try to create this outline by cutting from one side of the forehead to the other, you would almost certainly end up with one side longer than the other. The method given here is both quicker and more accurate. The length of the bangs can also be used as a guide for cutting the remaining two-thirds of the top.

ELEVATION

Elevation refers to how high or low you hold the hair that is being cut in relation to where it grows on the scalp. The following examples of low, high, and medium elevation will help you to understand the purpose and effect of using different elevations when cutting hair. This is one of the few hair shaping techniques that can be applied to short hair.

Low Elevation

As Figure 8.26 shows, the hair from the bottom third of the nape section is held at its lowest point, close to the neck. There is no elevation to the hair. The purpose of a low elevation is to produce maximum bulk at the perimeter or ends of the hair. This elevation is most effective when the hair is fine and thin and when the finished style requires hair that is all of the same length. None of the hair is layered.

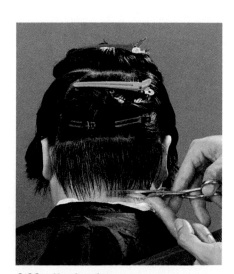

8.26   No elevation

◆ **Key Point** ◆

Elevation refers to how low or high you hold the subsection of hair in relation to the head. Low elevation creates bulk and high elevation creates layers. Medium elevation is used for blend.

High Elevation

In this example, the hair at the nape is parted vertically and lifted to the top of its section. Hair that is lifted to the top of its section results in the highest possible elevation. When hair is cut in this position, the shears must angle out from the head (Figure 8.27). Hair cut in this fashion will be layered (Figure 8.28). If you were to try to elevate the hair higher than its section, there would be too great a distance between the short hair and the long hair, and the hair would be too thin. A high elevation should be used on medium or thick hair, never on fine or thin hair.

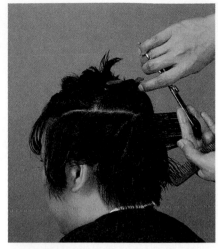

8.27   High elevation cut

Medium Elevation

To achieve a perfect medium elevation, the fingers must first be positioned flat against the head (Figure 8.29). The hair is lifted straight out from where it grows, and the fingers remain parallel to the head (Figure 8.30). The shears must follow the angle of the fingers. This cut gives you a perfect width of layered ends. In fact, the width of the ends will be the same as the width of the section from which the hair grows. The hair will fall softly, but it will not be too thin. A medium elevation can be used on all textures of hair.

Finished Styles Reflect Elevation

The finished style reflects the elevation used in the haircut. The model used for the medium and high elevations (Figure 8.31) has medium-textured, thick hair, yet the hair in both styles looks light and full.

Although different elevations can be used to achieve various looks, to be most successful the elevation used should match the texture and growth pattern of the hair.

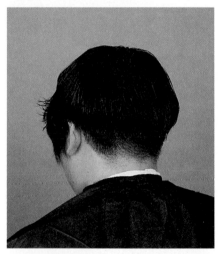

8.28   Finished layers

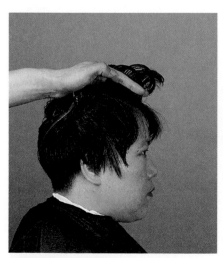

8.29   Position fingers

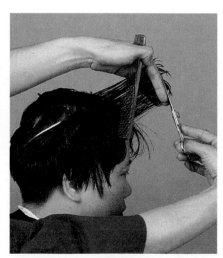

8.30   Medium elevation

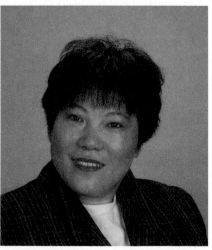

8.31

A MEDIUM-LENGTH HAIRCUT

This type of haircut is perfect for fine hair (Figure 8.32). **Medium-length** hair can vary in length from the chinline to just above the shoulders.

Materials

Shampoo cape and towel
Shampoo
Comb
Clips
Shears
Razor
Neck strip

Procedure for a Medium-Length Haircut

1. Wash your hands.
2. Drape the client and shampoo the hair (see Chapter 5).
3. Determine the basic sections, using the bone structure of the head.
4. Part the hair into four sections. For this particular style, notice that the top section has been divided in the center and that each half of the section has been combined with a side section (Figures 8.33 and 8.34). Figure 8.35 shows the nape section.
5. Part off the lower third of hair in the nape section (Figure 8.36) and clip the rest of the hair up out of your way. The part will extend across the nape from the bones behind each ear.
6. Comb the hair that is loose toward the center of the head. Hold your comb vertically from the protrusion of the occipital bone to the hairline to establish the middle of the section.

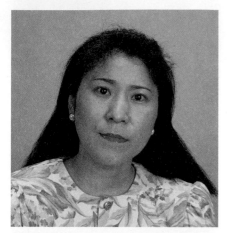

8.32

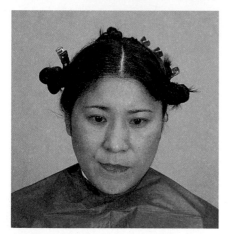

8.33   Part hair into four sections

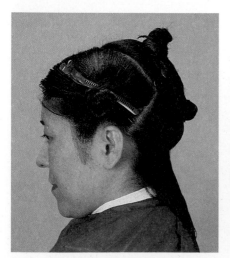

8.34   Side sectioning

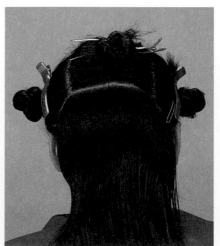

8.35   Back section

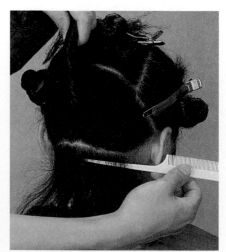

8.36   Part off lower third of nape

7. Hold the hair with your fingers, position your shears horizontally, and cut off at the desired length (Figure 8.37). Notice that the natural inverted curve has perfect proportions from the shorter center to longer sides (Figure 8.38). This is the result of using the bone structure of the individual head to determine the sections.
8. Part off the second third of the nape section (Figure 8.39).
9. Comb the hair to the center, using the first cut as a guide, and again cut straight across (Figure 8.40). The lengths should fall evenly. This helps to create weight and makes fine hair look thicker.
10. Let down the last third of the nape section and cut in the same manner.

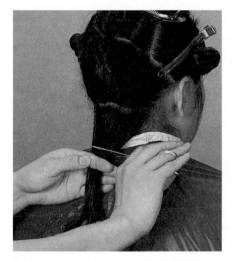

8.37   Cut guide straight across

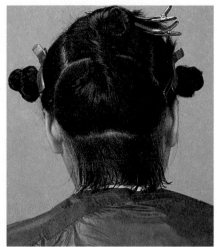

8.38   Hair falls in curve

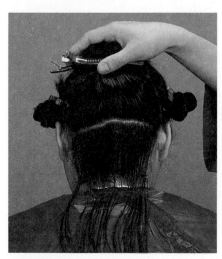

8.39   Part off second third

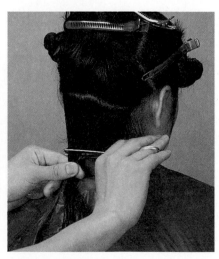

8.40   Cut straight across

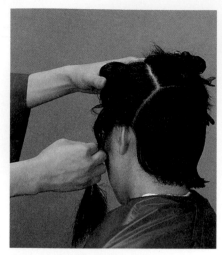

8.41   Part hair around ear

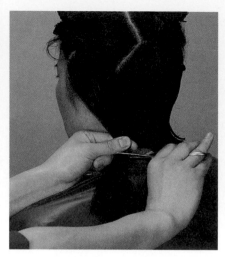

8.42   Cut section with back guide

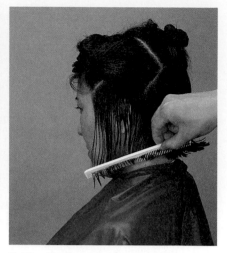

8.43   Side hair blends with back

11. Following the outline of the ear, part a strip of hair from the nape section to the front hairline (Figure 8.41).
12. Comb this strip, the guideline hair, back toward the nape section (Figure 8.42). Use the shears in a horizontal position and cut the hair to the same length as the nape section. This cut blends the sides and nape together and establishes the correct angle and length of hair to frame the face (Figure 8.43).
13. Comb down the rest of the side hair and all of the top section to blend in with the guideline just completed (Figure 8.44).
14. Cut the hair at the same length and angle as established in step 12 (Figure 8.45).
15. Continue cutting the top and the side section together using narrow, angled, vertical partings (Figure 8.46).
16. Cut the opposite side of the head in the same manner, repeating steps 11 through 15.

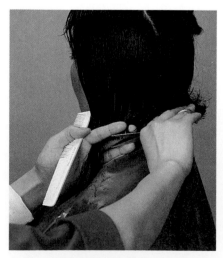

8.44   Comb down side hair

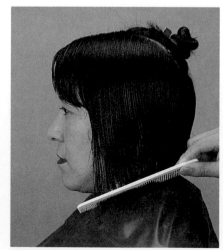

8.45   Cut side

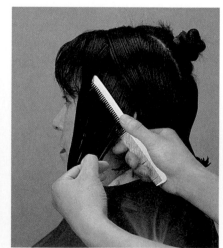

8.46   Cut top and side

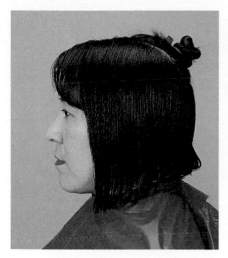

8.47   Side blends with back

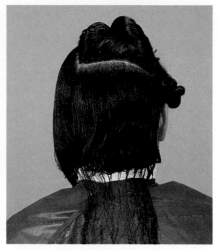

8.48   Part off bottom of crown

17. The finished side should blend evenly with the back. The top hair should be the same length as the guideline hair (Figure 8.47).
18. Part off a curved, narrow strip of hair across the bottom of the crown section (Figure 8.48).
19. Comb this strip of hair toward the center of the head (Figure 8.49). Hold the hair loosely without pulling against the scalp. Make a single cut as shown. The hair length and angle should follow the guide established in the nape section.
20. Continue cutting the crown section, using narrow partings and following the established curve.
21. The finished haircut should be the same length from top hair to nape and should follow a continuous line from back to front (Figure 8.50). This creates the weight necessary to give finer hair a fuller look (Figure 8.51).

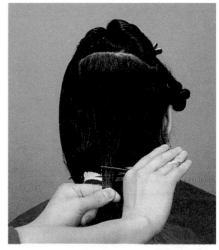

8.49   Comb hair to center

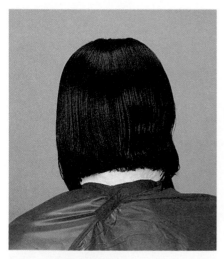

8.50   Finished line

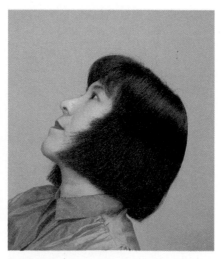

8.51

A LONG-LENGTH HAIRCUT

All the hair in this type of haircut is cut to the same length. The lengths and angles of the cut are determined by the size of the head. **Long-length** hair falls to the shoulder or below. The finished length can vary from medium-long to long, depending on the individual.

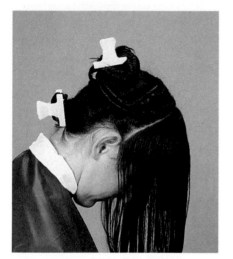

8.52   Part hair into four sections

Materials

Shampoo cape and towel
Shampoo
Comb
Clips
Shears
Neck strip

Procedure for Long-Length Haircut

1. Wash your hands.
2. Drape the client and shampoo the hair (see Chapter 5).
3. Determine the basic sections, using the bone structure of the head.
4. Part the hair into four sections. Half of the top section and the side section are treated as one section (Figures 8.52 and 8.53). This will ensure a smooth angle running from short hair around the face to long hair in the back. Figure 8.54 shows the crown and nape sections.
5. Part off a section of hair taken from the center front to be used as a guide. If the client has bangs, pull long hair from each side to the center of the face and cut below the point of the chin (see Figure 8.55). This will be the shortest point of the hanging length (see Figure 8.56). The bangs will be cut separately.

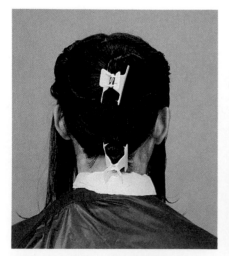

8.53   Half of top and side section are one

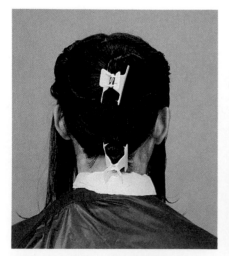

8.54   Crown and nape sections

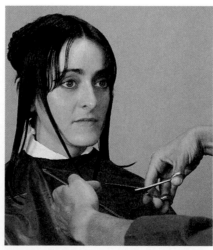

8.55   Cut guide

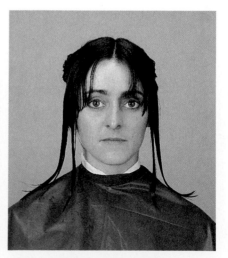

8.56   Shortest hanging length

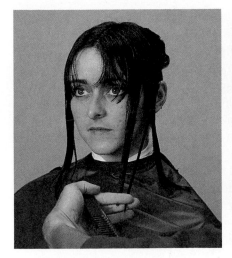

8.57 Comb first third forward

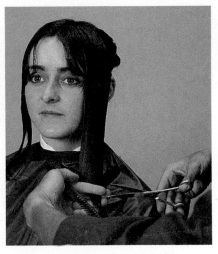

8.58 Hold fingers parallel to guide

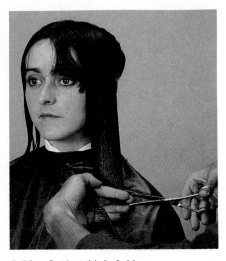

8.59 Cut last third of side

6. Comb the first third of the hair from the left side section forward (Figure 8.57) to the angle of the guide that was just cut.

7. Hold the hair forward so it continues to blend with the guide. Make the second cut just below the length previously cut. Notice that the scissors are held in a horizontal position to the jawline when making this cut. The angle of the completed cut is a result of the difference between the width of the section at the top of the head and the width of the section as it continues down the head.

8. Part off the second third of the side section and comb it down so it is distributed evenly with the section that was just cut.

9. Hold the first section as a guide for both the length and the angle of the second cut. Hold your fingers parallel to the guide and cut the hair the same length as the guide (Figure 8.58).

10. Comb down the remaining third of the side section and cut it in the same manner as the previous section (Figure 8.59).

11. Cut the right side of the head in the same manner, repeating steps 6 through 10. Notice, however, that your left hand holding the hair is in a different position because you are cutting on the opposite side of the head (see Figures 8.60, 8.61, and 8.62).

> ◆ **Key Point** ◆
> Long-length haircutting techniques are excellent for fine or extremely fine hair. Low elevation adds bulk to the perimeter or ends of the hair.

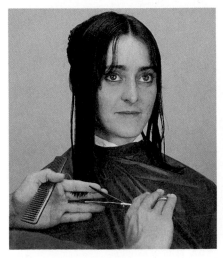

8.60 Cut first third of side

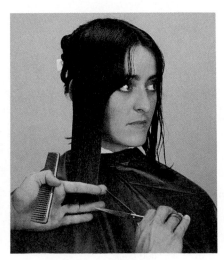

8.61 Cut second third

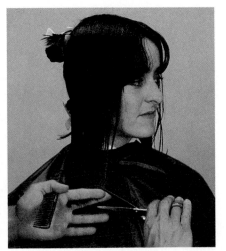

8.62 Cut final third

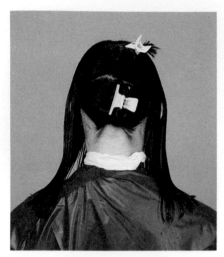

8.63   Check that sides are even

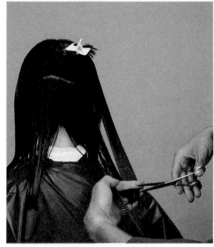

8.64   Cut guide for back

12. You are now ready to cut the nape section. Notice that the angle of the cut and the lengths of the side sections are even (Figure 8.63). This is the result of using the bone structure as a guide for the sections, ensuring uniform cutting lengths.

13. Divide the nape section in half. Comb each half to the side, blending the hair with the hair that has already been cut. Use the longest length from the side section as a guide for the back length. The cut is made on an angle to allow for more length at the center back (Figure 8.64).

14. Cut the other half of the back section in the same manner, again using the side section as a guide (Figure 8.65). Note the perfect symmetry that is achieved with two cuts of the shears when the hair is held at the correct angle (Figure 8.66). The outline for the haircut has been completed, and the nape section is blended with the side sections.

15. Part off the lower third of the crown section.

16. Comb the hair from the center of the back out to the sides. Using the hair cut previously as a guide, cut the crown hair to the same length (Figure 8.67).

17. Cut the other half of the section in the same manner. This lower portion of the crown section is cut in the same manner as the nape hair to give more bulk to the ends of the hair. This is particularly helpful when working with fine hair.

18. The remainder of the crown section is combed down and distributed evenly across the back of the head (Figure 8.68). In combing the hair, do not go beyond the projection of the parietal bones (Figure 8.69). The hair will not fall forward naturally beyond this point.

19. Starting at the side of the crown section, part off a 2-inch width of hair (Figure 8.70).

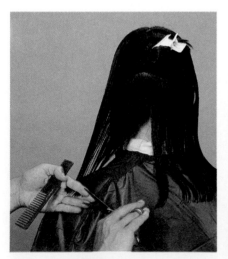

8.65   Cut left back

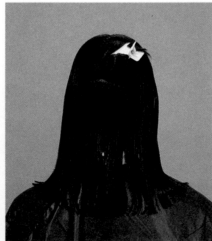

8.66   Finished back

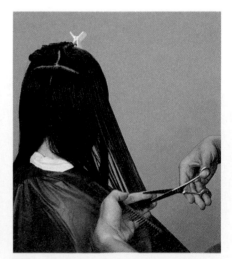

8.67   Cut crown hair

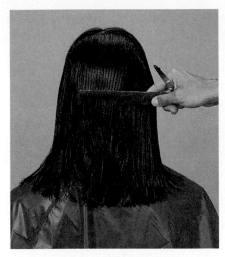

8.68 Comb down crown section

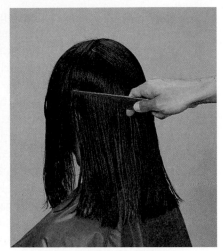

8.69 Stop combing at parietal bone

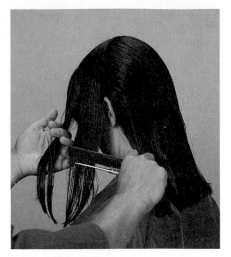

8.70 Part off hair at side of crown

20. Include the previously cut hair from underneath as a guide and roll up the fingers of your left hand.

21. From this position you are able to see the guide for the length and angle of the cut. Cut the center of the crown section to the same length as the guide hair (Figure 8.71).

22. Continue to use this technique as you cut the remainder of the crown section. Part off a 2-inch width of hair, roll up the fingers of your left hand, and cut using the previously cut hair as a guide.

23. The haircut has been completed (Figure 8.72). The hair is still slightly damp and is distributed naturally around the head. Notice that the ends are turning up slightly. This is the result of the overcutting technique (rolling the fingers of the left hand up before cutting) used when cutting the upper two-thirds of the crown section. If this overcutting technique had been used on all of the nape and crown hair, the ends of the hair would have been too thin. Figure 8.73 shows the completed style.

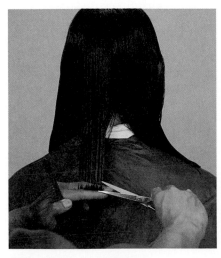

8.71 Cut center of crown

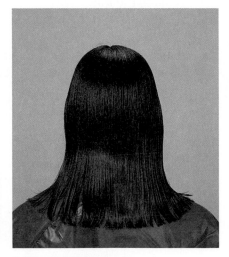

8.72 Finished cut

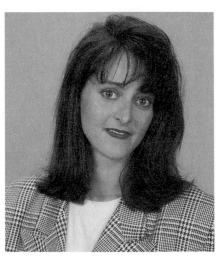

8.73

SUMMARY

The purpose of basic hair shaping is to provide a foundation for the style to be created. To master the art of hair shaping, you must be able to determine the shape and size of the head, and select the implement and the elevation which will give the desired effect.

Sectioning is the method you will use to determine the bone structure and the actual size of the head. Allow an appropriate section when the cut needs to fit in the nape or when creating a bang or fringe effect. Sectioning will also help you avoid cutting the ear area too short and will help you maintain even elevation.

Elevation is the angle at which you hold the hair from the head when removing length. Higher elevation will give you layers in the shaping while lower or blunt elevation will leave bulk at the ends for a thicker, one-length look. First, establish a subsection of hair as a guide for length, then hold the hair to be cut to that guide at the selected elevation. This cut hair becomes your guide for the next section, and so on until you have completed the shaping.

The implements you select for the hair shaping will make a difference in the finished look. Shears are used for a crisp, even line and are recommended for fine or thin hair. A razor can be used to create a soft, feather-edge effect. There are a number of implements that you can use to remove bulk rather than length, but thinning shears are especially designed for that purpose. Clippers are good for speed, and can be used to create sculpted looks on thick or coarse hair.

QUESTIONS

1. What are the basic hair shaping instruments and how is each used?
2. What effect do you get from each hair shaping instrument?
3. How do you hold the shears while combing the hair during a haircut?
4. How do you hold the comb while cutting the hair with a razor?
5. Why is sectioning important in hair shaping?
6. How does the texture of the hair influence the cut?
7. What does *composition* mean as it relates to haircutting?
8. What is meant by the term *length* in haircutting?
9. What is the *perimeter* of a haircut?
10. What are the three main levels of elevation and what is the purpose of each?
11. How would you give a medium-length haircut?
12. How would you give a long-length haircut?

1. On your mannequin, duplicate the sectioning patterns in this chapter. Practice until your sections are even and accurate.

2. Refer to the head forms you created in your anatomy projects. On these forms, you indicated the shape of the head and labeled the bones. Working with colored pencils, indicate the sectioning pattern you would use to compensate for the shape of the head for a long, a medium, and a short cut.

3. Analyze the head shape of at least six people. Keeping their finished style in mind, demonstrate the selected sectioning pattern. Have each verified by your instructor before proceeding with the cut.

4. On hair swatches, cut hair at no, low, medium, and high elevations. At each elevation, cut the hair with three different implements: shears, razor, and clippers. Observe the effect of each elevation and each implement on the hair ends.

5. Research at least five methods of thinning, or removing bulk from the hair. What implement should be used for each of the methods? Practice each method on your mannequin until you have mastered the technique of thinning the hair.

PRECISION HAIRCUTTING

CHAPTER GOAL

Precision haircutting is an advanced and refined technique for creating a style. After reading this chapter and completing the projects, you should be able to

1. Explain the procedures that make precision haircutting more advanced than basic hair shaping.
2. Describe the benefits of the classic bob.
3. Demonstrate the procedure for cutting a classic bob.
4. Explain the benefits of the short tapered cut.
5. Demonstrate the procedure for cutting a short tapered cut.

CHAPTER · 9

Precision haircutting evolved as an advanced technique during the 1960s. Vidal Sassoon is credited with advancing basic hair shaping into an artistry of precisely cutting tiny sections of hair so that a specific style was "sculpted" into the hair. Sassoon became best known for haircuts with sharp, crisp edges and geometric shapes.

As a haircutter, precision techniques will help you build your menu of services for your clients with active life styles. A precision haircut lends itself to a variety of quick and easy styling and finishing techniques.

The style is actually created by the cut. Pay close attention to the natural characteristics of the hair including its growth pattern, texture, and thickness. While in school, learn the principles of precision cutting and apply them to new styles introduced during your training. After you have graduated from school and received your license, you will have many opportunities to observe and practice precision haircutting. As a junior stylist, you will use a classic bob and a short tapered cut as the basis for other contemporary hairstyles. New and improved cutting methods are part of the quality advanced education available to the professional stylist.

Principles of Precision Haircutting

Precision haircutting is an advanced and refined method for shaping the hair that reflects the most up-to-date ideas in cosmetology. There are five basic rules to follow when giving a precision haircut.

1. *Cut the hair in very small sections.* In Chapter 8 we spoke about parting the hair off into large sections: the top, the crown, the nape, and the two sides. In precision haircutting we call these large blocks of hair **areas**, and we speak of the head as being divided into **basic areas**. Each area is then divided into very small sections. The sections in a precision haircut are generally no wider than $1/2$ inch. So when we speak about a section in a precision haircut, we are referring to a very small division of hair.

   Cutting small sections, rather than large blocks of hair, gives you much more control over the haircut. In addition, the margin of error is greatly reduced because mistakes can be corrected easily.

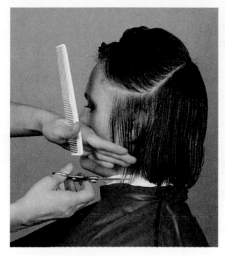
9.1 Blunt cutting

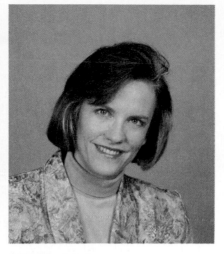
9.2 Classic bob

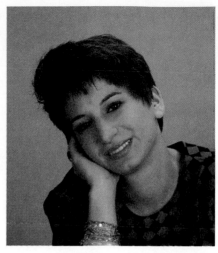
9.3 Short tapered cut

2. *Cut with straight, sharp lines.* In precision haircutting it is important that your cuts be straight. This is also called **blunt cutting**. The hair is cut straight across so that the ends are blunt (see Figure 9.1).

3. *Hold the hair taut and firm as it is being cut.* This will help to ensure that your cuts are clean and sharp. If there is slack in the hair, the ends will be ragged and not straight. But if the hair is taut, the cuts will be more precise.

4. *Elevate the hair where necessary for a graduated effect.* In Chapter 8 we spoke of elevation. Elevation refers to how high or low you hold the hair that is being cut in relation to where it grows on the scalp. Elevation is a basic principle of every haircutting method. However, in precision haircutting, elevation takes on new meaning. Because of the small sections used in this method, elevating the hair not only allows you to cut it shorter but also creates a graduated effect. The classic bob shown in Figure 9.2 appears to be a one-length cut, but in fact each small section has been elevated just slightly so that the hair is graduated. Since each section is barely shorter than the preceding one, the weight of the hair is distributed throughout the head instead of being all at the bottom. The finished style is swingy and bouncy.

   Elevating small sections also accounts for the close-cropped look of the short tapered cut shown in Figure 9.3. High elevation produces these sharp, dramatic lines.

5. *Cross-check many times during the cut.* Cross-checking is a step that allows you to reassess the hair cut and make any adjustments that might be necessary. To cross-check, you should move to a spot that will enable you to gather together a number of sections of hair that have been cut. The hair is then pulled in different directions so that the cut can be evaluated. For example, if you parted the hair into horizontal sections to cut it, part it vertically to cross-check. You should look for uneven ends, hair that has not been graduated enough, and any other imperfections.

> ### ◆ Key Point ◆
> Cutting the hair into subsections gives you control over the haircut. To ensure that the hair is evenly and sharply cut, hold the hair taut without stretching. Elevate the hair for a graduated effect.

A CLASSIC BOB

This timeless hairstyle will always be in fashion. A bob can be cut to any length; however, jaw length is most flattering. It will make a round face appear thinner and make a thin one look fuller.

Materials

Shampoo cape and towel	Shampoo Comb	Shears Clips	Neck strip (optional)

Procedure for Cutting a Classic Bob

1. Wash your hands.
2. Drape the client and shampoo the hair (see Chapter 5).
3. For this haircut, think of the head as being divided into five areas: the right back, the left back, the left side, the right side, and the portion of hair at the forehead that forms the bangs. Begin by parting the hair down the center of the back of the head from the crown to the nape (Figure 9.4).
4. Take the first ¼ inch section at the nape (Figure 9.5). The length of this section determines how long the finished style will be. Determine the length by your analysis of features and by your client's desires. Use your hand as a guide and cut the first back section, being sure that the cut is clean and straight.
5. Take the second ¼ inch section. Comb it over the first section and cut it to the same length.
6. Do the same with the third section (Figure 9.6), but after cutting it to the established length, elevate the third section of hair just slightly and cut it again so that all the hair is even. The elevation here is very low, not more than ⅛ inch from the head as shown in Figure 9.7.
7. Take another small section. Comb it down and cut it to match the preceding sections. Then elevate the hair slightly more than section 3 and cut it again in the elevated position (Figure 9.8).

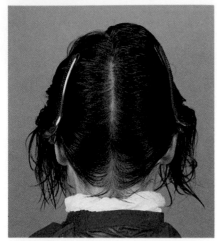

9.4   Part hair down center back

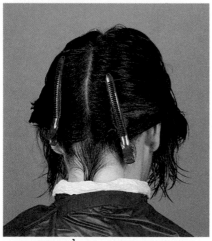

9.5   Cut first ¼ inch section

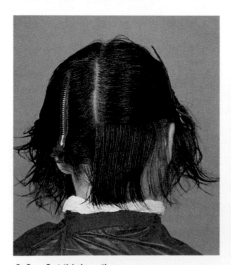

9.6   Cut third section

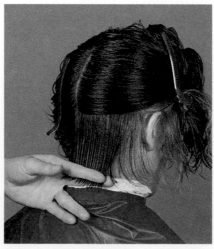

9.7   Cut at low elevation

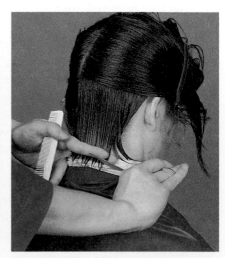

9.8   Elevate each section more

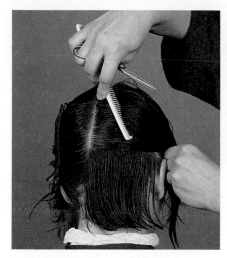

9.9 Cut sections up to crown

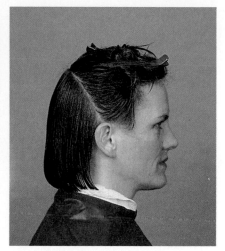

9.10 Finished left back

8. Continue cutting sections up to the crown, repeating the procedure in step 7 (Figure 9.9). Be sure to increase the elevation slightly with each section.

9. Figure 9.10 shows how the left back will look when it is cut. Notice how straight and even the line is. See how the hair is already falling into place. If each section were not graduated just slightly, the hair would not react this way.

10. Repeat steps 4 through 8 on the left back section.

11. To cut the side area on the left, take a small section and comb it over the ear. Hold the hair against the skin with your hand and cut a straight, even line to match the length of the back (Figure 9.11).

12. Notice in Figure 9.11 that the hair is not being stretched over the ear. If the hair is pulled too much in this section, the ear will be flattened; then, when the hair is released and the ear returns to its natural position, it will alter the line. The hair will be too short. To prevent that from happening, hold the hair somewhat loosely to make allowance for the ear.

13. Take a second section, comb it over the first, and recheck to be sure that the lengths of the side and the back are the same (Figure 9.12). Then cut the hair.

CLIENT TIP ◆◆◆◆◆◆◆

Allow any strong-growth (over the ears, cowlicks, bangs) hair to fall in its natural pattern. Then cut a precise line to the rest of the hair, using no tension. If you stretch hair that grows in a different direction or lifts at the hairline, the line will be uneven when the hair is dry.

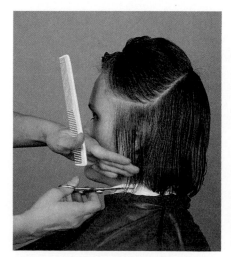

9.11 Do not stretch hair over ear

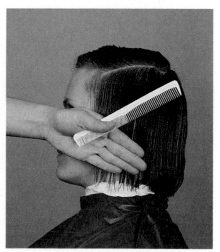

9.12 Comb down second section

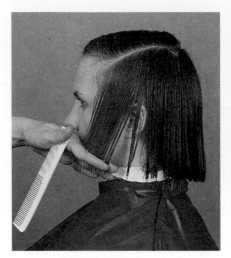

9.13   Elevate third section

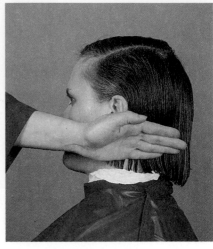

9.14   Hair falls in straight line

14. At the third section, elevate the hair slightly and cut it to match the first two sections (Figure 9.13).
15. The fourth section is also elevated when cut, but the angle of elevation is increased slightly. To be sure that the line is exact, comb the four sections that have just been cut behind the ear. Notice the straight line of the hair (Figure 9.14).
16. Continue cutting sections up to the center parting, always increasing the angle of elevation (Figure 9.15).
17. It is now time to cross-check the left side. This allows you to see if sections from the back and the side blend together. Take hair from the back and side areas and pull the combined sections straight out. Look to see if there are any ragged or irregular ends; if so, cut them so that they are even (Figure 9.16).
18. Now move to the right side of the head. Because this is a symmetrical hairstyle, the right side is cut exactly like the left. Extra care must be taken to be sure that the length of both sides is the same.
19. Follow steps 11 through 16 to cut the side area on the right side.

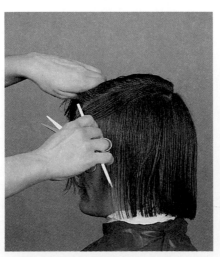

9.15   Elevate each section higher

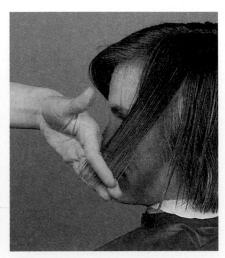

9.16   Check for uneven ends

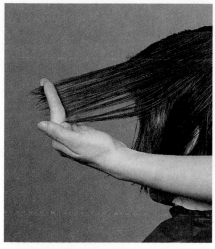

9.17 Cross check sides

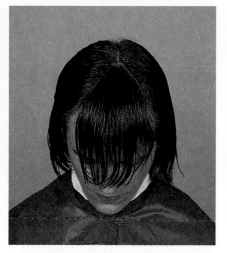

9.18 Triangle section for bangs

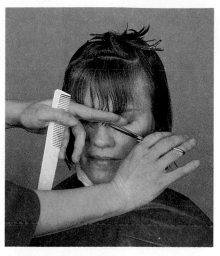

9.19 Cut first section

20. When you reach the center parting on the right side, carefully cross-check your work. Take hair from the back and side areas and look for uneven ends or hair that has not been graduated enough. Check to be sure that the left and right sides match. Look to see that the side sections flow into the back (Figure 9.17).

21. Now move to the area at the forehead to cut the bangs. As shown in Figure 9.18, the bangs are taken from a triangular portion of hair. Take a small section from the base of the triangle—the portion of hair nearest the forehead—and comb the hair down to see how it falls. Cut the hair to the desired length (Figure 9.19).

22. Take a second small section and cut it to match the length of the first section. Then elevate the hair just slightly as was done at the back and sides and cut the hair again. This graduation will prevent the bangs from being too heavy (Figure 9.20).

23. Do the same with the third section. Cut the hair to the established length, then elevate minimally and cut again.

24. Figure 9.21 shows the finished hairstyle. Notice how the ends are turning under. This is because the hair has been properly cut and graduated slightly. It is finished using a blow dryer and brush (see Chapter 11). Holding the hair very tautly as it is dried will help to remove any curl or wave and produce the sleek, smooth effect shown here and in Figure 9.21.

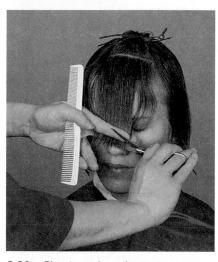

9.20 Elevate each section more

A SHORT TAPERED CUT

Many clients prefer to wear their hair short. This style is fashionable, contemporary, and well suited to all ages.

Materials

Shampoo cape and towel	Comb	Neck strip
Shampoo	Clips	Shears

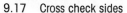

9.21 Finished cut

> ◆ **Key Point** ◆
>
> The first section cut is the most important; it establishes the length of the style and serves as the guideline for all other sections to follow.

Procedure for a Short Tapered Cut

1. Wash your hands.
2. Drape the client and shampoo the hair (see Chapter 5).
3. For this haircut, the head is thought of as being divided into ten basic areas, five on the left and five on the right (Figure 9.22). We will cut all of the areas labeled 1 and 2 from ear to ear. Then we will cut the areas labeled 3, 4, and 5, first on one side and then the other.

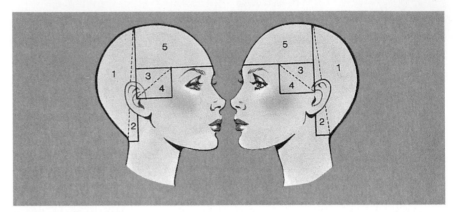

9.22   Sectioning pattern

4. Begin the haircut by parting the hair down the center of the back of the head from the crown to the nape (Figure 9.23).
5. The first section, not more than ¼ inch, is taken from both sides at the nape. This very first section is perhaps the most important of the entire haircut because it establishes the length of the style and is the guideline that all the other sections will follow. Using your hand as a guide, cut the hair. For this style, the hair is cut to a length of about an inch and a half (Figure 9.24).
6. Take a second small section. Comb it over the first and cut the hair to the same length. Now elevate the hair in the second section to a 90° angle and cut it again in this elevated position (Figure 9.25).
7. Do the same with the third section. First cut it to the established length, then elevate the hair of the third section and cut it again, but increase the angle of elevation slightly above 90°.

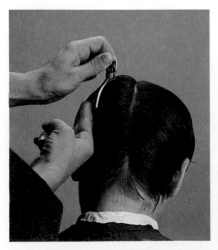

9.23   Part down center back

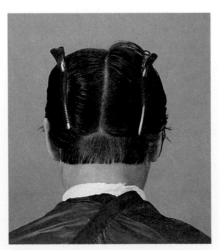

9.24   Cut guide

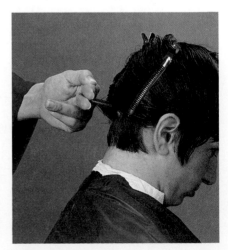

9.25   Elevate to 90°

8. Continue cutting sections up to the crown, repeating the procedure in step 7. As you move toward the crown, be sure to continue increasing the angle of elevation.

9. The portion of hair behind the ear (labeled area 2 in Figure 9.22) is cut next. For the first section, elevate and cut the hair as shown in Figure 9.26.

10. Section two is elevated when cut, as are sections three and four, but the elevation is increased each time (Figures 9.27, 9.28, and 9.29). Repeat these steps behind the right ear.

11. Now cross-check areas 1 and 2 that have just been cut. Make sure that all the sections blend together and that each has been cut properly (Figure 9.30).

12. The hair over the ear (labeled area 3 in Figure 9.22) is cut so that the entire ear is exposed. Using your hand as a guide, cut the first section (Figure 9.31). Be very sure to join this section with the hair behind the ear that has already been cut (Figure 9.32). Make certain that you take this section back far enough, or the hair will protrude from behind the ear.

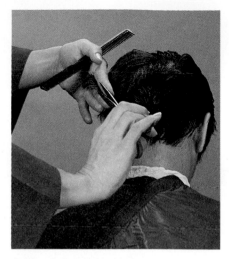

9.26   Cut area 2 behind ear

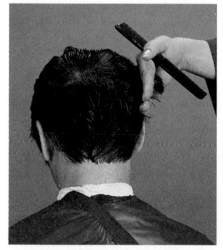

9.27   Cut second section

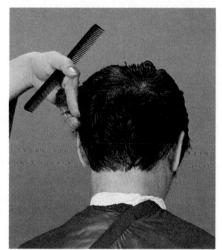

9.28   Elevate each section more

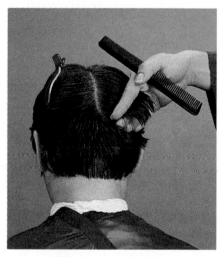

9.29   Cut last section behind ear

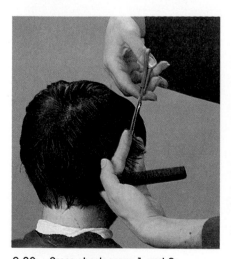

9.30   Cross check areas 1 and 2

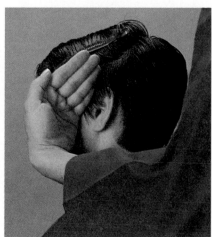

9.31   Cut guide for area 3

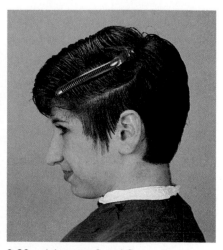

9.32   Join areas 2 and 3

13. The second and third sections in this area must be cut very carefully, because they form a corner—a point where the side and back meet. As shown in Figure 9.33, the hair in section two must be elevated to a 45° angle. It must be cut on that angle to blend with the hair behind the ear and the hair over the ear. The same is true for the third section, but the elevation is increased slightly (Figure 9.34). Cut the hair around the ear to blend with the back section (Figure 9.35).

14. The hair in front of the ear is labeled area 4 in Figure 9.22. Take a very small section at the top of the ear and comb it forward. Using your hand as a guide, cut a very straight line.

15. Comb a second section forward and cut it to match the established length. Then elevate the hair 45° and cut again. Do the same with the third section, but increase the elevation slightly (Figure 9.36).

16. Cross-check the sections that have just been cut. Move to a position that will enable you to gather together a number of sections and check to see if there are any uneven ends or sections that were left too long (Figure 9.37).

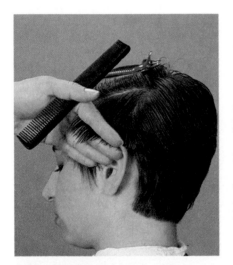

9.33   Elevate second section 45°

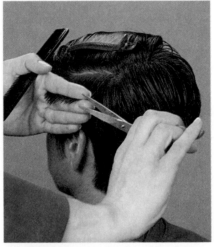

9.34   Elevate third section more

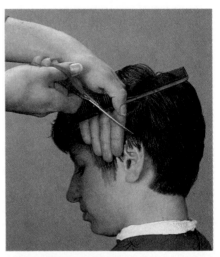

9.35   Blend hair around ear

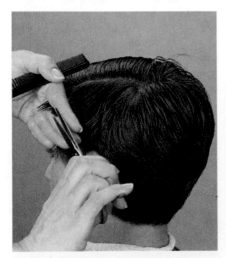

9.36   Cut area 4

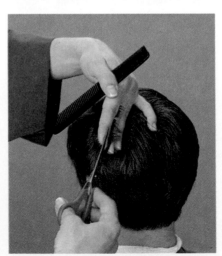

9.37   Cross check cut

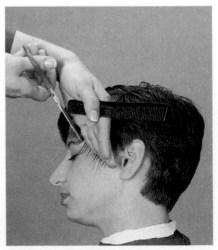

9.38   Comb area 4 forward

17. Comb all of the hair in area 4 forward in order to cut the design line along the face. First cut the hair closest to the ear using your hand as a guide (Figure 9.38). Then cut it to blend with the hair at the temple (Figure 9.39).

18. Elevate the second section slightly and cut it to match the first. Figure 9.40 shows the finished cut at the ear and side.

19. Now move to the right side of the head. The instructions for cutting the right side are the same as those for cutting the left side, but it is essential that you take special care to be sure that both sides are cut to the same length.

20. Continue cutting the right side, following steps 12 through 18. Be especially careful when cutting the hair over the ear. Make sure that this is the same length as the hair on the left side (Figure 9.41).

21. When the right side is completed, be sure to cross-check those sections (Figure 9.42).

22. To ensure that the front sections have been cut properly and that both sides are the same length, stand directly behind the client and grasp the hair of the left and right front sections. Comb this hair up with the hair in area 5. Cut the hair straight across (Figure 9.43). Continue this procedure back toward the crown. This will ensure that the front sections are properly graduated and will prevent the front area from being bulky.

23. Cross-check the entire head once more, and the cut is complete. You can finish this versatile style by brushing the front sections to either side or by combing them straight back. Figure 9.3 shows the hair brushed to the right.

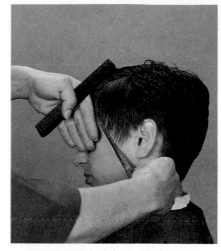

9.39   Blend hair with temple

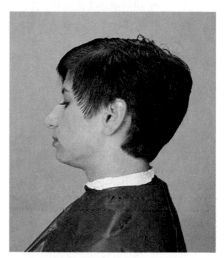

9.40   Completed hairline

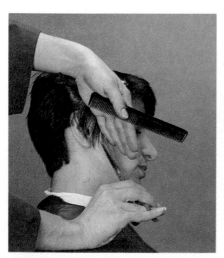

9.41   Cut right side

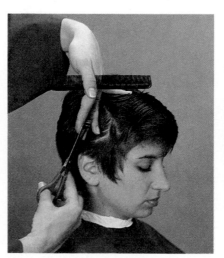

9.42   Cross-check right side

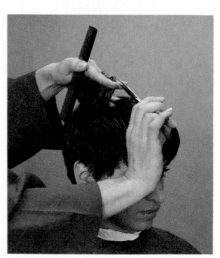

9.43   Cut top straight across

SUMMARY

Precision haircutting offers you the latest technology for shaping the hair. Always consider the shape of your client's face and head, his or her weight and height, and the texture and density of the hair. You will plan a style for a precision haircut with the hair in very small sections and along straight, sharp guidelines. Hold the hair taut and firm as it is being cut. Elevate the hair where necessary for a graduated effect.

QUESTIONS

1. What are the procedures that make precision haircutting more advanced than basic hair shaping?
2. What are the benefits of the classic bob?
3. What is the procedure for cutting a classic bob?
4. What are the benefits of the short tapered cut?
5. Why is the first section of a short tapered cut the most important?
6. What is the procedure for cutting a short tapered cut?
7. Why is cross-checking important for precision haircutting?

PROJECTS

1. Working with magazines, select at least six different styles that you determine might be best achieved with precision cutting techniques. Outline the sectioning pattern, the elevation, and the guideline for each.
2. Attach ¼-inch-wide strands of hair horizontally across the back of a head form. Fasten the strands ½ inch apart. Cut half of the head with the hair elevated vertically; one half with the hair elevated horizontally at the same degree. Compare the results and report the differences in class. When would you recommend each elevation type?
3. As directed by your instructor, give a classic bob and a short tapered cut to your mannequin. Have each area double-checked before you proceed to the next.

WET HAIRSTYLING

CHAPTER 10

CHAPTER GOAL

Wet hairstyling is the foundation for all styling techniques used in the salon. After reading this chapter and completing the projects, you should be able to

1. Explain how hair quality and hair growth patterns determine the styling process.
2. List the techniques and equipment available for wet hairstyling.
3. Explain the purpose of shapings and demonstrate the eight basic shaping patterns.
4. Demonstrate a finger wave formation over the entire head.
5. Describe the three parts of a pin curl and describe the function of each.
6. Demonstrate the construction of the various types of pin curls.
7. Demonstrate the use of rollers for on-base, half-base, and off-base placement.
8. List the functions of backcombing, lacing, smoothing, backbrushing, and wave stretching, and demonstrate how each is done.
9. Explain the recommended procedures for dressing long hair.
10. Demonstrate the procedure for French braiding.

Hairstyling, or the art of dressing hair, has its roots deep in ancient history. Virtually every civilization had beautification techniques that were recorded on cave walls, papyrus scrolls, or in detailed paintings. Hairstyling, as we know it, really developed around the turn of the twentieth century in France. There, barbers began to specialize in the making of wigs and hairstyling techniques for women. A barber with such expertise advertised his trade by hanging a large gilt ball to which a tuft of horsehair was attached in front of the doors to the shop.

Wet hairstyling techniques were advanced as the bob became popular during the 1920s. Wet hair was **molded** (made to conform) into waves, then dried for the fashionable "flapper" look. Next, hair was **carved** (shaped) out of moldings, wound into circlets, and attached with wire pins. It was a small step from rolling wet hair over mats of discarded hair to winding it around wooden pegs. Wire mesh was substituted to speed drying, and plastic rollers were introduced during the 1950s. Throughout this time of tool development, master stylists were developing techniques of molding, shaping, and winding to achieve specific styles.

As a professional stylist, you will mold hair into style lines. You will then carve subsections of hair to form pin curls and rollers to reproduce the results your client requests. Master comb-out techniques of backcombing and backbrushing to ensure your ability to finish hairstyles.

Principles of Wet Styling

Wet hairstyling is an art form. As any other art form, it is the result of a complicated set of rules, elements, and forces. In beginning your study of styling, it is important that you understand the characteristics of hair, and the tools that you have available to help you move and shape it. This is much like the clothing designer learning all about fabric, or the professional musician rehearsing scales before the concert begins.

Once you have mastered the basics of wet styling, you will want to apply them to every client. In Chapter 7, Elements and Principles of Design, you learned how to apply the principles of hairstyling for the best effects.

Hair Quality

The quality of hair is a determining factor in how it will perform. The performance of hair is dependent upon its texture, density, length, and condition, as well as the process or preparation used in styling it. Hair performance describes what the hair will or can do and the results that you can expect.

Texture and Density

Hair can be said to have a very fine, fine, medium, or coarse texture. It is further classified by its surface—whether it feels soft, wiry, or harsh and rough. Hair can be fine and soft, fine and wiry, or fine and harsh, and so on. The density of hair means that the hair is thin, medium, or thick, with any of the four textures. (See Chapter 16 for a complete discussion of hair texture and density.)

Hair that is thin and fine may be more difficult to style. Fine, soft, straight hair—cut short and permanent waved—will tend to appear fluffy, and give the appearance of being thicker.

Medium-textured soft hair and thick or dense soft hair is generally pliable and easy to style. It will also tend to hold a better curl.

Thin, wiry hair or thin, harsh hair has a hard surface (cuticle layer) that tends to make the hair slippery. This makes it difficult to work with. Depending upon how wiry the hair is, it may take a very tight curl or it may be difficult to get a curl or style to last.

Coarse, soft hair generally is easy to curl, and it is more manageable than other types. Hair that is coarse and wiry or harsh may be easy to manage if it is permanent waved. However, a lot depends upon the haircut, hairstyle, and method used to style the hair. Coarse hair gives the appearance of being thick. Thermal techniques, such as blow-dryer styling and iron curling, give good results on this type of hair.

Length

Hair length is important to hair performance. It has a tremendous effect on the finished style. Attempting a style on hair that is the wrong length is frustrating and sometimes impossible. In dressing longer hair, it takes more hair to go around a quarter-sized roller than to go around a dime-sized roller. It takes longer hair to make a double shaping (S formation) than it does to make a semicircular shaping (see Figure 10.1 on the next page).

Hair Condition

The condition of any type of hair is an important factor to be considered before styling. Hair that is weak and dry will tend to break, will have split ends, or may be very limp. It is difficult, if not impossible, to get this hair to retain a curl.

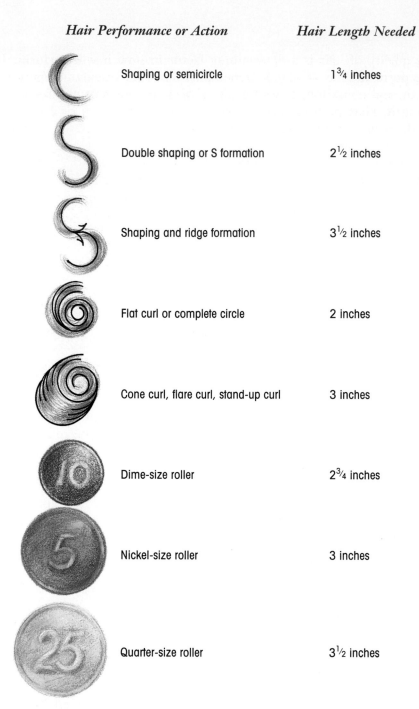

Hair Performance or Action	Hair Length Needed
Shaping or semicircle	1¾ inches
Double shaping or S formation	2½ inches
Shaping and ridge formation	3½ inches
Flat curl or complete circle	2 inches
Cone curl, flare curl, stand-up curl	3 inches
Dime-size roller	2¾ inches
Nickel-size roller	3 inches
Quarter-size roller	3½ inches

10.1 Length of hair necessary for various styling effects

Styling Process Used

The process or techniques used to style hair and the preparation of the hair before styling will vary according to the type of hair. Some hair should be wet before styling. Other types should be predried. Hair should be predried before it is iron curled. Long hair should also be partially predried before styling, in order to achieve a softer, more manageable curl.

Hair Growth Patterns

Peculiarities in hair growth should be considered before styling or cutting hair. This is an important factor in hair control and in the performance of the hair. A "peculiarity" is any odd or out-of-the-ordinary characteristic.

Cowlicks occur when the hair forms a pivot that distributes the hair from that point around in all directions. They are usually found in the crown area, but they may also be found along the hairline around the face and nape area.

On some heads, the hair recedes at the temple hairline. Irregularities may also occur at the nape, where the hair sometimes grows in toward the center or out toward the sides. The hair may also grow up from the nape, colliding with the hair growth from the crown.

A thorough understanding of techniques and principles will promote confident decisions. Once you understand why a particular hairstyle will suit your client's appearance and needs, you can decide which techniques to use to achieve that style. In this way, you can easily adjust to any situation and rapidly adapt to future changes in hairstyling.

Methods of adapting styles to your client's features are covered in Chapter 7.

> **◆ Key Point ◆**
> The styling technique you choose will be determined by the quality of the hair. Hair that is fine and thin is the most difficult to style. Coarse, soft hair is more manageable.

TECHNIQUES AND EQUIPMENT

There are two basic methods of styling hair. The first method is the traditional one and involves setting wet hair by one of the following methods:

1. Shaping (molding) the hair.
2. Finger waving.
3. Pin (pivot) curling or sculpture curling.
4. Roller setting.
5. Combining of these techniques.

The second method is called **thermal styling**. It involves dressing the hair by means of electric equipment or heat. We will discuss thermal styling in Chapter 11.

Equipment and Supplies

1. **Hairbrush** (Figure 10.2). A brush is used for brushing out a set, for removing tangles before a shampoo, or in giving a scalp treatment. Brushes which have natural boar bristles or synthetic bristles with rounded tips are best.
2. **Comb-out** and **lacing brush**. The small, narrow brush in Figure 10.2 is used to cushion or lace hair, smooth out a style, or lock hair in place. Brushes made from firm, synthetic, irregular bristles are best.

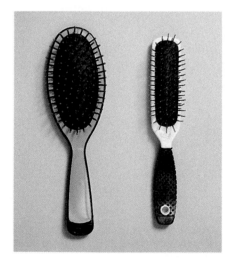

10.2

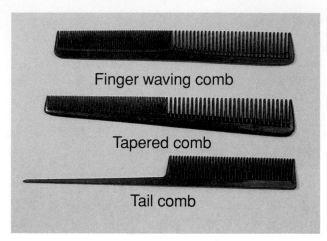

Finger waving comb

Tapered comb

Tail comb

10.3

3. **Comb-out comb**. A large comb used for teasing and locking the hair. Its large size aids in achieving hair control and manageability.

4. **Finger waving comb** (Figure 10.3). A 7-inch styling comb with teeth that will slide easily through the hair, moving scalp hair.

5. **Tail comb** (Figure 10.3). A shorter comb with evenly spaced teeth and a tapered tail at one end. It is used to part the hair into sections. The tail end aids in smoothing irregular hair lengths into the curl.

6. **Single-prong clips**. Used to pin curls that are small or for stand-up or stemmed curls on thin hair.

7. **Double-prong clips**. Used to pin flat curls, moldings, and shapings.

8. **Bobby pins**. These pins have either a smooth or crimped pattern. The smooth pins are best for pinning rollers and curls and may be aids in controlling hair shaping. The crimped pins are used for pinning and controlling long hair or hairpieces.

9. **Hairpins**. These double-prong pins are available in many lengths and sizes and are used for control in dressing wet or dry hair.

10. **Rollers**. Available in various standard sizes, from that of a dime to that of a half-dollar. Length varies from $1\frac{1}{4}$ to $2\frac{3}{4}$ inches.

11. **Setting lotions**. Available in liquid, mousse, or gel form and can be diluted to desired consistency. Gels are heavier and require a longer drying time. The selection of the proper setting lotion depends on the type, quality, and texture of the hair. These lotions are used to add body and firmness to preserve a hairstyle longer, and to provide better hair control and manageability.

12. **Hair sprays**. These products can be used to spray set hair before drying in order to obtain crispness, to hold hair during a comb-out, or as a light net to hold a hairstyle in place and to add body to the hair.

◆ **Key Point** ◆

Choose the tool to move hair according to its function, ease of use, and the effect you want to achieve.

SHAPINGS AND MOLDINGS

A **shaping** or **molding** in hairstyling is hair that has been formed into a pattern. A shaping has an open end and a closed end. The **open** end of the shaping is concave, and the **closed** end is convex (see Figure 10.4). The pattern can be a straight line (going vertically or horizontally, as in Figures 10.5 and 10.6) or a curved line going in a semicircular formation as in Figure 10.7.

A shaping can be placed anywhere on the head in a vertical, horizontal, or angular position. The angle of the comb and the action of the comb will determine the direction and the end result.

The shaping that you form will determine the size and direction of the curl. Establish each style by beginning each shaping right at the scalp and molding the hair into Cs.

When creating a style that is flat or close to the head, begin at the open end of the C shaping. This will avoid disturbing the shaping and will make it easier for you to work around placed pin curls, etc. If, however, you are creating a style that has volume or is raised from the head, begin at the closed end of the shaping.

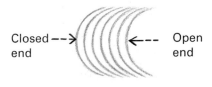

Closed end --→ ←-- Open end

10.4

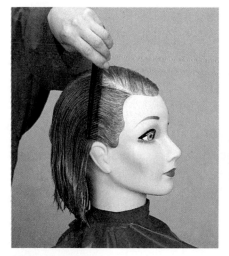

10.5   Vertical line

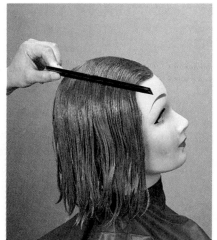

10.6   Horizontal line

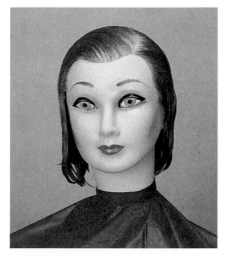

10.7   C-shaping

Shaping Technique

To mold the hair for a shaping, the hair is directed with the comb in lines first in one direction, then in the opposite direction. This leaves the hair in a curved, semicircular shape. Referring to Figure 10.7, notice that the hair moves from the open end *back* to the closed end, thus forming the top half of the letter C. The hair is moved from the closed end toward the open end to complete the C shaping.

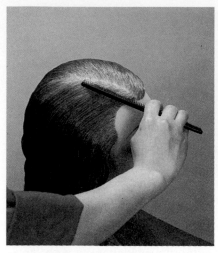

10.8   Comb is parallel to start

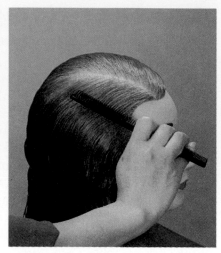

10.9   Comb to center of curl

Materials for All Shaping Techniques

Shampoo cape and towel	Setting lotion
Shampoo	Tail comb
Neck strip	Finger waving comb

Procedure of Shaping the Hair for Curl Structure

1. To form a C shaping, place the comb parallel to the starting point. In Figure 10.8, the starting point is the hair part.
2. Direct the comb back to the center of the shaping—that is, to the center of the size of curl you expect to make (Figure 10.9).
3. Place the index finger of the left hand horizontally above the comb. Hold the index finger in position to bind or hold the center of the shaping as the comb is turned teeth down (Figure 10.10).
4. Holding the shaping with the index finger, turn the comb down to mold the hair toward the face and then circle back to hold the shaping (Figure 10.11).

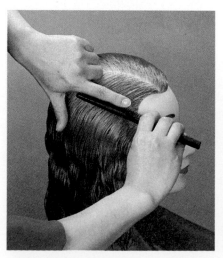

10.10   Place finger above comb

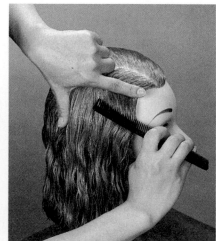

10.11   Mold hair toward face

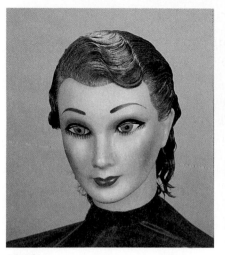
10.12

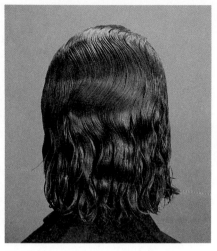
10.13

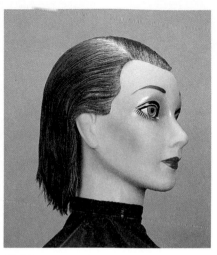
10.14

Purpose of Shapings

Shapings can be used for the following purposes:

1. As facings at the hairline, crown, and nape areas (Figures 10.12 and 10.13).
2. As outline guides in formulating designs (Figure 10.14).
3. As aids in distributing the hair (Figure 10.15).
4. As parts of finger waving (Figure 10.16).
5. As the bases of curls (Figure 10.17).
6. As guides for a row of pin curls.
7. As guides for roller placement.

> ### ◆ Key Point ◆
> The shaping determines the size and direction of the curl formed. Finished curls are placed in the center of the shaping.

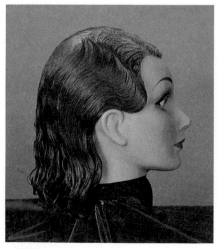
10.15

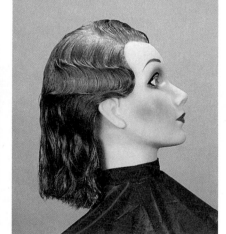
10.16

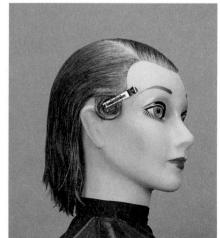
10.17

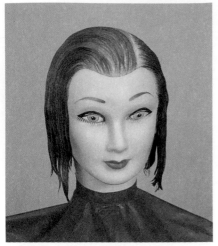

10.18

Shaping Exercises

Before proceeding to **finger waving**, which consists of straight vertical, straight horizontal, and curved shapings over the entire head, you should be able to perform the following shapings:

1. A curved shaping on top of the head (Figure 10.18).
2. A side curved shaping that ends at the temple (Figure 10.19).
3. A side curved shaping that ends in front of the ear (Figure 10.20).
4. A straight vertical shaping that ends above the ear (Figure 10.21).
5. A reverse straight horizontal shaping (Figure 10.22).
6. A forward straight horizontal shaping (Figure 10.23).
7. A curved crown shaping (Figure 10.24).
8. A forward and reverse straight horizontal shaping (Figure 10.25).

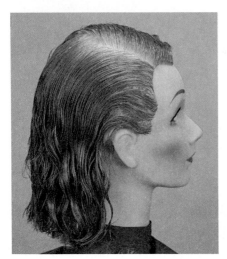

10.19

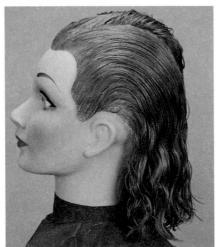

10.20

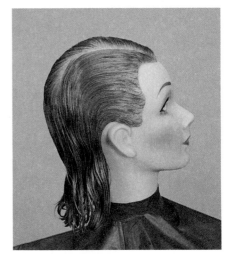

10.21

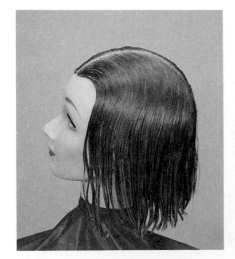

10.22

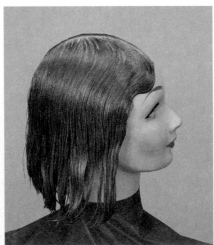

10.23

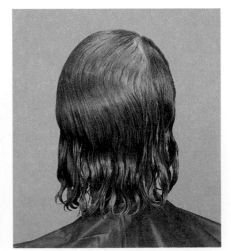

10.24

FINGER WAVING

The most basic method of styling, **finger waving**, uses only the fingers and comb to create a style featuring waves and ridges. Popular in the 1920s, this style or its variations come back into vogue from time to time. You should understand the concept of movement that finger waving requires. You will apply that theory in all wet styling and thermal techniques.

In finger waving, the scalp hair must be kept wet so that the hair will blend and mold easily. It is helpful to use a liquid wave set.

Use a seven-inch finger waving comb. The coarse teeth of the comb will move the scalp hair more easily. Begin by separating the hair to form a natural part. This is done by directing the coarse teeth of the comb from the hairline back to the crown (Figures 10.26 and 10.27). The teeth of the comb will groove the hair, and each groove will separate when the hair is gently pushed forward as shown in Figure 10.28. Strong hair growth or cowlicks will become more obvious and a more natural part will be exposed.

If you part the hair following its natural tendencies, you will find that it is easier to mold and will not tend to buckle or separate at the crown.

Finger Waving Fundamentals

The hair is evenly distributed away from the part in preparation for the first shaping that will surround the part (Figure 10.29). Begin on the **heavy side**, which is the side of the part where the most hair falls. Use the coarse teeth of the comb to form a forward shaping that is parallel to the part from the hairline. You are now ready to form the first ridge. For all finger wave services, you will need the same materials as for shaping techniques, as listed on page 182.

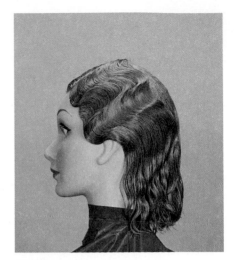

10.25

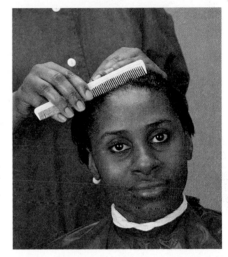

10.26   Separate hair to form a natural part

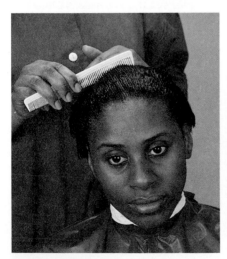

10.27   Direct comb to crown

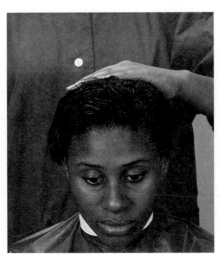

10.28   Push hair forward

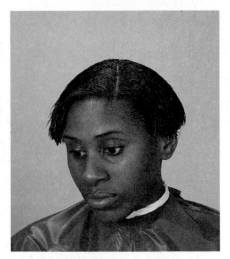

10.29   Hair is distributed evenly

Procedure for Forming Ridges in Finger Waving

1. The index finger is placed over the center of the shaping. The coarse teeth of the comb are placed below and parallel to the index finger. The teeth of the comb face toward the index finger (see Figure 10.30).
2. Direct the comb ½ inch away from the index finger following the direction of the hair (see Figure 10.31 and the dotted line in Figure 10.32a). Straighten the comb so that the teeth face toward the index finger.
3. With the teeth directed toward the scalp, move the comb straight up to the index finger (see Figure 10.33 and the dotted line in Figure 10.32b).
4. Move the comb slightly forward along the index finger to lock the hair, emphasize the ridge, and allow space between the ridge and the comb so that you can change finger position (see Figure 10.34 and the dotted line in Figure 10.32c).
5. Change finger position. Place the middle finger on the center of the shaping that you began with in step 1, and place the index finger under the ridge (Figure 10.35).

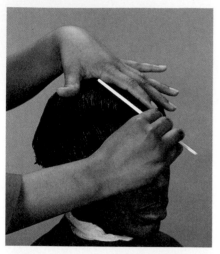

10.30   Finger over center of shaping

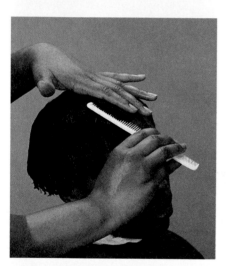

10.31   Move away from finger

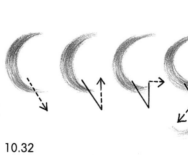

10.32

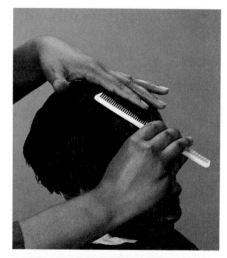

10.33   Move up to finger

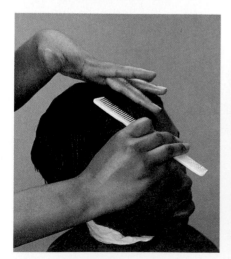

10.34   Lock the hair

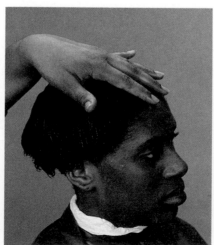

10.35   Place index finger under ridge

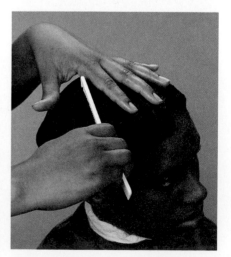

10.36   Direct hair away from ridge

6. Use the comb to direct the hair away from the ridge formation, moving diagonally in a direction opposite to that taken in step 2 (see Figure 10.36 and the dotted line in Figure 10.32d). This forms a complete ridge.

Procedure for Finger Waving

1. Preparation for finger waving begins with the hair surrounding the part. Distribute the hair evenly away from the part (Figure 10.37).
2. Make a forward shaping on the heavy side of the head.
3. Begin forming the first ridge on the heavy side of the head. Starting at the open end, pull the hair forward one inch (Figure 10.38).
4. Lay comb down flat to scalp, to form a ridge (Figure 10.39). Place your middle finger above the ridge and your index finger below.
5. Hold the completed ridge between your fingers and form a shaping for the second ridge (Figure 10.40). This shaping will circle the entire head.
6. The formation of the second ridge begins at the open end of the shaping at the hairline (Figure 10.41). This ridge circles across the crown (Figure 10.42) and continues along the heavy side of the head (Figure 10.43).

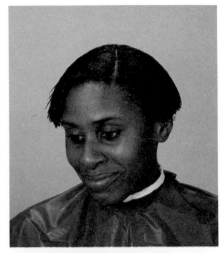
10.37   Distribute hair from part

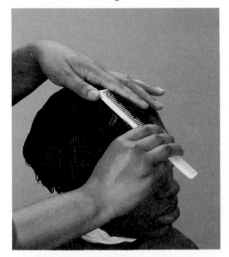
10.38   Begin first ridge

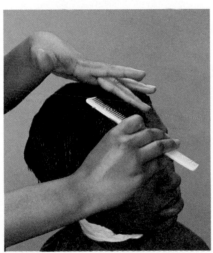
10.39   Lay comb flat to form ridge

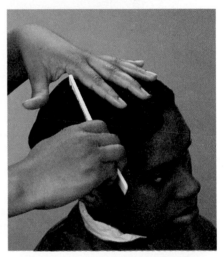
10.40   Form shaping for second ridge

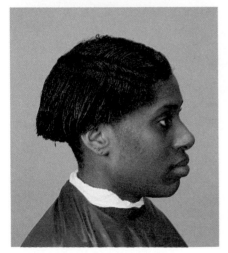
10.41   Second ridge begins at hairline

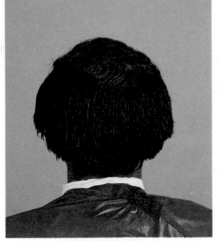
10.42   Ridge circles crown

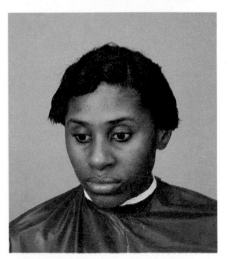
10.43   Ridge continues to heavy side

7. At the end of the second ridge on the heavy side of the head, a new ridge begins at the open end of the shaping (Figure 10.44). This ridge circles the crown (Figure 10.45), forming a completed finger wave (Figure 10.46), and continues to the light side of the head, ending again at the hairline (Figure 10.47).

8. The finger wave ridge formation continues in this way from the open end of the shaping across the crown to the heavy side and back again. Figure 10.48 shows the completed finger wave.

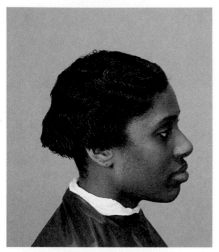

10.44 New ridge begins at open end of shaping

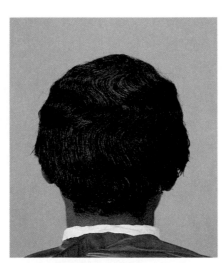

10.45 Ridge circles crown

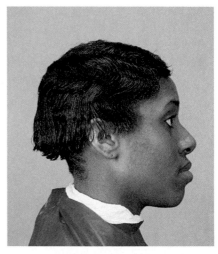

10.46 One completed finger wave

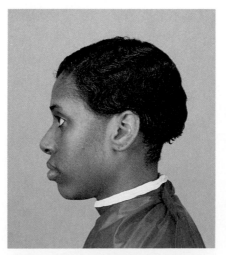

10.47 Completed finger wave on light side of head

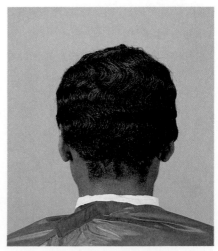

10.48 Completed fingerwave

PIN CURLS

Pin curls and the more advanced **sculpture curls** can be used anywhere on the head to create a variety of hairstyles. A sculpture curl differs from a pin curl in that it is built on a shaped base, but both types of curls are commonly referred to as pin curls.

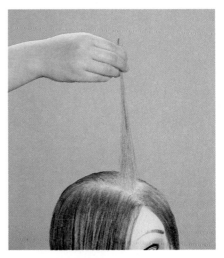

Circle

Stem

Base

Parts of the Curl

Every curl has three parts: the base, the stem, and the circle (see Figure 10.49).

The Base

The **base** is the foundation and the strength of the curl. The base can have many shapes, depending upon the type of curl you wish to create.

1. A **rectangular** base is used for an upswept effect and for forming flare curls (Figure 10.50).
2. A **triangular** base is used on the hairline to prevent splits in the finished style or to form stand-up curls (Figure 10.51).
3. A **square** base will produce a curly, long-lasting hairstyle (Figure 10.52).
4. A **C-** or **arc-shaped** base can be used anywhere on the head (Figure 10.53). This is the most common base used.

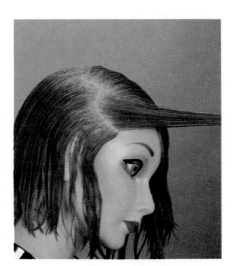

10.50   Rectangular base

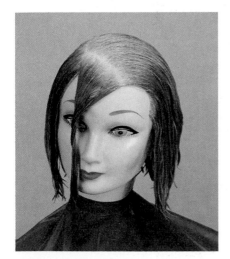

10.51   Triangular base

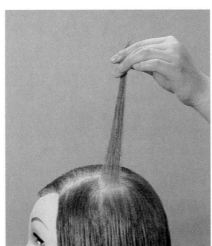

10.52   Square base

10.53   C- or arc-shaped base

The Stem

The stem controls the mobility of the curl. The length of the stem determines how much movement the curl will have.

1. A **no-stem** curl (Figure 10.54) means that the circle is placed directly on the center of the base. This will produce a firm curl with little movement.
2. A **half-stem** curl (Figure 10.55) means that the circle is placed half off its base. This kind of curl has more movement but less firmness.
3. A **full-stem** curl (Figure 10.56) is placed completely off its base and gives the hair the greatest mobility.

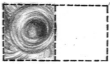 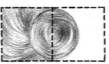 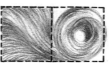

10.54   No-stem   10.55   Half-stem   10.56   Full-stem

The Circle

The **circle** creates the actual curl. The size of the circle determines how tight the curl will be at the ends.

Types of Curls

There are many different types of curls. They may be used for firmness on certain types of hair, for sculptured casualness, to create special effects, or as an aid in curling hair that is too short to place around rollers.

Methods and techniques are as varied as the types of curls. These different techniques are designed to help you achieve professionally controlled hair quickly and efficiently. They are also a source of the basic knowledge that will help you to become a successful hairstylist.

In addition to the forward and reverse curls, which you will be shown on the following pages, other types of curls include stand-up or cascade curls, cone-shaped curls, and flare curls. Each is used for a specific purpose.

Pin curls can also be used along with other wet styling techniques to create interesting effects.

Fill-in curls are used in the areas between shapings that frame the face and run around the crown (Figure 10.57). The hair between these shapings is left unset.

A **skipwave** is a hairstyle that combines pin curls and finger waving. When doing a skipwave, place the pin curls in every other finger wave formation (Figure 10.58).

Principles and Mechanics of Pin-Curl Construction

Curls may be said to be forward or reverse, clockwise or counterclockwise. Forward curls on the right side of the head are formed in a counterclockwise direction. Forward curls on the left side of the head are formed in a clockwise direction.

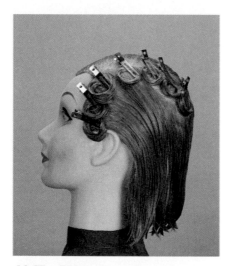

10.57   Fill-in curls

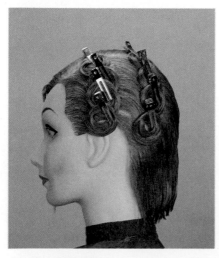

10.58   Skipwave

To achieve the same kind of curl on both sides of the head, the technique used to form a curl on the right side of the head must be mechanically different from that used on the left side. This is because you use the same hand to form curls on both sides of the head. If you are right-handed, you always use your right hand; if you are left-handed, you always use your left hand. If you are left-handed, you should use the procedure given for the right side of the head on the left side, and vice versa. Counterclockwise curls are formed away from your body position, whereas clockwise curls are formed toward your body position. Before going on to the curl formation procedures, review the Procedure for Shaping the Hair for Curl Structure on page 182 (Figures 10.8 through 10.11).

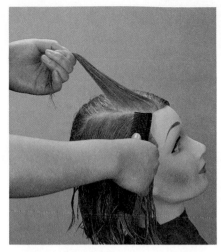
10.59   Part off base

Materials for All Pin-Curl Services

Shampoo cape and towel	Setting lotion
Neck strip	Tail comb
Clips	Finger waving comb

Procedure for Forming Forward Counterclockwise Pin Curls

1. Part off a section of hair for the base (Figure 10.59).
2. Insert the comb across the sectioned strand. Place the index finger of the left hand in the center of the strand and control the ends with the comb and the thumb of the right hand (Figure 10.60).
3. Begin to circle the strand forward with the comb while holding the base of the curl with thumb and index finger of the left hand (Figure 10.61).
4. Use the end of the comb to ribbon, or stretch, the hair forward, turning it in a counterclockwise direction. Be sure that the very ends of the strand are inside the circle (Figure 10.62).
5. Hold the formed curl with index finger and thumb of the left hand and insert a clip down the stem and into the curl to hold it in place securely (Figure 10.63).

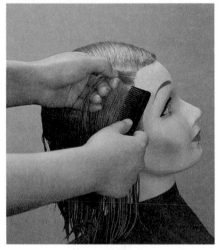
10.60   Insert comb across strand

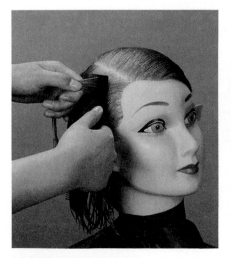
10.61 Circle strand forward

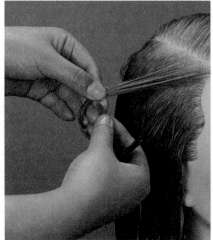
10.62   Ends are inside circle

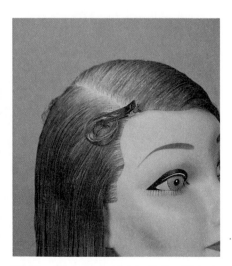
10.63   Forward counterclockwise pin curl

Procedure for Forming Forward Clockwise Pin Curls

1. Part off a section of hair for the base (Figure 10.64).
2. Insert the comb across the sectioned strand. Place the index finger of the left hand in the center of the strand and control the ends with the comb and the thumb of the right hand.
3. Turn the comb down a quarter-turn forward, so that the comb forms a twist at the base of the curl (Figure 10.65).
4. Using the end of the comb, ribbon—or stretch—the hair down along the index finger of the left hand. Continue to ribbon the hair upward, in a clockwise direction, to form a circle.
5. Complete the circle. Be sure that the very ends are inside the circle (Figure 10.66).
6. Hold the circle with the index finger and thumb of the left hand and insert a clip down the stem to the center of the curl (Figure 10.67).

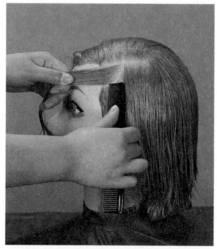

10.64   Part off base

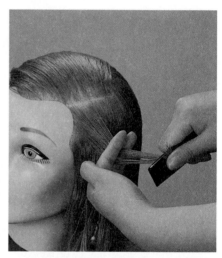

10.65   Form twist at base

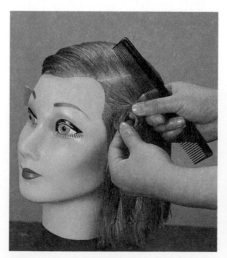

10.66   Complete the circle

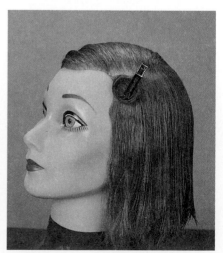

10.67   Forward clockwise pin curl

Procedure for Forming Reverse Counterclockwise Pin Curls

1. Part off a section of hair for the base.
2. Insert the end of the comb into the hair at the open end of the shaping and place the index finger of the left hand over the shaping to hold the hair (Figure 10.68).
3. Direct the hair back around the index finger at the base of the curl to bind the hair into a semicircle (Figure 10.69).
4. Ribbon the ends, holding the hair at the top of the circle that is formed. Turn ribboned ends to center and begin forming the circle. Control the hair between your index finger and thumb (Figure 10.70).
5. Place the circled hair down on its base. The ends are looped into the center of the circle (Figure 10.71).
6. Insert a clip through the center of the curl, pinning it from the open end of the shaping (Figure 10.72). This allows the curls to overlap.

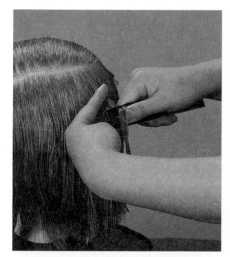

10.68   Place finger over shaping

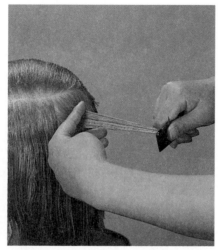

10.69   Direct hair around finger

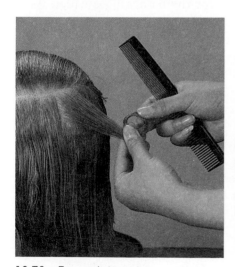

10.70   Turn ends to center

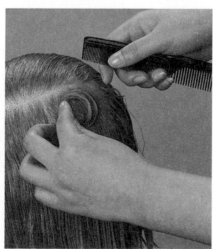

10.71   Place circle at base

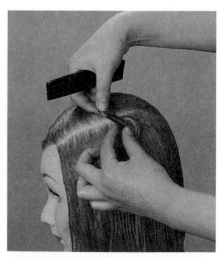

10.72   Reverse counterclockwise pin curl

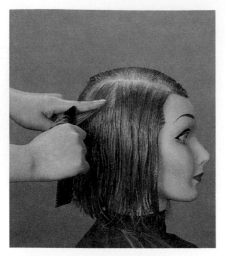

10.73 Turn hair up over finger

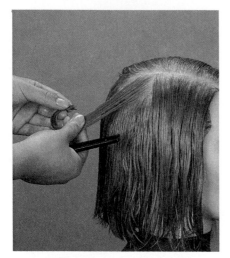

10.74 Ribbon hair to lock ends

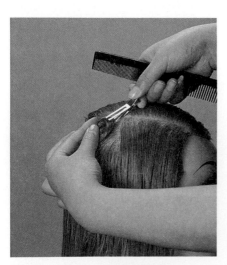

10.75 Reverse clockwise pin curl

Procedure for Forming Reverse Clockwise Pin Curls

1. Part off a section of hair for the base.
2. Insert the comb across the sectioned strand. Place the index finger of the left hand in the center of the strand and control the ends with the comb and the thumb of the right hand. Turn the comb down a quarter-turn at the base of the curl. This tightens the hair at the base of the curl and keeps it from buckling at that point.
3. Turn the hair up over the index finger and place the thumb of the left hand under the strand of hair to hold it in position (Figure 10.73).
4. Ribbon the hair and lock the ends together (Figure 10.74).
5. Place the completed circle over the base. Hold the curl with a clip as the ends are fitted into the center of the circle (Figure 10.75).
6. Insert the clip into the curl, pinning through the center of the curl. The clip is placed down the stem from the open end, so that it remains out of the way and allows the following curls to overlap.

ROLLER SETTING

Roller Bases

The **roller base** is the section of hair at the scalp that is parted off for a roller curl. The size of the base is determined by the size of the roller used. The base should be the same width and approximately the same length as the roller that you are going to use.

The diameter of the roller determines the amount of curl that will be set in the hair. If a roller with a small diameter is used, the section of hair parted off for the base will be narrower. Therefore, the finished style will have more curl. If a roller with a large diameter is used, the section of hair parted off for the base will be wider. As a result, less curl will be evident in the finished style.

Cosmetologists usually speak of roller bases as having three possible placements: off-base, half-base, and on-base. The base placement used is determined by how much lift or fullness is desired in the finished style.

Off-Base Roller Placement

An off-base placement gives only a slight amount of fullness. It should be used whenever the style requires closeness. It is also used when you are working from a fuller section to a flat or molded line. An off-base placement eliminates the splits or separations created between an on-base placement and flat sculpture curls.

Materials for All Roller Sets

Shampoo cape and towel	Setting lotion
Shampoo	Clips or bobby pins
Tail comb	Rollers of various sizes

Procedure for Off-Base Roller Placement

1. Part off a section of hair that is the same size as the roller that is to be used.
2. Comb the hair in the direction of the roller action, that is, the direction in which the hair will be rolled (Figure 10.76).
3. Smooth the ends of the hair around the roller and roll it down to the scalp. Use a clip or a bobby pin to secure placement of the roller to the scalp hair.
4. A roller placement off-base sits completely off the section of hair used for the roller (Figure 10.77).

Half-Base Roller Placement

A **half-base placement** gives a moderate amount of fullness and should be used only when the style requires a little lift or fullness. It is also used when you are working from a full or lifted movement to a closer line of design.

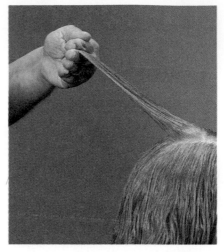

10.76   Comb hair in direction of roller action

Procedure for Half-Base Roller Placement

1. Part off a section of hair that is the same size as the roller that is to be used.
2. Comb the hair straight out from the scalp (Figure 10.78).
3. Smooth the ends of the hair around the roller and roll it down to the scalp. Pin the roller securely to the scalp hair.
4. A roller placement half-base sits halfway on and halfway off the section of hair used for the roller (Figure 10.79).

On-Base Roller Placement

An **on-base** (or **full-base**) **roller placement** gives maximum fullness or lift to the hair and should be used wherever you want the fullest part of the hairstyle.

Procedure for On-Base Roller Placement

1. Part off a section of hair that is the same size as the roller that is to be used.
2. Comb the hair in the direction opposite to that of the roller action (Figure 10.80).

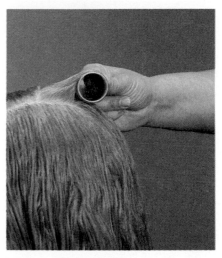

10.77   Off-base roller

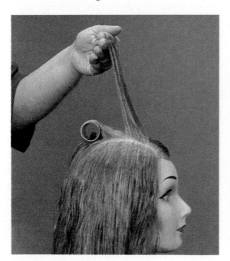

10.78   Comb hair straight out

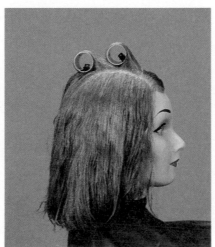

10.79   Half-base roller

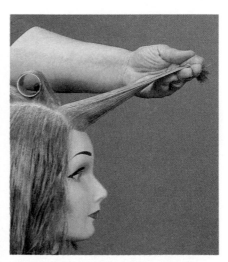

10.80   Comb hair in opposite direction from roller action

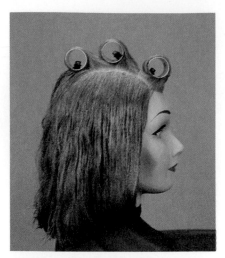

10.81   On-base roller

3. Smooth the ends of the hair around the roller and roll it down to the scalp. Pin the roller securely to the scalp hair.

4. A roller placement on-base sits on its own base with the section part showing on both sides of the roller (Figure 10.81).

Roller Placement for Spiral Curls

Spiraled placement is used to create a definite style. They are placed on a base shaped flat to the scalp, and the ends of the hair are rolled up completely to create fullness.

Procedure for Roller Placement for Spiral Curls

1. A forward shaping is made to form a semicircular guide. With the aid of a tail comb, section through the center of the shaping, following the line of the shaping (Figure 10.82).

2. Insert the comb into the hair, picking up all of the hair parted off for the roller. Without distorting the shaping, smooth the ends of the hair around the roller. Roll the hair up and place the roller in the shaping (Figure 10.83).

3. Notice that as the roller is rolled to the scalp, it is held at the same angle as the shaping. Hold the roller and insert a clip to secure it (Figure 10.84).

4. Notice that the forward shaping and the direction of the hair have not been disturbed. The hair from the shaping circles over the roller, giving the stem of the curl a forward action (Figure 10.85). If the hair is long enough, the curl action can unwind and create a wave line with volume or fullness.

Roller Placement for Directional Patterns

Directional roller placement creates a definite line or style, ranging from volume or fullness to indentation or closeness at the base of the roller. Rollers can be placed on rectangular, triangular, or diagonal bases. Volume is created by turning the roller under, whereas indentation is achieved by placing the roller on a flat base and turning the

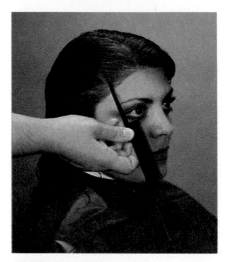

10.82   Section hair

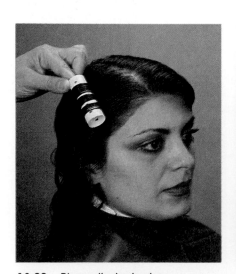

10.83   Place roller in shaping

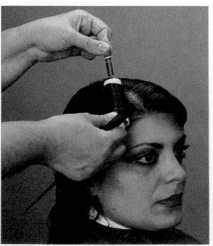

10.84   Roller is at angle of shaping

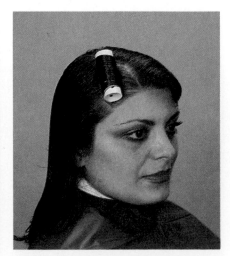

10.85   Hair circles over roller

ends of the hair up. Directional placement can be used to create the same effect as sculpture curls. To do so, you simply have to remember to direct the roller and the base of the section parted off for the roller just as you would direct a sculpture curl.

Procedure for Roller Placement for Directional Patterns

1. Direct the sectioned hair toward the face (Figure 10.86).
2. The hair direction (action) is reverse (Figure 10.87).
3. Direct the sectioned hair away from the face (Figure 10.88).
4. The hair direction (action) is forward (Figure 10.89).
5. The directional roller placement begins at the top with a forward curl. This is followed by a reverse curl, then another forward curl, and then another reverse curl, and so on. The direction of the curls is alternated in this manner down the side of the head. The partings are angled to follow the contour of the head. The single roller on the hairline can be forward or reverse at the same angle (see Figure 10.90). Figure 10.91 shows the completed setting pattern.

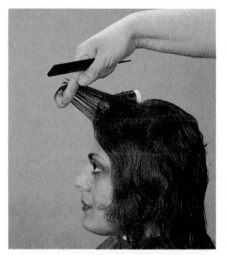

10.86　Direct hair to face

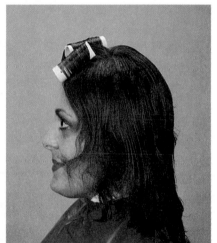

10.87　Curl action is reverse

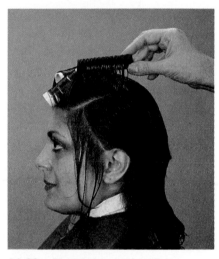

10.88　Direct hair away from face

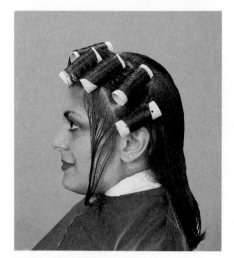

10.89　Curl action is forward

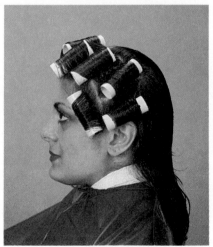

10.90　Single roller at hairline

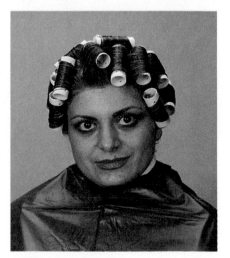

10.91　Complete set

Comb-Out Techniques

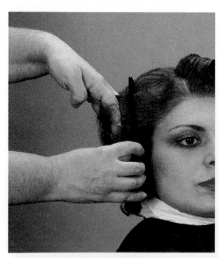

10.92   Brush curl

The comb-out is an important part of any hairdressing service. It is here that you can use your skill and artistry to create special effects. The procedures for the techniques used in combing out a hairstyle—**backcombing**, or **teasing**, **lacing**, **smoothing**, **backbrushing**, and **wave stretching**—are listed and illustrated in this section.

Although some of these techniques may seem dated, it is very important that you study and master them. In order to be a competent and well-rounded cosmetologist, you should be able to perform all of the services that your clients request. With the changing whims of fashion, it is more than likely that these techniques will once again be used in high-fashion hairstyling.

Materials Needed for All Comb-Out Techniques

Shampoo cape and towel	Comb
Neck strip	Hair spray
Brush	

Procedure for Backcombing or Teasing

1. Brush all the curl thoroughly (Figure 10.92).
2. Loosen the hair by combing it back (Figure 10.93).
3. Controlling the ends of the hair between the middle and index fingers, hold the comb vertically, combing from the hairline to the center of the shaping (Figure 10.94). Move the comb firmly back toward the base to create a cushion underneath the strand.
4. Turn the comb to loosen the surface hair and circle the ends forward toward the face (Figure 10.95).
5. Move back to the next section. Again, form a cushion by combing the hair back between the fingers (Figure 10.96).

10.93   Comb hair back

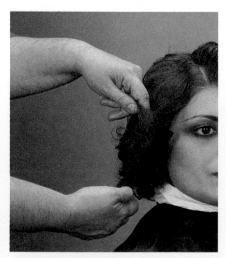

10.94   Hold comb vertically

10.95   Circle ends forward

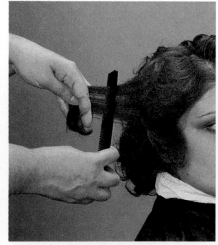

10.96   Form cushion of hair

6. Turn the comb to lift a thin section of surface hair (Figure 10.97).
7. Circle the ends forward (Figure 10.98).
8. The backcombing procedure continues in this way, as each thin section is peeled and then circled forward to form a fluff (Figure 10.99).

Procedure for Lacing

1. Brush out the curl following the direction of your set.
2. Hold the hair evenly between the index and middle fingers (Figure 10.100).
3. Place the side of the brush on the surface hair with bristles pointing upward (Figure 10.101).
4. Roll the brush down and toward the base. Direct it over the surface hair (Figure 10.102).

CLIENT TIP ◆◆◆◆◆◆◆

Make sure that the hair is thoroughly dry and cool before beginning the comb-out. If the setting lotion you selected makes the hair stiff when it's dry, comb through the hair with a large-toothed comb to avoid discomfort to your client.

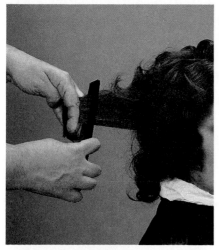

10.97   Left surface hair

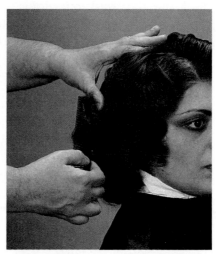

10.98   Circle ends forward

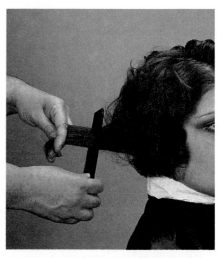

10.99   Backcomb next section

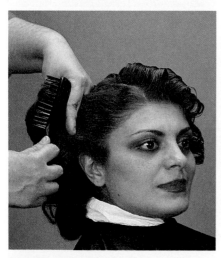

10.100   Hold hair with fingers

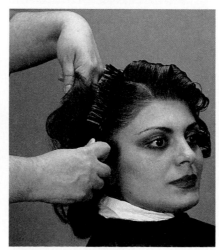

10.101   Point bristles upward

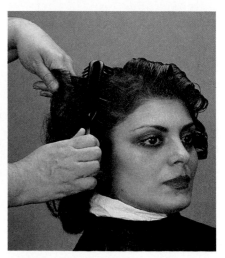

10.102   Roll brush down

5. At the bottom, turn the brush so that it is flat against the scalp (Figure 10.103). A thin section of hair has been meshed to the scalp (Figure 10.104).

6. Use the same procedure on the top of the head.

Procedure for Smoothing

1. Brush the surface hair back.

2. Keeping the hair in place with your hand, circle the brush down and forward (Figure 10.105).

3. This procedure results in a smooth, flared surface (Figure 10.106).

Procedure for Backbrushing

1. Brush the curl out and pick up a generous section of hair.

2. Holding the hair firmly, place the brush under the strand about two inches away from the scalp (Figure 10.107).

3. Rotate the brush toward the scalp, keeping it against the strand. Move the brush out along the strand and rotate it again, back-brushing the hair all the way to the ends. Back brush and smooth the top of the strand (Figure 10. 108).

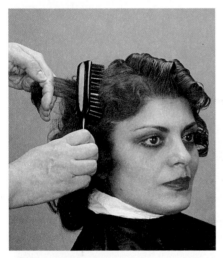

10.103   Brush is flat on scalp

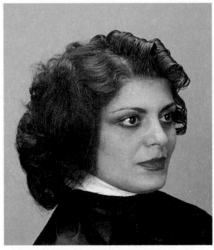

10.104   Hair is meshed to scalp

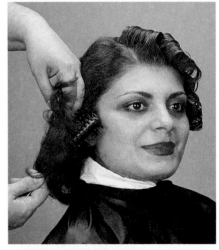

10.105   Circle brush down

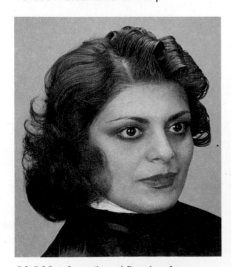

10.106   Smooth and flared surface

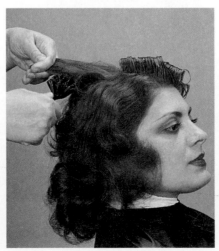

10.107   Place brush under strand

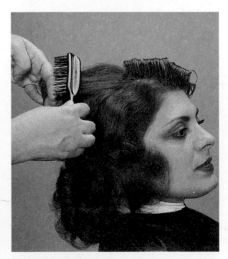

10.108   Smooth top of strand

4. Pick up another section of hair and combine it with the backbrushed hair.

5. Repeat the same backbrushing procedure until all the hair has been completed.

6. Backbrushing locks the hair with a soft, textured look.

Procedure for Wave Stretching

1. Brush out the wave pattern. The hair can be backbrushed to lock curl out and to give slight fullness and a smooth surface.

2. Begin the wave by placing the comb on the center forward shaping (Figure 10.109).

3. Place the index finger over the center forward shaping as the comb traces down to the center reverse shaping.

4. Move the index finger back and place it over the center reverse shaping (Figure 10.110).

5. Lift the hair ends and smooth them for fullness.

6. Circle the ends to finish the wave pattern (Figure 10.111).

7. The finished style shown in Figure 10.112 can be brushed smooth to give a more controlled, less fluffy look, as in Figure 10.113.

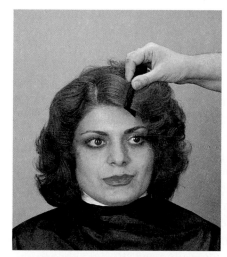

10.109   Comb in center forward shaping

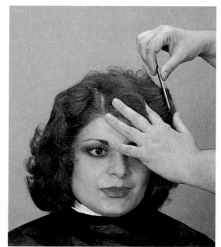

10.110   Index finger in center reverse shaping

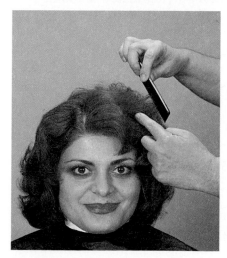

10.111   Circle ends

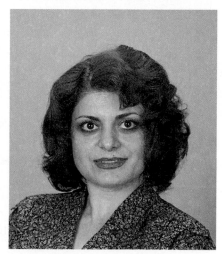

10.112   Finished style

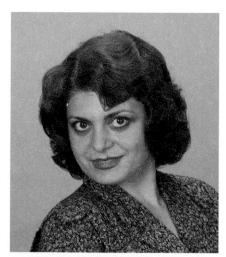

10.113   Finished smooth style

DRESSING LONG HAIR

Long hair can present many problems if it is not handled properly. This is particularly true if the hair is dry and tangles or breaks easily. Overdressing or underdressing long hair may result in frustration and hair loss. The following procedure for dressing long hair makes it easier to control the hair and will help you to achieve satisfactory results in a reasonable length of time. Note that the following procedure is different from that used on short hair.

1. Longer hair may tend to be dry or may have split ends, particularly if the hair has not been cared for by brushing, shampooing, conditioning, and so on. Long hair should be shampooed with a good conditioning, detangling shampoo. If necessary, a conditioner can be used after each shampoo. This will prevent the hair from splitting, will preserve a more even length, and will make combing the hair easier.

2. Blot the hair by placing a towel lengthwise under the hair at the nape and then folding each end of the towel to the center. Hold the folded towel at the nape and wring the hair to blot excess water and prevent dripping. Do not rub the hair with the towel. This could cause tangling or breakage.

3. Apply a quick-drying, detangling setting lotion to the hair. Concentrate on the scalp hair and comb it through the hair.

4. Divide the hair by parting it from the center front to the back. Loosely twist each section and pin it up.

5. The hair is predried for four to eight minutes, depending on hair length and density. This dries in the setting lotion and prevents the strong overdressing that would result if the hair were too wet.

6. In setting long hair, stick to simple setting patterns. If you do, the hair will be more manageable and you will achieve satisfactory results. For better manageability, be sure to set the hair in sections according to the style desired.

7. In setting long hair, rollers are generally used. Rollers absorb the length more readily, and the resulting style will not be too tight.

8. If the hair is to be blow-dried, predry the hair of excess water by loosely separating the hair and blowing it slightly. Then begin drying the hair for finish. Begin at the nape, drying one section at a time. By working up to the crown area, you will keep the finished dry hair out of your way (see Chapter 11).

> **◆ Key Point ◆**
> Remove excess water from long hair by blotting. Predry hair to avoid damage and overdressing. This greatly reduces drying time.

BRAIDING

Braiding is another technique for styling hair. As a cosmetologist, you will braid the hair in a design, and often you will teach your clients how to braid their hair at home. Styling with braids does not require long hair; some braiding techniques, such as corn-rowing, can be performed on hair of almost any length. Braiding requires the use of all of your fingers, and control of the hair for a smooth, even finish. You can achieve any number of effects, depending upon the size and the placement of your braids.

You can braid wet, partially dry, or completely dried hair. Use a light-weight styling aid for control. Curly hair is easier to braid if it is dry with a light-weight oil added to the hair for flexibility. The procedure that follows is for continuous braiding that begins at the scalp, commonly called the French braid.

Materials for Braiding

Shampoo cape and towel   Comb
Neck strip   Fastener for end of braid
Brush

Procedure for Braiding

1. Section off the hair to be braided. The size of the section will determine the finished look you achieve.
2. Divide the hair into three even subsections.
3. Grasp each outside subsection with your little fingers and control the center with the index and forefinger of your left hand (Figure 10.114).
4. Fold the right section over the center. Switch fingers so that your middle left finger controls the folded strand and your right little finger picks up the center strand now moving to the right (Figure 10.115).
5. With the index finger of your right hand, reach to the far left section, and fold it over the center (Figure 10.116).
6. With your fingers back in the original positions described in step 3, pick up a little more hair from the right subsection near the scalp with the little finger of your right hand. Fold the entire section over the center (Figure 10.117).

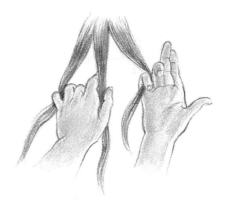

10.114

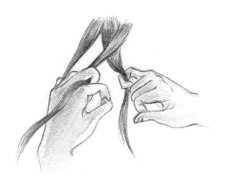

10.115

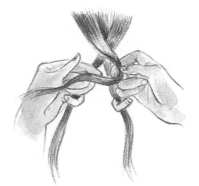

10.116

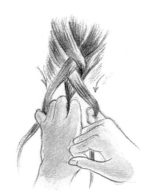

10.117

7. Position your fingers as described in step 4.
8. Pick up more hair from the left subsection near the scalp with the little finger of your left hand. Combine it with the left strand and fold over the center.
9. Continue in this manner, picking up more hair from the scalp with each little finger, combining it and then folding it over the center strand. When you reach the end of the hair, fasten the ends and finish the braid as desired.

◆ **Key Point** ◆

Braiding is an easy-care styling technique for long hair. Hair can be braided wet or dry. Use a styling lotion to help control the hair.

The size of the braid you create will determine the styling effect you achieve. For corn-rows, small braids are created all over the head, often in a pre-planned design. A corn-row is also the basis for a hair weave extension, discussed in Chapter 11. You can create the entire style with a single braid down the center of the head, commonly called the "fish tail" braid. The key to braiding skill is the dexterity in your fingers. Use all of your fingers and control the hair with moderate tension.

Summary

Hairstyling is the art of molding, shaping, and forming wet hair into a predetermined pattern. The shape of the base of a curl is selected by the function of the curl formed and the strength desired. The stem of the curl or roller will determine the mobility. It will also determine the direction in which the curl moves. The circle or the roller itself will determine the size of the finished curl. Hair should move around a roller $2\frac{1}{2}$ times to create a full wave pattern.

After the hair is thoroughly dry, brush to remove separations and then style. Comb-out techniques of backcombing and backbrushing create volume while lacing interlocks movements. Smoothing controls the surface and flares the curl; stretching extends the curl formation for a less fluffy look.

Before you can effectively style wet hair, you must analyze the qualities and the natural growth patterns of the hair. You will then create a design using the proper equipment and implements intended for the task. As a stylist, you will mold hair to prepare it for style execution. Carve hair out of those moldings and form even individual curls. These fundamental concepts of wet hairstyling apply to all hairdressing techniques. Your choice of implement to execute the concept will be based upon the current styles that your clients desire.

Questions

1. What characteristics determine hair quality?
2. Why should hair-growth patterns be considered before wet styling?
3. What equipment is available for wet hairstyling?
4. What is the purpose of shapings?
5. Can you demonstrate the eight basic shaping patterns? For what style might each be used?

6. What is a finger wave? How does it serve as a basis for current hairstyling techniques?
7. Explain how a finger wave formation is done over the entire head.
8. What are the three parts of a pin curl and where is each located?
9. How are pin curls constructed? Describe at least two types of pin curls and highlight the differences between the two.
10. Describe the placement of the roller for an on-base, a half-base, and an off-base placement.
11. What is an example of a style using rollers placed upon each of the bases?
12. What are the functions of backcombing, lacing, backbrushing, smoothing, and wave stretching? How is each comb-out technique done?
13. How is long hair dressed differently?
14. Describe how to complete a French braid.

PROJECTS

1. Select 10 hairstyles from magazines. Include a variety of short, medium, and long styles for men and women. Working with a photograph and your mannequin, mold wet hair into the shapings necessary to create the basic movements.
2. Continue from each molding in project 1, and finish the wet styling techniques to create the style look. Use rollers, sculpture curls, or any combination to duplicate the look.
3. Work each of the 10 styles into three comb-outs: the first with backcombing and placement, the second with backbrushing and soft design, and the third by stretching the wave movements and using finishing techniques. Describe the differences among the finished looks.
4. Working on your mannequin, complete and have your instructor check the following assignments: pin curls in a C shaping, pin curls in an S shaping, ridge curls, skipwaves, horizontal waves, vertical waves, and vertical roller placement. Repeat these exercises until your instructor indicates you have reached salon mastery.
5. Finger wave the entire head for approval at least six times. Find at least six photographs of present-day finger wave techniques. Share your findings with the class.
6. Practice French braiding on your mannequin. Work to master both the "fish tail" and the "corn row" techniques.

THERMAL HAIRSTYLING

CHAPTER GOAL

Thermal hairstyling is the most popular method of creating basic and advanced styles in today's busy salon. After reading this chapter and completing the projects, you should be able to

1. List the equipment used in thermal styling and demonstrate the technique required for each.
2. Describe the basic technique for blow drying the hair.
3. Explain the techniques for styling curly hair.
4. Demonstrate how heat lamps are used safely to dry hair.
5. Explain the function of hot rollers for the professional stylist.
6. Demonstrate the formation of a figure-eight curl, a barrel curl, and a figure-six curl.
7. Explain the function of hair pressing in the contemporary salon.
8. Demonstrate the procedure for hair pressing.
9. List the safety precautions for thermal hairstyling.
10. List and demonstrate the steps for maintaining nonelectric and electric thermal styling equipment.

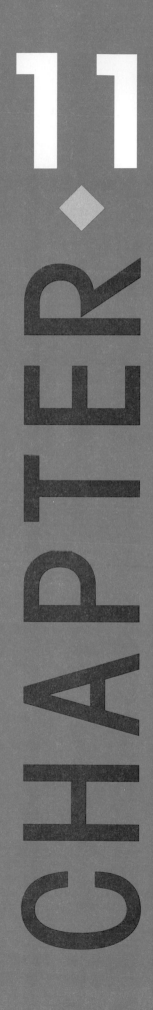

CHAPTER 11

Even the most primitive methods of styling the hair used thermal, or heat, techniques. Early records indicate that the sun was used to speed the process of early perms, lighteners, and colors as well as to dry the hair around sticks or reeds for a particular look. Thermal styling as we know it today uses hand-held equipment to direct the hair into a particular pattern.

The trend toward thermal styling followed the development of precision haircutting. The combination of the two drastically changed the way that professional cosmetology salons operated. In place of the weekly shampoo-and-set customers of the past are clients who come into the salon every four to six weeks to have their styles refreshed. In between, they style their own hair according to the directions given by their stylists.

It would be difficult to imagine a modern salon without thermal styling equipment. Yet, only a few years ago, thermal styling techniques were known as "quick service" methods. Thermal procedures are slightly faster; however, the same care must be taken with these techniques and the same principles applied as for wet styling. The key benefits are versatility and a soft, natural look.

As a professional stylist, you will greatly expand your hairdressing abilities by mastering the basic techniques of thermal styling. You must be able to select the thermal equipment that will best achieve the style on your client's hair type and use that equipment safely. You must know how to mold the hair close to the head with a styling brush. You must be able to direct the ends of the hair into the style line as you direct the air current down the hair shaft. You should know how to form curls with thermal irons, applying the concepts from Chapter 10. New equipment and procedures are constantly being developed, so stay abreast by attending seminars and trade shows.

TECHNIQUES AND EQUIPMENT

Thermal styling means dressing the hair by means of heat. Thermal equipment is used to

1. Style and dry the hair.
2. Curl or wave the hair.
3. Straighten the hair.

◆ **Key Point** ◆

Each piece of thermal equipment is designed with a particular styling technique in mind. Basic techniques that you must master are created with the blow dryer and the curling iron.

Equipment and Supplies Used in Thermal Styling

There are many types of thermal equipment available. Implements often follow fads in styling so you should be aware of currently preferred methods.

1. A **blow dryer** (Figure 11.1) is used for drying the hair and styling it at the same time. It can also be used to temporarily straighten wavy or curly hair. Hand-held blow dryers come in a variety of styles and usually have four heat settings.

2. A **diffuser** (Figure 11.2) is a special attachment for the blow dryer that is very effective in drying curly hairstyles. The air is directed over a wide area of the head, and the hair dries "naturally" without any loss of curl.

3. An **air waver** is used to style the hair. The effect is the same as using an ordinary comb, except that the hair dries as it is styled. Some air wavers also have hairbrush attachments. Air wavers are primarily used for platform and competition work. Your instructor may share methods of obtaining air waving effects with a standard blow dryer and a comb.

4. **Styling brushes** are used along with the hand dryer to create different styling effects. The various brushes are round and flat, with natural or synthetic bristles (Figure 11.3).

5. **Heat lamps** (Figure 11.4) help to speed up the time it would take for the hair to dry naturally. The lamps can be stationary or movable and have adjustable arms.

6. **Hot rollers** (Figure 11.5) are electrically heated rollers that come in a variety of sizes. They allow the hair to be roller-set without the inconvenience of sitting under a conventional dryer. Hot rollers are seldom used in the professional salon. As a stylist you may, however, use these tools for model or fashion-show work when your time and equipment are very limited.

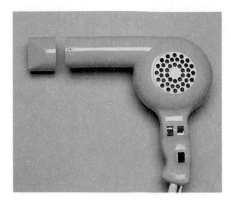

11.1   Blow dryer

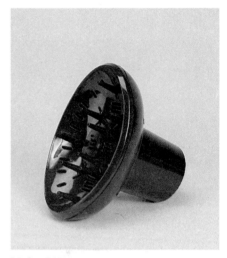

11.2   Diffuser

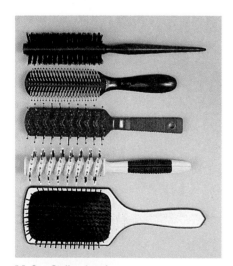

11.3   Styling brushes

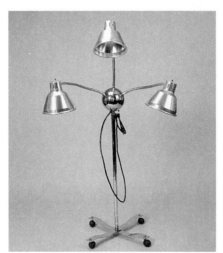

11.4   Heat lamp

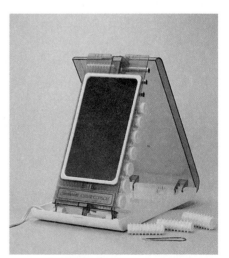

11.5   Hot rollers

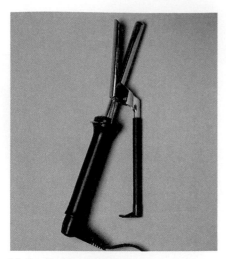

11.6 Electric curling iron

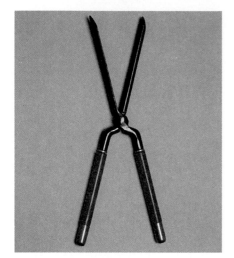

11.7 Nonelectric curling iron

7. **Curling irons** can be electric (Figure 11.6) or nonelectric (Figure 11.7) and come in a variety of sizes ranging from very small to jumbo.

8. **Hard rubber combs** should always be used with a curling iron because a metal comb could burn the client and a plastic one could melt.

9. **Pressing or straightening combs** can be nonelectric (Figure 11.8) or electric pressing combs (Figure 11.9) are used when giving a thermal press. The combs vary in size from those with 40 teeth (used on coarse hair) to those with 52 teeth (used on normal hair.) A temple comb has short, fine teeth and is used for the hairline and short neck hair.

10. **Electric heaters** (Figure 11.10) are used to heat straightening combs and nonelectric curling irons. The heaters are available in two sizes. The large size accommodates two combs or irons at one time. Only one at a time fits into the smaller heater. Electric heaters reach 500°F, which is far more heat than is necessary. Therefore, extreme caution must be used when heating the combs and irons.

11. **Pressing oil** or **cream** is applied to the hair before a thermal press. This allows the hot comb to glide through the hair and give the hair a gloss and sheen. Pressing oil or cream should be applied lightly, so that the hair does not become too heavy or oily.

12. **Scalp-and-hair conditioners** are essential. Because heat is applied directly to the hair, thermal techniques can be very damaging. Therefore, it is important to apply conditioners to keep the hair and scalp healthy. (See Chapter 6.)

13. **Styling aids** are also essential to protect the hair from heat damage and to make the set longer lasting. Styling aids come in liquid, foam, and spray forms.

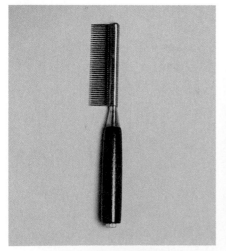

11.8 Nonelectric pressing comb

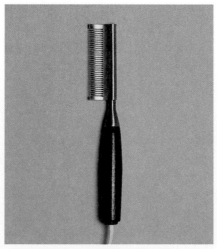

11.9 Electric pressing comb

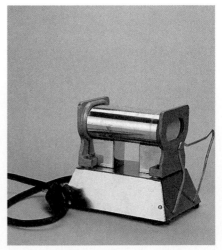

11.10 Electric heater

BLOW DRYING

Styling the hair with a hand-held blow dryer has become a standard hairdressing technique. At first it was considered a "quick service" method, but now it is used in almost every salon.

Blow drying involves using the hot air from the dryer and a brush to mold the hair into the style you wish to create. A blow dryer can also be used to temporarily straighten curly or wavy hair.

Using a **nozzle** on the dryer (Figure 11.11) will concentrate and intensify the flow of air. This will allow you to have more control over the hair and the style.

The procedure that follows will show you the basic techniques for blow drying. By using different brushes you can create a variety of styling effects. For example, using a narrow, round brush (Figure 11.12) will make the hair turn under in a tight curl. Using a wide-toothed brush will allow more air to flow through the hair and give it more volume and lift.

Best results are achieved on healthy hair that has been properly cut. Hair conditioners and styling lotions are used whenever necessary to give body to the hair and to help hold the style lines in place.

> ◆ **Key Point** ◆
> Apply the principles of wet hairstyling. First, mold the hair, then slice a section. Establish the base with brush and dryer. Follow the stem in the direction of the style and finish by creating a circle around the brush as desired.

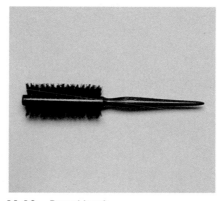

11.11   Blow dryer and nozzle   11.12   Round brush

Materials

Shampoo cape	Comb
Neck Strip	Brushes
Shampoo	Blow dryer
Towels	Nozzle for dryer
Styling aids	Clips

Procedure for Blow Drying: Basic Techniques

1. Hair is shampooed and partially towel dried before beginning the style line.
2. The hair is molded close to the head by using the brush on top of the section of hair (Figure 11.13). The air from the blow dryer is directed at an angle down the hair shaft and above the brush. Do not apply the flow directly to the scalp because it will be too hot.

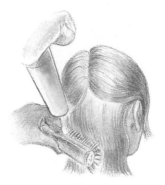

11.13   Mold hair to head

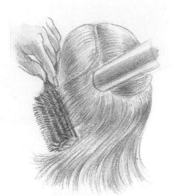

11.14 Brush underside of hair

3. The style is given some fullness by brushing the under side of the hair strand with a slight lifting motion (Figure 11.14). The air flow is directed down the hair shaft, while the ends of the hair are directed into the style line.

4. A roller formation is simulated by turning the ends of the hair under with a brush (Figure 11.15). The air flow is directed onto the top portion of the hair at the base of the curl; again, avoid a direct flow of air on the scalp.

5. A slight crown lift is achieved by using the brush to lift the hair at the scalp, slowly moving it out and then in a downward motion (Figure 11.16). The air flow is directed at the base of the formation.

6. To straighten the hair, the brush is used to stretch the hair gently while drying the base, shaft, and hair ends (Figure 11.17).

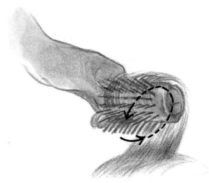

11.15 Simulate roller formation

11.16 Create slight crown lift

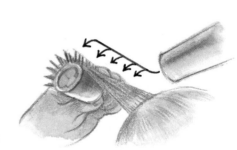

11.17 Straighten hair

The hair is continuously controlled during the drying and styling process by the use of the hairbrush and the blow dryer.

Work from the base of the style up to ensure placement of recently dried hair over hair previously dried. If you are creating a mid-length bob, for example, begin at the bottom as shown in Figure 11.13. Work the hair in sections up toward the crown.

As the hair dries, lower the temperature setting and the air control to low. Finish the style on cool, then wait until the hair is no longer warm before finishing with comb-out techniques.

Curly Hair Styles

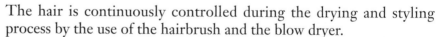

A diffuser is used to dry curly hair without removing or frizzing the curl. The diffuser is attached to the nozzle on the blow dryer (Figure 11.18). First, dry the hair nearest the scalp. Move the dryer as you lift the hair from the scalp with your fingers to avoid burning your client. Dry the lower sections first, then work your way up toward the crown, lifting the hair from the scalp as you go.

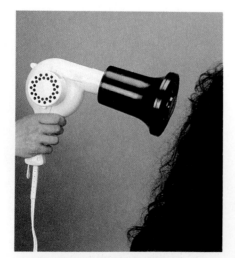

11.18 Dry curly hair with diffuser

Tousle the hair with your fingers gently. "Scrunch" the curl into place by gently squeezing the hair between your fingertips and palm. Place the hair into style lines as the hair dries. Continue up and around the head until all the hair has dried. Allow the scalp to cool, then lift the hair at the base with a pick for a finished look.

Infrared heat or white quartz lamps are also used to help the hair dry without disturbing the hairstyle. They are very effective when used on hair that has been chemically waved because none of the curl is removed and the hair does not tangle.

The client should be seated comfortably with the lamps directed at the head. Be sure that the lamps are at least 24 inches from the client. As each section dries, the lamps are rearranged and redirected to another area.

CLIENT TIP ◆◆◆◆◆◆◆

Remember to direct the lamps at the hair only, not at the skin. Move the lamps every few minutes so your client does not get too hot.

USING HOT ROLLERS

Electrically heated rollers are used the same way that ordinary rollers are used, but the time spent under the dryer is eliminated. Because they heat the hair directly, hot rollers have a tendency to dry out the hair. Therefore, be sure to apply a conditioner. Wrapping the hair with permanent-wave endpapers before rolling will help to prevent excessive damage.

Setting times vary with different equipment, so you should follow the manufacturer's instructions to see how long the rollers should be preheated and left in the hair. See Chapter 10 for the correct procedure for roller setting.

◆ **Key Point** ◆

Take care that you do not distort the curl pattern. If the curl is worked too much while dying, it will become frizzy and unmanageable. Work with a light styling aid so the curl is not weighted down.

◆ **Key Point** ◆

Electric rollers are not commonly used in today's professional salon. They are, however, an invaluable tool in your portable kit for location styling for fashion shows, photography sessions, TV productions, and guest appearances.

USING CURLING IRONS

Marcel Grateau perfected the curling iron and the technique for waving and curling hair with a hot iron in 1875. Because of his contribution to hairdressing, this technique was called marcel waving. Today it is more often called iron or thermal curling.

The success of any curl formed with a hot iron depends on the thickness of the hair strand, the temperature of the iron when applied to the hair, and the length of time the iron remains on the strand. Each of these factors must be carefully controlled.

Parts of the Curling Iron

The part of the iron used to curl the hair is constructed of two parts—the groove (or bowl) and the prong (Figure 11.19). The prong is the solid part and is perfectly round. The groove is hollowed out or curved to fit around the prong when the iron is closed. The edge of the groove nearest you is called the inner edge; the edge farthest from you is called the outer edge.

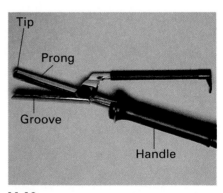

Tip
Prong
Groove
Handle

11.19

The thickness or size of the prongs vary from very small to medium, large, and extra large, or jumbo. The most common barrel sizes used are sizes of a nickel and a quarter. Smaller irons are used for tight curls, especially around the hairline. Jumbo irons are used for smooth looks or to curl just the ends (Figure 11.20).

The size of the iron used is determined by the area of the head to be worked on and the style to be achieved. Small irons are used for neckline hair or wherever curls of small circumference are needed. Jumbo irons are used in the crown area or in any area where volume in the style is needed.

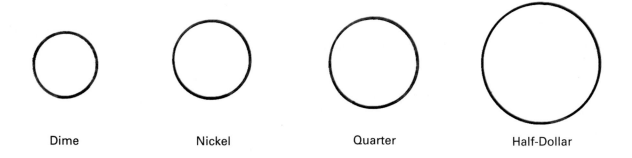

Dime   Nickel   Quarter   Half-Dollar

11.20

Types of Curling Irons

Nonelectric curling irons are usually imported from France and Germany. They are made of either blue or white steel so that they hold heat evenly. Irons are available with revolving or insulated stationary handles.

Tempering New Irons

Most new irons are factory tempered. This means they will heat evenly and so are ready for use when you receive them from the supply house or manufacturer. If a new iron has not been factory tempered, it must be treated in the following manner before it can be used: The iron is heated until red hot, then it is submerged in cold water, and finally it is dried and rubbed with linseed oil. After this treatment, the iron will hold heat evenly.

Most professional stylists prefer to use an electric curling iron. Usually these are designed with a freely revolving coupling at the end of the handle. This prevents the cord from twisting as you use the iron. These irons have an on-off switch. The temperature of the iron is constant and even. Cordless electric units are also available. The base unit heats the iron when it is inserted.

How to Hold the Curling Iron

1. With the iron held in the hand, the ring finger and little finger are used to control the opening and closing of the groove over the prong. The index and middle finger control the turning (rotating) of the iron. The thumb rests on the handle of the iron to provide support and balance while the iron is manipulated on the hair strand (Figure 11.21).

2. Although the basic position for holding the iron is shown in Figure 11.21, the entire iron, as well as the hair strand, must be rotated to create a professional-looking curl. Figure 11.22 shows the position of the hand and iron for this rotating action. Rotating the iron is the most important technique that you must acquire for iron curling. Practice holding, turning, opening, and closing the iron until the motions become natural.

3. A hard rubber styling comb is always used with the iron to produce curls and waves. Hold the comb in the hand at all times when working with the iron.

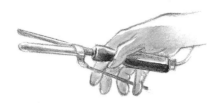

11.21　Basic hold for iron

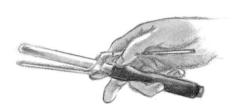

11.22　Hand position for rotating iron

Materials for Thermal Styling Using Curling Irons

Curling iron(s)　　Shampoo cape
Hard rubber comb　Neck strips
Styling aids

Procedure for Forming a Figure-eight Curl

This is the type of curl frequently used for longer hair. It produces a firm base near the scalp and is suitable for medium or long hair.

1. With a hard rubber comb, slice out a section of hair two inches long and about as wide as the diameter of the curling iron.

2. Test the iron against a white tissue or neck strip to determine the proper temperature. If the iron scorches the tissue, it is too hot to use on the hair.

3. Hold the strand between the index finger and the third finger.

4. Insert the iron close to but not touching the scalp, enough room to allow a one-quarter turn. The groove should be on top of the strand (Figure 11.23).

5. Immediately upon insertion, rotate the iron one-quarter turn toward yourself, directing the hair with the free hand toward the handle of the iron (Figure 11.24).

6. Open and close the iron rapidly (this is called "clicking" the iron). Turn one-half turn toward yourself (Figure 11.25).

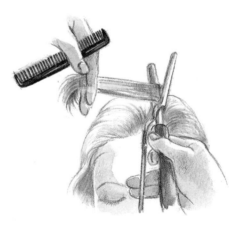

11.23　Use hard rubber comb with iron

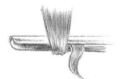

11.24　Turn iron toward you

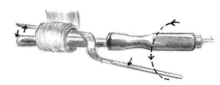

11.25　Click and turn iron

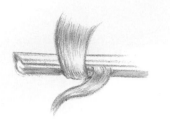

11.26   Direct hair toward iron tip

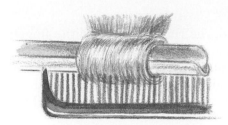

11.27   Protect scalp with comb

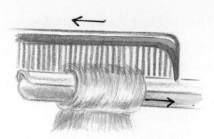

11.28   Slide iron out of curl

7. With your free hand, direct the ends of the hair toward the tip of the iron (Figure 11.26).
8. Continue to roll and click the iron until all the hair ends disappear around the iron. The ends will be inside the curl.
9. Insert the comb under the iron to protect the scalp (Figure 11.27).
10. Leave the iron in the curl until the ends are heated and they take the curl position.
11. Roll the iron to be sure the ends are free. Slide the iron out (Figure 11.28). If the iron does not slide out easily, the ends have not been properly manipulated. The iron needs to be rolled and clicked once or twice more.

Procedure for Forming a Barrel Curl

This curl is used on short to medium-length hair. It is not as firm as a figure-eight curl. Sometimes this curl is referred to as a styling curl.

1. Follow steps 1 through 4 of the figure-eight curl.
2. Begin to rotate the iron toward you while you direct the hair ends into the center of the curl with your free hand (Figure 11.29).
3. Open and close (click) the irons rapidly.
4. Continue to rotate the iron as you guide the ends into the center of the curl (Figure 11.30).
5. Place a hard rubber comb under the curl.
6. Hold the heat on the ends for a few seconds. Click the iron and rotate to free the ends. Slide the iron out of the curl (Figure 11.31).

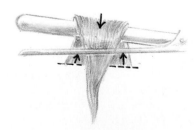

11.29   Rotate iron toward you

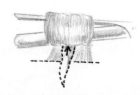

11.30   Direct ends to center of curl

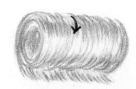

11.31   Slide iron out of barrel curl

Procedure for Forming a Figure-six Curl

This curl is used on short to medium-length hair. It produces a strong curl and is very popular in salon work.

1. Follow steps 1 through 4 of the figure-eight curl.
2. Rotate and click the iron one-half turn toward you while holding the end of the strand in your free hand. Direct the end toward the center of the curl (Figure 11.32).
3. Rotate the iron one-half turn toward you, directing the end of the hair toward the tip of the iron (Figure 11.33). Click the iron as you turn.
4. Rotate the iron a complete turn toward you as you click.
5. Open the iron and pass the end of the hair between the groove and rod (Figure 11.34).
6. Close the iron and rotate and click until the ends disappear into the center of the curl (Figure 11.35).
7. Rotate the iron several times to distribute the heat to the ends.
8. Place a hard rubber comb under the curl and slide the iron out.

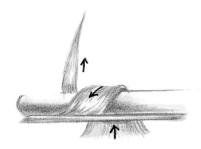

11.32   Direct hair to center of curl

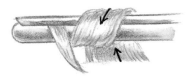

11.33   Direct hair to iron tip

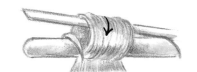

11.34   Pass hair between groove and rod

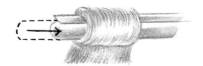

11.35   Rotate until ends disappear into curl

Forming Other Types of Curls

A **spiral curl** is similar to the barrel curl. The iron is held in a vertical position and the hair is inserted near the joint of the iron. The hair is fed into the iron so that it "spirals" toward the tip of the iron. All lengths of hair may be used, but this type of curl is usually best with long hair.

A **bob curl** is used with very short hair, $1\frac{1}{2}$ to $2\frac{1}{2}$ inches long. Grasp the hair ends with the iron and rotate them under or over until you come close to the scalp. Allow the heat to penetrate for about two seconds and slide the iron out.

Points to Remember When Iron-Curling

1. The hair should be dry before being treated with the iron.
2. Apply a protective styling aid to the hair before using the iron. The hair will not dry out and will have a glossy sheen after curling.
3. Use the same sectioning and subsectioning as in roller setting to style the hair.

◆SAFETY **P R E C A U T I O N**◆

Hair that has been lightened or hair that is naturally white or gray will discolor if the curling iron is too hot. Use a lower temperature setting and test the iron on tissue to be sure the paper does not turn brown before curling light hair.

◆ **Key Point** ◆

A curling iron is the thermal substitute for a roller. As in roller placement, slice out the section, establish the base, and wind the curl in the direction desired. Let hair cool before finishing with comb-out techniques.

4. The iron may be used on fine hair or on hair that has been lightened or permanent waved, but you should use less heat and should shorten the time that the hair is in contact with the iron.

5. Always keep the hair strand smooth on the iron; never twist the ends of the hair.

6. The thickness of the strand to be curled depends on the texture and condition of the hair and the amount of curl desired.

7. The hair strand and the iron must be turned at the same time to create the perfect curl.

8. When using the iron to refresh curls before recombing, brush the hair thoroughly to remove any hair spray that might stick to the hot iron.

9. To avoid frizzy curls, hair that is curled with an iron should be blunt-cut with little taper in the ends.

10. If the iron you are using has no built-in heat control, test the iron against a white tissue to determine the proper temperature. If the iron scorches the tissue, it is too hot to use on the hair.

Hair Pressing

Thermal hair straightening (pressing) is the process of temporarily rearranging the basic structure of extra curly hair into a straight form. When this is professionally done, it usually leaves the client's hair straight and in a satisfactory condition to be styled with curling irons in almost any style.

To become good at thermal hair straightening, the cosmetologist must acquire technical knowledge and expertise in the use of the pressing combs, curling irons, and electrical heaters.

Straightening combs are constructed of stainless steel, brass, or a combination of brass and copper (see Figure 11.8). Combs are available in different sizes. Some have more teeth than others, and some teeth are spaced farther apart than others. Combs with teeth very close together will produce a very smooth look. A small straightening comb is used for short ends and around the hairline. The following are the more commonly used sizes:

1. A straightening comb with 40 teeth is used for coarse hair or for long hair. These combs are available with or without a copper inlay. The copper inlay permits the teeth to bend if the comb is mistreated or dropped.

2. A straightening comb with 52 teeth is used for normal hair. These combs also come with or without a copper inlay.

3. A temple comb has short, fine teeth and is used for the hairline and for short neck hair.

Electric pressing combs are also available (see Figure 11.9). They have one temperature setting (usually about 212°F) and have a thermostat that maintains the temperature. They reach their maximum temperature about 15 minutes after they are plugged in.

Hair Analysis

The cosmetologist must be able to recognize individual differences in hair texture, elasticity, porosity, and flexibility or lack of flexibility of the scalp before using a straightening comb or curling iron.

Hair texture refers to the diameter of the hair—whether it is fine, medium, or coarse. Fine hair is small in diameter. Fine, soft hair that is extra curly requires very little heat. This type of hair also requires more care because it burns and breaks easily. Hair of a medium texture responds easily to pressing or straightening. Hair with a coarse texture can tolerate the greatest amount of heat, and it is the most difficult to press. The amount of natural oil present in the hair also affects the amount of heat used. Oily hair can withstand more heat, dry hair less.

Gray, tinted, and bleached hair require special attention. Tinted and bleached hair is more porous because of the chemical action of the haircoloring products, and thus more fragile. Frequently, it is too damaged to withstand much heat during a pressing treatment. Gray hair will scorch, so you should use less heat. More pressure may be necessary, depending upon the texture of the hair (gray fine, gray medium, or gray coarse).

You must test the hair to determine its elasticity. Always test for elasticity when the hair is dry. The hair will be pressed when dry, and so testing on wet hair will give inaccurate results. Too much pressure during the pressing treatment will destroy the elasticity of the hair and cause it to break. More pressure should be applied to the scalp hair than to the ends because the ends of the hair may have been pressed many times.

Pressing Cosmetics

Cream press or pressing oils are preparations that are applied to the hair before the pressing service. These products make the hot comb glide easily through the hair and give the hair a sheen or gloss. **Pressing oil** is a liquid or solid that deposits an oily film on the hair. If too much of this product is used, the hair strands will stick together, and soft, natural styling will not be possible. Some hairdressers use pressing oil when they are giving a hard press because it helps to keep the hair perfectly straight. If a customer perspires heavily, a pressing oil will help to keep the hair from reverting to the natural curl.

Cream press is a solid, waxy product that is more popular than pressing oil. It leaves the hair soft and pliable and makes it easy to style. Pressing oil and cream press should be applied after the shampoo and before the hair is dry. The water helps to distribute the product through the hair. Experience will teach you how much of these products to apply, depending on the quality, density, and length of the client's hair. Start with very little; you can always add more. If you start with too much, you will have to shampoo the hair to remove the product.

Scalp-and-hair conditioner is a cosmetic that is applied to the hair and scalp to prevent dryness. During a pressing and curling service, heat is applied to the hair close to the scalp. Sometimes the scalp becomes dry and flaky. If so, the conditioner is applied to the scalp very sparingly after the press, and the hair is brushed to distribute the conditioner into the hair. If the hair does not need the conditioner, apply it to the scalp only. This can be done after the hair has been styled with the curling iron, but before the comb-out.

Basic Hair Pressing Techniques

A hair pressing treatment exerts pressure on the scalp. Whenever possible, the hair should be pressed in the direction in which it grows. A client with a tense, tight scalp may have some discomfort during the pressing treatment. When you are pressing hair on a client with a loose scalp, it is difficult to apply pressure without burning the scalp. By using small sections and light pressure, you will obtain satisfactory results.

If irons or combs that are too hot are used, discoloration or breakage of hair may result on gray, tinted, or bleached hair. When pressing this type of hair and very fine hair, avoid excessive heat and pressure near hair ends. When you are pressing short, fine hairs along the hairline, do not use irons and combs that are too hot. Fine hair may be damaged easily. With practice, you will learn what the correct temperature for all pressing instruments should be. You will also learn the amount of pressure that different textures of hair can tolerate without resulting in hair breakage.

There are many definitions of what constitutes a hair-pressing service for extra curly hair. Some hairdressers use a hot comb, while others use a comb and an iron. Some press the top of the strand, while others press the bottom. Keep in mind that the effect you achieve depends upon the percentage of curl you remove. How much curl you remove depends on the texture and condition of the hair and the outcome you desire. Hairdressers usually speak of three types of pressing:

1. **Soft press**—removal of 60 to 70 percent of the curl.
2. **Medium press**—removal of about 75 percent of the curl.
3. **Hard press**—removal of 100 percent of the curl (this totally straightens the hair and leaves it in a weak condition).

Remember that it is the percentage of natural curl that is removed that gives the final result. You should not be concerned with how many times you pass the thermal comb through the hair or with whether you pass the comb through on the top or bottom of the strand.

Giving a Straightening or Pressing Service

Materials

Shampoo cape and towel	Hair spray	Electric heater (optional)
Neck strip	Pressing combs	Tangle comb
Shampoo	Curling irons	Brush
Pressing oil or cream press	Hard rubber tail and styling combs	Hair clips
		Hair dryer or blow dryer

Procedure for Hair Pressing

1. Wash your hands with antibacterial soap.
2. Drape the client.
3. Examine the client's scalp and hair. If there are any abrasions or injuries on the scalp, the pressing treatment should not be given. If an examination of the hair shows damage due to haircoloring, chemical relaxing, or improper pressing treatments, a series of hair reconditioning treatments should be recommended.
4. Shampoo, rinse, and towel-dry the hair. Use cool water for the last rinse.
5. Apply a small amount of pressing oil ($\frac{1}{4}$ teaspoon is ample for the average head) or cream press. Work it into the entire head of hair. Turn on the pressing comb or heater with comb inserted.
6. Use a regular dryer or a blow dryer to dry the hair. Clip the hair in small sections to keep it controlled. The hair will not be so curly and will be easier to press when this method of drying is used. Release the sections when the hair is almost dry. Be sure the scalp is completely dry to avoid steam burns.
7. Comb the hair with a styling comb and section it into four main sections. Clip only three sections, leaving a back section ready for subsectioning. Subdivide the section you are working on into smaller sections as you press the hair. The size of the section should be one-half the length of the comb and one-half the depth.
8. Test the temperature of the heated pressing comb on a white tissue or neck strip. If the paper or hair shows any signs of scorching, allow the comb to cool.
9. Starting at the top of the back section, subsection the hair with a hard rubber comb.
10. Hold the end of a small section of hair between the index finger and thumb. Hold the strand upward and away from the scalp.
11. Insert the teeth of the pressing comb into the top side of the hair section close to the scalp (Figure 11.36). Roll the comb until teeth face you while holding the hair strand firmly against the back rod of the comb (Figure 11.37). It is the back rod, or bar, of the comb that carries the heat and actually does the straightening.
12. Keeping the hair strand firmly against the back rod of the pressing comb and turning the comb slowly away from you, draw it up through the entire hair strand until the hair ends pass through the teeth (Figure 11.38). Hold the hair ends with your hand as you pass the hot comb through the section.

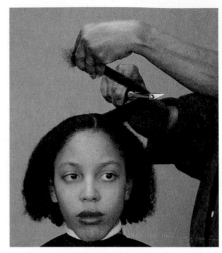

11.36   Insert comb in top of strand

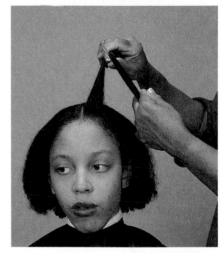

11.37   Roll teeth of comb toward you

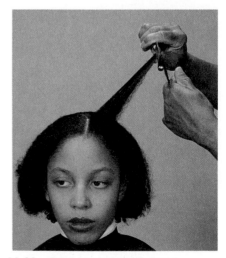

11.38   Draw comb through strand

13. Repeat this pressing motion on the top and bottom of the strand until you achieve the desired straightness.
14. Each completed subsection should be clipped up or to one side to keep it away from the working area.
15. Continue over the entire head until all sections have been pressed.
16. After all the hair has been pressed, cool the hair under a cold hair dryer for 3 to 5 minutes if the hair is fine.
17. If a haircut is to be given, this is usually done after the press and before the curl.
18. Comb the hair, style it with the curling irons (see the following section), and finish with an application of hairdressing or hair spray.

Hair Shaping Services

Hair that is thermally straightened needs to have shape and design, just as does hair that is wet-set or blown dry. The best results are usually obtained when the hair is straight. For this reason, the shaping is done on dry hair, usually with scissors. Shaping can be done before the shampoo if the client's hair is already 75 percent straight. It can also be done after the shampoo and press, but before the set.

Styling

Resection the hair for curling with an iron. The iron size is determined by the hairstyle. A large iron is used to produce a high and loose style. A medium-sized iron is used to make curls that will be tighter and more durable. The small iron is suitable for short hair on the neck.

After the hair has been curled, it should be cooled for 5 to 10 minutes before combing. If hair is combed while still warm, it may produce the same effect as combing out a wet set before it is completely dry. Hair may be styled in almost any style.

SAFETY PRECAUTIONS AND EQUIPMENT MAINTENANCE FOR THERMAL STYLING

Safety Precautions for Thermal Styling

1. Before pressing the client's hair, examine the hair and scalp thoroughly. Decide on the conditioner or pressing cream to be used. Recommend a good shampoo.
2. Avoid excessive heat and pressure on the hair and scalp during hair pressing.
3. Dry the hair completely after it is shampooed to prevent steam burns.
4. Do not use too much pressing oil on the hair. This can cause undesirable effects.
5. Give a reconditioning treatment to damaged hair before attempting to press the hair.

6. Avoid excess heat on gray, tinted, or lightened hair.
7. Apply protective cream immediately to any scalp or skin burn.
8. Do not use metal, celluloid, or plastic combs in connection with thermal waving and curling. Metal ones may become hot and burn the client, and plastic and celluloid ones may melt. Use only hard rubber combs.
9. To prevent burning the scalp when giving a thermal waving and curling service, place a comb between the scalp and the iron.
10. Do not allow the pressing comb to overheat. This may cause the metal to lose its temper.
11. The pressing comb should be kept free and clean of carbon at all times. Remove loose hairs before reheating the comb.
12. Adjust the temperature of the pressing comb to the condition and texture of the client's hair.
13. To cool hot irons, place them in a spot where people will not come in contact with them and burn themselves.
14. Do not place the handle of the iron too far into the heater. This will damage the handle of the iron, and you may burn your hand when you remove the iron.
15. Balance the iron properly in the heater to prevent it from falling.
16. Avoid smoking the hair or burning the hair during the pressing service.
17. Use a small pressing comb at the temple area. Use a moderately warm comb at the temple area and the back of the neck.

<table>
<tr><td>

◆ **Key Point** ◆

Always handle thermal irons and pressing combs carefully to avoid burning yourself or your client. Regulate the heat so you can achieve desired results without hair damage.

</td></tr>
</table>

Care of Nonelectric Irons and Straightening Combs

It is necessary to clean the irons and combs regularly to remove the carbon (a chemical substance that forms on the steel) and buildup of burned hair. To do this:

1. Remove all hair from the irons and combs.
2. Pour a commercial cleaner or a solution of 28 percent ammonia (full-strength) into a clean glass jar. If the combs and irons are to be cleaned at the same time, it will be necessary to have jars of several different sizes.
3. Be sure that only the teeth and neck of the combs are immersed in the ammonia. The solution will damage the handle of the comb.
4. A taller jar should be used for irons. Again, only the metal parts of the iron should be immersed in the solution.
5. Allow the combs and irons to remain in the ammonia solution overnight.
6. Remove the combs and irons from the solution. Use fine steel wool to remove the remaining carbon. A knife blade or similar instrument can be used to help loosen the carbon from between the teeth of the combs. The cleaning process may be hastened by holding the implements under running water while using the steel wool.
7. Dry the irons thoroughly and apply a thin coat of oil before putting them away.

Care of Electric Irons and Pressing Combs

Electric thermal equipment should be cared for to prevent electric shock and cleaned after each use. To do this:

1. Check cord as it enters the iron and the plug to see that the plastic sheath is not wearing or cracking. Avoid wrapping the cord tightly around the iron when storing to avoid damage.
2. Do not handle electric equipment with wet hands and be sure you are standing on a dry surface.
3. After use, unplug the iron and let cool. Remove any hair that may be caught in the joint. Clean the surface of the iron with cotton saturated with 70% alcohol or an approved disinfectant that will not harm metal. Allow the alcohol to evaporate naturally.

Summary

Thermal styling services are the mainstay of the contemporary salon. Thermal services are slightly faster than wet-setting techniques. Many stylists feel that the results of thermal styling are softer and more versatile. Thermal styling can be used to simply dry the hair in its natural configuration, or to add or remove curl from the hair.

Thermal pressing is an alternative to blow-drying and iron-curling for extra curly hair. While the blow dryer and the curling iron can be used to style curly hair, some clients prefer the smooth look achieved with a pressing service. Pressing combs are electric or can be heated in a stove especially designed for that purpose. The hair is worked smooth, section by section, then thermal-ironed into the desired style.

In any thermal technique, use caution that the client is not uncomfortable from the heat and that burns do not occur. Allow the hair to cool before finishing with comb-out techniques.

As a cosmetologist, it is essential that you choose the correct equipment for the client's hair type and the style desired. You must use the equipment correctly for the style while executing proper safety measures so you do not burn yourself, your client, or the hair. Your success in thermal hairstyling will depend on how you combine the techniques of blow drying and the principles of shaping and curl formation.

Questions

1. What are four pieces of equipment frequently used in thermal styling? Perform a hairstyling technique with each tool.
2. Perform the basic technique for blow drying hair.
3. What are the techniques used for styling curly hair?
4. How are heat lamps used to dry hair safely?
5. What function do hot rollers serve for the professional stylist?
6. Form a figure-eight curl, a barrel curl, and a figure-six curl on your head form.
7. What function does hair pressing serve in the contemporary salon?
8. What types of combs should be used with thermal styling equipment? What can happen if you use the wrong combs?

9. What is the procedure for removing carbon buildup from non-electric thermal hairstyling equipment?
10. How do you care for electric thermal hairstyling equipment? What are the two goals of maintenance for electric equipment?

1. Refer to the first project in Chapter 10, and recreate each of the 10 selected styles with thermal styling techniques. Report the differences in effects and the similarities in techniques to the class.
2. Research the styling aids available in your school. Note the features and benefits of each. Indicate the styles for which each product could be used.
3. Use thermal techniques to create the following: a finger wave, a pincurl, a ridge shaping, on-base volume, half-base volume, off-base volume.
4. Press at least four heads of curly hair. After the curl is removed, thermal-style for a contemporary look according to each client's request.

Projects

WIGS AND HAIRPIECES

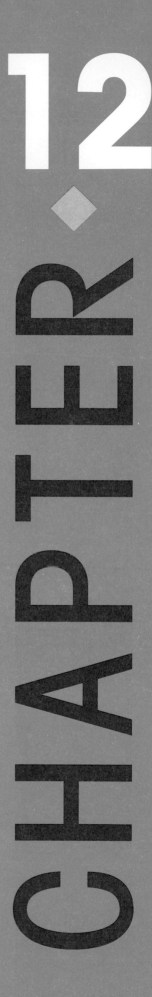

CHAPTER GOAL

Wigs and hairpieces serve many practical as well as cosmetic purposes. After reading this chapter and completing the projects, you should be able to

1. List the purposes for which wigs are worn.
2. Describe the construction of wigs and materials most often used.
3. Describe the types of hairpieces available.
4. Demonstrate how to measure and fit a client for a wig and a hairpiece.
5. Outline the maintenance of synthetic and human-hair wigs.
6. Describe the purposes of special-effect hair additions.

Wigs are fun! Wigs come and go as a fad of fashion. The Egyptians first recorded the use of wigs 6000 years ago. The twentieth century witnessed the extensive use of wigs in the 60s and early 70s with specialty wig shops popping up everywhere. As the 70s progressed into the natural-is-best 80s, wigs declined in popularity. The early 90s saw a resurgence of wigs for fun and hair extensions and weaves for glamour.

Wigs and hairpieces serve a practical purpose for people who have experienced temporary or permanent hair loss. Hairpieces and extensions are an important dimension of the services that you will offer as a professional cosmetologist. You will be able to measure and fit a hair addition of the correct color. You will be able to care for hairpieces and wigs in the salon and instruct your client about care at home. You will also be able to attach hair additions and style them to meet your client's needs.

WHY WIGS AND HAIRPIECES ARE WORN

◆ **Key Point** ◆

Wigs and hairpieces serve replacement purposes in cases of temporary or permanent hair loss due to genetic factors, illness, or medical treatment such as chemotherapy.

People choose to wear wigs for several reasons—mostly for convenience and a quick change of style. There are also people who wear wigs because a medical condition has caused a temporary or permanent loss of hair. Women wear hairpieces to create special styles; many men who are unhappy with balding wear toupees. Wigs are used extensively in theatre, music, and movie productions to create characters, time periods, and other special effects. Wigs are also worn to cover temporary or permanent damage done to the hair, which can result from incorrect chemical application. Hairpieces are often worn just for fun as a clip-on addition for a party or other special occasion.

MATERIALS AND CONSTRUCTION

Wigs and hairpieces are constructed of human or synthetic hair. Recent improvements in synthetic wigs have made them look and feel very natural. Hairpieces sometimes incorporate animal hair, although these pieces are primarily used for theatrical purposes. The demonstration swatches used in many schools are available in human or synthetic hair.

Human hair wigs and hairpieces are the most expensive. They can be arranged in a variety of styles, colored, and sometimes even permanently waved. The feel of a human hair wig is usually slightly softer than wigs made from animal or synthetic hair. With proper care they can last for years. Much of the human hair used for hairpieces and wigs comes from the Far East. Hair of any type can be processed and colored as needed for hair offering various textures, amounts of curl, and color.

Synthetic wigs and hairpieces are the most popular. They are more natural looking than ever before. They are prestyled and hold that style very well if they are cleaned and dried properly. The style cannot be changed in most instances, although specialists in theatrical work have been successful with thermal techniques.

A "match test" will help you determine if a wig is made of human hair or of a synthetic fiber. Place a small section of hair cut from the wig in an ashtray and light it with a match. Human hair burns slowly and gives off a strong odor. Synthetic hair burns very quickly, almost melts, and will leave tiny hard beads.

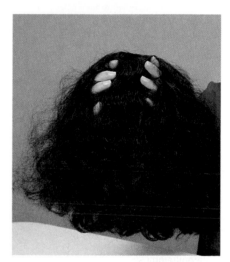

12.1a   Wefting inside a wig

Bases Used for Wigs and Hairpieces

Most wigs are made of rows of wefting sewn to strips of elastic (see Figure 12.1). A **weft** is a thin strip of hair, woven together with thread. This type of wig is very light in weight, cool, and stretches to conform to the wearer's head.

Wigs are generally available in one standard head size of 22 inches, although petite and large wigs are also available. An adjustment band of elastic is sewn into the area that will touch the nape of the neck.

Hairpieces are constructed on a more solid base. The shape of each base is determined by the size and the function of the piece. The base is usually made of a meshed material and finished at the edges with a sewn tape. A comb is attached, usually at the top, so that the hairpiece can be secured.

Toupees (too PAYS), hairpieces for men, have a similar construction. These pieces come in a variety of sizes and shapes and are often custom made to the individual pattern of baldness. These pieces often have open meshwork at the front, known as lace fronts, a thin plastic "skin" insert, or a style made into them so that the appearance is as natural as it possibly can be.

12.1b   Wefting allows ventilation

Construction of Wigs and Hairpieces

All wigs and hairpieces can be made by machine or by hand. The machine-sewn wigs are less expensive. However, hand-knotted pieces are the most natural looking. Many of the most popular wigs and hairpieces today are a combination; they are machine sewn, but hand finished at the crown and facial hairline. This makes the wig or hairpiece more affordable, and still gives it a natural look around the face, at the crown, and where the hair is typically parted.

You should help your client find the most natural-looking hairpiece possible by examining it closely. Check that the amount of hair is not excessive. An overly thick piece looks artificial and you will need to remove the excess hair when styling. Check to see that the

> **◆ Key Point ◆**
> Today's wigs are made with very fine wefts of hair. The hair may be crimped at the base to add volume. Wefts are attached to elastic for comfort and fit.

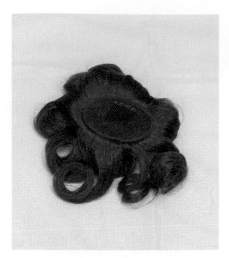

12.2 Wiglet

wefts of the wig are close together, but that only a thin section of hair is sewn to each weft. Avoid wigs or hairpieces that attach the hair in definite patterns. Most good wigs will have rows of wefts that match the patterns of natural hair growth. Avoid wigs that have wefts sewn in a circle around and around the head and ending in a clump of hair at the crown. This "ponytail" looks very artificial and is extremely difficult to cut and style into an attractive look. The more natural hairpieces look on your clients, the happier they will be with their purchases.

TYPES OF HAIRPIECES

Hairpieces come in many shapes, sizes, styles, and colors. Talk with your clients to determine what their needs are. Explain the effects that are possible with each hairpiece.

Wiglets

Smaller hairpieces for women are known as **wiglets** (Figure 12.2). They can have various sizes and shapes of bases, depending upon the effect desired and the amount of hair added. A small wiglet contains about $1\frac{1}{2}$ ounces of hair that is 5 to 7 inches long. A larger wiglet will contain 3 to 5 ounces of hair that is usually longer—about 10 to 12 inches. Cascade wiglets have an oblong base and longer hair. These are often designed to be worn on the back of the head, attached at the crown.

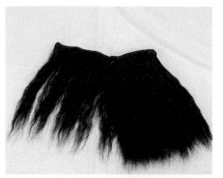

12.3 Hair sewn into a headband

Falls

Longer-hair looks can be achieved by using a **fall**. These machine-made pieces are often hand finished at the front of the base where it attaches behind the hairline. Another variety, shown in Figure 12.3, is machine sewn onto a bandeau, or headband. This more casual look is finished by covering the seam with a colored headband or scarf. Falls come in several lengths from 10 to 26 inches. The amount of hair also varies from 5 to 10 ounces.

Switches

Long hairpieces that are wefted to a small base or attached to a loop in three strands are known as **switches** (see Figure 12.4). These long pieces are usually attached for a dramatic or evening look and can be styled as a braided ponytail, a chignon, or a French twist.

There are also many types of specialty curls and small hairpieces that can be clipped into place as needed. These are usually made must for fun and often are worn in contrasting colors. They can, however, be used to cover a specific problem area such as a patch of baldness. In those cases, the hairpiece is glued with spirit gum rather than clipped into place.

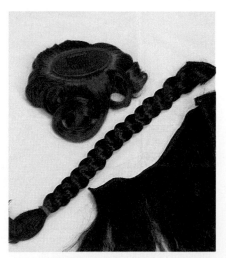

12.4 Switch

Toupees

Hairpieces that are custom designed to fit a man's pattern of baldness are known as **toupees**. These pieces are made to exactly fit the hairless area and are custom colored to match the client's remaining hair. Although these pieces were once almost exclusively human hair, synthetic hair is growing in popularity as the manufacturing methods make it look and feel more natural. Figure 12.5 shows samples of toupees.

Measuring and Fitting a Wig or Hairpiece

Proper fit of hairpieces and wigs is essential to achieve a natural look. Your clients will be more satisfied when wigs and hairpieces fit properly and feel comfortable.

Measuring for a Wig

To ensure a comfortable and secure fit, measure your client's head before ordering the wig. Machine-made wigs come in few sizes, the most common cap size is 22 inches. Petite and extra-large wigs are also available. Measuring your client will help you greatly when you begin to adjust the wig after it is purchased. Custom-made wigs are manufactured to the exact specifications that you give.

Materials

Cape	Measuring tape
Towel or neck strip	Record card and pen
Brush	Haircutting shears
Bobby pins	Scotch tape

Procedure for Measuring

1. Seat your client comfortably at your styling station.
2. Sanitize your hands.
3. Drape your client.
4. Brush your client's hair back and away from the face. Secure with pins so that the hair will be as flat to the scalp as possible and away from the hairline. If the hair in the back is medium length or longer, brush it up and toward the crown. Twist the hair into a roll up the back and secure as flat as possible at the crown.
5. Measure the **circumference** (the distance around) of the head with a tape measure. Place the end of the tape measure slightly behind the front hairline. Wrap the tape around the head, above the ears, and below the bulge of the occipital bone in the back of the head (see Figure 12.6). Record this measurement on your record card.

> ◆ **Key Point** ◆
> Hairpieces come in a variety of sizes and shapes for every need and occasion. Hairpieces are styled with and into the client's own hair for the most natural look.

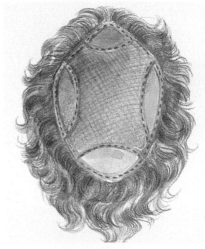

12.5a

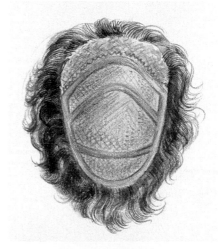

12.5b

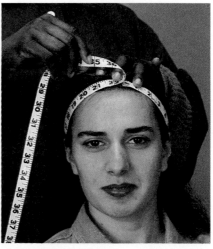

12.6 Around the head

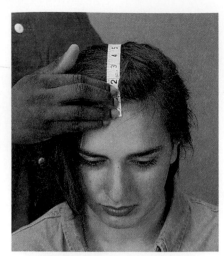

12.7   Front to back

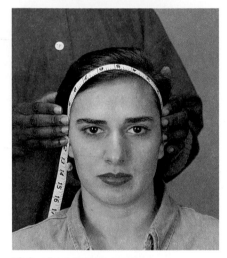

12.8   Front hairline length

6. Measure the distance from the center front hairline straight back to the center of the nape hairline (Figure 12.7). Record this for the volume of the wig.

7. Measure from ear to ear just behind the front hairline as in Figure 12.8 and record.

8. Next, measure from ear to ear, across the top of the head (see Figure 12.9). Your tape should stop about $\frac{1}{2}$ inch above each ear.

9. Last, measure the back hairline across the nape of the neck (Figure 12.10). This is a very important measurement for you to record because this is where you will most often make adjustments to your client's wig.

10. Clip a very small sample from the front, the side, and the back of your client's hair. Attach these samples to the record card and clearly mark from where each was cut. If the wig is to be custom made, you will include these with your order so the wig can be properly matched. If you are ordering a machine made wig, you will most likely order the color swatch closest to that of your client's natural hair color. The color ring is shown in Figure 12.11. Keep the samples with the record card to adjust the color as necessary to suit your client.

11. If your order is for a custom made wig, you will also record details of styling such as the location of the part, bangs, length, and quantity of hair.

12. Send a copy of the record card with your order and file the original until your client's wig arrives. You can then make the basic adjustments necessary before the client arrives for a fitting.

Fitting a Wig

Once the wig arrives, you will want to schedule your client for a fitting. Determine whether the client will leave the salon wearing the new wig, or would prefer styling of the natural hair following the fitting.

Carefully drape your client before fitting the wig. Brush the hair back and away from the hairline, pinning it as you did when measuring. You may also choose to secure the hair under a fine mesh net.

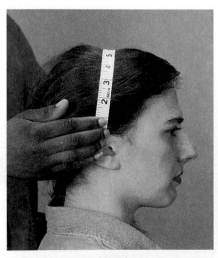

12.9   Across top of head

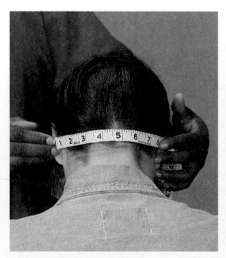

12.10   Hairline at nape

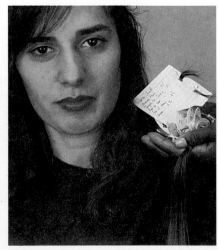

12.11

Place the front of the wig at the client's front hairline. Hold the wig at the hairline with one hand and with the other, pull the wig securely down and back to the nape. Adjust both sides, making sure that the ear tab is in place at the temple and that the client's ears are free. Run your index finger under the front edge of the wig so that the bangs are free and the edge is flat and smooth. Comb and adjust the style on the client for the best results.

Adjusting a Wig

Machine made wigs can be adjusted for a better fit. A wig should fit snugly, but should not bind. The most common adjustment is to the elastic strip located at the nape of the neck (see Figure 12.12). Today's wigs feature a small plastic hook that can be inserted into the correct slot for a smooth, snug fit. If further adjustment is necessary, you may need to take tucks in the wig. Refer to the measurements that you have recorded on the client's card and loosely sew tucks as necessary in the back or at the sides (see Figures 12.13 and 12.14). After you have retried the wig to ensure that the fit is correct, permanently sew the tuck, keeping the seam as smooth and flat as possible. Fold tucks up at the top of the head and down at the sides for the best fit.

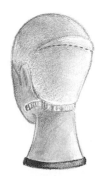

12.12   Elastic strip at nape

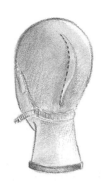

12.13   Tuck sewn in back

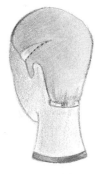

12.14   Tuck sewn in side

Blocking

Human hair wigs can be stretched or shrunken slightly. Only very minor adjustments should be made by this method and it is only effective when the cap of the wig is made primarily of cotton. This method, known as **blocking**, adjusts the size of the wig temporarily. The procedure that follows lists the most common method of blocking a wig to size.

Materials

Towels	Grease pencil or magic marker
Canvas wig block	T-pins (T-shaped pins)
Plastic bag	Completed record card

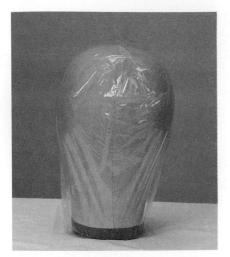

12.15   Canvas wig block

Procedure for Blocking

1. Referring to your client's record card, select a canvas wig block (a head form covered with cloth) whose size is the closest to the circumference measurements recorded (Figure 12.15).
2. Cover the wig block with a plastic bag and secure at the back.
3. According to your record-card measurements, mark where the hairline of the wig should be placed for a proper fit.
4. Turn the wig inside out and spray the cap thoroughly with warm water (Figure 12.16). Completely saturate the cap. Allow the excess water to run off.
5. Fold the wig in half, then fold in half again, and squeeze gently (Figure 12.17).
6. Open the wig so that it can lie flat against a towel. Place it on the towel, a few inches from the edge.
7. Fold the edge of the towel over the wig then roll the wig in the towel (Figure 12.18). Apply gentle pressure to remove as much water as possible without distorting the shape of the wig.
8. Pin the wig on the block with T-pins at the front, side, and back markings. Secure the crown with T-pins and add additional pins along the hairline.
9. Proceed with styling and drying.

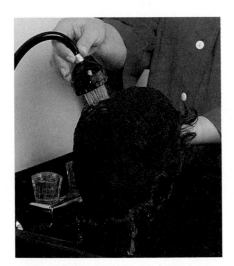

12.16   Spray cap with warm water

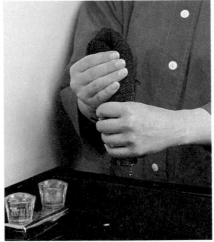

12.17   Squeeze gently

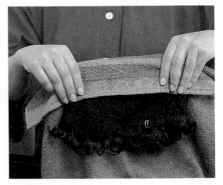

12.18

Removing a Wig

To remove a wig from your client, first check that no hair pins have been used at the edges to secure it. Then simply grasp the front hairline of the wig while holding the back in place. Simply move the wig up and away from the face, sliding it off the back neckline. Store the wig on a styrofoam® headblock.

Choosing and Attaching a Wiglet

It is quite simple to determine the correct hairpiece to order for women by the style desired. When you are considering a wiglet to cover a thinning area, the base of the piece ordered should be just slightly larger than the area to be covered. That way, you can use some of the normal hair surrounding the area to make a base to which you will secure the wiglet. Balding is unusual in women. More common is the thinning of the hair at the top of the head. A wig is the best solution for thinning that gradually occurs all over the head. There are very rare cases where a woman might have pattern baldness. In those cases you may choose to use the toupee techniques discussed next or refer to the weaving section of this chapter.

Attaching a wiglet is quite easy. Most have a comb attached at the front of the base to provide a secure fit. To attach the hairpiece, first make a large pin curl in the crown and fasten with bobby pins. Slip the hairpiece comb under the pin curl and fasten the base of the hairpiece with additional pins.

Making a Toupee Pattern

For a man's hairpiece or toupee to look natural, the measurement and ordering are critical. You will want to cover the bald spot exactly, without having the base of the toupee cover any of the remaining hair. As a specialist, you will eventually be able to do this with tape measurements alone. To begin building that expertise, let's see how to make a pattern.

Materials

Plastic wrap	Tape measure
Scotch tape	Cape
Marker	Neck strip
Haircutting shears	

Procedure for Making a Toupee Pattern

1. First, sanitize your hands.
2. Seat your client comfortably.
3. Drape the client.
4. Tear off about 2 feet of plastic wrap and place on top of your client's head. Twist the ends to conform as much as possible to the shape of the head. Either have your client hold the ends or clip them firmly to the remaining natural hair.
5. Take strips of adhesive tape (the type with a dull surface is better for writing), and completely cover the bald area (Figure 12.19). Try precutting the strips to the approximate length of the area to be covered by hair. Have strips ready and adhered to the edge of your station.
6. Determine where the front of the hairpiece should be. Make a dot with the marker in the center front on the plastic wrap (Figure 12.20).

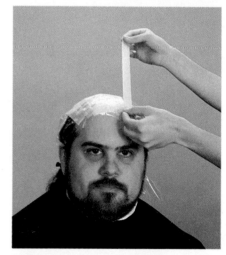

12.19   Apply tape over plastic

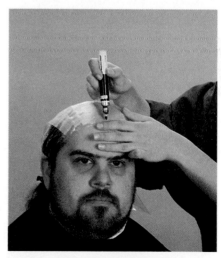

12.20   Mark front of hairpiece

CLIENT TIP ◆◆◆◆◆◆◆

For a front hairline to look natural, it should not be too low. As a general rule, place three fingers above the eyebrow, directly in line with the center of the nose.

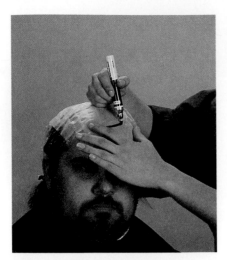

12.21 Connect dots with marker

7. Mark a dot on each side, at the front hairline where the piece will meet the client's own hair.
8. Make dots at the back of the bald spot, straight back from the nose, and at each side where the piece will blend with the client's own substantial growth.
9. Connect the dots by drawing a curving line with the marker as in Figure 12.21. Ignore minor growth and sparse areas as you mark this perimeter of substantial growth.
10. Mark the front and the back of the pattern and remove it from your client's head. Cut around the edges with scissors, replace over bald area to check that it covers all of the area desired but does not overlap normal hair growth.
11. Cut small samples of the client's hair from the side and back. Clearly mark them and attach to the sample as shown in Figure 12.22.

Send this pattern off with your order, specifying the type of hairpiece you want. For example, a lace-front toupee often looks more natural, especially if the hair is styled off the face. You can also specify that the piece be made with a side part if your client prefers. A flesh-toned plastic is inserted and the hair is sewn in the proper directions.

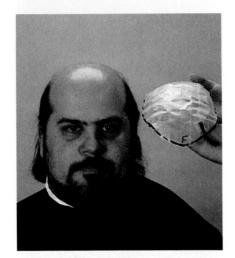

12.22 Finished pattern

Applying a Hairpiece

When the hairpiece arrives, double-check that all the specifics of your order have been met. Then, schedule your client for a styling session. You will want to shampoo the hair, apply the toupee, custom cut as necessary, and style.

Materials

Cape and neck strip	Spirit gum	Alcohol
Haircutting implements	Small applicator brush	Blow dryer
Comb, styling brush	Solvent	Shampoo
Double-sided hair tape	Cotton	Towels, one lint-free

Procedure for Applying a Hairpiece

1. Sanitize your hands.
2. Seat and drape client.
3. Shampoo hair, trim if necessary, and blow dry.
4. Remove any surface oils from the bald area with cotton dampened with alcohol.
5. Remove any fine hairs on scalp where tape or lace is to be attached. Your instructor will advise you about the best method of hair removal for your clients.
6. Attach strips of double-sided tape to reinforced parts of the foundation at front, sides, and back (Figure 12.23).

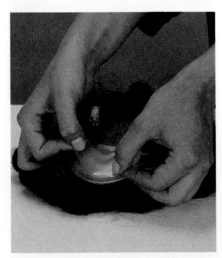

12.23 Apply toupee tape

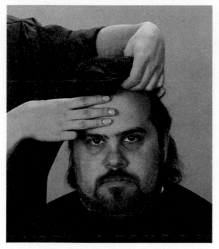

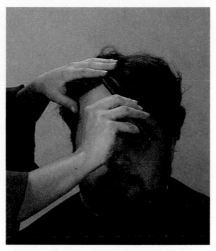

12.24   Apply hairpiece   12.25   Styling a toupee

7. Establish the desired front hairline by again placing three fingers above the eyebrows. Press front of hairpiece firmly into place (Figure 12.24).
8. Press the other taped areas firmly into place with a rolling motion.
9. Cut, taper, and blend the hairpiece into the client's own hair. (Figure 12.25).

Procedure to Apply a Lace-Front Toupee

Lace-front toupees should be applied in the following manner for best results. Do not apply tape directly on a lace-front toupee. Instead, follow steps 1 through 5 of the preceding procedure, then do as follows:

6. Attach tape strips to the sides and back at reinforced areas. Trim lace at front to within ¼ inch of the hairline (Figure 12.26).
7. Establish front hairline location.
8. Lift lace and brush spirit gum sparingly on scalp immediately under base. When gum is tacky, press down the lace with a moist linen cloth.
9. Cut, taper, and blend as necessary to create the desired style.

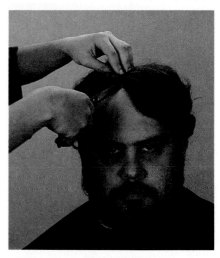

12.26   Trimming the lace front

Removing a Hairpiece

To remove a client's hairpiece, simply insert fingers under the base, where tape was applied. Lift up and back, away from the face. To remove a lace-front toupee, soften the spirit gum under the lace by applying solvent with cotton or a brush. Allow the solvent to loosen the hairpiece from the scalp, do not pull or stretch the lace.

> ◆ **Key Point** ◆
> When measuring for a hairpiece, make sure that the entire bald and receding area is covered until you reach an area of substantial hair growth. Before applying the hairpiece, shave any stray tufts of hair from the area to be covered to ensure your client's comfort.

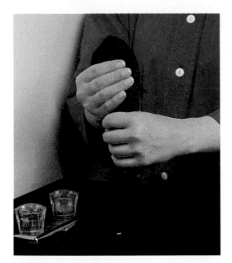
12.27 Rinse wig

CARE AND MAINTENANCE OF WIGS AND HAIRPIECES

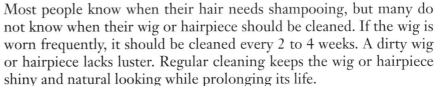

With the correct care, wigs and hairpieces can offer clients years of trouble-free convenience. Human-hair wigs usually last longer than the synthetic ones, which is part of the reason they cost more. However, if they are not properly cared for, they will be short-lived and very expensive.

Proper care and maintenance of wigs and hairpieces involves cleaning, conditioning, shaping, styling, and coloring. Synthetic wigs do not need and will not absorb conditioning treatments, nor can they be treated with any chemical service.

Cleaning

Most people know when their hair needs shampooing, but many do not know when their wig or hairpiece should be cleaned. If the wig is worn frequently, it should be cleaned every 2 to 4 weeks. A dirty wig or hairpiece lacks luster. Regular cleaning keeps the wig or hairpiece shiny and natural looking while prolonging its life.

Synthetic hair goods should be shampooed in cool water with a mild shampoo that has been diluted. Care should be taken that the wig is not rubbed, but that you use your fingers to gently separate the strands and work the shampoo through all of the hair fibers. With your fingers, gently cleanse the hairline band, especially at the front, to remove oil and makeup. Clean the wig in a large glass bowl so you can dip and swirl the wig to improve cleansing without damaging the wefting.

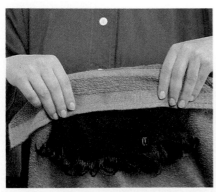
12.28 Gently squeeze wig

To rinse a wig, gently turn it inside out (Figure 12.27). Use lower pressure and cold water to thoroughly rinse the wig. When rinsing longer hairpieces, first thoroughly rinse the base from underneath, then follow the hair from the base to the ends to ensure that all the shampoo is removed.

Let excess water run from the wig, then fold it in half. Fold in half again and gently squeeze (Figure 12.28). Unfold the wig to half and lay the wig on a towel. Fold the edge of the towel over the wig, continue to roll, and press out excess water gently (Figure 12.29). Do not wring. Remove the towel and shake the wig gently so the preset curls will fall into place. Place the wig on a plastic-covered wig block. Using the T-pins, anchor the wig to the block at the ear tabs, in the center of the back, and at the front hairline. Let the hair completely dry **without heat** for 48 hours. Then simply brush the hair into its preset style. Do not use hair spray on a synthetic wig.

Human hair can be cleaned with acid-balanced shampoos designed for chemically treated hair. Some manufacturers still recommend that human hair wigs be cleaned with a special cleanser.

12.29 Fold towel over wig

Use special caution with a **liquid dry cleaner** as the chemicals are irritating to the skin and the fumes should not be inhaled. Always wear gloves and work in a well-ventilated area. Better yet, consider alternate cleansing solutions that are safer. Follow your manufacturer's directions for best results.

Conditioning Wigs and Hairpieces

Synthetic hair goods should not be conditioned. Since the fiber cannot absorb the conditioner, the ingredients will build up on the surface and dull the wig.

Human hair goods need both protein and moisture conditioning with each cleansing, especially if a dry cleanser is used. After the hair is rinsed and blotted, apply a small amount of conditioner and work it through the hair. You may choose to spray a liquid formula for ease of application. In either case, select a conditioner that can be left in the hair. Do not overuse the product or the hair will be dull and lifeless and lose its set rapidly.

Shaping Wigs and Hairpieces

Ideally, all hair shaping should be done when the customer is wearing the wig or hairpiece. Mistakes made on a wig are permanent in nature. Take special caution where the wig blends into the customer's own hair and around the hairline. Remember that the band of a wig sits just behind the hairline so that bangs and face line hair should be left longer.

Today's wigs are much more natural looking, but they still have too much hair sometimes. This "wiggy" look can be eliminated by careful use of thinning techniques. Again, use care as the hair will not grow back! Your instructor will guide you in the best techniques to avoid any lines within the hairpiece.

Styling Wigs and Hairpieces

Synthetic hair goods do not have to be styled. The selected style is permanently set into the hair. You can refresh that style in an older wig by drying (without heat please) the hair on rollers one size smaller than the curl you wish. If you work with theatrical pieces, you will learn techniques with limited heat that can also alter the style of synthetic pieces.

Human hair goods require setting each time they are cleaned. While you can achieve virtually any style you choose, a few precautions will help you avoid problems. See Chapter 10 for a complete study of setting techniques.

1. Carefully plan the front hairline to avoid splits. Unless you plan to use the client's front hair, the wig should always be styled with soft forward shapings that extend just beyond the wig cap.

2. Use arc-shaped bases at the hairline to avoid splits. Clip rollers at the back of the roller, away from the face. Use pin curls at the side and nape hairlines. With all clips, use care not to damage the wefting or netting.

3. Use a softer setting lotion so the wig does not set too tightly.

Coloring a Wig or Hairpiece

Only human hair goods can receive any chemical service, and then special cautions should be taken. It is usually more effective to work with temporary or semipermanent tints. If a permanent tint is selected, strand-test very carefully because wigs will take color and process faster than you might expect. Use special care to avoid getting color material on the base; it will permanently stain it and weaken the stitching. It is not recommended that a wig or hairpiece be lightened.

> ◆ **Key Point** ◆
>
> Today's wigs are easy to clean with diluted shampoo of good quality. Always make sure that the wig is thoroughly rinsed so the hair does not become dull.

SPECIAL EFFECTS WITH ARTIFICIAL HAIR

Many special effects can be obtained with artificial hair. All of the areas briefly discussed here are opportunities you could have with advanced training.

Weaving

Weaving is a special technique with many applications. It can be used to camouflage thinning or balding hair. It is a service frequently used by performers to give their hair dramatic effects. When the natural hair has been severely damaged or pulled from the scalp, weaves can provide a useful cover-up while the client's hair grows back.

Weaving involves the sewing or gluing of wefts of hair in tracks of the client's own hair. Most professionals prefer sewing-in the tracks if the purpose of the weave is to let the client's own hair regrow

Materials

Hair wefts	Brush
Shears	Curved needle
Clips	Cotton thread
Comb	

Procedure for Weaving

1. Cut wefts of hair slightly longer than the parting where you will attach the hair.
2. Lay the first "track" by making a tiny French braid all along the part (Figure 12.30).

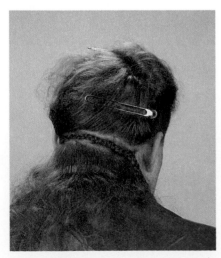

12.30 Track

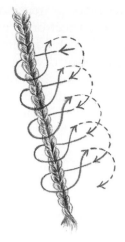

12.31 Lock-stitch

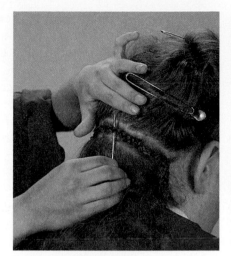

12.32 Lock-stitch in track

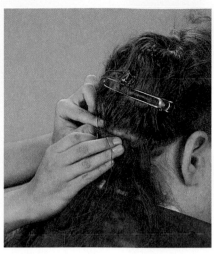

12.33 Attach weft

3. Secure the braid by lock-stitching the braid with cotton thread and a curved needle (Figure 12.31). To lock-stitch, insert the needle behind the braid at the bottom and push up around the braid. With the index finger of your free hand, hold the thread to make a loop. Bring the needle back over the braid and through the loop with every stitch. Work from side to side, securing the end of the track with a knot (Figure 12.32).

4. Attach the weft by stitching it to the track (Figure 12.33). Work from side to side, using a blind stitch. Knot securely. Work back across in the opposite direction, crossing your stitches. Knot the thread and cut off excess.

5. Continue to lay tracks and attach wefts until the desired amount of hair is obtained.

Both synthetic and human hair is available for weaving, but human hair is usually preferred. Human hair gives the stylability required and looks much more natural.

Extensions

Extensions are also used to increase the length and volume of the hair. The added hair, however, extends the natural hair in a particular style. Extensions can be sewn onto the client's hair, but are more commonly braided in or woven into coils, usually for ethnic styling. Caution must be used in extensions for young children, as excess tension can cause baldness around the hairline. This traction baldness, caused by pulling, is common if extensions are not properly applied.

Hair Ornamentation

Competition or show work that is done on a platform could very well introduce you to the artistry of hair as ornamentation. Flowers, bows, and garlands made of hair can be used to create intricate hairstyles.

> ◆ **Key Point** ◆
>
> Special effects can be created either as a corrective or an ornamental technique. All special effects with artificial hair will require that you receive specialized training. Practice until your fingers are very limber and you can add hair so smoothly that the seam between natural and artificial hair cannot be seen.

SUMMARY

Wigs come and go as fashion statements. Hairpieces, extensions, and weaves will always be used in some manner to correct or to camouflage undesirable hair loss. As a cosmetologist skilled in the techniques of artificial hair, you must be able to measure, color-match, and fit the artificial hair to the area needing to be covered. You must properly attach the appropriate hairpiece with the greatest comfort to the client. You must also be able to clean and style the artificial hair and explain to your client what he or she must do to maintain the hair between visits.

QUESTIONS

1. For what reasons do people wear wigs?
2. What are the two main methods of wig construction? What are the two most common materials used in the making of wigs?
3. What types of hairpieces are available?
4. What is the primary purpose for each type of hairpiece?
5. How would you measure a client for a wig? How would you fit the wig?
6. How do you make a toupee pattern?
7. How do you specify color for a toupee? How do you attach it?
8. What are the basic steps for maintaining a synthetic wig?
9. How do you care for human-hair wigs?
10. What is the purpose of special-effects hair additions?
11. What are three different hair additions in style today?

PROJECTS

1. Analyze the hair of three different wigs to determine whether they are made of human or synthetic hair. Explain your answer.
2. Measure three people for wigs, noting measurements and color samples on record cards.
3. Using construction paper, create balding areas of various shapes and attach them to mannequins. Then, measure for, and make patterns for toupees.
4. Check to see if there is a "Look Good...Feel Better" program available in your community. Report back to the class on the benefits available to patients and the process by which a stylist can become certified in the program.
5. Braid tracks and attach wefting to your mannequin until your instructor indicates you have reached salon mastery.

CHEMISTRY FOR COSMETOLOGISTS

CHAPTER GOAL

The basic chemistry of hair, skin, and nails is the fabric on which you perform salon services. After reading this chapter and completing the projects, you should be able to

1. Define key terms of the science of chemistry.
2. Explain the two types of chemical bonds that occur.
3. Outline the differences between physical and chemical changes and give examples.
4. Describe the characteristic that makes water unique. List at least three ways you take advantage of this characteristic every day in the salon.
5. Outline the importance of pH to a professional cosmetologist.
6. Describe the chemical structure of the hair, listing the six bonds found in the hair and the function of each.
7. Explain how chemistry makes hairstyling possible.
8. List the four basic chemical services offered in the salon and briefly explain the activity of each.
9. List at least six categories of chemical agents used in the salon and describe their functions.

The study of cosmetic chemistry grew from the industries creating materials for clothing. The most similar protein to hair is wool. The huge industry for wool processing, based in Australia, has provided valuable research. Cosmetic chemists have been able to adapt those findings for human hair to produce permanent waves, hair color, lighteners, shampoos, and conditioners. Similarly, study of the tanning of leather lead to original formulas for skin care products. Later developments have come from the medical and especially dermatological professions.

What does chemistry have to do with your study of cosmetology? Why should you learn chemistry? As a cosmetologist, you will be mixing ingredients and watching for chemical reactions during salon services. You also will be recommending products to your clients that will help them maintain their nails, skin, and hair at home. Knowledge of chemistry will help you understand the structure of hair, nails, and skin as well as guide you in the safe use of products in the salon. That means you will be able to anticipate problems and have more success with your services. Chemistry will be another important tool that you can use to meet your client's needs. So, why should you learn chemistry? Only to be successful, to be a cut above, to give yourself a competitive edge in today's progressive salon.

The Science of Chemistry

Before we begin to study chemistry, let's take a moment to see just what it is. We've heard chemistry is hard to understand, but is that really true? Very simply, **chemistry** is the study of matter—its composition, structure, and properties—and the changes it may undergo. The key in our definition is **change**, as this is what gives us the ability to alter the properties of matter. And what is matter? **Matter** is anything that occupies space and has weight.

Matter Makes the World Around Us

Look around right where you are reading this. You will see many things and they are all matter: the desk, your chair, this book, even you! Chemists group matter into three major categories: solids, liquids, and gas.

Solids have definite weight, volume, and shape. Take your desk as an example. It weighs a certain amount. It has volume, or takes up space, which you would know if you walk into it. Lastly, your desk has a definite shape. There probably is a flat top, and legs to keep it stable. Other examples of solids would be scissors, hair, and permanent-wave rods.

Liquids have a definite weight and volume, but they have an indefinite shape. Pour water into a glass and you notice that it has weight. It has volume—it will take up space in the glass—but it does not have definite shape. It will take on the shape of the glass into which you pour it. When you pour water, it will run until it is either blocked or absorbed by a solid. You'll work with many liquids in the salon: shampoos, permanent-wave lotion, nail polish, and hair color.

Gases have definite weight. The volume and shape of a gas are indefinite. Blow out your breath and you can see that your breath does not have shape nor does it occupy a certain area of space. But if you blow into a balloon, your breath will take on the size and the shape of that balloon. We use gases in the salon to propel liquids, for example, the agent in an aerosol activator for acrylic nails or the air forced through your pump hair spray when you push down with your finger.

The Basic Building Blocks of Matter

All forms of matter have components or parts. The simplest form of matter that exists is called an **element**. Elements are stable and cannot be broken down into any simpler substance. There are over a hundred different elements. Some of the more common ones are gold, silver, copper, and neon. Each element in the chart (see Figure 13.1 on the next page) is assigned a symbol, a sort of chemical shorthand. The more important elements found in the human body and their symbols are listed for you in Table 13.1.

TABLE 13.1   Some Important Elements in the Human Body

Element	Symbol
Oxygen	O
Carbon	C
Hydrogen	H
Nitrogen	N
Chlorine	Cl
Sodium	Na
Sulfur	S

An **Atom** is the smallest part of an element. An atom can be broken into smaller pieces, but when this happens it no longer exhibits properties of the element.

Periodic Chart of the Elements

Group	1A	2A	3B	4B	5B	6B	7B		8B		1B	2B	3A	4A	5A	6A	7A	INERT GASSES
Period 1	1 H 1.01																	2 He 4.00
2	3 Li 6.94	4 Be 9.01											5 B 10.81	6 C 12.01	7 N 14.01	8 O 15.99	9 F 18.99	10 Ne 20.18
3	19 Na 39.10	19 Mg 39.10											13 Al 26.98	14 Si 28.09	15 P 30.97	16 S 32.06	17 Cl 35.45	18 Ar 39.95
4	19 K 39.10	20 Ca 40.08	21 Sc 44.96	22 Ti 47.90	23 V 50.94	24 Cr 51.99	25 Mn 54.94	26 Fe 55.85	27 Co 58.93	28 Ni 58.70	29 Cu 63.55	30 Zn 65.38	31 Ga 69.72	32 Ge 72.59	33 As 74.92	34 Se 78.96	35 Br 79.90	36 Kr 83.80
5	37 Rb 85.45	38 Sr 87.62	39 Y 88.91	40 Zr 91.22	41 Nb 92.91	42 Mo 95.94	43 Tc (97)	44 Ru 101.07	45 Rh 102.91	46 Pd 106.4	47 Ag 107.87	48 Cd 112.41	49 In 114.82	50 Sn 118.69	51 Sb 121.75	52 Te 127.60	53 I 126.90	54 Xe 131.30
6	55 Cs 132.91	56 Ba 137.33	57 La 138.91	72 Hf 178.49	73 Ta 180.95	74 W 183.85	75 Re 186.21	76 Os 190.2	77 Ir 192.22	78 Pt 195.09	79 Au 196.97	80 Hg 200.59	81 Ti 204.37	82 Pd 207.2	83 Bi 208.98	84 Po (209)	85 At (210)	86 Rn (222)
7	87 Fr (223)	88 Ra 226.03	89 Ac (227)	104 Ku (260)	105 Ha (260)													

58 Ce 140.12	59 Pr 140.91	60 Nd 144.24	61 Pm (145)(147)	62 Sm 150.4	63 Eu 151.96	64 Gd 157.35	65 Tb 158.93	66 Dy 162.50	67 Ho 164.93	68 Er 167.26	69 Tm 168.93	70 Yb 173.04	71 Lu 174.97
90 Th 232.04	91 Pa 231.04	92 U 238.03	93 Np 237.05	94 Pu (2)	95 Am (243)	96 Cm (247)	97 Bk (247)	98 Cf (251)	99 Es (254)	100 Fm (257)	101 Md (258)	102 No (259)	103 Lr (2)

13.1

A **Molecule** is two or more atoms joined together by a chemical bond (Figure 13.2). If all the atoms are the same, the molecule is an element. Different atoms joined together become the smallest part of a compound.

Compounds are the result of the chemical combination of two or more elements. A compound is always an entirely new substance with properties of its own and is totally different from the original elements. As an example, think about the element hydrogen. It is represented by the symbol H and is a gas. Then consider oxygen, another gas represented by the symbol O. When these two elements are combined in the right proportions, two parts (or atoms) hydrogen to one part (or atom) oxygen, water is formed. Water, represented by the formula H_2O, is completely different from its parts. It is a liquid now with properties of its own. It is very important that we understand how this joining together of atoms works. So let's analyze it deeper.

Structure of the Atom

Even the tiny atom can be broken down into smaller parts or pieces. But as we have just learned, the identity of that atom as an element is gone once it is broken down. We'll take a brief look at the parts of the atom here. We don't intend to be chemists; we intend to be cosmetologists. But by understanding how atoms work—how they combine with other atoms to make substances we work with every day and how they can change a substance like hair—we can understand how to change the properties of the hair to satisfy our clients.

Atoms have three basic parts: **protons**, **neutrons**, and **electrons**. Each part of an atom gives it special properties.

Protons are found in the center, or nucleus of the atom. They have a positive electrical charge. It is the proton, or the number of protons, that identifies the atom. If it has one proton, it is hydrogen; if it has eight, it is oxygen, and so on. Look again at the chart of the elements in Figure 13.1 and you will see the atomic numbers at the top of each box. Locate the protons in Figures 13.3 and 13.4.

Neutrons are also found in the nucleus of the atom. They have no electrical charge. A chemist will combine the protons and the neutrons to find the weight of an atom. This is called the molecular weight. Molecular weight is important to us as cosmetologists. We need to know if a conditioner, for example, has small enough molecules to penetrate the hair and repair it, or if it will only coat the cuticle to make it feel smooth.

Electrons are the smallest part of an atom. They are located in orbits or shells (Figures 13.3 and 13.4). Electrons are in constant motion within those shells, circling around the nucleus. They have a negative electrical charge. It is the electron that gives the atom its ability to unite with other atoms. Chemists call this ability **valence** (**VAY** lens)—the combining capacity of an atom. The valence is determined by the electrons in the outermost orbit or shell. An atom will always try to complete its outer shell. When an atom gives up or gains an electron by transferring or by sharing it, bonding occurs.

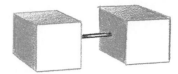

Molecule of like atoms

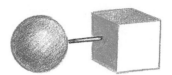

13.2   Molecule of different atoms

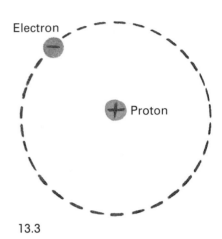

13.3

Electron

Proton

Nucleus

Electron shells

13.4

◆ **Key Point** ◆

Atoms have three parts. The positive protons identify the atom and give it an atomic number. The neutrons combined with the protons give it molecular weight. The negative electrons determine if it can combine with another atom.

CHEMICAL BONDS

When atoms join to form molecules, they are held together by forces known as **bonds**. All bonds are the result of a chemical reaction. This means that both atoms are changed and that the identity of each atom is lost and a new substance is made. The electrons will determine what type of bond is formed.

Covalent Bonds

Co means "together." A covalent bond occurs when atoms combine by sharing electrons in their outer shells. But why would atoms want to share electrons? Let's take a look at the most common covalent bond, water, to see why.

Hydrogen is a flammable gas. As we learned earlier, it has 1 proton with a positive charge. Hydrogen also has 1 electron with a negative charge. Electrons hold the key to the ability to bond because an atom will always try to fill its outer shell with all the electrons it can hold. The outer shell of hydrogen would be full with 2 electrons. Since hydrogen only has one electron, it will constantly try to gain a second or give up the electron it has.

Oxygen, also a gas and combustible, is a larger atom, having 8 protons, 8 neutrons, and 8 electrons. Its first shell holds 2 electrons, and its second shell would be full with 8. Since there are only 8 electrons total, the outer shell of oxygen has 6 electrons and needs 2 more to be complete.

When water is formed, one oxygen atom shares an electron with two hydrogen atoms as Figure 13.5 indicates. This completes the outer shells of all the atoms with the maximum number of electrons that they can hold. Since the electrons are shared, the bond is **covalent**, and quite strong. The chemical formula representing this union is H_2O. We can also see that the characteristics of each atom were lost in making this molecule. What used to be a flammable element (O) and a combustible element (H) have been combined into a completely non-flammable and noncombustible compound. What used to be two gases combined to create a liquid—one that is even used to put out fires. So we can see that the identity of each atom was lost and that a completely new substance—water—was formed with all new properties.

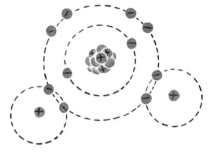

13.5   Water molecule

Ionic Bonds

An ionic bond occurs when electrons completely transfer from one type of atom to another. Remember that atoms are always trying to have complete outer shells. In covalent bonds, atoms complete their outer shells by sharing electrons. But in an ionic bond, electrons from one kind of atom are completely transferred to another atom. When an atom gains or loses electrons it becomes an **ion** (EYE on), or charged atom. Atoms that gain electrons become negatively charged and are called **anions**. Atoms that lose electrons become positively charged and are called **cations**. Positively and negatively charged atoms are attracted to each other. Since "opposites attract," the cation and anion are pulled together by their electrical charges and an ionic bond is formed. Ionic bonds commonly occur when salts are formed, so they are sometimes called salt bonds.

Sodium is an element represented by the shorthand Na. It has 11 protons (see Figure 13.6). When we look at the electrons in the outermost shell, we find only one. Since atoms are always trying to have a complete outer shell, sodium wants to give up its outermost electron. The electron is far from its nucleus, and since atoms are constantly in motion, this electron can easily be pulled from the atom altogether. When this happens, the sodium atom becomes a positively charged cation. But now, how did that electron get pulled from its orbit?

Consider chlorine (Figure 13.7), a gas that is represented by the shorthand Cl. It has 17 protons and neutrons in the nucleus. Seventeen electrons are arranged in three shells that orbit the nucleus. The outer shell of this atom, however, only contains 7 electrons and is constantly in search of an extra electron to complete its shell. Since it is so close to having a full shell, it can pull an electron into it. When that happens, it has more negative charges from its electrons than positive charges so the atom has a negative charge and is an anion.

Positive and negative charges attract one another. So the Cl$^-$ atom will unite with the Na$^+$ atom due to an exchange of electrons to complete the outer shells. What has just happened is another chemical change. A metal and a gas just combined to form a solid which we know as common table salt—NaCl (Figure 13.8).

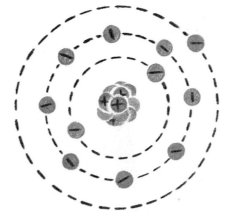

13.6   Sodium atom (Na)

THE POSSIBILITIES OF CHANGE

They say, "Love makes the world go round." They also say, "Nothing is constant except change." It is certain that change is what makes us love our cosmetology world because change is what makes it possible. When we add the fact that everyone seems to want what they don't have to the possibilities for change that chemistry provides, the exciting industry of cosmetology is created. Let's take a look at change and apply the technical terms we have just learned to our own chosen profession.

Some changes are temporary, others are permanent. In the world of chemistry these are referred to as **physical** and **chemical** changes.

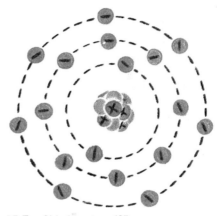

13.7   Chlorine atom (Cl)

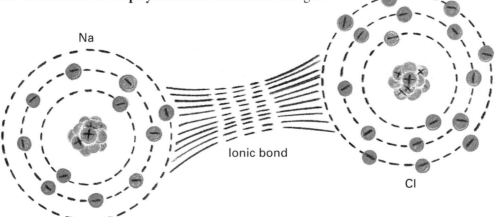

13.8   Table salt molecule (NaCl) forming

Physical Change

A physical, or temporary, change can occur when two different forms of matter are combined. This is known as a **mixture**. In a mixture, each component, or part of the mixture, retains its individual characteristics and can be separated back out of the formula. No bonding occurs during this temporary change. You can mix together, for example, vinegar and oil. Just after you shake the bottle, you have a nice salad dressing. If you let it stand for a short period of time, however, you will notice that the oil will separate and float to the top and the vinegar will stay at the bottom. Common mixtures that you will use in the salon are shampoos, conditioners, and setting lotions.

Another form of temporary, or physical, change occurs when we alter the state of matter. An ice cube is solid, for example. It is composed of H_2O. If we leave it out at room temperature, it will melt into the liquid form of water. And if we put it in a pot over a hot burner, it will change into the gaseous state—steam. Physical change occurs in the hair when we wet the hair with water, disturbing some of the bonds that we will discuss soon. After we shampoo the hair, we can blow it dry or set it into a certain shape or style. This physical change will last until the hair is again dampened, thus destroying our temporary change. In the salon, physical changes are those that you as a stylist can make without the aid of chemicals.

Chemical Change

A chemical change occurs when one substance is changed into an entirely different one. Bonding always occurs during this type of change as we saw in the example of common table salt formed from the bonding of the gas chlorine and the metal sodium. Another example of a chemical change would be baking a cake. You have a mixture of flour, water, eggs, and whatever else it takes to make your choice of cake. But then a chemical change takes place because you pour this liquid into a pan and place it in a hot oven. Once that cake is baked, there is nothing that you can do to turn it back into its ingredients. It is a chemical change that you might just as well eat!

In the salon, chemical changes are made in the interior layers of the hair. We use a chemical product to control the onset of these changes. These changes occur when we color, lighten, permanently wave, or chemically relax the hair; or when we mix the powder and liquid to build an acrylic nail.

Let's take a look at haircolor. If you have a client with gray hair, he or she probably wishes it wasn't there. What can you do? Well, you can mix haircolor of the correct shade with a developer, such as hydrogen peroxide. Hydrogen peroxide is known to chemists by the formula H_2O_2. If you look at the formula, you can see that it is a combination of water and oxygen. If this mixture is added to an alkali (a liquid with a pH above 7.0), or is exposed to heat or light, it will break down into its component parts. Hair tint is alkali, so when you mix the two together and put them on your client's hair, changes occur. First, the peroxide breaks down. The oxygen released, with all of its electron shells looking to complete themselves, combines with the pigment into a giant molecule that is trapped within the hair and permanently colors it. Voila! No gray hair! You have a happy client who pays you for looking younger so you can put gas in your car to go see a movie with your friends.

See how chemistry works?

CHEMISTRY OF WATER

Of all the chemical substances, water (H_2O) is the most abundant and probably the most important for a cosmetologist. As we discussed earlier, one molecule of water is made by covalent bonds— electrons shared between two atoms of hydrogen and one atom of oxygen.

In the special case of water, this sharing is not equal. The shared electrons are more strongly attracted to the oxygen atom, making it a little bit negative and the hydrogen atoms a little bit positive. This lopsidedness is called electrical **polarity** (poh **LAR** i tee) and it works much like a very weak magnet. Hydrogen atoms that are a little bit negative will attract other oxygen atoms that are a little bit positive and the whole situation results in a field of oxygen and hydrogen atoms that are constantly changing the electrical attractions among each other. This gives water the ability to dissolve things mixed in it.

So many of the products that we use can be dissolved by water that we call it the **universal solvent**. These special **hydrogen bonds** that result between different water molecules due to their polarity, hold water together in drops (see Figure 13.9). They also occur inside the hair as we will see shortly.

This characteristic of changing electrical charges, or polarity, makes water a very active chemical molecule. Molecules are always in motion, but the molecules of water are constantly changing between positive and negative poles. This makes water a perfect solvent, as

> ◆ **Key Point** ◆
>
> It is important to know the characteristics of the water in your area. If you live where the water is "hard," metallic ions are dissolved in the water. This can interfere with the ability of water to rinse products from the hair and can cause problems when perms or color react with the minerals in the water rather than with the hair.

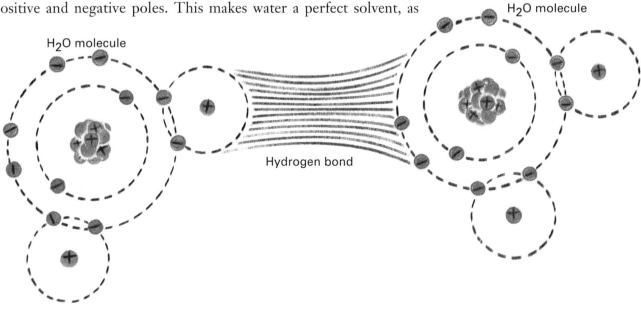

H₂O molecule

H₂O molecule

Hydrogen bond

13.9

the activity within the compound itself will dissolve many other substances. We take advantage of this characteristic to remove products from the hair, to dilute chemicals to their proper strength, and to carry chemical compounds inside the hair. Water is unique in that it will take on the positive or negative electrical charge of anything that is dissolved in it. This is especially important when we discuss pH, coming up next.

pH

What on earth do these two letters mean? We hear about pH all the time. One shampoo is supposed to be good for the hair because it is "pH balanced," while the other one is harsh because its pH is not. Chemicals used in salon services, such as relaxers, can be damaging because they have a high pH. What is this mystery pH, and why is it so important to what we do? Read on only if you want to be a top-notch stylist.

Actually, **pH** is the answer to a complicated chemical formula in which pH stands for **potential hydrogen**. It tells us the amount of acid that is present in any water-based liquid.

Because there are so many different kinds of substances, chemists have a tendency to group items that have similar characteristics. Acids are one such group. Acids all have similar characteristics: they taste sour, they harden, and they shrink and constrict other substances that they contact. A common example of an acid is lemon juice, with its tart, sour taste. Try biting into a lemon; it will certainly constrict your lips! Acids are commonly used in the salon as ingredients for instant conditioners to remove tangles from the hair, or as final rinses (known as acidifiers) to finish a chemical service.

An opposite group of substances, alkalis, have different properties. They soften, swell, and expand whatever they contact, and have a bitter taste (of course chemicals in the salon are never tested by taste). Common alkalies used to affect the interior layers of the hair are haircolor, relaxer, and permanent waves.

CLIENT T I P ◆◆◆◆◆◆

Hair tangles when its acid mantle is lost from harsh shampoos, etc., making the hair alkaline. The cuticle will lift and catch on other hair. Fix the problem by using an acid rinse, which restores the pH mantle and lightly coats the cuticle to make it smooth.

The pH Scale

The **pH scale** is used to determine the strength of acids present in a water solution. Even though the alkali content cannot be measured by pH, it can be deduced by knowing the acid content. **Both acid and alkali are always present in anything dissolved in water because of its polarity.**

The pH scale measures the concentration of **hydronium** (high **DROH** nee uhm) or acid H_3O^+ ions in water. The scale ranges from 0.0, having the highest concentration of acid, to 14.0, having the least. The center of the scale is chemically neutral, having equal amounts of acid and alkali. Pure water is neutral. The hair itself has no pH since it is a solid, but the **protective mantle** of the hair has a pH that ranges from 4.5 to 5.5 on the scale (see Figure 13.10).

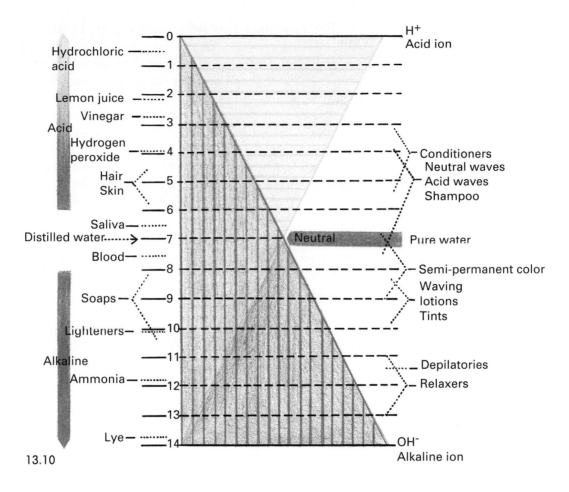

13.10

Anything that you apply to the hair that is below 4.5 will act as an acid. It will harden, constrict, and shrink the hair. Anything that you apply that is above 5.5 will act as an alkali and soften, swell, and expand the hair. The protective mantle of the hair should be returned to a pH of 4.5 to 5.5 after any service that you offer. This will make your services last longer and will make your client's hair more manageable.

pH and Cosmetology

pH, then, becomes another tool to use in the salon to achieve the results you and your customer want. If you need to affect the interior of the hair (for example, changing the curl or the color), use an alkaline product. If, on the other hand, you want to correct damage from chemical services or protect the outside layer of the hair, choose an acidic product. It is also important to know the ingredients of products you use in addition to their pH. If you know both, you are well on your way to fame, fortune and—well at least your license and a position in a good salon.

Water, as we mentioned previously, is very important to pH. First of all, we cannot measure the degree of acidity without water. Hair, which is a solid, has no pH that we can measure. If the hair is dampened, however, we can test the pH of the protective mantle of the hair or of the conditioning and styling products that are on it. **Because water is the universal solvent, it will take on the pH of whatever you mix into it.**

> ### ◆ Key Point ◆
> The normal range of pH for the hair and skin is 4.5 to 5.5. To change the surface, you often use a lower pH. To change the interior, you choose a higher pH. Always finish salon services by ensuring that the protective pH, 4.5 to 5.5, has been returned.

The last thing that we should say about pH is that chemists count each increment, or measure, of pH in multiples of 10. This means that the difference between 4.5 and 5.5, the normal range to protect the hair, is not one but ten! In other words, a pH of 4.5 is 10 times more acidic than a pH of 5.5. A permanent wave (Figure 9.2–9.4) is not a difference of four from the normal pH of hair, but a difference of 10x10x10x10 or 10,000. No wonder hair is more prone to tangling after a perm—unless, of course, you know what to do about it. Returning the hair to its protective pH and telling your client how to care for the hair at home can make the difference between chemical damage and chemical success.

THE CHEMICAL STRUCTURE THAT IS HAIR

The chemical definitions, categories, and conditions can be applied to the subjects you really want to learn about—hair, skin, and nails.

The protein of hair, skin, and nails is made up of a number of elements. Sulfur, nitrogen, oxygen, carbon, and hydrogen are present in the greatest amounts. Hair is a solid, protected by liquids with a pH of 4.5 to 5.5. It is the bonding between atoms that makes up a very complex chemical structure of the human body. Since these proteins are going to affect your livelihood, let's take a closer look and see what they really are all about.

The Building Blocks of Protein

Hair and nails are composed of a protein called keratin. Skin is a softer protein, known as collagen. All proteins are built from amino acids, and the protein of hair—keratin—contains over a dozen different amino acids. These amino acids join together, by covalent bonding, to form the unique structure of hair. That bonding gives hair its properties. Adjusting the bond chemically allows us to change those properties according to our clients' whims and fancies.

Peptide Bonds

When the hair begins to form within the follicle, two amino acids bond together. They form a **peptide (PEP** tide) bond (Figure 13.11). Whenever this happens, one molecule of water is lost, so that the hair becomes more dehydrated, or keratinized.

The second type of bond to be formed as the hair moves up the follicle is the **polypeptide** bond (Figure 13.12). The prefix *poly* means "many." This is a bond that connects many peptides lengthwise in a chain. Long chains of thousands of amino acids can be formed in this way.

As the newly formed chains move up through the hair follicle, further bonding occurs. Each time a bond is formed, one molecule of water is lost so that the hair becomes harder as it goes. It also forms into a special configuration called a **helix (HEE** licks) (see Figure

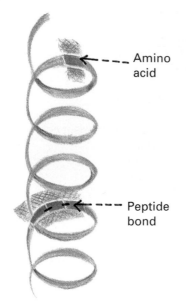

13.11 Peptide bonds

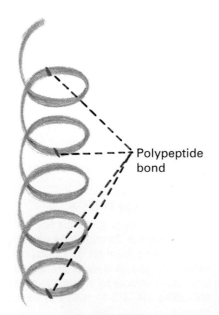

13.12 Polypeptide bonds

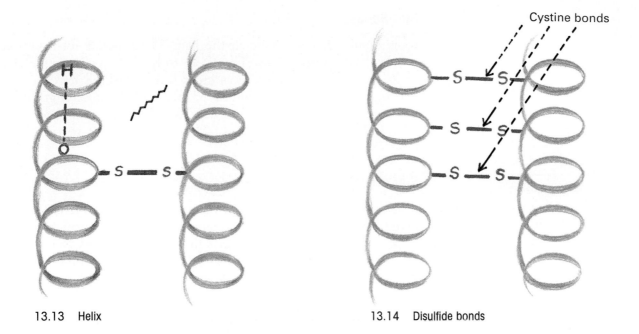

13.13   Helix

13.14   Disulfide bonds

13.13). A helix is a spiral shape with a straight backbone, like a spiral staircase or the back of your spiral notebook.

This spiral makes the finished hair very strong. It also permits bonding to occur across the polypeptide chains, much like rungs on a ladder.

Disulfide Bond

One bond that occurs across polypeptide chains is the **disulfide** (die **SUHL** fide) bond. In Figure 13.14, the disulfide bond has a cross-link occurring between an atom of sulfur on one polypeptide chain and an atom of sulfur on another. The bond forms the amino acid **cystine** (sis **TEEN**). Because it occurs between two sulfur atoms, it is sometimes referred to as the sulfur bond. The disulfide link adds toughness and abrasion resistance to the hair. This is the bond that determines the natural curl configuration of the hair. Genetic factors determine whether this bond is straight across polypeptide chains or not. If the bond is straight, so is the hair fiber. If it is at an angle, the hair is wavy. If the bond is at an extreme slant, the hair is very curly. This is the covalent bond that we change during permanent waving and relaxing, as we will see shortly.

Hydrogen Bond

Other bonds form between and among polypeptide chains as they move up through the follicle. Another bond important to you as a cosmetologist is the **hydrogen bond** (Figure 13.15). This bond is formed between hydrogen and oxygen atoms from different parts of the same protein chain or from one chain to another. This bond preserves and strengthens the helix shape. The hydrogen bond is responsible for 35 percent of the strength of the hair and 50 percent of its elasticity. These bonds are not very strong and are broken whenever the hair is shampooed. They are also disturbed in any chemical service to the hair.

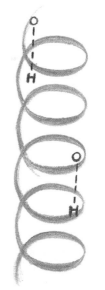

13.15   Hydrogen bonds

Salt Bonds

Ionic bonds are also found in the hair. These bonds form between positive and negative ions. They help to hold the polypeptide chain in its helix. They also serve as cross-links, working together with hydrogen bonds by contributing 35 percent of the strength of the hair and 50 percent of its elasticity. Salt bonds are broken during chemical processes and must be reformed in order to restore the moisture balance of the hair.

Sugar Bond

A last bond that forms a cross-link between polypeptide chains is an **ester** (or **sugar**) **bond**. We do know that this bond occurs between amino acids in two different protein chains. We think that it forms simply as a side effect of keratinization. This bond may add some abrasion resistance to the hair. At present, its function is unknown.

How Bonds Form Hair

Bonding changes the hair from cells to the solid form that we see and feel. Amino acids are joined by peptide bonds. Peptide chains are linked end to end by polypeptide bonds. Polypeptide chains coil into a helix, and three of these coils or helices twine together to form a protofibril. Seven to eleven protofibrils then twist together to form a microfibril; many microfibrils join together to form a macrofibril. Thousands of macrofibrils twist around each other to form the cortex. All of this occurs in the follicle at the same time that cuticle layers are being formed. It all occurs around a soft, spongy tissue, the medulla (see Figure 13.16). For a more in-depth view of the formation of skin, hair, and nails, see Chapter 2.

> ◆ **Key Point** ◆
>
> The hair is a complex structure created by chemical bonds. By understanding its structure and knowing the chemicals that alter the bonds, you can use the tools to change hair. By applying chemistry, you can make changes without damaging the hair.

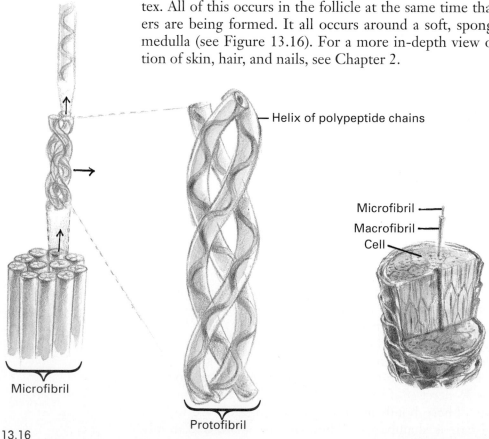

Helix of polypeptide chains

Microfibril
Macrofibril
Cell

Microfibril

Protofibril

13.16

SALON PROCEDURES USING PHYSICAL CHANGES

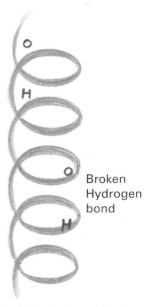

Let's move on further into the practical world of the salon. The bonds that we have discussed give the hair its **tensile** (**TEN** sill) strength. Tensile strength is the resistance to forces trying to pull any material apart. This strength keeps hair from breaking when it is combed and brushed. When we do salon services, we never want to break all the bonds in the hair. Instead, we use chemicals that affect specific bonds.

Water breaks the salt and the hydrogen bonds, and that is why you wet your client's hair before styling it. When you shampoo the hair, more of these bonds are broken and the hair will stretch further so that the protein backbone of the hair can be straightened or moved into the position that you desire (Figures 13.17 and 13.18). As the hair dries (Figures 13.19 and 13.20), the hydrogen and salt bonds

Broken Hydrogen bond

13.17   Broken hydrogen bonds

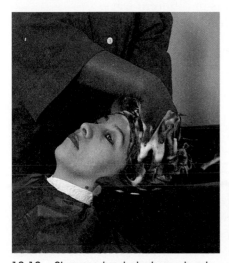

13.18   Shampoo breaks hydrogen bonds

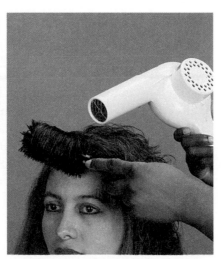

13.19   Bonds reform into new shape as hair dries

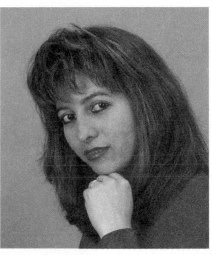

13.20   Bonds will retain new shape until they are broken by water

are reformed into this new shape and will stay that way (Figure 13.21) until the bonds are again disturbed by water. When the hair is wet, it is more fragile. Take extra care not to stretch it beyond its capacity to return to normal.

Water has no effect, however, on the peptide, the polypeptide, or the disulfide bonds. To break these, first of all you need to penetrate into the inner regions of the hair. Chemists carefully formulate solutions to color, lighten, curl, or relax the hair so that the cortex is penetrated without breaking the peptide bonds. If this were to happen, the hair would literally fall apart.

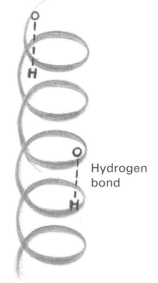

Hydrogen bond

13.21   Reformed hydrogen bonds

CHEMICAL CHANGES FROM SALON SERVICES

When a more permanent change in the hair is desired, suggest that your client receive a chemical service. That way, the service that you recommend (such as a permanent wave or a tint) will last and not have to be repeated with every shampoo. There are two chemical reactions that are used for chemical changes in cosmetology. They are **reduction** (re **DUCK** shun) and **oxidation** (ox i **DAY** shun).

Reduction

Reduction is a chemical reaction that forces a compound to gain an electron. This reaction is most commonly caused by the addition of hydrogen atoms to a compound. Hydrogen atoms, with their one electron looking for a second to fill the shell, cause molecules to break apart and rearrange themselves in different ways.

Reduction is used in the salon to break the disulfide bond between polypeptide chains. Common reducing agents are the processing lotion of a permanent wave lotion and chemical relaxer. Both of these agents alter the amount of natural curl in the hair. We'll take a look at how these salon services work in just a moment.

Oxidation

Oxidation is a chemical reaction that forces a compound to lose electrons. It is most commonly accomplished by forcing oxygen atoms into a compound. Oxygen atoms, lacking two electrons in their outer shells, will pull electrons to themselves inside that compound. This again causes rearranging of the bonds in that compound.

Oxidation is used in the salon to reform bonds, to join together artificial pigment molecules in color, or to lighten the natural color pigment in the hair. The most common oxidizing solution used in the salon is hydrogen peroxide (H_2O_2).

Oxidation and reduction always occur together. In our practice of cosmetology, we use one term to describe the action that we desire. For example, the permanent-wave processing lotion **reduces** so we call it the reduction agent because it adds electrons to the hair. The processing lotion also undergoes a chemical change. It gets **oxidized** since it loses electrons. Once this has happened, it will no longer work as a processing lotion.

On the other hand, hydrogen peroxide **oxidizes** the hair. It will pull electrons to itself. Hair color, for example, also changes chemically. It gets **reduced** since it has gained electrons and is no longer effective.

Salon Services

This section will examine each chemical salon service to see what effect it has on the hair.

◆ Key Point ◆

Oxidation and reduction always happen at the same time. This means that both the hair and the chemical product you put on it are changed. Water is always formed in this reaction.

Permanent Waves

The active ingredient in most cold permanent waves is **thioglycollic** (theye oh **GLEYE** kol ick) acid. It is a reducing agent. It is typically combined with ammonia, or another **amine** (**AYE** mine) to increase the pH of the lotion to approximately 9.3. This gives the processing lotion the ability to penetrate the hair rapidly while the reducing agent is still active. Once inside the hair, ammonium thioglycolate reduces the disulfide bond (Figures 13.22 and 13.23).

Once the test curl (Figure 13.24) is satisfactory, the processing lotion residue is removed from the hair. This is followed by the application of an oxidizing solution—usually hydrogen peroxide or a bromate mixed with conditioners and water. This step reforms the disulfide bonds in cystine so that the curl is reformed (see Figure 13.25).

When these chemical activities are combined with the physical activity of wrapping the hair around rods, a new physical and chemical shape is formed in the hair (see Figure 13.26). This example shows how typical cold waves work. There are, however, other waves such as those called "acid" that work in a similar fashion but use different ingredients. "Exothermic" (*ex*=outside; *therm*=heat) perms add activators that create heat so that the lotion can enter the hair rapidly without needing to be quite as alkaline. Chapter 16, Chemical Waving, discusses selection of the correct perm for your client.

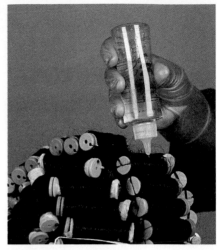

13.22 Apply lotion to hair

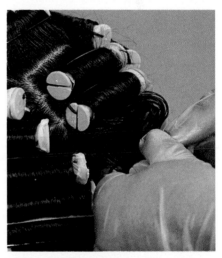

13.23 Check test curl

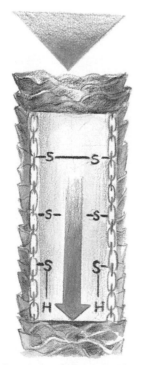

13.24 Lotion reduces disulfide bond

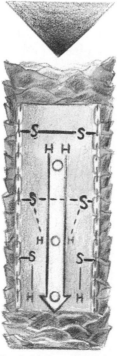

13.25 Oxidation reforms bonds

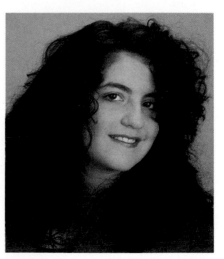

13.26

Chemical Relaxing

There are two types of chemical relaxers. The first is a "thio" relaxer. It is cream formula that works exactly like the permanent wave, except that rods are not used. Instead, physical pressure of combing is used to reduce the curl present. Because of the damage that can occur when combing *any* chemical through the hair, and because the amount of curl that can be removed is small, thio relaxers are seldom used to relax hair in today's progressive salon. Instead, thio formulations are used for curls; perm formulations for extra curly hair. The pre-wrap gel or cream is typically a mild thio relaxer.

Sodium hydroxide relaxers are much more common in the salon because they work very well. They are a heavy cream formula, whose active chemical agent is NaOH, a reducing agent. "No-lye" and calcium relaxers work in the same fashion with slightly different ingredients. Hydroxide relaxers are used because they are fast in their action and can remove curl from the hair without physical damage to the hair from combing. How do they work?

After alkaline cream penetrates the hair (Figure 13.27), the disulfide bond is broken as Figure 13.28 shows. When this happens, the hair will smooth out and curl will be reduced.

The cream should be rinsed *very thoroughly* from the hair with warm water. The next chemical step takes place during a shampoo with an acid-balanced (4.5–5.5) shampoo. You will notice a strange smell, much like rotten eggs, that comes from the hair. This is the reaction of the acid in the shampoo with the residue of the relaxer.

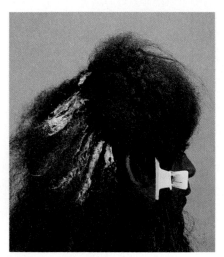

13.27   Apply alkaline cream to hair

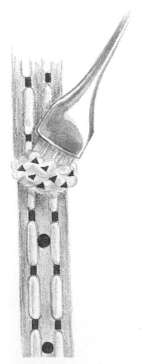

13.28   Relaxer breaks disulfide bond

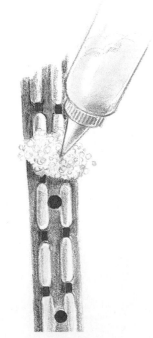

13.29   Shampoo forms lanthionine

The hair should be rinsed again and again until the hair foams well; it should then be rinsed again.

During the shampoo to remove the relaxer, a new bond is created in the hair called **lanthionine** (lan **THEE** oh neen). Notice in Figure 13.29 that it is a monosulfide bond with only *one* sulfur atom. This bond cannot be reduced any further, nor can it be oxidized. This is why an oxidizer is NOT necessary in a relaxing service and can actually cause extensive damage. This is also why you do not reapply relaxer to the same hair, or give it a reconstruction curl service.

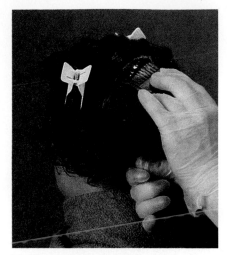

13.30   Applying tint to hair

Permanent Color

Permanent color can be achieved by several different means: mineral dyes, vegetable tints, or compound dyes. All of these methods are very harsh and can create extreme problems. The one remaining method, that of **aniline** (**ANN** i lynn) **derivative tints**, is used in the professional salon. These compounds, derived from coal-tar byproducts, offer almost endless options in coloring services. Shall we see how they work?

Permanent color is available in many forms: liquid, cream, or gel. All sorts of formulas are available that will give you the entire range of natural hair colors. The correct color formula for the desired results is combined with a developing agent. The most common of these agents is hydrogen peroxide.

When color mixed with a developer is applied to the hair (Figure 13.30), several things happen. First, the alkalinity of the color allows it to penetrate the hair. Second, the H_2O_2 oxidizes the color by pulling electrons to itself. When this happens, the individual molecules of the tint are bonded together (Figure 13.31) and become trapped within the cortex fibers.

The excess color formula should then be removed with water and shampoo. The last step is to acidify the hair so that the molecules will remain trapped inside and the hair has its natural protection returned.

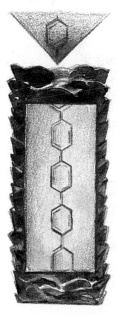

13.31   Tint molecules bond together

Hair Lightening

We remove color from the hair whenever we want a lighter, brighter effect. This can be done all over the head, or in small sections for special effects. Whatever the result desired, hair lighteners work in the same way.

A chemical compound is used, usually a powder or a cream, that contains alkalis and lightening compounds. It is activated by the addition of an oxidizer, usually H_2O_2. The alkalinity of the mixture allows for penetration into the hair. Once there, the formula attaches itself to the pigment in the hair. Again, electrons are pulled from the pigment to the lightener.

CLIENT   T I P   ◆◆◆◆◆◆◆

Hydrogen peroxide is the most common activator for lighteners. But new developers, enzymes, ozone, etc. are constantly being introduced. Learn the properties of each so you can choose the best developer for your client's hair condition and the result desired.

The natural pigment, melanin, is surrounded and transformed into oxymelanin—a lighter pigment compound (see Figure 13.32). If you decide to continue the lightening process, so many electrons will be lost that the larger (oxymelanin) pigment granules will break down even more and scatter into tiny molecules that reflect little or no color (Figure 13.33).

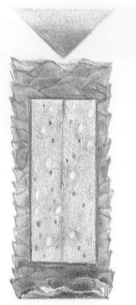

13.32   Oxygen surrounds pigment

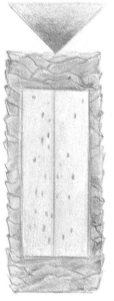

13.33   Diffused pigment molecules

KEY CHEMICAL AGENTS USED IN THE SALON

There is an almost unlimited array of chemicals that can be used in the salon, but many of them work in the same way. We will group chemicals into the primary families and the activities associated with each grouping. Your instructor can refer you to a number of reference books that can help you research further any specific chemical ingredients that interest you.

Cleansers

Soaps, shampoos, facial cleansers, and even some of the products you use for sanitizing the salon contain cleansers as their primary ingredient. To a chemist, a cleanser is a **surfactant** (sir **FACT** ant), or a surface active agent. A surfactant is any compound that affects the surface tension when it is dissolved in water. What? Imagine that you are driving in your car. Your windshield isn't exactly clean and it begins to rain. The first few drops of rain will "bead up" on the glass because they are sitting on top of oils and dirt. If you only turn on your wipers, what will happen? A streaky mess! But if you first push your washer button, a liquid solution containing surfactants will squirt onto the glass. The solution will reduce the tension between the oil and water and make them mix. When the wipers pass across, your windshield will be cleaned and you'll be able to see where you're going.

When your client's hair is soiled, dirt and hair spray are attached to the oil and that makes the acid mantle of the hair. If you only rinse the hair, the hair will not be cleaned because the oil—holding the dirt—and the water don't mix. But if you then add shampoo, its primary surfactant ingredient will reduce the surface tension between the two. One part of the shampoo molecule, often called the head, will turn the dirt, oil, and water into an **emulsion** (eeh **MUHL** shun). The second part, sometimes called the tail of the shampoo molecule, is attracted to water. It will pull the head and attached dirt from the hair during the rinse, leaving the hair clean in the process.

Some cleansers are harsh and some are gentle. Today's chemist can formulate cleansers so that they are acid-balanced to that of the skin and hair, 4.5 to 5.5. This ensures that the hair is not over cleaned and left open to damage. Sodium laureth sulfate is an example of such a surfactant. Special shampoos are formulated for chemically treated hair that also incorporate conditioners, natural oils, and so on. Your instructor can guide you in the selection of products to suit particular needs.

Conditioners

This huge family of chemicals consist of **emulsions**. An emulsion is a mixture of oil and water. A chemist can combine these in very exact proportions, and also stabilize them so they do not separate. Natural oils such as essential fatty acids add **lubricity**, or lubrication, to the hair. Conditioners can also contain specialized ingredients like **hydrolized** (**HIGH** droh lyzed) protein that is broken down into a small molecular weight so it can penetrate the hair or skin. "Oil free" conditioners have been formulated with ingredients that moisturize or add strength without leaving oils behind. You might want to refer again to Chapter 6 to refresh your memory about the different types of conditioners available to the professional hairstylist.

Conditioners are also available for the skin. They contain **humectants** (hyoo **MECK** tants) such as sodium PCA that carry moisture and bind it inside the skin. They often contain collagen, the protein of the skin, in order to protect it from harsh elements such as sun and wind that cause the skin to age prematurely. A further discussion of skin conditioners is found in Chapter 18, and covers facials and skin treatments.

Alcohols

Alcohols are a group of organic (carbon-based) compounds. They are often used as sanitizing and disinfecting agents due to their ability to kill or retard the growth of bacteria. Glycerine is another alcohol that is used very frequently in cosmetics. It is harmless to people and is found in many foods as well. Glycerine will pick up and hold water, so is also used as a humectant in hair and skin conditioners.

Amines

We have referred to amines in this chapter, when we were discussing the processing lotion of a permanent wave and again when we were analyzing how haircolor works.

Amines are alkalizers—ingredients added to formulas to help them penetrate the hair. They are compounds that consist of nitrogen and hydrogen. Ammonia, NH_3, is a common amine used in chemical preparations for the hair. A benefit that ammonia has over other amines is that it is a gas in its natural form. Being a gas, it will dissipate (or evaporate) from the hair as it is dried and cause no further harm.

Other amines used in cosmetic formulations are usually advertised as having "no ammonia." Be careful when using these compounds to use the conditioner provided to ensure that these particular amines are neutralized.

CLIENT TIP ◆◆◆◆◆◆◆

Maintenance shampoos should be acid balanced (4.5 to 5.5) to protect the hair. Special ingredients are added to make the shampoo right for certain hair types (moisturizers for dry hair, extra cleansers for oily hair, etc.). To remove product buildup from the hair, use a special shampoo that is more alkaline or has harsher cleansers. Restore the pH balance to the hair at the end of your service for protection.

CLIENT TIP ◆◆◆◆◆◆◆

Recommend conditioners according to the type and amount of hair damage. Light conditioners are used to maintain healthy hair or to correct slight damage. Heavy conditioners are for more severe damage and also used during chemical services. Waxes only coat the hair and are seldom recommended. Use polymer conditioners for extreme damage when parts of the hair structure are completely missing.

CLIENT TIP ◆◆◆◆◆◆◆

Even though you may think of alcohol as drying, chemists can formulate "alcohol free" products that eliminate the drying effect. Alcohol is not always bad for hair and skin.

Esters

These very complicated compounds are formed when an acid reacts with an alcohol. They usually have a pleasant odor, so they can be used in the formulation of ingredients to mask or perfume other ingredients. Esters are also good solvents. Ethyl acetate, for example, is used in nail polish removers and also in some nail polishes.

Quaternary Ammonium Compounds

Commonly called "quats," these compounds are used for a variety of reasons and in many professional products. The positive charge of the quat molecule enables it to easily attach to or penetrate the hair or skin. Whether it will penetrate depends on the size of the molecule, the molecular weight of the particular quat, and the condition of the hair. Badly damaged hair, for example, with a lifted or broken cuticle, will allow larger molecules to penetrate. Badly damaged hair is also more alkaline and actually attracts the positive quats to the damaged areas.

Chemists identify quats by number. Quaternium-23, for example, is a conditioning agent that makes it easier to comb the hair and improves its sheen, but it can build up on the outside of the hair. Consult an ingredient dictionary and your instructor to lead you through the maze of quaternary ammonium compounds.

Some quats are used as sanitizing agents; however, they are usually combined with other antibacterial agents to improve their effectiveness.

PEGs

Polyethylene glycols (pol ee **ETH** i leen **GLEYE** calls) are another complex family. They consist of large molecules that form chain polymers. Specific PEGs are followed by identification numbers such as PEG-20 or PEG-40. They are used as softeners and humectants, lubricants, and as bases for cosmetics.

Ingredient Labels

Your instructor can assist you greatly in analyzing products and determining what is in them. There are a variety of cosmetic ingredient dictionaries and other references that can give you basic information on the source of ingredients and their effects. When you read an ingredient list on a label, components are listed in the order of their concentration or activity. So, the first ingredient listed makes up the largest portion of the product, the second is next in concentration, and so on. Manufacturers must list all **active** ingredients that are present in a concentration of 1 percent or more.

Chemistry is a complicated and often difficult subject, but don't let it get the best of you! Instead, use it as a professional tool to achieve results without adverse side-effects.

♦ Key Point ♦

Read the ingredient lists on product labels so you can recognize potentially harmful ingredients. Be aware of the way chemists can combine ingredients to maximize thier good effects and minimize harsh side effects.

Chemistry is the study of matter and the changes it can undergo. Matter can be a solid, a liquid, or a gas. Each form of matter has special properties. As a cosmetologist, you will deal with solid substances—hair, nails, and skin—and usually treat them with penetrating liquids.

Matter is composed of atoms. An atom is the smallest unit that can retain the identity of the element it represents. Molecules are combinations of different atoms. They combine chemically to form compounds such as hair. Atoms can react with each other, and the electron is responsible for this ability. Oxidation, the loss of an electron, and reduction, the gain of an electron, are the primary chemical reactions and especially important in cosmetology.

Chemical bonds create the world in which you live and work. Covalent bonds are shared electrons. They are very strong and are responsible for the composition of hair and skin. Ionic bonds are electrical attractions between positively and negatively charged ions.

Change can be either physical (a temporary alteration in the form or the description of an object) or chemical (an alteration resulting in an entirely new object with characteristics all its own). You will cause a physical change when you shampoo and style your client's hair. A chemical change occurs when you alter properties inside the hair such as the natural curl pattern or color.

Water is an important substance in our lives. Because it is the universal solvent, water is used in all cosmetology services. Another critical tool you will use as a cosmetologist is pH. This is a mathematical formula that tells you the potential acid activity of liquids with which you work. You will use alkaline substances to penetrate the hair to change it. You will use acids to protect the cuticle layer of the hair and to return the hair to normal after a chemical service.

The hair itself is formed by a series of chemical bonds. Key bonds occurring in the hair are the hydrogen, salt, peptide, polypeptide, and disulfide bonds.

Reduction, the addition of an electron via hydrogen, occurs during permanent waving or relaxing when bonds in the hair are broken. Oxidation, the loss of an electron via oxygen, occurs when you reform bonds in permanent waving and also when you color or lighten the hair.

The understanding of chemical activity and specific ingredients is important to you as a professional cosmetologist. You will determine when a chemical process is necessary by recognizing which aspects of hair chemicals can alter. The chemical descriptions of hair products will help you estimate the products' effects. Chemistry offers you the possibilities to safely and successfully complete your service with the maximum of customer satisfaction!

QUESTIONS

1. Define the following terms: *matter, element, atom, compound, molecule, valence.*
2. What two types of bonds can occur?
3. What is the difference between a physical and a chemical change?
4. Give an example of each type of change in the cosmetology salon.
5. Why is water unique as a molecule? List at least three uses that we make of water as a result of this unique quality.
6. Why is pH important to a professional cosmetologist?
7. What are the pH ranges of six salon products? Why is that pH best?
8. What are the six chemical bonds found in the hair and what is the function of each?
9. What happens in the hair chemically when you shampoo and style a client?
10. What are the four basic chemical services offered in the salon?
11. Briefly explain what happens to the hair chemically when each chemical service is performed.
12. What are the categories of chemical agents that are available to you in the salon? In a general sense, explain how each works and give one example of an ingredient in each category.

PROJECTS

1. Test the pH of products available with a pH meter or with pH paper. Estimate the activity each product will have on the hair, based on its pH.
2. Using the same products as in Project 1, analyze the ingredients of each and estimate their effects on hair.
3. Combine the information gathered in Project 1 and Project 2 to predict the effect that each product will have on the hair. Based on this information, explain the actions of the products on the chemical bonds in hair.
4. Working in pairs with a fellow student, list each step of a permanent wave. Describe which are physical and which are chemical. Outline what activity occurs inside the hair with each step.

HAIR COLORING

CHAPTER GOAL

Changing the color of hair is an art that offers return business and financial rewards for the skilled professional colorist. After reading this chapter and comparing the projects, you should be able to

1. Explain the principles of color, including primaries, secondaries, and complements.
2. List the classifications of hair color and indicate the advantages and disadvantages of each.
3. Outline how the correct color formula is selected.
4. Demonstrate how a client is prepared for a hair coloring service. Include draping, patch test, and preliminary strand test procedures.
5. Demonstrate at least five different techniques for coloring hair.
6. List safety measures which must be observed by anyone working with chemicals in the salon.

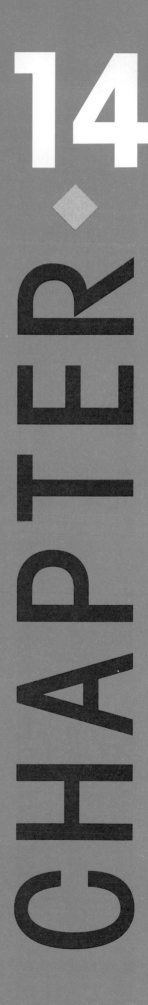

CHAPTER 14

Color is dynamic. It can be used to express personality, mood, fashion, and time. Hair coloring has been with us since the beginning of the written history of cosmetology. In ancient Egypt, henna was used to color the hair red. In Europe, indigo, sage, and chamomile were used to change the color of hair. During the Middle Ages, blond or black hair was favored, while red was disliked. Throughout history, color choice of the rich and famous has often set the tone for the rest of the population.

In this century, hair coloring has moved from the difficult and messy techniques of former ages to ones that are much more simple. Today's array of chemicals provides you, the professional colorist, with an almost endless palette of colors. In addition to colors, a huge menu of techniques gives you the ability to duplicate nature—even improve it! As a professional colorist, you will analyze the natural level and tone of your clients' hair, and the level and tone of the desired color. You will determine the correct product and ideal application technique according to your consultation.

BASIC PRINCIPLES OF COLOR

The first step to becoming a first-class colorist is to learn just what color is all about. The *Color Key Program* you learned in Chapter 1 was a step to understanding how color can enhance your client's features. Before we tackle the details of hair coloring, let's first analyze how color works. The theory of color that we will study in this chapter is that of pigment, or solid color.

Primary Colors

All color begins with three **primary colors**: blue, red, and yellow. A primary color is an elementary color not obtained by a mixture. Each primary color has certain characteristics.

Blue is the dominant primary color (Figure 14.1). The characteristic, **dominance**, means that the properties of blue will add depth, or darkness, to a color tone. Blue is described as cool; it recedes from the eye. The effect of blue is calm and soothing. Even though blue is the dominant pigment, it is the first to be lost when exposed to sunlight, harsh chemicals, or oxidation. Think about your jeans. They may be very dark when you first buy them, but will fade with every washing, especially if they are dried in the sun or washed with bleach.

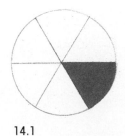

14.1

Red is the medium primary color (Figure 14.2). Red gives warmth and provides highlights. Red has a stimulating effect; it excites, and is used for warning. Red color tones are the second to fade, but are much more resistant than blue.

Yellow is the third primary color, and the weakest one (Figure 14.3). Yellow adds lightness and brightness to a color tone. Yellow advances to the eye, and seems larger than it really is. Yellow is the last pigment to be lost. Yellow reflects light, adds highlights, and shows detail. You probably have noticed how dramatic yellow appears against a black background.

Try setting the hair on a brown and a blond mannequin in exactly the same style, dry the hair, and then comb it out. When you place them side by side, you will notice that the blond mannequin looks larger and closer to you than the brown one. You will also notice that you see the outside shape of the brown mannequin more clearly, but notice the inside lines of design on the blond one.

When we mix the primary colors together in unequal proportions, we make the color brown. There is an almost limitless number of brown shades, depending upon the amount of each primary present. Take a look around where you are right now and find all the different colors of brown. Now, look more closely. Look at the differences and the quality of each brown. Knowing that blue makes brown dark, red makes it warm, and yellow makes it bright, try to estimate the amount of blue, red, and yellow in each of the colors. Compare your estimates to Figures 14.4 through 14.6 to test your primary color knowledge. Remember that all three primaries must be present to make the color brown.

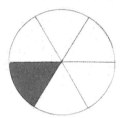

14.2

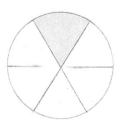

14.3

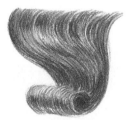

14.4   Golden brown

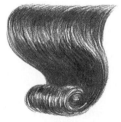

14.5   Warm brown

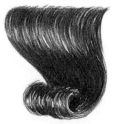

14.6   Dark brown

Secondary Colors

When you mix two primary colors together, you make a new color called a **secondary color**. When you mix primary red and primary yellow, you make the secondary color orange. The combination of primary blue and primary yellow make the secondary color green. The combination of the primaries red and blue make the secondary color purple (or violet). While purple, green, and orange might be fad party hair colors, they are seldom the tones desired by the majority of our clients. Secondary colors can be used to change **tonal** value or to correct color mistakes. **Tonality** refers to the warmness (visible red and gold) or the coolness (visible blue) of a color. The *Color Key Program* in Chapter 1 shows the relationship of different tonal qualities.

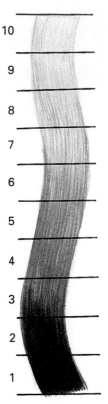

14.7   Color level

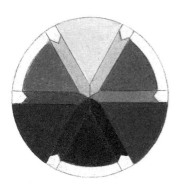

14.8   The color wheel

Value is a term used to describe the depth of a color—its darkness or lightness. While all color has value, it is easiest to understand by looking at the color black. Black is a combination of all the primary colors in equal proportion. Look at Figure 14.7. At the bottom you see the color black. As white is added, the black lightens until at the top of the graph there appears just a hint of black (what we call the color gray). In hair coloring, depth is described by the **level** of the color. The darkest level is 1, and depending upon the manufacturer of the color you use, either 10 or 12 is the lightest level.

If you look again at black, you will see the dominance of blue. Even though all primaries are represented, the depth, darkness, and coolness of blue is most noticeable.

Complementary Colors

Complements are pairs of colors that are located exactly opposite each other on the color wheel (Figure 14.8). Another way to determine complementary pairs is to think about the primary colors once again. A complementary pair consists of a primary and a secondary color. The secondary color of the complementary pair is a combination of the other two primary colors. Consider yellow. It is a primary color. What are the other two primary colors? Red and blue combine to make the secondary color violet. Violet is the complement of yellow. Try green. It is a secondary color, right? It is made up of primary blue and primary yellow. What's missing? Red, which is the complement of green. We have not discussed blue. Is it primary or secondary? What are the other two primaries? What is the complement of blue?

Complementary colors interact in an interesting way. When they are placed side by side, they accent each other and each color appears more intense. Take a look at the complementary pairs and you can see holiday and advertising colors: red and green, yellow and purple, and blue and orange.

When you mix complementary colors together, they *neutralize* each other and produce a shade of brown. This is very important to the hair colorist. Imagine a client who originally liked the hair color you applied, but now thinks it has become brassy. How would you correct this problem and return it to the color that was satisfactory? Well, think about it. What is brassy? Is it orange? What is the complement or orange? Orange is a secondary color made up of red and yellow. The missing primary, located directly opposite on the color wheel, is blue. If you add blue to the client's hair, you will neutralize the brassiness of orange and have a satisfied customer. Now think one step further. The client in question was pleased when the hair was first colored. But then what happened? The hair was exposed to light and perhaps a harsh shampoo. As a result, pigment was lost from the hair. What is the first pigment to be lost? You're right: blue. The addition of blue to the hair solves the problem of brassiness. Refer to Chapter 6, *Hair Damage and Treatments*, for methods to help prevent fading of hair color.

The Effect of Light on Color

Most color work is done in the salon under artificial lighting. The truest test of colors is always natural daylight—what artists call north light—not direct sunlight. The best time of day to get this true color is between 11:00 A.M. and 3:00 P.M., depending upon the season. Direct sun casts a golden light that intensifies color and changes its tonality, increasing the warmth. It is important to have lighting in the salon as close to natural light as possible so that you can accurately analyze results. Table 14.1 describes the effect of incandescent and fluorescent light on hair color. The closer the lamp is to the hair, the more intense these effects will become.

TABLE 14.1 Effects of Artificial Light on Hair Color

Color Series	TYPE OF LIGHT	
	Fluorescent	*Incandescent*
Ash	Ash colors appear more drab than they really are. Your ash color may not be as ash as you want. Ash-blond colors may take on a greenish tone.	The bluish tones of ash colors are neutralized. Ash colors appear less drab. If the color is not ash enough, the color will take on either red or gold tones, depending on the intensity of the light.
Gold	Gold colors are neutralized somewhat and appear more ash than they really are. Gold colors do not appear to have the desired brightness.	Gold colors take on an added brightness. Both the red and gold tones are intensified.
Red	Red colors lose their brightness. Red colors appear more brown than red. Theoretically, the blue light should create a purple tone, but actually the color appears to have a red-brown cast.	The red and gold tones of red colors are brightened and intensified.
Smoke	Smoke colors already have a bluish tone, and so the blue tone is intensified. Silver and platinum blonds may take on a greenish tone.	Smoke colors are neutralized. Silver and platinum colors lose their bluish tone and take on a gray tone.

Many progressive salons combine incandescent and fluorescent lighting to balance the effects of light on color. "Daylight" fluorescent lighting is now also available. Discuss lighting with your client during the color consultation. If you client complains that the hair is too drab, determine whether this is the case in natural, fluorescent, or incandescent lighting. Is it really drab, or is it the lighting where your client usually sees the hair color. What can you do to correct it? Refer to Table 14.1 and to your study of complementary colors and see what you would suggest.

> **◆ Key Point ◆**
> The key to hair coloring is the understanding of brown—*a mixture of all three primaries*. You can create the color you want and correct tonal problems by applying the law of complements to create brown.

CLASSIFICATIONS OF HAIR COLOR

Hair coloring is classified according to how long it lasts on the hair. This characteristic, **color fastness**, is affected by the product formulation as well as the porosity of the hair. Color will penetrate deeper if the cuticle is raised and the hair is porous. Color will also last longer on more porous hair in most cases. Extremely porous hair, with the cuticle severely damaged or missing, will absorb a deep color; but will not usually hold it because the color molecules cannot be trapped inside the hair.

Temporary Color

Temporary hair color is designed to coat the hair shaft until the hair is shampooed. It has no lasting effect on the natural hair color. Temporary colors cannot lighten; they can only add color to the hair and blend tones together (Figure 14.9). Temporary hair coloring is available in a variety of shades and in several forms.

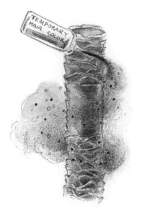

14.9

Types of Temporary Color

1. **Rinses** are prepared with **certified colors** (colors approved for use by the Food and Drug Administration), water, and usually a mild setting agent. Rinses coat the hair and remain until the hair is shampooed. Color rinses are also available as creams and gels.
2. **Color shampoos** consist of shampoo mixed with color pigment to blend color tones or neutralize unwanted shades. Many are violet, for example, to neutralize unwanted yellow in white or gray hair.
3. **Color sprays**—usually bright, party colors—are applied directly to dry hair.
4. **Crayons** and **mascara** are used for facial makeup. Temporary hair color crayons are also used in the theater.

Uses of Temporary Color

1. Toning down unwanted color.
2. Adding a different color.
3. Blending gray.
4. Creating special temporary effects.

Advantages of Temporary Color

1. Neutralize any unwanted tones in the hair.
2. Enhance and add brighter tones to dull hair.
3. Correct faded color until the client arranges for a more permanent solution.
4. The chief advantage of temporary hair coloring is that it does not alter the structure of the hair, nor does it affect the client's own natural color.
5. In most cases, temporary color does not require a patch test.

6. Temporary color is quick and easy to apply.
7. Temporary colors shampoo easily from the hair.

The Disadvantages of Temporary Color

1. It must be reapplied after every shampoo.
2. Color results may be uneven, especially if enough rinse is not applied. The color itself will run with moisture or perspiration, will rub off on pillows and clothing, and will flake off when the hair is brushed or combed.
3. If the hair is damaged, temporary color will penetrate the hair cuticle layer and uneven color will be evident, after the hair is shampooed.
4. Temporary rinses can only deposit color, they cannot lift or lighten color.
5. Often hair that is colored in this manner is dull and lacks sheen.

Semipermanent Color

Semipermanent color lasts longer than temporary color, yet fades gradually without affecting the natural pigment in the hair. Semipermanent colors are formulated to last through four to six shampoos and are gradually removed from the hair.

Traditional Semipermanent Color

This type of semipermanent color works by coating the cuticle and slightly penetrating it (Figure 14.10). Semipermanent hair color was first popular in the days of weekly shampoos and sets. Now that many clients shampoo every day, semipermanent tints have been reformulated to last longer. These new colors are one of the fastest growing categories of hair color today.

Activated Semipermanent Color

Many semipermanent colors are mixed with a chemical activator supplied by the manufacturer to make the color effects last longer. These semipermanent colors bridge the gap between color that washes out with each shampoo and permanent color. When an activator is used, the color molecules are trapped within the cuticle imbrications (or scales) and last longer.

Activated semipermanent colors are used to blend gray into the natural color, and can also be effective in coloring it. The effectiveness of semipermanent color depends upon the hair's porosity. Activated semipermanent colors can be used to blend larger amounts of gray, especially if it is evenly spread. Activated semipermanent colors are very effective in adding highlights and sheen to otherwise dull hair. Today's stylist often combines semipermanent color with another salon service so that the color lasts longer with minimum damage to the hair. Services such as lightening or chemical relaxing that increase the porosity of the hair, encourage the semipermanent color to penetrate the cortex and therefore last much longer without additional damage to the hair.

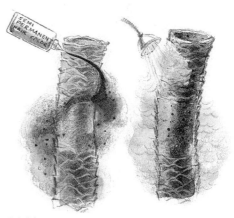

14.10

CLIENT **T I P** ◆◆◆◆◆◆◆

Suggest that your hair relaxing client also receive a translucent color service. This will add depth and sheen to the newly processed hair and increase stylability.

CLIENT **T I P** ◆◆◆◆◆◆◆

Advise your newly graying client to try a semipermanent color. This will enhance the hair by adding sheen and blending gray for a youthful effect. Your client can enjoy the vibrancy provided without worrying about regrowth.

Translucent Semipermanent Color

The last type of semipermanent color is translucent. This color is applied directly to clean, damp hair and processed under a dryer. The result is a sheer color addition that enhances the client's natural color. Translucent color is very effective on chemically processed hair, especially on hair that has been relaxed. It is available in a variety of colors as well as a clear gloss.

The Advantages of Semipermanent Color

1. The structure of the hair is not affected. Even though some small amounts of swelling may temporarily occur, the interior cortex layer of the hair is not affected.
2. Semipermanent color can be very effective in blending gray hair, and is an especially good way to introduce a client to more permanent methods of hair coloring.
3. Semipermanent color can enhance natural hair color by adding tone and depth.
4. These colors are also formulated as toners for prelightened hair.
5. Many semipermanent colors do not contain paraphenylenedi- amine (a color molecule made from coal tar) and are safer to use on clients with sensitive skin and scalp.
6. Those that do not require an activator can provide an alternative to permanent hair colors for use on clients during pregnancy.

The Disadvantages of Semipermanent Color

1. Limited shades of the older formulas.
2. The color is not long lasting unless activated, and may need to be repeated as often as every week, depending on the frequency of shampoos.
3. A patch test is necessary on some types of semipermanent color.
4. If the hair is very porous, the effect of semipermanent color is longer lasting; however, the color often fades to off-shades after several shampoos.
5. Semipermanent hair color rarely provides sufficient coverage on gray hair.
6. Semipermanent color cannot lift hair color; it can only deposit pigment.

Permanent Color

As the name indicates, **permanent color** is designed to remain in the hair until it grows out. Both the hair's natural color and the applied color undergo a chemical change. Almost any shade desired can be achieved with a permanent color. If the color selected is very different from the natural tone, a line of demarcation will be evident as the hair grows out.

Vegetable Tints

Permanent hair coloring is derived from a variety of sources. The earliest recorded hair coloring in history is that of staining with plant derivatives. As a coating color, henna was most commonly used, although indigo, sage, and chamomile were also applied. The plant methods are still used today, although they are messy and time consuming. The plant extracts build up on the outside of the hair, and usually preclude any other type of chemical service.

Metallic or Mineral Dyes

Mineral-based colors and compound products, combined with plant extracts, are another type of permanent color. These agents are *never* used professionally because the damage to the hair can be quite severe, the range of colors extremely limited, and the hair is left unfit for further chemical service.

If you suspect that your client may have used a metallic color, test the hair before you proceed with a chemical service. *Test for metallic salts*: Cut off a strand of the colored hair. Place it in a solution of one ounce of 20-volume hydrogen peroxide and 20 drops of 28% ammonia for 30 minutes. Remove the strand from the solution and let it dry. Look for the following reactions:

1. *Lead*. The strand will lighten as soon as it is placed in the solution. The dry strand will not break when stretched.
2. *Silver*. There will be no change in color because the solution cannot penetrate the coating. There will be no breakage when stretched.
3. *Copper*. The strand and solution will become very hot within a few minutes, and you will detect a disagreeable odor. The strand will break when pulled.

Oxidation Tints

The primary ingredient of today's penetrating permanent color is an aniline derivative. These tint molecules, derived from coal tar, combine with the developer to form giant molecules within the cortex layer of the hair (Figures 14.11 and 14.12). These colors can both **lift** (make lighter) and **deposit** (add color) so that the range of shades possible is almost endless.

◆SAFETY **PRECAUTION**◆

Do not offer chemical services to clients who have used metallic or progressive dyes. Your services will not be successful and may cause severe hair damage. The hair must be removed by cutting.

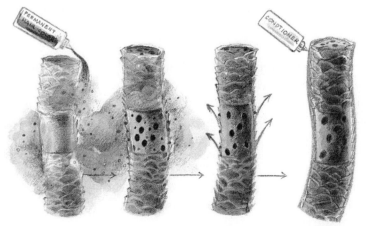

Tint plus developer on hair

Tint mixture enters cortex

Tint pigments formed

Cuticle closed to trap pigments

14.11

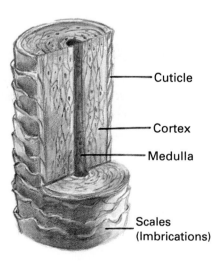

Cuticle

Cortex

Medulla

Scales (Imbrications)

14.12

The Advantages of Oxidation Tints

1. Any natural shade can be duplicated. These colors are permanent, and visible growth requiring a retouch is often not evident for a month or more.
2. Tints can lift or deposit so that you can give clients any result they desire.
3. Tints can blend or totally cover gray in any percentage.
4. The hair is not coated and can receive other chemical services.
5. Since the tint penetrates to the cortex layer of the hair, color results appear very natural.

The Disadvantages of Oxidation Tints

1. A patch test must be given prior to every application.
2. The hair undergoes a chemical change so that the hair must be reconditioned and carefully maintained.
3. The natural pigment of the hair is altered. In most cases, the pigment is lifted. Over time, the hair may become brassy.
4. In order to remove the effects of a tint, you must use a tint remover (which can also lighten natural pigment), retint to camouflage results, or cut the hair to remove the tinted portion.
5. The hair color can fade with time and shampooing, to off-color or harsh tones.

SELECTING THE CORRECT FORMULA

How do you decide on the formula that will give you the results your client is requesting? Is there a formula to give you all the answers to your questions? The key is your confidence with the knowledge and techniques you develop. The enthusiasm and excitement that accompany this phase of artistry grow with each experience.

Consider a plan to gather information from which you will make your decision, or conclusions, that will result in a formula. You will find, as you read further, there are simple things you should do, and ways you can train your eye to develop your professional instinct.

The Consultation

The most important step in correct color selection and application is the consultation you have with your client. This is a time when listening skills are critical. Analyze the condition of the scalp and the hair so that you can perform the service without damaging the hair. Record all of your observations on the client record card.

Explain the release statement to your client; obtain client's signature and file the release for future reference. If the client is under the age of 18, the form should be co-signed by a responsible adult. The release provides documentation that the client was made aware of the processes of the service.

Check the scalp for abrasions. Do *not* perform a coloring service if there are irritations on the scalp. To do so would increase the risk of an allergic reaction, further irritation of the scalp, or even an infection. Aniline derivatives can often cause allergic reactions, so you must perform a patch test. Follow manufacturer's directions for patch test timing.

Carefully analyze the condition of the hair. Check it for elasticity, for moisture, and for strength (see Chapter 6). Healthy hair will give you the most successful results and the most natural looking color. If the hair is severely damaged, suggest postponing the coloring service until you give the necessary reconditioning treatments. Or, your instructor may advise you to incorporate conditioning treatments into the color service if the damage is less severe. Recommend a mild shampoo (low pH) and conditioner for your client to use at home after the coloring service. Proper maintenance will protect the client's hair and chemical service results.

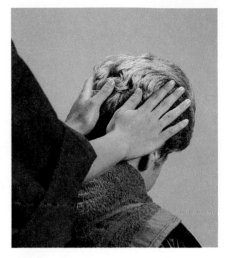

14.13

Client's Natural Coloring

Look at your client. Observe the tone of the skin, and the color and depth in the iris of the eye. Check the natural hair color. Note the amount of red, yellow, and blue present in the natural shade. Use your knowledge of the *Color Key Program* when selecting a hair color for your client (see Chapter 1). All hair colors are represented in both *Color Key* palettes. The correct palette is selected by the under-tone of the hair color. Blond hair in the *Key 1* palette has blue or ash (green) undertones. Blond hair in the *Key 2* palette has warm, golden undertones. Red hair in *Key 1* has pink to wine undertones; in *Key 2* they have rust or golden undertones. The brown hair in *Key 1* has smoke or ash undertones, while in *Key 2*, brown hair has gold or red-gold highlights.

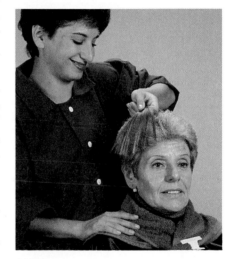

14.14a

Check the hair for color **concentration**—the quality of depth, or darkness. Think of concentration in terms of levels ranging from 1 to 10. Level 1 is the darkest (black); level 10 is the lightest (pale blond). Figure 14.7 will help you determine the level of your client's present color.

Part the hair in the back and observe the hair near the scalp at the nape of the neck (Figure 14.13). This is the area where the color is darkest, and it will let you know how difficult lifting color may be. Push the hair with the palm of your hand back toward the part. This will let light through the hair so that you can determine the natural depth of color. The natural pigment, melanin, is known as **contributing pigment**. Keep this formula in mind: Contributing Pigment + Color Formula = Final Hair Color Result.

Now, you are ready for an exciting color experience! Listen carefully as your client discusses hair color. Working with photographs will let you know how your client sees color and enable you to avoid any misunderstanding. Your client may think "strawberry blond" is much brighter or lighter than your understanding of the shade. Make sure your client is reacting to the hair color, not to the model's face. Once you have settled on a hair color in a photo, try to find similar color in your own setting, or work with color swatches. Be sure to spread the swatches to let light through (Figure 14.14). This way, you can be sure that your client is able to see the *actual* color (in addition to the photo).

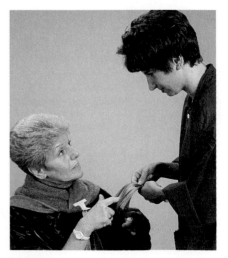

14.14b

Try to determine your client's life-style. If your client is in the sun often, any color you apply will fade or lighten. If the client has a very busy life, choose the application technique that will last the longest with the minimum of upkeep.

Consider the client's age when selecting hair color. Select a color two or three shades lighter for a gray-haired client who wants to go back to natural hair color. As the skin tones have lightened along with the hair, the lighter hair color will be softer and appear more youthful.

The Color Formula

To arrive at the correct color formula, you will be calculating depth and color tone. Determine the level (1–10) of the natural hair color. What primaries make up the color you see and in what proportion? Are the natural highlights red or yellow? Record your observations.

Go through the same analysis of the desired color. What level is it? What are its primary colors and highlights? Let's say, for example, that the client's natural color is level 2, very dark brown. If your client wants to be a level 6 redhead, you will need a level to provide enough lifting capability. Select a color level that will give you that ability. Manufacturers provide information indicating how much each color can lift. In most cases a level 8 color would give you the lift you need for this example. Once you have decided the correct level of the formula, you need to decide the correct tone.

Select the tone for your color formula by comparing primaries in the present color and primaries in the color your client wants. If you are going *darker* you will need to *add* primary colors to the natural hair. If you are going *lighter*, as in the previous example, you will be *removing* primary colors from the natural hair. Be sure you compensate for the lifting action that will take place on the hair's natural pigment. Sometimes a tone that you want retained will be removed in the lifting process. Remember that blue is first to go, then red, and finally, yellow. You may need to add a small amount of primary pigment to your final formula to replace lost tones.

When you have determined your formula, you will then review the hair coloring products you have available. Select the type and level of color according to your formula. Ask your instructor to explain the codings on the bottle or tube of color, so that you will become familiar with identifying the base colors of red, yellow, blue, or a combination. Table 14.2 lists the codings that indicate the base of the color. Refer to color swatches or charts to see how color is produced when applied to white hair with standard (20 volume) peroxide (developer), and the changes in the final result when the same formula is applied to blond, brown, and brunette shades of hair.

An alternate method of formulating recommended by some manufacturers is to select the color desired based upon your consultation. Calculate the correct volume of peroxide (or alternate developer) according to the number of levels you want to lift. If you want to lift one level, use 10 volume peroxide; to lift two, use 20 volume; for three, select 30 volume, and so on. If you are going from a lighter level to a

◆ Key Point ◆

The basic rules of color selection are

1. Determine the natural color level.
2. Determine the color level you will need.
3. Determine the tonal value.
4. Determine lightening and depositing action.

TABLE14.2 The Tone Factor

Tone is the visible warmth or coolness of a color. The tone of the final color depends on the predominant base in the color formula used. The base is coded by the manufacturer. For example:

N	Refers to neutral tones that carry an equal blend of the primary colors.
G	Refers to predominant gold base.
R	Refers to a predominant red base. Some products use a pink-red with this designation.
R-O	Refers to a predominant red-orange base.
R-V	Refers to a cool red base. This color contains some blue.
V	Refers to a violet base.
A	Refers to an ash base that may contain gray, green, blue, or a combination.
B	Refers to an ash base that contains primarily a blue or blue-gray base.

darker one, use a reduced volume, such as 10. In this system, it is assumed that for every 10 volume of developer used, you achieve one level of lightening action. The color you select will determine the amount of deposit achieved and the color value of that deposit.

Selecting the correct color formula is the key to good results. Use the procedure that follows to select a color formula for the strand test.

Materials

Cape	Wide-tooth comb
Towels	Photographs
Neck strip	Color swatches (optional)
Brush	

Procedure for Selecting the Color Formula

1. Seat client comfortably at your station.
2. Wash your hands.
3. Observe how the colors your client is wearing affects his or her complexion. Select the client's Color Key palette.
4. Drape the client.
5. Brush the hair lightly to remove tangles.
6. Part the hair with a wide-tooth comb and check the scalp for abrasions, redness, or irritations.
7. Analyze the integrity (condition) of the hair.
8. Determine the natural color level.
9. Determine the color tone present.
10. Determine the level you wish to achieve.
11. Determine the color tone desired.
12. Considering all factors, estimate color formula.

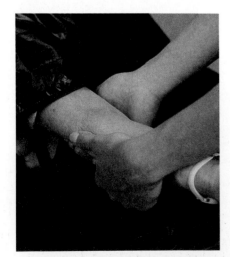

14.15

14.16

14.17

PREPARATION FOR HAIR COLORING

Your key to successful hair color is to follow each step in this working plan. After the analysis and consultation, you are ready to begin the actual color application.

The Patch Test

A preliminary patch test to determine a possible allergic reaction is required if you are using any aniline derivative color. Mix a small amount ($\frac{1}{2}$ tsp) of the chosen formula with developer according to the manufacturer's directions. Apply a small amount with a cotton tip applicator behind the ear or in the fold of the elbow. Leave undisturbed for time recommended by the manufacturer (24–72 hours), to determine if the client is allergic to this type of hair coloring.

Materials

Protective gloves	Towel	Peroxide or developer
Cape	Spray bottle	Small glass or plastic
Neck strip	with water	mixing bowl
Mild soap	Cotton swab	Measuring spoon
Cotton	Selected color	

Patch Test Procedure

1. Seat client comfortably at your station.
2. Wash your hands.
3. Drape your client.
4. Cleanse a small area behind the ear or in the fold of the elbow with mild soap (low pH) and water. Remove cleanser with cotton saturated with water.
5. Mix $\frac{1}{2}$ teaspoon of selected color with peroxide, according to manufacturer's directions. Blend thoroughly.
6. Apply color to cleansed area with a cotton swab (Figures 14.15 and 14.16)
7. Advise client not to touch the patch-test area.
8. Check for any indication of redness, swelling, or irritation after the recommended time (Figure 14.17). Note results on the client's record card. If the patch test shows signs of irritation, suggest an alternative coloring product to which the client does not react.

Draping the Client

Draping the client properly for the hair coloring service will protect the skin and clothing from stains.

Materials

Neck strip (optional)
2 towels
Large clip
Tint cape
Brush

Procedure for Draping

1. Seat client.
2. Cleanse your hands.
3. Ask client to remove earrings and neck chains.
4. Turn the client's collar to the inside; make sure it is straight and will not get wrinkled.
5. Place a towel folded diagonally across the client's shoulders so that at least a quarter of the width of the towel is resting across the neck. Bring the ends together and overlap in front of the client, under the chin (Figure 14.18).
6. Place the center of the neck of a tint cape directly over the center of the overlapped towel. Bring both sides of the cape around to fasten in the back. Check that the cape is not directly touching the skin (Figure 14.19).
7. Fold the towel over the neck of the cape and adjust as necessary to ensure your client is comfortable and protected. Use a second towel for a "double drape," according to your instructor's recommendation (Figure 14.20).
8. Remove any pins or clips from the hair.
9. Gently brush the hair to remove any tangles, avoiding contact with the scalp.

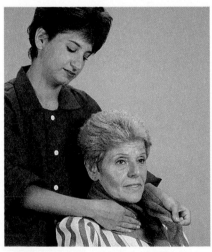

14.18

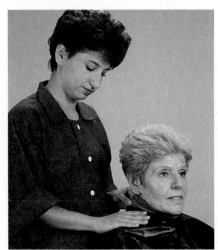

14.19

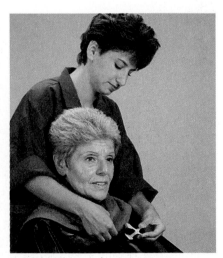

14.20

Preliminary Strand Test

Now that you have created a custom color formula, try it out on a small strand of hair. A preliminary strand test will let you know how the hair will react to the formula and how long the formula should be left on the hair. Perform the strand test after the hair is completely prepared for the coloring service.

Materials

Plastic clips	Glass or plastic	Spray water bottle
Towels	mixing bowl	Shampoo
Protective gloves	Mixing spoons	Aluminum foil or
Record card	Selected tint(s)	plastic wrap
Tint brush or bottle	Developer	

Procedure for a Preliminary Strand Test

1. Assemble materials.
2. Put on protective gloves.
3. Mix a small amount of formula according to manufacturer's directions.
4. Part off a ½ inch square in the lower crown (Figure 14.21). Use plastic clips, as necessary, to fasten other hair out of the way.
5. Mix ½ teaspoon of the selected color formula with the amount of developer recommended by the manufacturer (Figure 14.22).
6. Place the strand over the foil and apply the mixture. Follow the application method for your color procedure (Figure 14.23).
7. Check the development at 5-minute intervals until the desired color has been achieved. Note the timing on the record card.
8. When satisfactory color has been developed, remove the protective foil. Place a towel under the strand, mist it thoroughly with water, add shampoo, and massage through. Rinse again by spraying with water. Dry the strand with the towel and observe results (Figure 14.24).
9. Adjust the formula, the timing, or the application method, as necessary and proceed to color the entire head.

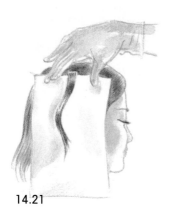

14.21

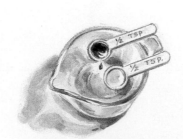

14.22   Mix tint and developer

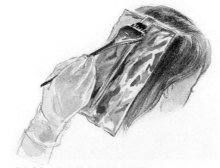

14.23   Apply tint to strand

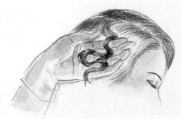

14.24   Observe results

TECHNIQUES FOR THE PROFESSIONAL COLORIST

There are many exciting options in the world of hair coloring. Here, we will present the basic color application techniques and a few of the established methods for creating special effects. Trends in hair coloring change frequently, but each technique you learn will increase your ability as a colorist. The secret to a successful hair coloring service is to combine the right formula with the technique best suited to the client.

Temporary Color Application

Temporary color is the easiest to apply. Follow the manufacturer's directions and ask your instructor for guidance with your first few applications.

Materials

Neck strip	Applicator bottle, if necessary
Shampoo cape	Towel
Shampoo	Wide-tooth comb
Selected color rinse	Protective gloves (optional)

Procedure for Temporary Color Application

1. Drape your client and seat at shampoo bowl.
2. Shampoo, rinse, and towel dry the hair.
3. Apply 1 to 2 ounces of color rinse, starting carefully at the hairline and follow through to the ends (Figure 14.25).
4. Comb through for even saturation (Figure 14.26). Add more color product as needed.
5. Towel-blot and proceed with styling.

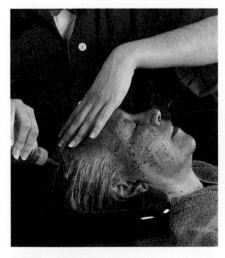

14.25   Apply color rinse

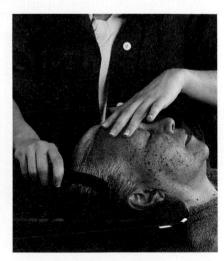

14.26   Comb color through

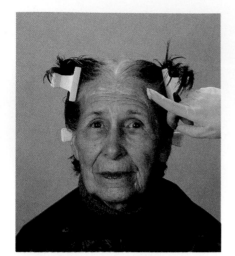
14.27 Apply protective cream

Semipermanent Color Application

There are a variety of semipermanent colors available to you as a professional stylist. Some are self-penetrating and do not require a developer. Some require a predisposition, or patch test. Become familiar with the semipermanent hair color products that are available. Study the features and benefits of each. Consult with your instructor before you begin application on your client. The following is the basic procedure.

Materials

Towels	Timer	Plastic cap (optional)
Tint cape	Wide-tooth comb	Record card
Protective cream	Plastic clips	Stylist's smock
Protective gloves	Cotton	(optional)
Applicator bottle or	Mild shampoo (low pH)	
plastic or glass bowl	Selected semipermanent	
and tint brush	color(s)	

Procedure for Applying Semipermanent Color

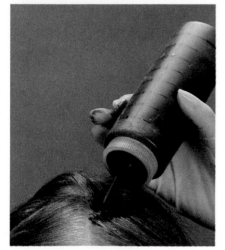
14.28 Apply color at scalp

1. Seat client and drape.
2. Check results of patch test, if required, and record on client's card.
3. Shampoo the hair, rinse, and towel-blot. Dry hair if recommended by the manufacturer.
4. Apply protective cream around hairline and over ears (Figure 14.27).
5. Put on protective gloves.
6. Mix the formula according to the manufacturer's directions.
7. Begin application where the most color change is desired (Figure 14.28) and apply from scalp to ends (Figure 14.29).
8. Work the color through to the ends with your hands. Saturate the hair thoroughly (Figure 14.30) without massaging into the scalp. Pile the hair loosely on top of the head.
9. If required, place a plastic cap over the hair (Figure 14.31).

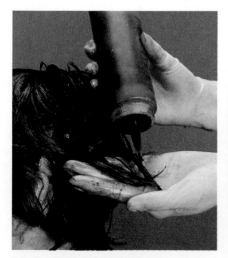
14.29 Apply color to ends

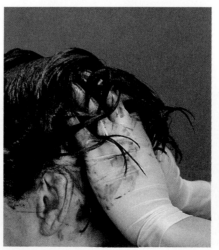
14.30 Work through hair

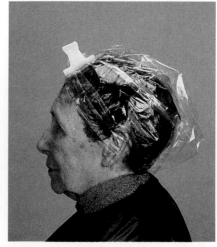
14.31 Plastic cap over hair

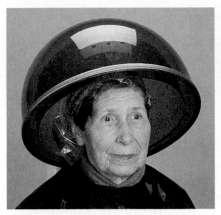

14.32 Place client under dryer

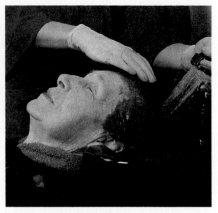

14.33 Rinse thoroughly

Secure with a plastic clip, and place you client under a preheated dryer to activate the color (Figure 14.32).

10. Follow the manufacturer's directions for timing and for removal of the color from the hair. Some semipermanent colors contain shampoo in the original formulation and additional shampoo may not be necessary.
11. Rinse thoroughly and carefully cleanse the hairline area. Shampoo excess color from the hair (Figure 14.33) if needed.
12. Condition and moisturize the hair with a mild acid product for two to five minutes and remove by rinsing.
13. Fill out record card.
14. Style client's hair. Use less heat and tension if you are thermal styling.
15. Recommend the appropriate retail products for the client to use at home.
16. Clean up styling and shampoo areas.

CLIENT **T I P** ♦♦♦♦♦♦♦

Suggest semipermanent tints to introduce your client to color.

Permanent Tint Application

Aniline derivative tints give the greatest range of hair coloring options. This is the type of color you will apply most often. Permanent color involves a chemical reaction inside the hair. For best results, mix the color just prior to application (oxidation begins immediately). Apply the color quickly and thoroughly, beginning where the color is needed most, or where the hair is more resistant. Be aware of the timing as you work to complete the coverage. The standard procedures for an application to virgin hair (hair not previously colored) and a retouch application follow. Become acquainted with the manufacturer's recommendations for the color product you are using, and consult with your instructor before proceeding.

Materials

Towels	Timer	Mild acid conditioner
Tint cape	Plastic clips	Moisturizer
Protective gloves	Cotton	Spray water bottle
Protective cream	Mild shampoo (low pH)	Stylist's smock
Applicator bottle or	Tint product	(optional)
plastic or glass bowl	Developer	
and tint brush	Client record card	

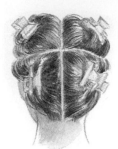

14.34   Section hair

Procedure for Applying Tint to Virgin Hair

1. Seat your client comfortably and drape.
2. Check the results of the patch test for any signs of redness or irritation. Proceed only if the skin is clear.
3. Shampoo the hair if necessary, or as guided by your instructor or manufacturer. Use caution; avoid any scalp manipulations during the shampoo.
4. Apply conditioning treatment if indicated by your analysis. Ask your instructor if a clarifying treatment should be given to neutralize any coating or chemical buildup on the cuticle of the hair.
5. Perform a strand test as outlined on page 282.
6. Section the hair into four equal sections (Figure 14.34).
7. Apply protective cream around the hairline and over the ears.
8. Put on protective gloves.
9. Mix formula according to strand test results and manufacturer's directions (Figure 14.35).
10. Apply the tint, starting in the most resistant area.
    a. If you are going lighter, this will be the darkest area. Begin applying at the midshaft.
    b. If you are going darker, it will be the lightest, or most gray area. Begin application at the scalp, outlining the section first.
    Part off a ¼- to ½-inch horizontal subsection (Figure 14.36). Apply the color to the midshaft area, beginning ½ inch from the scalp (at the scalp if going darker) and continuing up to, but not through, the porous ends. Lift the subsection up and apply to the bottom of the hair (Figure 14.37). Lay the hair up toward the crown and proceed to the next ¼- to ½-inch subsection. Work quickly and rhythmically for best results. Lift the hair from the scalp and gently turn sections back over. Avoid packing the hair against the scalp (Figure 14.38).

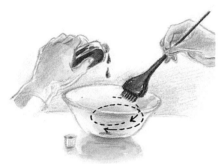

14.35   Mix color formula

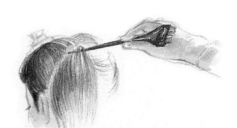

14.36   Part off subsection

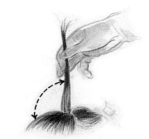

14.37   Apply color under strand

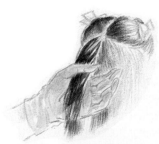

14.38   Apply to mid shaft

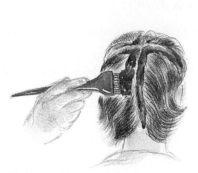

14.39　OUtline section

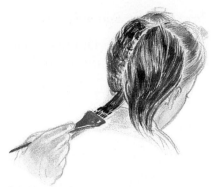

14.40　Apply to next section

11. Quickly move to the next section, outlining it if the application is going darker (Figure 14.39). Apply color, lift the hair from the scalp, and turn it over to the original position (Figure 14.40).
12. Set your timer according to your strand test results.
13. Cross-check each section by gently making vertical partings and adding more color formula, as necessary (Figure 14.41). While you are cross-checking, make certain color does not contact the scalp. If it does, gently blot with a damp towel.
14. Check timing by removing color from a subsection five minutes before timer indicates (Figure 14.42). Mist the subsection with water and towel dry to evaluate results. If color is not complete, resaturate subsection and continue timing.
15. When the center strand (going lighter) has developed according to your strand test results, apply color to the scalp area up to the midshaft.
16. Again, according to your strand test results, work the tint formula through the ends and time (Figure 14.43).
17. Take a final strand test to confirm your timing and the results you desire.

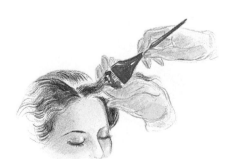

14.41　Cross check

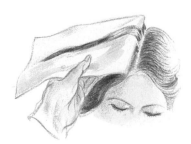

14.42　Check timing

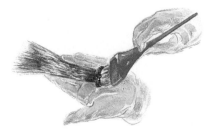

14.43　Apply tint to ends

Procedure for Removing Tint From The Hair

When you are certain that the strand test is indicating the color you want, remove the tint from the hair.

1. With the client at the shampoo bowl, rinse the hair lightly with lukewarm water (Figure 14.44). Emulsify the color by gently massaging with the palms of your hands (Figure 14.45). Rinse thoroughly.
2. Pour a small amount of acid-balanced (pH 3.8–4.5) shampoo into the palm of your hand. Work the shampoo with your hands and apply to the client's hair, beginning at the hairline. Massage gently, working with your fingers underneath the hair to avoid tangling (Figure 14.46).
3. Rinse and repeat as necessary until all excess color and protective cream has been removed from the hair and scalp (Figure 14.47).
4. Towel blot excess moisture (14.48).
5. Acidify the hair (Figure 14.49). Work product through the hair and time as directed.
6. Rinse and towel blot.
7. Moisturize according to your analysis of the hair (Figure 14.50).

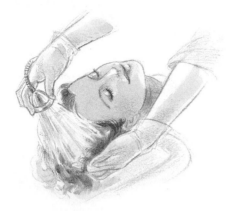

14.44   Rinse hair

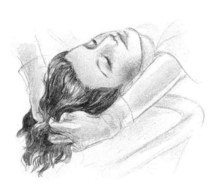

14.45   Gently massage hair

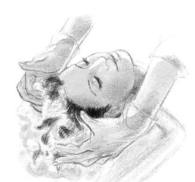

14.46   Shampoo hair

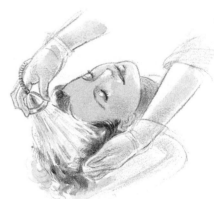

14.47   Rinse shampoo

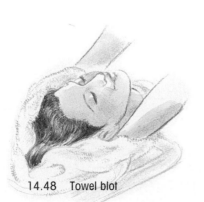

14.48   Towel blot

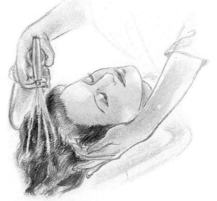

14.49   Acidify hair

14.50   Moisturize hair

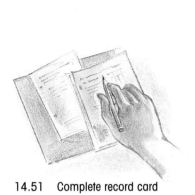

14.51 Complete record card

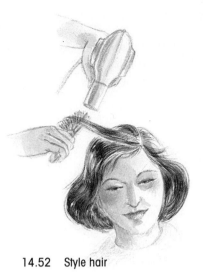

14.52 Style hair

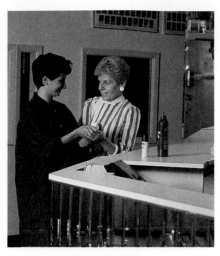

14.53 Recommend products

8. Make all notations on the client record card (Figure 14.51).
9. Towel blot and proceed with styling. If you decide to thermal style the hair, use a lower heat setting and less tension with your brush (Figure 14.52).
10. Recommend the appropriate retail products so the client's hair can be maintained in excellent condition at home (Figure 14.53).
11. Clean up working areas.

Styling Tinted Hair

Special precaution should be taken when styling freshly tinted hair. Avoid high heat and use as little tension as possible to obtain the styling results you desire. If you are setting your client's hair and drying it under the dryer, use a lower temperature setting. If you are thermal styling your client, first remove at least half of the moisture with your dryer on a cool setting. Finish the style with natural-bristle brushes and less tension. Use a styling aid to protect the cuticle of the hair. A leave-in conditioner may also be desired for smooth results. Refer to Chapter 11, Thermal Hairstyling, for techniques that produce results without damaging your client's hair.

Tint Retouch

Hair grows approximately $\frac{1}{2}$ inch per month. If the client has all-over-the-head hair color, expect to do a retouch every month. For certain styles and colors, it will be necessary to retouch the hair more often. Color results are always best when the hair has not been permitted to grow a long new growth or "root" area. A patch test is required prior to the retouch application. Check the manufacturer's instructions for the length of time a patch test will take.

CLIENT TIP ◆◆◆◆◆◆◆

Schedule the next retouch application before your client leaves the salon. Advise your client that color results are best when hair is retouched regularly.

CLIENT TIP ◆◆◆◆◆◆◆

If the previously tinted hair is dry or damaged, lightly apply liquid protein conditioner with a spray bottle. Comb through for even distribution.

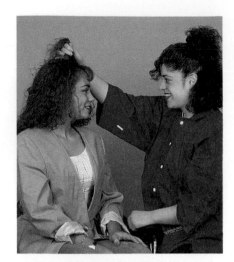

14.54   Analyze hair condition

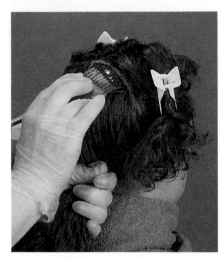

14.55   Apply color to regrowth

Materials

Client record card	Selected color(s)	Timer
Mild shampoo (low pH)	Developer	Protective cream
Mild acid conditioning	Wide-tooth comb	and gloves
solution	Plastic clips	Stylist smock
Moisturizer	Color applicator bottle	(optional)
Towels	or glass or plastic bowl	
Tint cape	and tint brush	

Procedure for a Tint Retouch

1. Seat client and drape.
2. Analyze the condition of the hair and the color results from the last application. Discuss the client's satisfaction with their color and be prepared to make minor changes to the formula if necessary (Figure 14.54).
3. Prepare the hair as necessary. Refer to the *Procedure for Applying Tint to Virgin Hair*.
4. Check the results of the patch test.
5. Section the hair into four equal parts.
6. Put on protective gloves and mix the formula according to record card and your analysis. Strand test if you are changing the color formula.
7. Begin color application where the hair is most resistant or where previous color faded the most. Apply from the scalp to the line of demarcation (Figure 14.55). Do not overlap color as this could produce off-color results and breakage.
8. Outline the parting of the first section (Figure 14.56). Apply color to horizontal subsections ¼- to ½-inch deep (Figure 14.57). Quickly work from section to section, outlining as you go. Lift each subsection from the scalp to apply underneath (Figure 14.58). Turn hair of each section back over to original position as you complete the application.

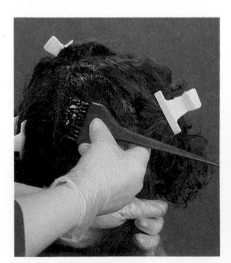

14.56   Outline first section

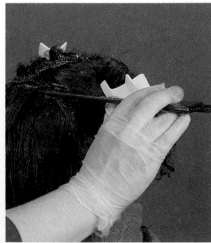

14.57   Apply to subsections

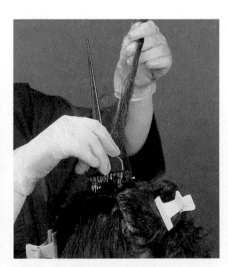

14.58   Apply color under hair

9. Cross-check color application by parting vertically and adding more product as necessary. Time according to your record card, and strand test as necessary to confirm development.

10. Dilute remaining color formula with conditioner, shampoo, or water as needed or directed by your instructor. Work it through the ends only to refresh existing color (Figure 14.59). Time 5 to 10 minutes and begin removal of color as outlined in *Procedure for Removing Tint from the Hair*.

Continue styling your client's hair. Advise your retouch client about home care. From your analysis of the hair and color, you will know if the hair faded because of the formulation or as a result of life-style or styling damage. Encourage your client to use the correct shampoo and conditioning products at home and to protect tinted hair from excess sun.

Specialty Techniques for Hair Coloring

Application techniques for hair coloring are unlimited. Most specialty techniques involve coloring only selected strands of hair, rather than the entire head. These techniques can be done alone, or can be performed on colored hair for custom color effects. Partial coloring techniques are recommended for clients who are extremely active, looking for special effects, or inexperienced with hair coloring. The basic techniques of specialty application are described in Chapter 15, Hair Lightening. Any of these specialty techniques can be used with permanent tint.

Another significant way to vary the results of hair coloring is to change the value of the peroxide (see Table 14.3). Lower volumes of peroxide (20 volume and below) increase the deposit you can get from a selected color. Higher volumes (20 volume and above) increase the potential lift. Check with your instructor and with the manufacturer for directions regarding the effects of peroxide volume on color.

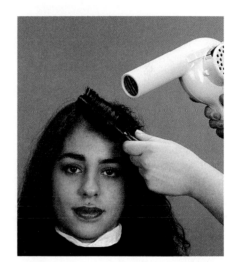

14.59 Work color through ends

14.60

TABLE 14.3	The Effects of Peroxide Volume
2–5°	Deposits color only. Can be effective on soft, white hair or soft, fine hair. Excellent for use as the developer for toners.
10°	Deposits color with a minimum of lift. Increases depth of levels 1–6. Excellent for deposit on gray hair.
20°	Provides both lift and deposit. This is the standard volume used by manufacturers to create the effects indicated by color charts and swatches.
25–30°	Provides lift and some deposit. Does not fully develop deeper color tones. Effective on virgin extra curly hair and resistant gray. Increases the lightening action of high lift tints.
40°	Provides lift and less deposit. Increases the lift capability of tints level 6 and higher. Can effectively lighten coarse, textured hair. Can cause cuticle damage. Should be used with care on hair that undergoes other chemical services.

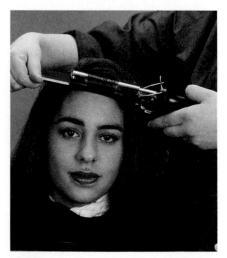

14.61

Alternative Developers

New developing agents for activating permanent hair coloring have recently been introduced to the market. **Enzyme activators**, for example, claim to produce color results faster and without the damage of oxidation from hydrogen peroxide. Consult with your instructor regarding alternative products.

Dimensional Color Techniques

As a color specialist, you should carefully observe how nature distributes color and how technicians alter it. Hair is usually lighter around the face and at the top of the head due to greater exposure to sunlight. As we mature, the hair in this area is usually the first to fade and then gray. You can take advantage of this by applying a lighter formula using a higher volume of peroxide on the top and front sections. You can highlight other areas with small-strand techniques such as slicing or weaving (see Chapter 15).

From your analysis of hair color, you know that hair is naturally darkest in the nape area. You can take advantage of this and make your hair color look more natural by adjusting your formula for this area of the head. Specialized color techniques can also be used to draw attention to the style. Remember that lighter colors draw attention while darker colors define the outside shape. You can highlight a wave pattern, for example, or define a bob line with a darker color. Subtlety is the secret to effective hair coloring. Observe television personalities and photographs of models in magazines to see how subtle hair color effects must be to look natural.

Highlighting Shampoo Tint

Also known as a soap cap, the **highlighting shampoo** tint is a color technique that gives highlights, blends in faded areas, covers gray slightly, lightens the hair slightly, and is a good introduction to hair coloring. The formula for the soap cap is usually a level 6 or lighter tint, developer, and shampoo. This technique is especially effective on naturally blond or fine hair.

Prepare the client as for any color service (Figure 14.62). At the shampoo bowl put on your protective gloves and mix the formula desired. Apply the mixture to damp hair. Massage gently for distribution using special caution not to irritate the scalp (Figure 14.63). Time for 10–15 minutes (Figure 14.64), rinse, and remove color as outlined on page 288 (Figure 14.65).

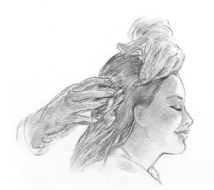

14.62　Prepare for color service

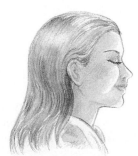

14.63　Massage gently

14.64

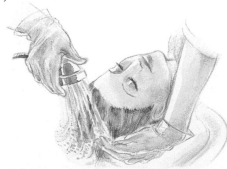

14.65

Color Stain

This specialty technique involves the use of a permanent color without developer. Rather than mixing the color with peroxide, a cream protein conditioner is used. Consult the manufacturer to ensure that the color product you use is compatible with this technique. On clean, damp hair, quickly apply the stain. A low volume peroxide can be added to increase color fastness (retention) or to help blend gray.

Place a plastic cap over the hair and seat client under a warm dryer for 15–25 minutes. Rinse and shampoo excess color from the hair.

This technique actually works as a semipermanent color, but is often longer lasting. It adds highlights and color to the hair, requires no maintenance, and produces incredible sheen. This technique is not effective if the hair is more than 10 percent gray. Color stains can also be mixed with hot water. A mixture of tint and hot water can be effective as a filler (see following section) during corrective color procedure. When tint is used as filler, the hair is not processed under a dryer.

Fillers

A **filler** is a product used to deposit color on damaged or porous hair so that the overall color is even. A filler can be a conditioner which will equalize areas that are overly porous, or it can be a color filler that adds base pigment to the hair and also evens the porosity before the color process.

If more than 50 percent of the natural pigment has been removed from the hair, it is necessary to replace the missing warm (red) pigment before the hair can be tinted back to a darker level. Apply fillers to clean, damp hair. Process according to manufacturer's directions, blot the excess from the hair, and proceed to apply desired color directly over the filler product.

Coloring Gray or White Hair

When the hair loses pigment, whether from age, trauma, or illness, it can be more difficult to color. Unwanted yellow tones can be evident, or the gray hair will be more resistant to coverage by the coloring product. If the amount of white or gray is small, you can obtain good color results by selecting a base N or neutral color from the correct level. The larger the percentage of gray, the more warm tones will need to be added to the N base color you select.

If the hair is soft in texture, try using a lower volume of peroxide in your color formula. When the hair is resistant or glassy, however, you may find that higher volume (25–30) peroxide is necessary. Since deposit decreases with higher volumes of peroxide, increase the depth of the color formula. Consult with your instructor and strand test for best results.

Presoftening and Prelightening

Presoftening, the application of a product to increase the porosity of the hair, and **prelightening,** the partial removal of pigment from the hair prior to tinting, are seldom used in today's professional salon. While these techniques were necessary in prior years to treat resistant hair, today's products and methods are more advanced and make hair coloring possible for a large percentage of your clientele.

There may be occasions when you want more lightening action than you can obtain from the tint you desire. You may elect to use a higher volume of peroxide or you may choose to do a two-step application in which you lift the hair color with a mild lightener or a high lift tint, then apply a second tint to complete the process and achieve the desired tone.

Hydrogen peroxide used alone is ineffective as a prelightener or as a presoftener. Hydrogen peroxide is an acidic solution that must be activated, or alkalized with ammonia or some other alkaline solution before its softening and lightening characteristics can be achieved.

Tinting Back to the Natural Shade

Occasionally a client who has had lightened hair will decide to return to the natural hair color or go to a darker shade. These techniques are known as **tint backs** and can be the test of your professional talent. Your client should be advised of the drastic difference in appearance that darker hair will create. Carefully analyze the condition of the hair. Pay special attention to the porosity and the elasticity of the hair. The technique you select must treat hair damage caused by previous color services as well as replace pigment.

To develop a color formula for a tint back, determine which of the primary colors must be added to create natural looking brown tone. For example, imagine that you have a client with light blond hair who complains that it is too difficult to maintain. The client wants to return to the natural easy-care medium brown shade. What to do?

Analyze the present color. The hair is primarily a level-9 yellow. It is dry and has some protein loss. The regrowth is an ash brown at level 5. Since ash is green, if you simply applied ash brown color, the result would have a strong green tone. In addition, the color would be very dark because the hair is damaged. A professional colorist will first deep condition the hair with a cream protein. Do this step alone, or add the missing primary—red—as a color filler. Process the hair until it is a medium orange. Now add blue—the other missing primary. It is blue that you will add to the brown color with an ash base. Process with a low volume peroxide and check frequently so the color does not become too dark. Finish by acidifying and moisturizing the hair.

It is usually better to return to darker hair in a gradual fashion. You may want to consider reverse frosting (see Chapter 15), where strands are pulled through a cap or woven, filled, or tinted to a darker shade. Any of the weaving techniques can be effective, and offer a more subtle return to the darker shade. If you decide that a total tint back is the best method, carefully recondition the hair. Use a color filler to replace missing primaries and finish the process with a tint mixed with low volume peroxide. Carefully monitor the condition of the hair as it grows. Replace the warm tones as necessary with a staining technique until enough hair has regrown that you can cut the formerly lightened hair.

Materials

Tint cape	Conditioner	Timer
Towels	Selected tint color(s)	Moisturizer
Record card	and filler	Stylist's smock
Mild shampoo (low pH)	Glass or plastic bowl	(optional)
Protective cream	Tint brush	Comb
and gloves	Acidifier	Clips

Procedure for Tinting Back to the Natural Shade

1. Seat client comfortably and drape.
2. Carefully analyze condition of the hair and scalp (Figure 14.66).
3. Condition the hair according to your analysis.
4. Analyze the primary color present in the lightened hair.
5. Analyze the primary pigments and the concentration of the desired color.
6. Apply protein conditioner to the hair if it is damaged. Comb through for even distribution.
7. Section the hair into four quadrants.
8. Apply appropriate color filler or custom formula of conditioner and color to replace missing primaries, especially the warm tones. (If conditioner filler is used, eliminate step 6.) Part the hair into ¼-inch subsections and apply filler where needed (Figure 14.67). Time according to manufacturer's directions (Figure 14.68).
9. Towel blot excess filler (Figure 14.69), and perform a strand test with the suggested color formula.

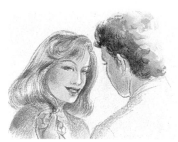

14.66   Analyze hair

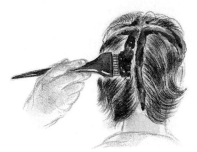

14.67   Apply filler

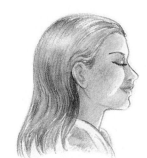

14.68   Time application

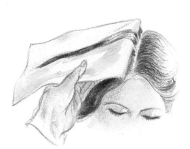

14.69   Towel blot filler

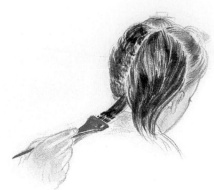

14.70 Apply color formula

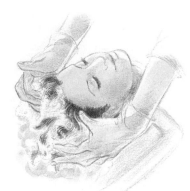

14.71 Shampoo hair

10. Carefully monitor development and record all results on the record card. Rinse the strand, dry, and analyze results.
11. Readjust formula and repeat strand test until you have the results you desire.
12. Apply color formula to entire head (Figure 14.70), carefully monitoring development. Strand test frequently.
13. With client at shampoo bowl, rinse hair gently with lukewarm water. Apply acid-balanced (low pH) shampoo and carefully massage underneath the hair to avoid tangling (Figure 14.71).
14. Acidify the hair for 5 minutes.
15. Recondition as necessary and finish by moisturizing the hair.
16. Record all results on the client record card, clean work areas, and proceed with styling.
17. Use a styling aid to protect the cuticle layer of the hair, and use as little heat and tension as possible. It is usually best to wet set the hair rather than use thermal styling.
18. Schedule your client for a series of reconditioning treatments.
19. Suggest that client purchase the correct products for care of the hair at home.

Tint Removal

When the color deposit on the hair is very heavy, or color products have built up on the hair, you may decide to use a tint remover. This is a specialty technique to be used only after careful consideration has eliminated any other corrective coloring technique.

Tint removers are solvents that lift the artificial pigment within the hair. They also lighten the hair's natural pigment. The pH of these products is very alkaline, so you must consider the damage done by the coloring procedures as well as estimate the damage that will be done to the hair during the removal process.

Safety Measures for the Professional Colorist

Whenever you are working with chemicals—shampoos, conditioners, or chemicals that penetrate the hair—observe safety practices. This will reduce the risk of injury to you and your clients and protect you from possible lawsuits. The chemicals you work with are not dangerous if handled, stored, and used properly. The following is a summary of safety precautions recommended for the professional salon offering coloring services.

Storing Color Materials

All hair coloring materials should be tightly capped. This prevents the color from oxidizing in the bottle from exposure to the air. Hair coloring products should be stored in a cool, dark place so the color is not prematurely activated. Partial bottles of color should be used first. Be aware of the expiration date stamped on the outside of each color bottle. When you select a bottle that has been previously used, check the surface of the color through the bottle. If you see a ring of developed color, discard the bottle and select a fresh supply. If your school uses tube color, protect it from exposure to air by carefully folding the bottom of the tube as color is used. Keep tubes tightly capped.

Peroxide and other developers should also be stored in a cool, dark cabinet. Do not store color materials in direct sunlight, or near the furnace or hot water heater. Color materials should be stored on shelves clearly marked with OSHA information.

OSHA and You

The Occupational and Safety Hazards Act requires that chemicals in any business be stored with evident markers indicating content and effects on the human body. Do not be intimidated by the information, but use it to protect yourself and your client. Use common sense when handling chemicals. Do not smell them. Avoid standing directly over the color bowl when you are mixing a formula, so that you do not inhale the potent fumes created when the chemicals interact. Wear protective gloves and protect your client with cream and cotton where necessary. Discard any unused color formulas by rinsing containers immediately so that they cannot accidentally spill on clothing and cannot be picked up by inquisitive people, especially children.

Additionally, OSHA requires that a manual be available that describes chemicals used in your salon or school, antidotes if they are accidentally spilled or ingested, and general safety precautions. Remember, the guidelines are for raw chemicals; you work with solutions that are diluted.

Record Cards

The record card is your primary reference as a professional colorist. It tells you the exact condition of your client's hair and scalp, the desired results, the formula and timing, the actual results, and the retail items purchased by your client. Client records can also be stored on disk in computer systems. This way, you can store service data as well as pertinent marketing information such as birthdays, anniversaries, names of children, occupation, and much more. Update the record every time you service your client and use the "comments" section to fine-tune future color services.

Release Forms

A release form protects both you and your client. Your client's signature on the release form indicates your client is aware of the procedures and risks involved in the hair coloring service. Many insurance carriers require that you obtain such a release from your clients. In the rare event that you are involved in a malpractice lawsuit, the release form provides documentation of professional practices.

> ◆ **Key Point** ◆
> Proper storage of color materials will keep your workplace safe and guarantee fresh products for your client.

Hair Coloring Glossary

The following list contains common hair coloring terms. You may wish to add to this glossary those terms your instructor gives you for specific hair coloring products available in your school.

- **accent** A concentrated formula that can be added to the color formula to intensify or tone down the color.
- **activator** A specialized developer used to increase development of color (see also **activator** in Chapter 15, Hair Lightening).
- **base** The combination of colors that make up the tonal foundation of a specific hair color.
- **brass** A term used to describe undesirable tones of either red or gold that make the hair color too intense.
- **color refresher** **1.** Color applied to midshaft and/or ends during the service to replace the pigment lost by oxidation. **2.** Specialized shampoo used to balance color between salon services.
- **color remover** Specialized product that removes artificial pigment from the hair. Also known as a "stripper."
- **contributing pigment** Natural or artificial pigment present in the hair before the coloring service.
- **coverage** In hair coloring, a term used to describe the success of coloring gray or white hair.
- **deposit** The addition of color to the hair to make it darker.
- **depth** The lightness or darkness of a color.
- **developer** An oxidizing agent, usually hydrogen peroxide, that chemically reacts with artificial hair coloring products and the natural pigment to produce a change in hair color.
- **drab** Color containing no red or gold. Ash.
- **eumelanin** A type of natural melanin pigment found in black, brown, and blond hair.
- **fade** To lose color through exposure to the elements, etc.
- **intensity** Used to describe the strength of a color's tone, its warmth or coolness.
- **level** The value of the depth of color on a scale of 1 to either 10 or 12. The darkest level is 1.
- **lift** The action of a hair lightening product on the natural pigment of the hair.
- **line of demarcation** An obvious difference between natural and colored hair.
- **melanin** The natural color pigment.
- **nonammonia color** Color that does not contain ammonia. Also, color that does not lift, only deposits.
- **pheomelanin** A type of melanin. The natural pigment found in red hair.
- **shade** A gradation of difference between one hair color and another.
- **tone** A word used to describe the warmth or coolness of a color.
- **tyrosine** The amino acid essential for the creation of natural melanin.
- **value** The lightness or darkness of a color. Also known as "level" or "depth."
- **volume** The relative strength of peroxide. Its capability to release oxygen (when mixed with certain chemicals) and thereby lift color.

The exciting world of the professional hair color technician offers unlimited challenges and high financial returns. Cosmetologists who want to master the art of hair coloring may choose to specialize.

A professional hair colorist must have a clear understanding of the laws of color. The primary colors—red, yellow, and blue—have characteristics of warmth, highlight, and depth. When two primary colors are mixed in equal amounts, a secondary color is created. Red and blue make violet, blue and yellow make green, and red and yellow make orange. All three primary colors must be present to form brown.

Hair coloring is classified according to color fastness (or retention). Temporary colors last one shampoo only; permanent colors, or tints, last until there is new hair growth; and semipermanent colors last from four shampoos to several weeks, depending upon the type selected. A patch test is required for all aniline derivative colors, regardless of their classification.

As a professional colorist, you must be able to analyze the level (darkness) of the natural hair color and of the color desired. You must note the tone (warmth or coolness) of the color present and the color desired. With this information, you will select the hair coloring and the ideal formula to achieve the results your client wants. Choose the application technique which will suit your client's lifestyle and give the best results.

Before you color, you should drape your client for protection and perform a patch test if the color you use is aniline based. Perform a strand test to double-check your formula before you apply it to the entire head. Record all consultation and color process information on a permanent file in the client's name.

SUMMARY

QUESTIONS

1. What are the three primary colors?
2. What are the secondary colors?
3. How do complements interact? What is their importance to the professional colorist?
4. Explain the three classifications of hair color. Indicate the advantages and disadvantages of each.
5. How is correct color formula determined?
6. How is a client prepared for a coloring service? What special precautions should you take when draping?
7. What is the importance of a patch test? How is it performed?
8. How is a strand test performed? How do you determine whether you have selected the correct color formula?
9. Name at least five different application techniques available to the professional colorist.
10. What safety measures should you use when storing hair coloring chemicals?
11. What is the impact of OSHA on the salon?
12. What key items should you list on the client's record card?
13. What is the value of having a release form signed prior to color services?

PROJECTS

1. Working with gel food coloring, create a color wheel using only primary colors.
2. Working again with only the primaries, create brown and black.
3. Mix complementary pairs and place them side by side to compare results.
4. Research the classifications of hair coloring products available at your school. List the features and benefits of each.
5. Experiment at least five times with each type of hair coloring product. Use your mannequin, fellow students, or clients.
6. Select at least three photographs from magazines for each of the following hair colors: brown, red, blond, and gray. Analyze the primaries and the highlights in each photograph.
7. Working with the same magazine photographs, select any pair and propose a color formula to change the hair color in photograph #1 to the hair color of photograph #2. Try several examples and review your results with fellow students and your instructor.
8. Arrange a sequence of photographs to represent the levels of hair color.
9. Find at least six photographs from magazines which illustrate different specialty hair coloring techniques. List the procedures you would need to follow in order to achieve the results in each photograph.
10. Research the MSDS (Material Safety Data Sheets) available for the hair coloring products in your school. Discuss with your classmates steps you can take to avoid injury to yourself and your clients, and the proper way to store chemicals.

HAIR LIGHTENING

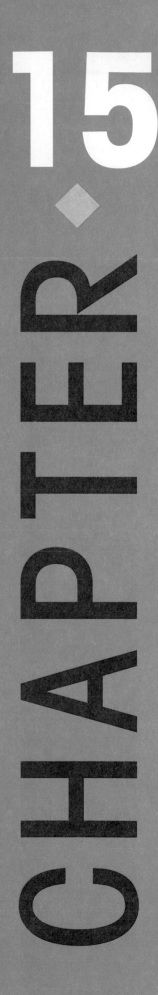

CHAPTER GOAL

Mastering the art of creating healthy and beautiful blonde hair will build your list of happy, repeat clients. After reading this chapter and completing the projects, you should be able to

1. Describe lighteners available and explain their effects.
2. Explain the effect of oxidation on the hair shaft and the two methods of peroxide measurement.
3. Demonstrate how to prepare a client for the lightening service.
4. Outline the procedures for lightening virgin hair and for retouching.
5. List at least six problems that can occur with lightening. Explain the causes of these problems and what you would suggest to solve them.
6. Demonstrate at least six special-effects techniques and explain the results of each.
7. Explain safety measures to protect the client, yourself, and the salon during the lightening procedure.

Hair lightening.is a specialty art. While the lightest shades of blond are often dictated by fads of fashion, blonding of one sort or another is always in style. The artistry of lightening can be subtle or dramatic; you, the professional cosmetologist, will decide.

The Romans used a variety of native minerals combined with old wines and water to lighten the hair. They left the mixture on at least overnight and more commonly six or seven days. The effect was a reddish-gold shade. Next, the painter Titian popularized the golden-red shade through his paintings. Women of Venice achieved this desirable effect by pulling their hair through the brim of a hat and applying a solution of rock alum, black sulfur, and honey. This technique became the rage in sixteenth-century France.

The discovery of hydrogen peroxide by Louis Thenard of France in 1818 made lightening quicker and somewhat less messy, although it was still mixed with harsh and sometimes even dangerous chemicals. By the Paris Exposition of 1867, a revolutionary lightening technique using three percent (10°) peroxide had been developed. The modern era of hair lightening had begun.

Based on your consultation with your client, select the appropriate procedure for hair lightening. Choose, prepare, and apply chemicals in the correct manner. Practice all safety techniques.

LIGHTENERS AND THEIR EFFECTS

Hair lightening is the process of permanently making the hair lighter than its natural shade by changing pigment in the cortex layer. This process can be done all over the head, or in small sections for special effects. Whatever the result desired, hair lighteners work in the same way.

Lighteners are alkaline chemicals that are most commonly available as powders or creams. They are mixed with acidic hydrogen peroxide to start a chemical reaction. When the lightener mixture is applied to the hair, it penetrates into the cortex. There, the natural pigment melanin is changed. Melanin is a dark pigment granule responsible for the brown tones that we see in hair. When it is *oxidized* by the lightener mixture, a new pigment, oxymelanin is formed. If you decide to continue the process, oxymelanin granules can actually break down until the hair is pale yellow or almost white.

The changes inside the cortex caused by lighteners are permanent. When the hair grows, the new growth has to be lightened in a similar fashion. With today's lighteners, a little or a lot of pigment can be removed from the hair without significant hair damage. Today's blond shades are soft and natural looking without the garish "peroxide blond" tones of the past.

When the hair is lightened, it goes through seven stages of lightening from black up to an almost white color. Those stages are black, brown, red, red-gold, gold, yellow, and pale yellow.

If you can remember the color theory discussed in Chapter 14, you will understand how this occurs. What is the first pigment to be lost? Blue. As blue, then red, and finally yellow are lost from the overall hair color, it goes through the seven stages shown in Figure 15.1. As red is lost from the hair, the pigment molecules in the hair begin to disintegrate and to diffuse throughout the cortex layer. Even though pigment is still present in the hair, the granules are so small that little or no color is reflected back to the eye.

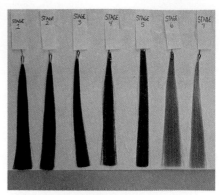

15.1   Seven stages of lightening

Lightening, as any chemical service, will make the hair more porous. This means that it will absorb liquids more rapidly and is more prone to damage. Counteract this side effect at some point during the service so that the hair will remain in good condition and you will obtain the desired tonal results.

Types of Lighteners

Modern lighteners evolved out of the use of hydrogen peroxide mixed with ammonia water. The ammonia water was needed to make the mixture alkaline so it could penetrate the hair and lift color. Of course, the liquid formula was very messy and difficult to control, so magnesium carbonate (soap flakes or "white henna") was added to thicken the mixture. Other lightening and conditioning compounds were added until the formulations in use today were developed. These lighteners are most often available as a cream or a powder.

Cream lighteners contain thickeners, conditioners, and emulsifiers. They are a very popular lightener and are most often used for application at the hair closest to the scalp. They are easy to control because there is no running or dripping. Cream lighteners are easy to use for retouch applications and can be used for both brush and bottle methods.

Oil lighteners are seldom used alone because they are slow and very messy. Oil lighteners can be used for special effects lightening or as additives to other formulas.

Powdered lighteners are also known as "quick lighteners." They were originally developed for off-the-scalp application such as frosting, but many powder lighteners are now gentle enough to be used near the scalp. Powder lighteners are usually faster in their activity, are often slightly more alkaline, and can be drying to the hair. Powder lighteners must be kept moist to continue working; if the mixture dries, the action will stop.

Accelerators are not actually lighteners, but are additives to speed the process. Also known by names such as protinators, boosters, and activators, they are added to hydrogen peroxide prior to mixing it with the chosen lightener. Accelerators are most commonly available in prepackaged packets that accompany lightener selected.

◆ Key Point ◆

Lighteners to permanently remove color from the hair are available as cream, powder, or oil formulations.

They are crystallized oxidizers that increase the strength of the peroxide chosen. Follow the manufacturer's directions and be sure that the activator is totally dissolved in the hydrogen peroxide before adding the lightener.

Color Additives are also used in lighteners to add color tones to the hair that will offset the harsher tones as the hair loses color. Some lighteners contain blue additives that subdue the orange tones. Many of today's powder lighteners come in a variety of colors so that a base tone can be added to the hair as the hair is lightened.

Color Removers are a corrective form of hair lightener. They are similar to powder hair lighteners, but have the ability to also break down artificial pigment that has been added to the hair. These products are mixed with peroxide or water. Reconditioning is necessary after color removal to ensure that satisfactory color results are obtained without excessive damage.

Advantages of Hair Lighteners

1. Hair lighteners allow the professional cosmetologist to lighten the hair through all seven stages, from very dark brown or black to almost white or pale yellow.
2. Hair lighteners offer much greater lifting power than tints.
3. Lighteners can be used for corrective work when previously applied colors are no longer desired.
4. Lighteners can quickly remove color from hair for special effects in a single process, providing that the natural color is not too dark.

Disadvantages of Hair Lighteners

1. Hair lighteners can be damaging to the hair if the proper precautions are not followed.
2. Lightening processes that require toning take more salon time to accomplish desired results.
3. The hair needs more reconditioning on a regular basis since the hair-lightening process creates more porosity in the hair shaft and decreases sheen on the surface.
4. Thermal styling options are restricted.

OXIDATION

The primary chemical activity that takes place in all lightening procedures is **oxidation**. Chapter 13 will help you understand how this process works technically. During the lightening service, oxidation breaks down and diffuses the pigment in the cortex layer of the hair. The tiny pigment granules become much lighter or barely visible to the eye. The hair will be lighter in color, or may even appear to be colorless.

The chemical that activates this process in the hair is **hydrogen peroxide**. Hydrogen peroxide is typically available today as a liquid, cream, or gel in strengths of 10, 20, 30, and 40 volume. Other volumes are available or can be made by diluting from a very strong liquid formula. Volumes higher than 60 are not used often. The American system of measuring peroxide is by volume; the European method is by percentage. Let's see what these mean and compare them.

Volume is a measurement of capacity (the amount of space occupied). The volume (°) of peroxide indicates the potential the peroxide has for lightening the hair. One liter of 10° H_2O_2 (the chemical formula for ten volume hydrogen peroxide), for example, can release 10 liters of free oxygen gas. One liter of 20° H_2O_2 can free 20 liters. The amount of oxygen gas liberated indicates the lifting or lightening capacity of the liquid.

The **percentage** method of measuring hydrogen peroxide indicates the amount of active ingredient. In a 3% solution, 3% of the content is active oxygen gas; the other 97% is water and other inert ingredients. Each percent of peroxide in the European method of measurement is equal to 3.3 volume of peroxide in the American method.

Table 15.1 outlines the effect of hydrogen peroxide in various strengths. *Deposit* indicates the use of H_2O_2 in a tint formulation; *lift* indicates that H_2O_2 is mixed with a high-lift tint or a lightener.

TABLE 15.1 The Effects of Peroxide Volume	
2–5°	Deposits color only. Excellent to use as the developer for toners and stains.
10°	Used with some powder lighteners for subtle high-lights. Used as a developer of midrange toners. Deposits color with a minimum of lift. Increases depth of levels 1–6. Excellent for deposit on gray hair. Used for lift on relaxed hair.
20°	Provides both lift and deposit. This is the standard volume that is used with powder and cream lighteners. Used by manufacturers to create the effects duplicated in color charts and swatches.
25–30°	Used with lighteners on resistant hair. Speeds quick lighteners for off-the-scalp applications. Provides lift and some deposit. Does not fully develop deeper color tones. Effective on virgin overcurly hair, resistant gray, and to increase the lightening action of high-lift tints.
40–60°	Used as a speed lightener for some freehand techniques. Can be used with a cream lightener with less protinators or activators than directed. Used for spot lightening and corrective work. Provides lift and little deposit. Increases the lift capability of tints level 6 and higher. Can be effective on over curly, coarse-textured hair. Can cause cuticle damage. Should be used with caution if hair undergoes other chemical services.

Hydrogen peroxide is a mild acid (pH 4.0) and must be alkalized in order to begin its activity. This is typically done by the addition of lightener, color, and other alkalines. If hydrogen peroxide is used alone, it must be alkalized to be effective either as a presoftener or as a lightener. Do not allow peroxide to come in contact with metal—violent chemical reactions could occur. Always store hydrogen peroxide in a cool, dark place.

The volume of peroxide or many other liquids can be measured with a **hydrometer** (heye **DRO** mi ter). To measure, pour liquid H_2O_2 into the measuring tube and float the indicator. Read the volume of peroxide on the indicator at the top of the peroxide. Hydrometers, also known as peroxometers, can only reliably measure liquid formulations since the indicator must float freely.

Cream or gel formulations of hydrogen peroxide are also available. These thicker formulas offer more control in application, especially for freehand techniques. Many cream or gel peroxides also contain buffers to help prevent scalp irritation.

Higher volumes of peroxide are seldom used as the possibility of damage is high. When you mix activators with lighteners, you effectively raise the working volume—sometimes above 70°. High volumes of peroxide should be used with great care and only after you have achieved salon-level mastery.

Altering Volumes of Peroxide

Stronger volumes of peroxide can be diluted to make the strength you desire. Dilute peroxide *only* with distilled or **deionized** (dee **EYE** oh nyzed) water (water without an electrical charge). Tap water contains metallic elements and will react, sometimes violently, with peroxide. This reaction is dangerous and could cause severe injury. Ensure the accuracy of your dilution by checking the volume with a hydrometer. Tables 15.2 and 15.3 will serve as guides for the dilution of peroxide.

PREPARING FOR LIGHTENING

A consultation prior to chemical services is vital. Determine your client's commitment to the upkeep of the hair after lightening. Select a lightening process based on your client's willingness to care for the more delicate lightened hair and the results you want to achieve.

The Consultation

During the consultation, you will select the color, examine the scalp, analyze the condition of the hair, and arrange for a preliminary strand and patch test if necessary. You may want to refresh your memory of the detailed procedure for a consultation in Chapter 14, Hair Coloring.

> ◆ **Key Point** ◆
> Oxidation is the primary chemical reaction that causes lightening of the natural pigment, melanin.

TABLE 15.2 Peroxide Chart—High Volumes

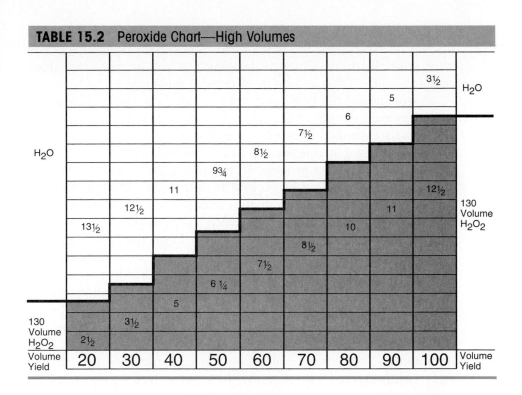

Volume Yield	20	30	40	50	60	70	80	90	100
H₂O	13½	12½	11	9¾	8½	7½	6	5	3½
130 Volume H₂O₂	2½	3½	5	6¼	7½	8½	10	11	12½

TABLE 15.3 Peroxide Chart—Low Volumes

Volume Yield	2½	5	7½	10	12½	15	17½	20
H₂O	14	12	10	8	6	4	2	
20 Volume H₂O₂	2	4	6	8	10	12	14	16

The color selection process in hair lightening is more simple than that of one-step hair coloring. In lightening, the manufacturer will guide you to the level or stage of color removal that you should obtain prior to application of the toner to get desired results. Or, with many of today's lighteners, you will only use one application, and will decide the color of lightener to apply to neutralize undesired tones and/or deposit color highlights.

CLIENT TIP ◆◆◆◆◆◆◆

Use the consultation time to educate your client about the processes and maintenance involved. At the same time, analyze the hair to determine whether you can achieve the results your client wants.

Be honest with your client about the processes involved, the upkeep necessary, and the cost of the total service. Remember, you want your client committed to keeping the hair in the same salon-perfect condition that you create. Consider this story:

A woman had her hair lightened and loved the result. Two weeks later, however, she called the salon to express her unhappiness. She was greatly disturbed because she could see dark hair at the scalp. She was surprised by this because her stylist had explained that lightening was a permanent process. To this client, permanent meant forever. As hard as it might be for you to believe, she thought that she was a blond for life! She was invited back to the salon and the entire procedure was explained to her. Once understanding for the first time what was really involved, this client knew that she could not afford the time nor the money for the upkeep that was necessary. So then what happened? The salon decided to tint her hair back to its original shade, at no expense to the client. This misunderstanding could have easily been avoided with just a few more minutes of conversation until the stylist was sure that the client understood and the client was sure that her desires were going to be met. She could then have chosen an alternative blonding service better suited to her life style and budget. Unfortunately, in a corrective service with an unhappy client, the salon had far fewer options.

Give your client a realistic estimate of the cost of maintenance on a monthly or quarterly basis. If the cost of upkeep is prohibitive for your client, suggest an alternative method that will give reasonable results within the client's price range. You might offer one of a number of partial lightening techniques or a hair coloring option. Even if the idea of lightening is abandoned altogether, you will have an informed client who will value your advice and honesty and certainly return to you for future services. The following basic care guidelines should always be discussed:

1. Use a quality shampoo designed for lightened hair.
2. Have a deep conditioning treatment once a week.
3. Arrange for retouches every three to five weeks.
4. Take care to protect lightened hair from the sun.
5. Cover the hair with a bathing cap when swimming.
6. Avoid swimming in chlorinated water.
7. Use caution with thermal styling. Avoid excessive heat and stretching.

The Record Card

As with all chemical services, maintain an accurate record card for each client. Be sure to record the condition of the hair and scalp, and the results of the preliminary strand and patch tests. When you perform the full service be sure to include:

1. The type of lightener used, and the formulation and timing.
2. The degree of lightness obtained.
3. The toner (if any) and the formulation and timing.

◆ **Key Point** ◆
The consultation ensures that you are communicating with your client and the hair is in good condition. Confirm your analysis with a patch and a strand test.

CLIENT TIP ◆◆◆◆◆◆
Applying a penetrating conditioner during the lightening process minimizes damage and leaves the hair in the best possible condition.

4. Conditioners or treatments performed during the service.
5. Results obtained and any corrections suggested for the next appointment.

◆ **Key Point** ◆

Preparation for a lightening service should include a consultation, an analysis, and a strand test. Follow manufacturer's directions regarding patch tests. Record all observations.

The Patch Test

A patch test may be required for many toners used in the salon. Consult the manufacturer's instructions to see if a preliminary test to determine allergy to the toner is necessary. If so, this should be performed at least 24 hours prior to each lightening service. It is easy to perform the patch test when you have the original consultation.

Materials

Cape	Towel	Peroxide
Neck strip	Spray bottle with water	Small glass or plastic mixing bowl
Mild shampoo	Cotton swab	Measuring spoon
Cotton	Selected toner	Client record card

Procedure for a Patch Test

1. Seat client comfortably and drape.
2. Cleanse your hands.
3. Cleanse a small area behind the ear or at the fold of the elbow with mild shampoo.
4. Rinse and gently blot dry.
5. Mix ½ tsp. of selected toner with the correct amount of peroxide as directed. Apply with a cotton-tipped swab and leave undisturbed for at least 24 hours (see Figure 15.2).
6. Gently cleanse patch-test area and examine for any signs of redness, swelling, or irritation (Figure 15.3). Continue with the lightening and toning service only if your client had no reaction to the patch test. Note results on client's record card.

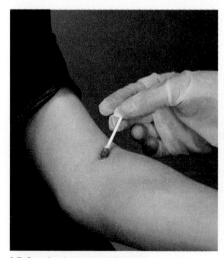

15.2   Apply toner with swab

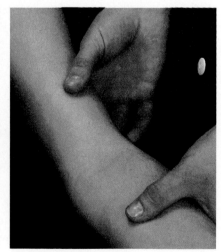

15.3   Check for reaction

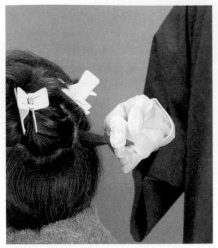

15.4 Part off section

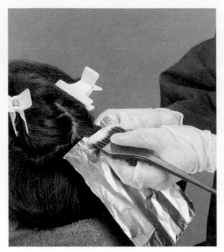

15.5 Apply to mid-strand

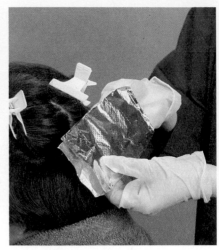

15.6 Fold foil over strand

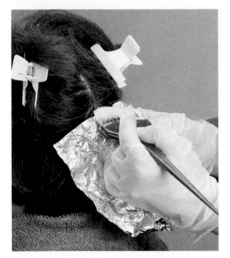

15.7 Apply to hair near scalp

The Preliminary Strand Test

A strand test is a necessary step in a professional lightening service. The strand test helps you select the correct formula, estimate timing and avoid hair damage during the procedure (Figures 15.4–15.8). You will most frequently test a strand of the client's hair on the day of the service. For a strand test you will need all the materials for a patch test plus your selected lightening formula, tint brush, clips, and foil. If you determine that more testing is necessary, reschedule the lightening service and do the following: Part off a $\frac{1}{4}$ to $\frac{1}{2}$-inch section of hair from the client's head. Prepare a small amount of lightener in a glass or plastic bowl. Apply this mixture to the mid-strand and carefully observe timing and results obtained. After the mid-strand has lightened halfway to the shade you desire, apply lightener to the hair near the scalp. Replace foil and monitor results. When the desired shade has been reached, shampoo the strand, rinse it in lukewarm water, dry, and tape it to the client's record card. Be sure to record the formula and the timing on the card.

LIGHTENING THE HAIR

After you have finished these preliminary steps, you are ready to begin the lightening process. We will first discuss the techniques for lightening virgin hair, that is, hair that has had no prior chemical services. You will not have many clients in need of this particular approach, but you must know how to get them started on a regimen of healthy, lightened hair.

15.8 Check results

Lightening Virgin Hair

Materials

Towels	Cotton	Shampoo
Protective cape	Timer	Acidifying solution
Applicator brush	Wide-toothed comb	Conditioner
or bottle	Plastic clips	Client record card
Glass or plastic bowl	Selected lightener	Spray water bottle
Protective cream	and activator(s)	Plastic cap (optional)
Protective gloves	Hydrogen peroxide	

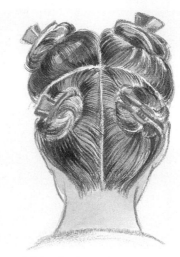

15.9   Section hair

Procedure for Lightening Virgin Hair

1. Cleanse your hands.
2. Seat your client comfortably and drape for a chemical service. Have your client remove ear and neck jewelry.
3. Analyze scalp and hair. The lightening service should be avoided if there are abrasions or inflammation of the scalp. Do not brush the hair.
4. Section the hair into four equal parts and clip out of the way (Figure 15.9).
5. Apply protective cream around hairline and over ears.
6. Put on your protective gloves and mix the lightening formula according to the manufacturer's directions.
7. Begin applying the lightener. Start in a section where the hair is darker, usually in the back. Make a thin parting across the section that is ⅛–¼ inch deep and apply lightener to the center of the subsection, from 1 inch away from the scalp up to the line of porosity but not through the porous ends (Figure 15.10).
8. Continue the application through the entire section, working quickly. Make sure that all hair is covered. The lightener must be reasonably thick for best results (Figure 15.11).
9. Continue application in all four quadrants. Your instructor may suggest that you place cotton on the scalp at partings to prevent irritation.

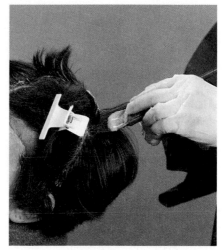

15.10   Apply to mid-shaft of hair

10. Cross-check each quadrant with vertical partings. Apply more lightener as needed and loosely pile hair on head. Do not pack hair to scalp.
11. Test for lightening action. Make the first check after about 10 minutes. Consult the manufacturer's directions for approximate total time. With a damp towel, remove the mixture from a small subsection where first applied. Analyze the progress of the lightening action. If it is half way, proceed to the next step. If not, reapply lightener and continue processing. Apply a plastic cap over hair, if desired, to speed processing.
12. When the center of the hair shaft is lightened half way to the stage desired, remove excess lightener by towel blotting. Mix fresh lightener and apply from the scalp out to (but not through)

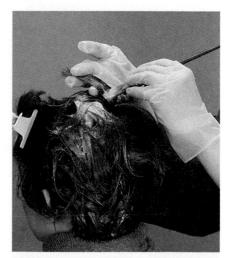

15.11   Complete section

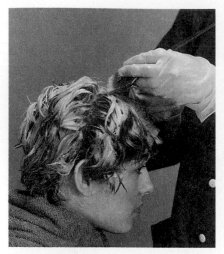
15.12 Apply at scalp

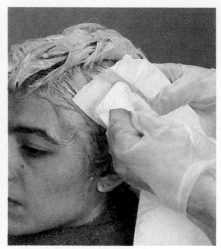
15.13 Blot a test strand

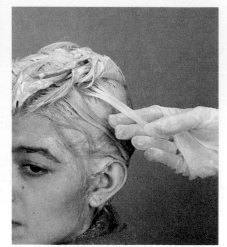
15.14 Check progress

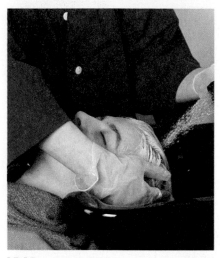
15.15

the ends (Figure 15.12). Remove any cotton between partings. Cross-check your application vertically, apply more product as needed and lift the hair from the scalp to permit oxidation. *Note*: Your instructor may direct you to apply fresh lightener to the scalp area without blotting the center shaft.

13. When the subsection is equally lightened from scalp through center, work the lightener through the ends of the hair. Add more lightener as necessary.

14. Strand test frequently. Blot a small subsection free of the lightener, towel dry and observe progress (Figure 15.13). If the hair is not light enough, reapply product and continue timing. When desired lightening is achieved (Figure 15.14), note timing on the client's record card and proceed to removal of the lightener at the shampoo bowl.

Procedure for Removing the Lightener from the Hair

1. Seat client comfortably at the shampoo bowl. Double-check that all nape area hair is inside the bowl and that the client's protective draping is adequate.

2. Rinse the hair thoroughly with cool water. Check the temperature on your wrist to make sure it is not too cold. Add just enough hot water for the comfort of your client. Use mild pressure to rinse the hair. Separate the hair with your gloved hand so that every section of hair is well rinsed. Pay special attention to the nape area (Figure 15.15).

3. Shampoo gently with a mild shampoo. Keep fingers underneath the hair to avoid tangling (Figure 15.16). Use only mild manipulation to prevent scalp irritation. Again, rinse thoroughly.

4. Towel blot. Examine the hair to ensure that the correct level of lightening has been achieved.

5. Apply a conditioner that can both acidify the hair and replace lost protein. Comb through hair with a wide-toothed comb, time, and rinse.

6. Fill out record card and proceed to toning, if desired.

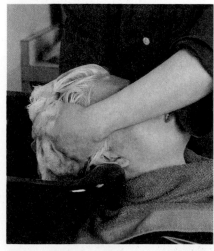
15.16 Shampoo gently

Lightening Very Dark Hair

Dark hair may require more than one application of lightening mixture to reach the pale yellow stage. Consult with your instructor to see if it would be preferable to use a powder, or quick lightener on the resistant midshaft area. Heat, with the hair covered by a plastic cap, can also speed processing, or a higher volume of peroxide can be used. Of course, any of these techniques should consider the condition of the hair and the client's comfort.

Lightening Retouch

The new growth at the scalp will of course be darker than the lightened hair, and will be quite obvious. It is best to perform a retouch application when the regrowth is slight, usually in 3–5 weeks. Consult the record card for the technique of the original lightening. Ask your client if he or she was satisfied with the original service.

Procedure for a Lightening Retouch

1. Assemble the same materials as for a virgin lightener.
2. Prepare the client in the same manner as for a virgin lightener.
3. Section the hair into four quadrants. Fasten out of the way with plastic clips.
4. Put on gloves and apply protective cream to the hairline and over the ears (Figure 15.17).
5. Mix the lightening formula according to manufacturer's directions.
6. Begin the application in the area where your record card indicates hair is most resistant. Apply in narrow $\frac{1}{8}$- to $\frac{1}{4}$- inch subsections, parting off carefully with the tail of the brush or the tip of the bottle to avoid scalp irritation (Figure 15.18). Apply lightener from the scalp up to (but not over) the line of demarcation (Figure 15.19).
7. Do not overlap. When lightener is applied or swells onto hair previously lightened, the hair becomes overly porous, bands of color are evident, and hair breakage can occur.
8. Process lightener until desired level is reached. Note all information on the client's record card regarding timing, formulation, and results obtained.
9. Follow the steps previously outlined in *Procedure for Removing the Lightener from the Hair.*

Toner Application

In most cases, a toner is applied to finish the lightening process. In all cases, analyze the condition of the hair and the scalp before continuing with the toning process. If the scalp is irritated, or if the hair is in damaged condition, you will want to perform corrective treatments prior to toning. In the case of scalp irritation, you may need to use a

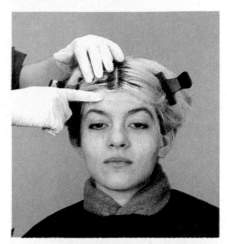

CLIENT TIP ◆◆◆◆◆◆

Make sure that your client is comfortable. If your client is sensitive, do not offer caffeinated drinks which could cause scalp irritation.

15.17 Apply protective cream

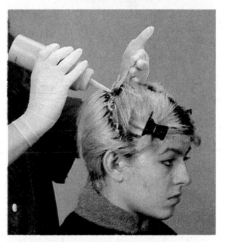

15.18 Apply in small subsections

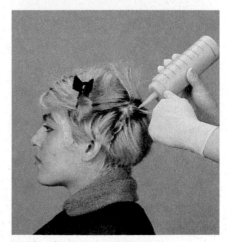

15.19 Apply to regrowth only

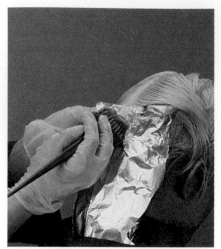

15.20 Apply toner to strand

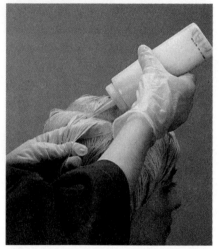

15.21 Begin at crown

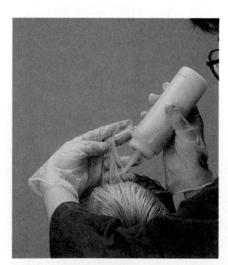

15.22 Apply toner gently

protective base, or postpone the toning service until the condition is healed. Most toners contain aniline derivatives, so a patch test is required at least 24 hours prior to application. You will perform the patch test prior to the lightening process and check results before proceeding with the service.

Materials

Towels	Protective cream	Record card
Protective drape	Timer	Mixing spoons
Applicator bottle or brush and bowl	Wide-toothed comb	Spray bottle of water
	Selected toner and peroxide	Aluminum foil or
Protective gloves	Mild shampoo	plastic wrap
Plastic clips	Conditioner	

Procedure for Toner Application

1. Check client draping to see that protection is adequate.
2. Spray the hair with a liquid penetrating conditioner to protect it during the toning process.
3. With a wide-toothed comb, section the hair into four equal quadrants.
4. Part off a ¼- to a ½-inch square subsection in the lower crown for a strand test. Use plastic clips to secure other hair out of the way if needed.
5. Put on your protective gloves and mix ½ tsp. of selected toner with peroxide as manufacturer directs.
6. Place the strand over the foil or plastic wrap and apply the mixture selected (Figure 15.20).
7. Check the development at five-minute intervals until the desired color has been achieved. Note the timing on the record card.
8. When satisfactory color has developed, remove the protective foil. Place a towel under the strand, mist it thoroughly with water, add shampoo, and massage through. Rinse by again spraying with water. Dry the strand with the towel and observe results.
9. Adjust the formula, the timing, or the application method as necessary and proceed to tone the entire head. Apply a heavy conditioner or protective cream to the strand so that it will not be recolored during the following application.
10. Apply protective cream around the hairline and over ears.
11. Mix toner according to strand-test results and manufacturer's directions.
12. Begin application in the back section of the crown. Use ¼- to ½-inch horizontal partings so that application will be quick and accurate (Figure 15.21).
13. Apply toner quickly from the scalp to the ends (Figure 15.22). Apply to entire head, then go back and cross-check each quadrant with vertical partings. Add more toner as necessary and separate hair so that hair is not packed to scalp (Figure 15.23).

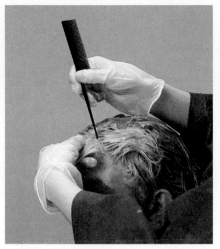

15.23   Separate hair

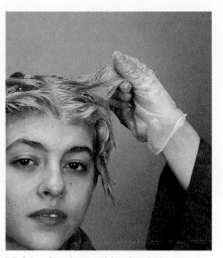

15.24   Check strand for development

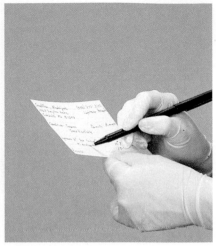

15.25   Complete record card

14. Process according to strand-test results. Verify development by removing toner from a small strand and observing color development (Figure 15.24).
15. Remove toner by adding a small amount of water and emulsifying the toner into the hair. Work around the hairline gently. Then, rinse with comfortably cool water. Use low pressure to avoid hair damage and tangling.
16. Add a mild shampoo and gently lather hair. Work lather into and around hairline to remove toner at scalp. Work with your fingers underneath the hair to prevent tangles. Rinse and repeat.
17. Rinse the hair thoroughly, lifting the hair from the scalp to make sure that all toner is removed. Pay special attention that all toner is removed from the nape area.
18. Towel blot and apply an acidifying solution or conditioner. Time as directed and rinse if necessary.
19. Apply a moisturizing conditioner. Rinse as directed.
20. Proceed with styling. Use less heat and tension when styling the hair.
21. Complete record card, clean work station, and suggest products for your customer to purchase for at-home maintenance (Figure 15.25).

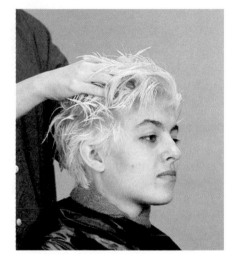

15.26   Apply deep conditioner

Toner Retouch

Whenever you schedule your client for a retouch lightening treatment, you will automatically do a toner retouch. Check the condition of the hair and incorporate deep conditioning into the retouch procedure (Figure 15.26 and 15.27). A patch test is necessary at least 24 hours prior to each application if an aniline-derivative toner is used.

Procedure for Toner Retouch

1. Assemble materials as for the toner application.
2. Gently towel blot the hair after lightener retouch and apply cream conditioner to the previously toned hair.

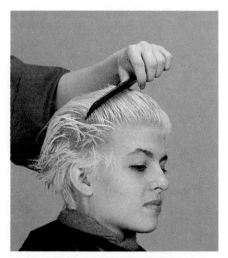

15.27   Comb conditioner into hair

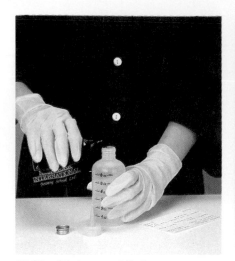

15.28 Mix toner and H_2O_2

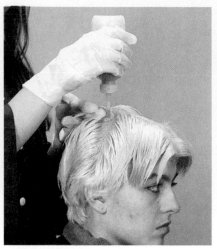

15.29 Apply toner to regrowth

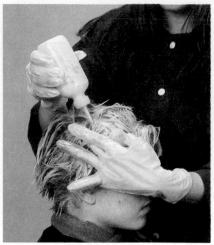

15.30 Cross-check application

◆ **Key Point** ◆

Lightening is typically a two-step process. First, the color is removed to the correct level. Next, a toner is applied to neutralize harsh gold tones and soften the blond color.

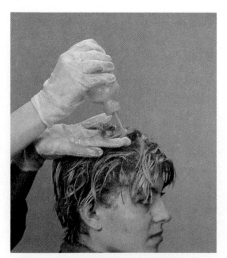

15.31 Work diluted toner to ends

3. Check the results of the patch test and examine the scalp for any sensitivity.
4. Apply protective cream around the hairline, and over the ears. Put on your protective gloves.
5. Part the hair into four sections. Strand test if color change is desired.
6. Mix toner with low-volume peroxide according to manufacturer's directions (Figure 15.28).
7. Make ¹/₂-inch partings and rapidly apply toner to former regrowth area (Figure 15.29).
8. Complete all 4 sections and then cross-check vertically. Add more toner as necessary. Avoid packing hair against scalp (Figure 15.30).
9. Time according to record card. Strand test to ensure desired results.
10. Work diluted toner through the ends to refresh color as necessary (Figure 15.31). Strand test to check even development.
11. Remove toner, acidify, and recondition the hair prior to styling.
12. Clean up work area, complete record card, and suggest products for your client to purchase.

HAIR LIGHTENING PROBLEMS AND SOLUTIONS

Hair lightening, as any other chemical service, can cause problems in the hair structure. Most of these problems are the result of insufficient lightening or incorrect toner selection. These can be corrected by proper strand testing and a change in the formula. Some hair lightening problems, however, do not result from improper toner selection and require more detailed analysis. Consult with your instructor before determining a course of action. Read the manufacturer's instructions and technical information available for any product you plan to use. The following situations are common hair lightening problems.

Excessive Porosity

Symptoms: The hair feels dry, rough, and strawlike.

Cause: Excessive lightening. Overlapping during the retouch application. Using too high a volume of peroxide in the toner formula. Failure to incorporate conditioning treatments into the lightening procedure.

What to do: Schedule the client for a deep conditioning treatment. Review products in use at home and recommend changes as necessary to correct prescription. Apply cream reconditioner to ends prior to retouch application. Do not pull lightener through ends and use special caution to avoid any overlapping. Use a low-volume peroxide toner or a stain, mixing the toner with conditioner rather than peroxide. Trim extremely damaged ends. Avoid thermal styling.

Elasticity Loss

Symptoms: Hair stretches excessively when wet, breaks easily when dry. When hair is wet, it feels soft, almost mushy.

Cause: Failure to correct porosity damage. Harsh handling and styling of the hair when wet. Overprocessing.

What to do: Immediate deep conditioning. Depending upon the level of elasticity damage (refer to Chapter 6, Hair Damages and Treatments), a polymeric conditioning treatment may be necessary. Find an alternative to further lightening until the damage is corrected or the hair in question is removed by cutting. Do not use thermal styling. Do not backcomb or backbrush the hair.

Toner "Grabs" Too Dark

Symptoms: Ends of the hair are significantly darker and show the base of the toner (blue or purple).

Cause: Repeatedly retoning the ends. Using peroxide of too high a volume in the toner. Porosity damage.

What to do: Always recondition the ends while the regrowth is processing. Use a low-volume peroxide toner or use a staining technique. Decrease toner processing time. Adjust toner formula. Do not apply toner to ends during retouch procedure.

Toner Does Not Hold Color

Symptoms: Excessively light and damaged ends.

Cause: Repeatedly lightening the ends during retouch applications. Using a toner with too high a volume of peroxide. Combing lightener or toner through hair, causing excessive damage. Harsh thermal techniques.

> **CLIENT   T I P** ◆◆◆◆◆◆◆
>
> Educate your client so that these typical damage problems can be avoided by regular conditioning.

What to do:	Deep-condition ends between and during every retouch treatment. Use a low-volume or a staining (low lighting) toner technique. Remove ends by cutting. Use end papers when styling the hair. Avoid thermal, and especially round-brush, styling techniques.

Hair Lightens to a Brassy Stage and No Further

Symptoms:	Hair, especially the midshaft, lifts to the red-gold stage and no further. Application of fresh lightener or extension of timing have little, if any effect.
Cause:	Metallic element inside the hair interfering with chemical activity.
What to do:	**Chelate** (**KEY** late) the hair with a product designed to inactivate metals in the hair. Apply lightener only to areas needed for spot lightening. Consider the use of a darker toner.

Insufficient Lightening

Symptoms:	Dark spots visible in the hair. Hair does not accept toner. Hair is darker than strand test indicated.
Cause:	Insufficient timing of lightener before removing. Failure to remove colored lightener. Improper application.
What to do:	Spot-lighten where necessary for even decolorization.

Gold Band

Symptoms:	A visibly darker gold tone shows at the line of demarcation after a retouch application.
Cause:	Usually insufficient lightening in the previous retouch or failure to apply lightener close enough to the line of demarcation. Can also be caused by overlightening the hair at the scalp, causing the regrowth to be totally colorless, and the center shaft darker.
What to do:	Recondition hair and carefully spot-lighten the gold band. Use a gentle lightener and low volume of peroxide as hair may be quite brittle. Use more caution in future applications to ensure that all hair is covered and overlapping does not occur.

> ### ◆ Key Point ◆
> Problems in hair lightening can be eliminated with analysis and preventive treatments. Record all results and corrective measures to avoid future problems.

LIGHTENING FOR SPECIAL EFFECTS

In today's professional salon, more and more color and lightening services are customized for each client. These techniques range from subtle to avant-garde, and give you great freedom to express your artistic talent while also satisfying your customers. Most of today's special effects techniques are subtle—imitating nature but improving upon what she offers. Special effects techniques can be used with lighteners or haircolors. You will be limited only by your imagination and technical skills.

Special effects techniques are almost limitless. You can add lighter tones (highlights), or you can add darker tones (lowlights).

What will be presented to you here are the most reliable techniques in use today. Add new techniques to your special effects repertory by consulting your instructor and attending trade shows and continuing education seminars. In addition to the materials needed for lightener application, you will need special implements for each of these special effects procedures.

The Cap Technique

For **the cap technique**, classically called **frosting**, strands of hair are pulled through perforated holes in a cap with a hook. The amount of highlighting can be adjusted by using alternate holes, pulling through smaller amounts of hair, using larger or smaller hooks, or pulling hair through holes in predetermined areas only (Figure 15.32).

If the density of the hair varies (is thinner around the hairline, for example), lessen the amount of hair pulled. If the hair is styled away from the face, your instructor may direct you to avoid pulling through right on the hairline.

If the hair is very long, pull the hair through in loops ½ to 1 inch long. After the desired amount of hair has been pulled into loops, comb it gently with a wide-toothed comb until the full length of the hair is through the cap.

Once the hair has been pulled through, comb it gently to remove any tangles. Apply lightener to the strands (Figure 15.33). Process until the desired level of lightening is achieved. Remember that lightener will only remain active when it is moist, so make certain the hair does not dry during processing. Remove lightener as necessary and apply fresh product until the desired lightness is obtained. Always lift the strands after application so that the hair is not packed at the cap, interfering with oxidation. You instructor or the manufacturer's directions may advise you to cover the hair with a plastic cap and place the client under a preheated dryer to speed processing (Figure 15.34).

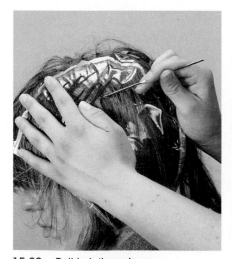

15.32   Pull hair through cap

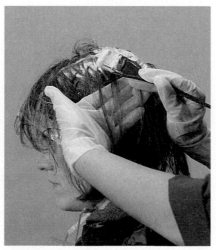

15.33   Apply lightener

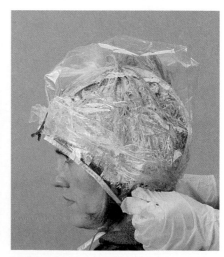

15.34   Cover hair with cap

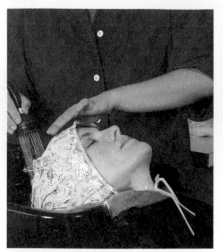

15.35   Rinse lightener

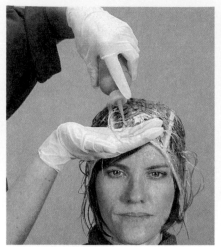

15.36   Apply toner

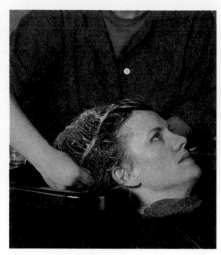

15.37   Remove cap

When the desired level of lightening is achieved, proceed to remove the lightener from the strands (Figure 15.35). Do *not* remove the cap from the head at this point. Rinse the lightener with cool water, shampoo the lightener gently from the hair, and rinse thoroughly. Normalize the pH of the hair prior to proceeding and/or apply conditioner as your analysis of the processed hair indicates.

At this point you are ready to tone the hair, if necessary. For most applications, especially if peroxide is used, you will want to apply the toner before you remove the cap from the head. Mix toner with low-volume peroxide as directed, apply it to the strands, and process as necessary (Figure 15.36). When processing is complete, remove the toner from the strands. Gently pull the cap from the head, working from the hairline toward the crown (Figure 15.37). The cap will pull more easily on long or porous hair if you apply an instant conditioner to the strands first. Now rinse, shampoo, condition as necessary, and proceed with styling. As always, make notes on the client's record card so that you can reproduce results.

Foil Techniques

A **foil technique** can be used to lighten selected strands of hair or to add subtle color tones to lightened hair or as a coloring technique. The technique provides many of the same results as the cap technique, but gives you more control over the placement of the lightener or color.

Weaving

Weaving uses strips of foil, paper, or transparent plastic to control placement of color or lightener on alternating strands of hair. These strips are commercially available, but you may prefer to make your own. The weave technique also places the lightener or color with the finished style in mind. Around the hairline, you will want to pay special attention to the finished style planned so that the placement of the weave will best enhance the style. Your instructor may direct you to style the hair first and then proceed to the weave.

CLIENT TIP ◆◆◆◆◆◆◆

Foiling techniques are the best choice for those clients who wish to disguise any evidence of hair coloring services.

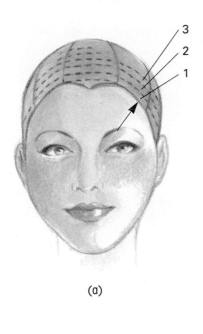

(a)

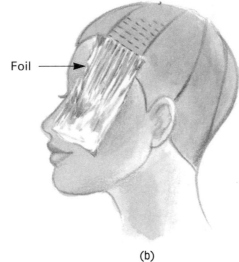

Foil

(b)

15.38　Sectioning for a weave

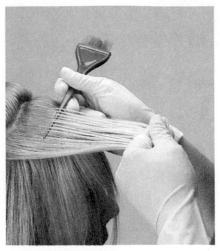

15.39　Weave strands from slice

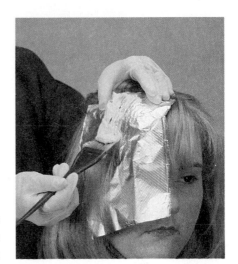

15.40　Apply lightener

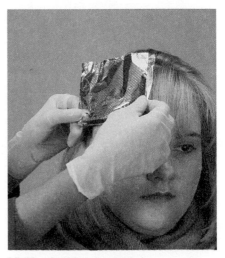

15.41　Fold foil over strand

Procedure for Weaving

1. Section the hair uniformly to provide the pattern you have designed. The best designs follow the hairline and consider the finished style. You will apply color or lightener to hair woven from every other section (Figure 15.38).
2. Begin weaving at the hairline by slicing a narrow subsection from the hair. With a tint brush or comb, weave tiny strands from the slice (Figure 15.39).
3. Place a strip of foil or transparent plastic under the woven hair. Apply selected lightener over the foil (Figure 15.40). Seal the edges to prevent seeping. Fold the strip in half from the ends toward the scalp and, depending upon the length of the hair, fold in half again (Figure 15.41).
4. Proceed in this systematic manner upward to the crown. Begin the next section at the hairline and work up to the crown in the same manner. Speed and accuracy of weaving are very important to the success of this technique.
5. Process to the desired shade. With client at the shampoo bowl, gently pull the foils from the hair.
6. Rinse and shampoo to remove all product.
7. Tone with a nonperoxide toner if desired.
8. Complete record card; indicate weave pattern.
9. Style hair.

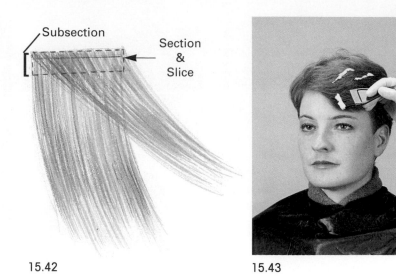

Subsection

Section & Slice

15.42

15.43

Slicing

Slicing is another foil technique, similar to the weave. The result is slightly more chunky than foiling, so the amount of lift should be only a few shades lighter than the client's natural color.

Presection and plan your slice as outlined for the weave technique. Begin at the hairline and work toward the crown.

Work with a fine-tail comb and slice paper-thin partings from a subsection (Figure 15.42). Place the foil under the slice and apply lightener. Working quickly, seal the edges, fold the strip, and proceed to the next slice. It is usually best to switch to the weave technique around the facial hairline and the design part so that the effect will be more subtle.

Painting

Painting is another fun way to create highlights. With this technique, a color brush or an artist brush is used to apply thin lines of lightener to dry prestyled hair (Figure 15.43). Use your artistry to accentuate the crest of a wave, to work very thin strips of lightener through the front, or to accent the uplift at the sides.

Choose the painting technique when you want subtle results with low maintenance. Select your formula so that the painted hair will be no more than two shades darker or lighter than the rest of the hair.

Scrunching

Scrunching is an alternative technique to painting, more suitable to curly or textured hair. Apply lightener to your gloved hands and scrunch the surface and the ends of the hair. You can control the amount of product placed on the hair by applying it to the palms of your hands or to the fingers only. You can also trace a particular line with your fingertips, just like fingerpainting.

The Comb Technique

There are various special application tools available that are used to "comb" color or lightener onto the hair. You may also use a conventional wide-tooth comb or rake for this technique. Prestyle the hair and carefully plan where you will place the lightener. Dip the applicator into the lightener or place lightener at the base of the teeth with the color brush or bottle (Figure 15.44).

Comb the product onto the hair where it will enhance the design of the style or cut. *Apply color or lightener once only* (Figure 15.45). Do not recomb the area once product has been applied. Process as directed, remove from the hair, condition, and style. On your record card make notes or include a sketch of the application pattern.

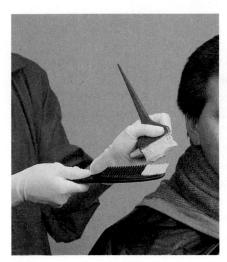

15.44

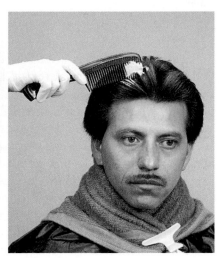

15.45

Optical Illusions

The creative colorist will also learn how to use lightening or coloring to enhance the shape of the client's face. The technique of using optical illusion to mask imperfections of the facial structure is called corrective coloring. Chapter 7, Elements and Principles of Design, explains line, proportion, and balance, so you can determine and achieve the best style for your client. In this section, we will discuss the proper placement of highlighting for various facial shapes.

The round face is full or moon shaped. It needs a lightening process that will enlarge the top and crown area, yet remain small at the sides. Using a short side part, frost or weave the hair on top and the top sides (above the temple) quite heavily. Frost very lightly above the ears to create an area of blend. Leave the lower sides the natural color. Use a light toner above the temple and a darker toner at the sides (Figure 15.46).

The square face applies the same theory as the round.

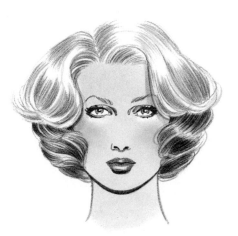

15.46

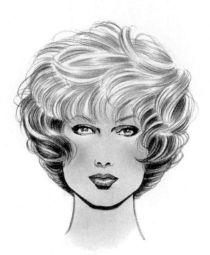

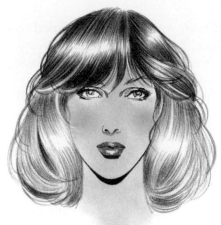

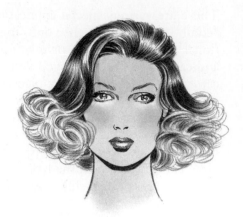

15.47   15.48   15.49

A diamond face has a narrow forehead and chin line with more width to the central facial region between. Frost or weave heavily in the narrow areas while avoiding the center facial region. This facial type also works well with dimensional coloring or lightening, which we will discuss shortly.

The triangle or pear-shaped face has narrowness at the forehead area and considerably more fullness in the jaw. Frost or weave the top area heavily. Gradually decrease the amount of hair lightened at the center sides, and leave the lower side fronts the natural color. Tone the top and top sides a light color. Tone the center sides a darker shade (Figure 15.47).

The inverted triangle or the heart-shaped face has a broad forehead and a narrow chin. Frost the lower sides heavily. Gradually decrease the amount of hair lightened as you work up to the eyebrow line. Use lighter toners on the bottom and middle sides at the front and a darker toner on the top sides (Figure 15.48).

The oblong face is long, narrow, and usually angular. Frost or weave the sides more heavily. Use little or no frosting on the top of the head. If longer bangs are worn, lighten the tips only. Use a light toner on the sides and a darker toner on the tips of the bangs (Figure 15.49).

Dimensional Hair Lightening Techniques

Dimensional lightening or **shading** is very striking when the colors blend well with a base shade that is compatible with the client's skin tones. Dimensional techniques use colors from the same tonal family and change gradually, without visible lines. Dark and light toners can be used against lightened hair, or a combination of tints and toners can be chosen. The hair can be lightened evenly all over, or the nape and lower back area can be left at a lower stage. Here are but a few suggestions to spark your imagination.

Blond-on-Blond

Blond-on-blond effects were a fad in the early 70s and then faded from popularity. With the onset of weaving and slicing techniques, however, we are seeing a return to multiple shades of tone on one head. There are two ways to achieve multiple blond tones. The first method incorporates weaving or slicing techniques with various strengths of lighteners or high-lift tints. This technique can be especially effective when the client's natural shade is a light brown or dark blond. If lightener is the lifting agent, use a nonperoxide toner after the foils have been removed to blend all colors.

The second method of achieving blond-on-blond tones is to lighten the entire head of hair to the desired stage and then use a foil technique (weaving or slicing) to apply various shades of toner. For best results with either of these artistic techniques, the base of the tints or toners must be compatible and the difference between the tones should be subtle.

Tricolor Blonding

Tricolor blonding is similar to the blond-on-blond techniques, but the various shades of color graduate in sections from the darkest to lightest according to the structure of the head. The nape is one section, the central area from the temple over the crown is a second, and the curvature of the top is the third section. Plan a *subtly* different shade of blond for each section. Another possibility is to leave the nape section at its natural shade, apply a medium tone in the central section, and the lightest tint at the top of the head. It is critical that the selected color tones blend and that there is no obvious jump in the level of tones selected.

Prior to special effects lightening, consult with your client to make sure that all colors selected are compatible with his or her skin and eye tones. Subtle variation of tones is best for believable color and for ease of retouch.

> **◆ Key Point ◆**
> Special effects lightening challenges your ability as a cosmetologist. Develop your technique, knowledge of color, and awareness of fashion to excel in this creative field.

SAFETY MEASURES FOR THE LIGHTENING EXPERT

Good safety practices protect you, your client, and your school or salon. Make safety a habit.

Safety Measures to Protect Your Client

1. Perform a patch test at least 24 hours prior to the use of an aniline derivative tint.
2. Do not use a lightener or toner if there are abrasions or irritations on the scalp.
3. Do not brush or massage the scalp prior to lightener application.

4. Cover your client with protective draping.
5. Apply protective cream around the hairline and over the ears before beginning lightener application.
6. Gently wipe any product from the scalp with a damp towel.
7. Maintain accurate records of each lightener service you perform.
8. Obtain a release statement from your client stating his or her awareness of the risks involved.
9. Make a preliminary strand test(s) to ensure successful results.
10. Avoid overlapping in any lightener retouch procedure.
11. Mix accelerators with peroxide before adding lightener to prevent burns to the scalp and to ensure proper mixing.
12. Do not apply lightener to hair treated with a metallic dye.

Safety Measures for Your Protection

1. Read and follow directions from the manufacturer and your instructor.
2. Wear protective gloves when mixing and applying lighteners and toners.
3. Read MSDS information from the manufacturer concerning health risks associated with certain products.
4. Post poison-control and other emergency numbers in the event of an accident or reaction to chemicals.
5. Mix lightener and toner with the bowl or bottle tilted away from you and your client so fumes will not be inhaled.
6. Mix lightener and toner *only* in a glass or plastic bottle or bowl. Never use metal containers—a drastic chemical reaction could occur.
7. Carefully recap bottles to prevent spilling and to preserve the strength of the chemicals.
8. Measure lightener, toner, and peroxide accurately.

Safety Measures for the Salon

1. Store all lightener, peroxide, and toners in a cool, dark place.
2. Keep all bottles clearly labeled and stored on shelves.
3. Wipe any spills of chemicals immediately.
4. Obtain and file a release form, and update the record card for each client and service.
5. Keep all lightening materials tightly capped.
6. Use partial bottles of toner and peroxide first. Take note of any expiration dates stamped on bottles. Do not use contents after expiration.
7. Discard any unused formula immediately.

> ◆ **Key Point** ◆
>
> Follow OSHA and state board guidelines for your protection and that of your clients. Store and mix chemicals safely. Observe manufacturer's recommendations for shelf life.

Hair lightening is an exciting option when you want more dramatic effects, or when lighter, blonder tones are the dictates of fashion. To take advantage of the option of hair lightening, you must be able to select the type of lightener and the level of oxidation necessary. Oxidation is the release of oxygen gas, usually caused by the addition of hydrogen peroxide to the formula. Hydrogen peroxide comes in various strengths, or volumes. The most common strength and the one at which color charts are developed is 20° H_2O_2. Higher volumes produce more potential lift, lower volumes provide more deposit. As a color specialist, you will select the correct volume based on your consultation and then dilute it with distilled water to the proper strength.

Lightener application is very important. Virgin applications always begin in the area where the hair is darkest, and on the center of the hair shaft. You will then process according to your strand test results and apply lightener to the scalp area and then the ends. You will lighten the hair to the stage required for the toner desired. Toners are applied to offset any harsh gold and to deposit the end color wanted. You will select the correct toner for your client's skin tone and apply it to the lightened hair.

Foiling techniques such as weaving and slicing are very popular in the contemporary salon. You must master these techniques in order to offer your clients the latest color services. Painting, scrunching, and the comb technique are but a few of the techniques that you will do for subtle effects that require no touch-ups at all. You will place these lightened areas to highlight the style you have created. The successful cosmetologist also creates optical illusions with lighteners, using the principle that light colors are larger and advance to the eye. Your analysis of facial shapes and the correct placement of lightener will enhance your professional career.

1. What lighteners are available in today's salon? What are the benefits and the effects of each?
2. What effect does oxidation have on the hair shaft? What are the two methods of measuring peroxide oxidation?
3. How would you prepare your client for a lightening service?
4. What is the procedure for lightening virgin hair?
5. How does a retouch differ from the application of lightener to virgin hair? What special precautions should you take?
6. How would you treat excessive porosity? What problems in lightening can this condition cause?
7. How would you correct dark spots or bands in the lightening service? How could you prevent them from happening?
8. What can happen during the lightening service if the hair has poor elasticity? How can you avoid this problem?
9. What special effects techniques are available to you as a professional colorist? What results can you expect of each technique?
10. What safety measures protect your client during the lightening service?
11. How would you protect yourself, the school, or the salon as a professional colorist?

PROJECTS

1. Research the lighteners you have available in your school. List the features and benefits of each; explain how they work and how they are mixed properly.
2. Working with a high-volume peroxide, mix 40, 30, 20, 10, and 5 volume peroxide with distilled water. Check each with a hydrometer for accuracy of volume.
3. Give at least three virgin applications of lightener to your mannequin, fellow students, or clients.
4. Give at least five retouch lightener applications.
5. Select at least six photographs from magazines showing special effect lightening techniques. Duplicate these procedures on your mannequin. Explain what the effect would be if you opted to use haircolor in the technique rather than a lightener and toner.
6. Research the treatment products available in your school. Explain which would be most effective for problems in hair lightening and explain why.
7. Research the MSDS (Material Safety Data Sheets) available for the hair lightening and toning products in your school. Discuss their hazards with your classmates, how you can avoid any damage to yourself and your client, and how these chemicals should be stored safely.

CHEMICAL WAVING

CHAPTER GOAL

Chemical waving is the most requested service in the salon to alter the curl of the hair. After reading this chapter and completing the projects, you should be able to

1. Explain the importance of hair analysis to a successful perm service.
2. List at least three different types of rods and explain the effect you create in the hair with them.
3. Describe the function of sectioning and demonstrate at least two wrap patterns.
4. Give at least eight characteristics of a well-wrapped perm and demonstrate a correctly wrapped perm.
5. Explain the chemical activity that takes place during a permanent wave.
6. Demonstrate the chemical wave procedure.
7. Explain at least two custom perm techniques and demonstrate at least three methods of wrapping long hair.
8. Describe the differences between soft or reconstruction perm waving and a regular permanent wave.
9. Explain the safety precautions you should observe during the perm process.

CHAPTER

Permanent waving is the most popular chemical service in the salon. It has been in great demand since the early Roman and Egyptian civilizations. Then, the attempts were quite primitive and not always permanent. Egyptian men were the first in recorded history to receive "permanent" waves. They would weave their beards between sticks, apply muck from the bottom of the Nile, and then bake in the sun for one to three days.

The first real progress came in 1905 when Charles Nessler demonstrated his invention, the permanent wave machine, in London. This machine applied heat, from clamps attached by wires, to curls wound on rods and soaked in borax. Nessler recommended that the hair first be cut to a length of three feet and that the hair be waved only around the hairline.

In 1929, a technique called the preheat method was introduced. It was similar to the machine method, except clamps were preheated and then placed over the curlers. It was no faster than the machine, taking all day to give one perm. The weight of the clamps, combined with the strong alkaline solution used, often caused severe hair and scalp damage.

In 1932, hairdressers could finally leave their machines behind with the invention of the so-called machineless perm by Ralph Evans and Everett McDonough. This method was also called a cold wave, to distinguish it from the heat methods then in use. The active ingredients were ammonia and thioglycolic acid. This perm, the forerunner of what we use today, became the largest income generator of the modern salon of the 1950s. Since then, ingredients have been improved to make perms less alkaline and more gentle. The newest perms use heat that is either chemically generated or externally applied.

Chemical waving, the process of either forming curl or reducing natural curl, uses physical and chemical methods. You will analyze the curl present and the amount desired and select the correct rods. You will determine the appropriate chemical formula to apply to the hair you have wrapped. You will process the hair according to your analysis of your client's hair condition.

HAIR ANALYSIS

The success of any chemical service you give in the salon depends on two key things: First is your knowledge of the hair, the chemicals involved, and your physical ability to perform the service. Second is the condition (integrity) of the hair. No permanent wave can be any better than the condition of the hair. Careful analysis of the condition of the hair and scalp will help you select the proper perm for the individual client. As you make your analysis, record all the information on the client's record card (see Figure 16.1).

Permanent Wave Record Card

Name .... Phone ( ) -
Address ....
City .... State .... Zip ....

Analysis of Hair
Porosity .... Elasticity ....
Texture .... Condition ....
Length .... Other chemicals ....

Perm Selection
Rods used ....
....
Perm solution ....
Additives or special instructions ....
....
Processing time .... Neutralizing time ....
Results ....
....
Date .... Stylist ....

Date	Perm Used	Results	Stylist

16.1

Chapter 6, Hair Damage and Treatments, contains detailed information for giving a hair analysis and for correcting any damage that you determine could interfere with your permanent wave service. Here we will discuss how analysis guides your selection of the correct permanent wave formula.

Client Consultation

Every perm client has a different idea of what the chemical service will offer. Listen carefully to what he or she expects. Ask about the client's life style and commitment to maintaining the hair. Work with photographs if necessary, but point out how the curl will look on your client. Use other clients or co-workers as examples. Once you know what the client wants and expects, determine what can actually be done with the hair. Compromise, if necessary, so that both of you will be happy with the finished service. Ask your client to sign a release form. This guarantees the client is aware of the procedures and risks associated with the perm service and agrees to them.

Scalp Condition

Check the scalp for abrasions, irritation, and open sores as you gently remove tangles from the hair with a wide-tooth comb. Take special care not to scratch the scalp as you are combing. If there is any scalp

CLIENT TIP ◆◆◆◆◆◆◆

Use an analysis instrument to determine hair condition. This professional approach is more accurate, impresses your client, and helps you retail the correct products.

problem, suggest that your client postpone the perm until the condition has healed. The chemicals used in the process could irritate the condition and be most uncomfortable for your client.

Hair Texture

The **texture** of the hair refers to its degree of fineness or coarseness. Hair is said to be coarse, medium, or fine, depending upon the diameter of each individual hair shaft.

Texture also refers to the way the hair feels. Whether it is smooth or rough is determined by the amount of natural curl present in the hair. Texture is a natural characteristic and should not be confused with hair damage or porosity.

The texture of the hair will help you determine the correct roller or rod size and the processing method to get the results you want. Fine-textured hair, for example, is often more difficult to curl. The cortex of fine hair is smaller so there are fewer bonds to change with the perm. You can use a smaller rod, or you can alter the service by such specialized techniques as transfer perming or air oxidation that we will discuss later in this chapter.

Hair texture is also a factor when you determine the correct processing formula. Considered with porosity, texture will help you estimate the processing time required.

Hair Porosity

If you look at a natural sponge, you will see that it is full of holes. When the sponge is immersed in water, it will absorb water very quickly. This characteristic, the ability to absorb liquid, is known as **porosity.** In the hair's natural state, the number of cuticle layers and how tightly they overlap each other determine the absorption of water. As the hair goes through temporary and permanent services, the cuticle layer is lifted and the hair becomes more porous.

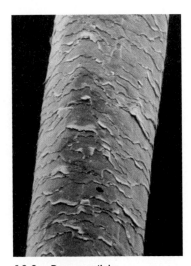

16.2   Porous cuticle

Hair that is resistant has a tightly compacted cuticle. This hair will process more slowly, and may even need to have heat applied to speed processing. Some people of Asian and African descent tend to have more cuticle layers due to genetic tendencies that will slow processing. Consider the natural characteristics of hair as well as the surface condition to determine porosity.

Hair that is porous or overporous is damaged. Its cuticle layer is lifted from the shaft and the defensive properties of the hair are gone (see Figures 16.2 and 16.3). You must use care when selecting the formula for porous hair and treat the damage during the service in order to get good results. If the porosity is extreme, postpone the perm service until your client has received conditioning treatments to correct the problem.

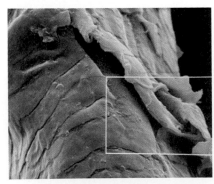

16.3   Severe cuticle damage

Hair that has received a prior chemical service is automatically more porous. Check the integrity of the hair; combine conditioning with an adjusted formula for a perm that will not damage the hair further. Your instructor may direct you to apply a liquid conditioner before processing, before neutralizing, or both. There are wrap techniques that also adjust for chemically treated hair such as the cushion wrap discussed in this chapter. Manufacturers provide formulas for different hair types; read and follow their directions for best results.

Elasticity

Without elasticity, it is impossible to get a good perm. **Elasticity** is the ability of the hair to stretch and return; it is what gives the hair the ability to spring into the curl pattern desired. Test to make sure the hair has 20 percent elasticity when dry before proceeding with the service. If it does not, the perm will not "take." Further, you risk severe damage to the hair such as breakage and soft, spongy ends. Test elasticity by stretching a single hair strand and observing return or by using an analysis instrument.

Density

The thickness of the hair, or the amount of hair per square inch, is referred to as **density.** In permanent waving, density will help you determine the correct blocking, or sectioning, pattern. Density will also help you decide how large each subsection should be for the rod selected. Normally, the subsection is as long as and as thick as the diameter of the rod you select. If, however, the hair is especially thick, you may need to make smaller subsections. Excess hair will slow or stop absorption of the lotion and neutralizer, so there cannot be too much hair on each rod. If the hair is extremely thin, adjust your technique so the subsections are slightly larger. Otherwise, the hair will be overexposed to the chemical solutions.

Hair Length

Standard permanent wave rods are designed to be used on hair that is 6 inches or less in length. This is so the hair can wrap around the rod at least 2 ½ turns and a wave pattern can be formed. If your client has longer hair, choose a wrap pattern or a specialty rod that permits even curling along the length of the hair.

If the hair is short, use a rod smaller than the curl you actually want and adjust the processing method to change the curl results. These techniques are discussed in Transfer Perms on page 351.

Hair Growth Pattern

The last factor to consider in a careful analysis of the hair is the natural **growth pattern.** Examine the crown area for hair growing in a "swirl" pattern. In most cases, crown hair grows toward the face while the rest of the hair grows in a slightly circular configuration to one side or the other. For the most natural looking results, and to avoid hair breakage, wrap the hair in the direction of its natural growth.

For those perm effects where you want to go against the natural growth, to get chemical lift (volume), or to combat a cowlick, you will have to balance the effect you want against the damage you might cause. Wrapping the hair to achieve a style (style wraps) also goes against the natural growth pattern of the hair. Share the results of your analysis, especially that of texture, with your instructor to decide if the result you want is worth the risk. It is usually more effective to perm in the natural growth pattern and style as desired rather than trying to achieve a style by chemical means.

Preperm Test Curls

If you are unsure of the hair condition or of achieving desired results, give test curls before perming the entire head. Select an area where you can wrap and process two or three rods that will not be noticeable. Perform the entire process and evaluate results.

ROD SELECTION

The **perm rod** determines the size and the shape of the curl. Neither the chemical chosen nor the amount of time that the lotion processes can change the shape of the curl. Selecting the right size rod is one of the most important decisions you will make during the perm service.

Rods are usually made of light-weight plastic. The ideal rod is slightly flexible so the hair can swell against it without damage during processing. The hollow core of the rod prevents excess lotion from becoming trapped and permits lotion applied from inside the rod to reach the ends of longer hair. Wooden rods go in and out of style, but can cause some damage because they swell during the process. Wooden rods are more difficult to clean and less resistant to water damage than plastic rods.

Rod Size

Permanent wave rods come in a variety of sizes, ranging from extra large ($\frac{3}{4}$ inch) to small ($\frac{1}{8}$ inch). Select the rod by the size of the curl desired and the length of the hair. In order to obtain a good curl, the hair should be long enough to wrap around the rod two and a half times. Think about a wave, or S pattern. The top curve of the S is formed by going around the rod one full turn, the bottom curve by the second. Only if the hair begins another circle around the rod will you see a full wave pattern. The **size** of that wave pattern will be determined by the size of the rod. Rods are color-coded by diameter.

Perm rods also come in various lengths: One-half, three-quarters, and full. Select rod length according to the size of the client's head and the width of each section. One-half-inch or short rods are sometimes easier to control if the hair is very short. They are often helpful around the hairline, especially at the neck, where the hair does not grow across the full width of your subsection. One-half-inch rods are also used for style wrapping. Three-quarter-inch rods usually fit the head best. Especially when wrapping in a pattern to imitate natural curl, three-quarter-inch rods fit the subsections and

◆ **Key Point** ◆

The condition of the hair will determine the success of your perm service. Select the perm solution and your technique according to the condition of the hair.

CLIENT **T I P** ◆◆◆◆◆◆◆

The rod determines the size of the curl. Hair must go around the rod at least two and one-half times for full curl development.

give close-to-the-head results. Full-length rods are helpful if the head is very large, or if you use a sectioning pattern that is long. Full-length rods are often used for special effects wrapping such as spiraling.

Rod Shape

During the chemical process of the perm, the hair is softened until it conforms to the shape of the rod. The shape of the rod you choose will determine the shape and pattern of the finished curl (see Table 16.1).

Straight rods are one uniform size in diameter. The rod is just as large at the ends as it is in the center. This rod is used to create an equal wave pattern across the entire subsection and from the scalp out to the ends. The straight rod is chosen by professional perm artists to imitate natural curl.

Concave rods are larger at the ends, and smaller in the center. These rods produce a curl that is larger at the scalp and tighter at the ends. Additionally, the wave pattern varies from larger to smaller across the subsection. Concave rods were initially designed for longer hair or for end curls so that the practitioner could get bouncy curls on the ends and a looser wave nearer the scalp. Concave rods can be used on slightly longer hair, but keep in mind that the curl diameter (especially the center) is enlarging as you wrap toward the scalp.

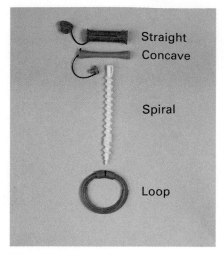

16.4

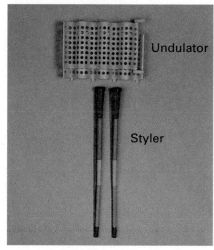

16.5

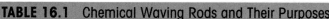

TABLE 16.1	Chemical Waving Rods and Their Purposes
Straight rod	Even curl from scalp to ends Even curl across rod Curl true to rod size (Figure 16.4)
Concave rod	Tighter curl at ends, softer at scalp Tighter curl in center of rod Curls vary in size (Figure 16.4)
Spiral rod	Elongated spiral curl (Figure 16.4)
Loop rod	Soft wave or spiral curl Curl larger than loop selected (Figure 16.4)
Triangular rod	Crimp curl
Square rod	Squared curl
Zigzag rod	Defined wave Crimped pattern
Undulator rod	Wave impression Soft, loose curl (Figure 16.5)
Crimper rod	Crimped wave pattern
Folding rod	Soft crimp pattern
Styler rod	Soft wave pattern Curl gradually becomes smaller or larger. (Figure 16.5)

Spiral rods are designed to produce a springy, visible curl pattern on long hair. The rod features a groove that runs around and around the rod at an angle. When you wrap the hair into the groove from scalp to ends, you can get special effects on long hair. This same effect can be achieved with straight rods, but some practitioners feel that special rods are easier and faster.

Perm loops are not rods at all but tubes of soft plastic that can be attached to themselves end to end. This is an alternative tool for perming long hair. The benefits of perm loops are that the wrapping is faster than traditional methods for long hair and does not put undue weight on the hair which could cause breakage. The disadvantages of perm loops are that the curl obtained is often soft and ill-defined. Test curls as an indication of progress are more difficult to evaluate because you distort the curl as you unwind it.

Specialty rod shapes go in and out of use. Two of the more common examples are triangular and spiral-shaped rods. Triangular rods give a curl with a crimp effect, for example, while spiral rods give a defined long curl. Specialty rods are usually a response to a fad, but do have their place in the progressive salon. Typically, they are used on hair that is more than 8 inches long. Some specialty rods drag on the hair and cause damage; others trap lotion against the scalp or within the strand. And some are just gimmicks that could cost you extra money for supplies in the salon. Be aware of the features and benefits of any permanent waving tool you may select.

SECTIONING PATTERNS FOR PERMANENT WAVING

There are several different ways of blocking or sectioning for a permanent wave, and no one sectioning pattern will be appropriate in all cases. Consider the growth pattern of the hair as well as the size and contour of the head when sectioning. Specialty wrapping techniques require different sectioning methods. In this section we will discuss the basics: the natural, nine-section, and straightforward wrapping patterns. We will also discuss dropped-crown and bricklayer patterns that can be used in a section or all over the head.

Natural Wrap Pattern

In classical permanent waving, every effort is made to wrap with the growth pattern. This "natural" technique is the kindest to the hair during the chemical process. Since it simulates natural curl, it is the wrapping pattern that provides a base for the largest variety of styles. The natural wrap permits any type of styling immediately after the perm and shows no splits or partings around the hairline. The natural wrap (see Figures 16.6–16.8), provides a basis for the longest lasting curl and is suggested for any close-to-the-head styling.

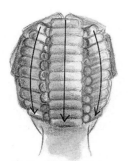

16.6   Back view

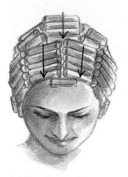

16.7   Front view

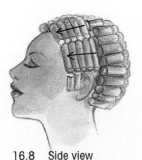

16.8   Side view

From the natural growth swirl in the crown, the hair is wrapped down and toward the hairline. To best simulate natural curl, use three-quarter-length rods and off-base wrapping techniques. If the hair is fine and you wish to avoid band marks, insert flat plastic straws under the bands or use bandless rods.

The wrap begins in the center back section, at the center of the growth swirl. Part off a section from the crown to the nape hairline that is as wide as the rod is long. Wrap the hair down and under until you reach the nape. The rods should be almost touching each other. Then roll the front crown straight down and toward the face. This subsection is the length of one rod. Next, wrap each side back section. Part the subsections so that each rod end almost touches the center back section rods. The first three rods will stagger slightly and will not be in a row. Now part the front hair down the middle. Wrap each section down and to the hairline. If your client has a widow's peak, a point of hair in the center front, you will have a single rod there. Finish the wrap by placing rods at an angle on each side. You may need to finish with a second row of half rollers or with a single rod rolled down, depending upon the growth pattern at the ear.

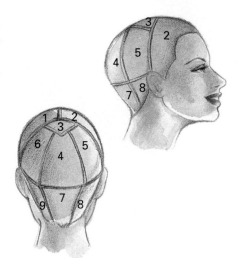

16.9   Nine-section wrap

Nine-Section Wrap Pattern

Sometimes called the **single halo** wrap, this pattern (see Figures 16.9 and 16.10) was developed for the preheat permanent wave. Some state boards still require it as the pattern during your practical exam, but it is seldom used in today's progressive salon. The primary reason is that the single halo wrap does not follow growth of the hair. The resulting curl shows splits along the hairline and especially at the center front. Since the pattern does not necessarily follow the contour of the skull, you may need to use varying lengths of rods to fit the section.

Begin by parting the hair in the middle. Then, beginning at the hairline, measure a section that will be the length of a permanent wave rod by placing the rod along the part with one end at the hairline. Section 3 is a pie shape taken out at the crown. The back is sectioned into thirds, and each long section is split at the center back (occipital) area.

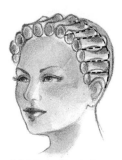

16.10a   Front view

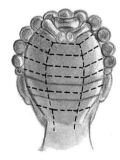

16.10b   Back view

Straight Forward Pattern

This pattern is similar to the natural wrap pattern, but the shape of the head is not taken into consideration. A panel is parted from the crown to the forehead the width of the length of a rod (see Figure 16.11). This section can be wrapped straight down and forward, or the three rods at the hairline can be wrapped down and the rest back toward the crown. This wrapping method toward the crown produces volume, but can be damaging to more fragile hair types and cause breakage at the scalp. The back is divided into three sections, and each side front is wrapped down and under. The straight forward pattern eliminates the problem of a split at the front, but produces visible splits on the side. Some stylists prefer it for speed of wrapping.

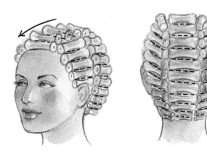

16.11   Straight forward wrap

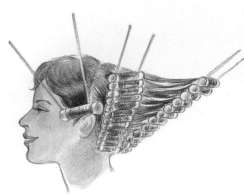

16.12 Stack wrap

Dropped Crown or Stack Pattern

This is not a pattern so much as a specialty method for longer hair. However, if you are giving such a perm, section the back of the head into three equal sections. Make a section on each side and adjust the front and top to meet the styling needs of your client. A dropped crown is an older technique also known as end curling. The stack technique (Figure 16.12) fastens the rods over sticks in a controlled pattern and produces even curl in a definite line from the crown. The stack pattern requires a bit more practice to master wrapping and test curling. Use a permanent wave solution that is blotted rather than rinsed from the hair prior to neutralizing. Rinsing a stack perm would be very uncomfortable for your client and would distort the pattern.

Bricklayer Pattern

This is not really a sectioning pattern, but a method to overlay rods much like bricks in a wall (see Figure 16.13). The theory is that splits between rods are not visible when doing a spiral or a style wrap. Bricklayer patterns can be in a section, such as the nape, or over the entire head for a spiral wrap.

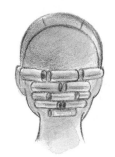

16.13 Brick layer pattern

If you are wrapping a spiral perm (see page 353), begin at the hairline. Part each section according to the diameter of the rod and the density of the hair. Wrap an entire layer across the hairline. Then move up a layer and stagger your partings so that an overlapping pattern is begun. Continue in this manner until you reach the crown. Then return to the side hairline and continue wrapping. Bricklayer patterns require time and organization. Plan your overlap so that the hairline growth pattern is also considered.

WRAPPING

Wrapping is the procedure you will use to wind the hair around the rod toward the scalp. As simple as it might seem, wrapping will require more of your practice time than any other procedure. The wrap is the single most important factor in the success of the chemical wave. When it comes to wrapping, "what you see is what you get."

There are five basic wrapping techniques—each with a specific purpose. Wrapping techniques are characterized by the placement of the **end** or **protective papers**. The purpose of using end papers in the permanent wave is to protect the hair, evenly spread the lotion and neutralizer, and control hair placement. Keep the end papers damp, but not wet, as you wrap.

◆ Key Point ◆

The wrap will determine the pattern of the curl. A natural wrap will best imitate natural curl with minimal damage.

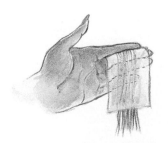

16.14 Single flat wrap

Wrapping Techniques

The **single flat** wrap uses one end paper and is most effective with straight rods. The end paper is placed lengthwise (see Figure 16.14) on top of the subsection. The method was introduced for shorter hair and increased speed.

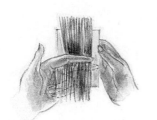

16.15   End paper under strand

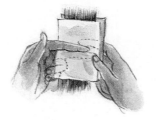

16.16   Double flat wrap

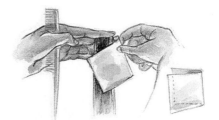

16.17   Bookend wrap

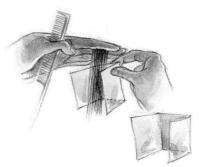

16.18   Trifold wrap

The **double flat wrap** is the most common wrapping technique in today's progressive salon. It protects the ends and gives you great control when wrapping, especially with straight rods. One end paper is used on top of the strand; the second is placed below (see Figures 16.15 and 16.16). The papers are then moved until they extend approximately ¹⁄₂ inch past the ends and the hair is wound around the rod.

The **bookend wrap** (Figure 16.17), originally designed for end curls, converges the hair ends to the center of the rod. This makes it the method of choice for those who prefer concave rods. With the hair ends combed together, the paper is placed horizontally so that one half of the paper is on top of the subsection. The paper is then folded under to protect the bottom of the strand and the hair is wound around the rod.

The **trifold wrap** is used primarily for specialty techniques on long hair. The paper is folded into three sections (see Figure 16.18) around the converged ends. That amount of paper around the ends can restrict absorption of lotion. Many technicians prefer to fold the paper lengthwise to ensure good curl on the ends. This technique should only be used when you need to peak the ends together for spiral wrapping. If used for conventional wraps, the ends will not be evenly curled as lotion cannot penetrate the paper.

A **cushion wrap** should be used if your client has damaged or chemically processed hair. Begin the wrap just as you would a double-flat wrap. Insert additional paper (see Figure 16.19) on the top of the strand as you wind so that the hair is totally protected. Tuck a new paper under the top end of the hair when no more the ¹⁄₂ inch remains unwound to avoid excessive paper that could interfere with processing.

CLIENT   T I P ◆◆◆◆◆◆

Use a cushion wrap if the hair is porous due to sun or salon lightening.

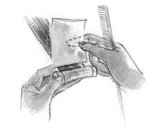

16.19   Cushion wrap

Selecting the Base

As in any other styling service, the base you select determines the amount of lift and movement that you get from the resulting permanent wave. Ideally, the chemical processes of the perm should be used to give the desired curl with a minimum of damage. You will then create your style needs after the perm is completed. There are times, however, when you might elect to create a style chemically with the perm. When you determine that your client's hair is in condition for this technique, the base you select will make a difference to the finished look.

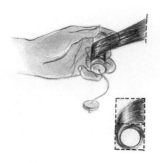

16.20   Off-base wrap

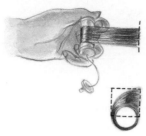

16.21   Half-base wrap

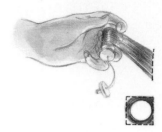

16.22   On-base wrap

Off-base wrapping is the most protective of the hair. Hold the hair at the angle of its natural growth of 45 degrees. Wrap the hair around the rod so the stress on the hair is equal throughout the entire subsection, preventing breakage. If the hair is subsectioned into parts no larger than the size of the rod, one rod will rest on the base below it and touch the next rod. This pressure curls the hair all the way to the scalp and produces the most natural looking, close-to-the-head curl. It also provides the greatest mobility (Figure 16.20).

Half-base wrapping has the very same purpose that it has in any other style technique, that of blending. When you elect to wrap a permanent wave rod half on its base, you stress the bottom part of the subsection by combing the hair against the direction from which it grows. Comb the hair at 90 degrees or straight up and out from the head. With any half base design you will get some volume, some movement. If the hair is damaged or fine, you risk breakage at the bottom of the subsection (Figure 16.21).

On-Base wrapping is selected when you want maximum volume and the client's hair is of excellent integrity and coarse texture. The stem of the curl is straight so that volume is achieved. The hair is held at 135 degrees or forward from the bottom of its base so that the wrapped rod is completely placed within its base parting (Figure 16.22).

Winding the Hair

Proper winding of the hair is critical to the success of the permanent wave. Winding is the process which includes establishing the base, placing the end papers, curling the hair, establishing and maintaining control, and securing the rod. The following procedure describes an off-base double-flat wrap. You can adjust the procedure simply by changing the angle at which the hair is held away from the head or the placement of the papers. All of the other techniques apply in all cases.

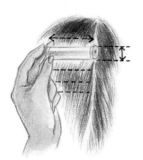

16.23   Measure subsection

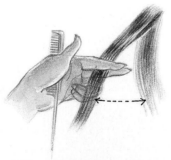

16.24   45° angle from part

Procedure for Winding the Hair

1. Establish the desired sectioning pattern.
2. Part off a subsection of hair that is equal to the length and diameter of the rod (Figure 16.23).
3. Comb the hair smooth, establishing a base 45 degrees away from the bottom parting (see Figure 16.24). Make sure that you comb only the top of the strand once the base is established. Comb the

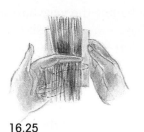

16.25

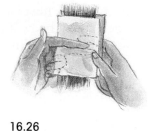

16.26

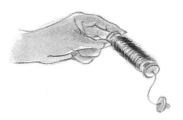

16.27 Wind hair in rod

hair so it is equally spread across the base and hold between your index and middle finger.

4. Position an end paper beneath the strand as shown in Figure 16.25. Position the paper so that it is above the ends and hold between fingers as shown in Figure 16.25.

5. Position a second paper above the strand. With both hands, slide the papers down (Figure 16.26) until they extend about ½ inch below the ends.

6. Place the rod at the ends of the papers, parallel to the base parting. Turn the rod with one hand while directing it with the other (Figures 16.27 and 16.28). The first turn of the rod should only wrap the end paper to prevent fish hooks or crimped ends.

7. Continue winding the rod with one hand and controlling it with the other. Wrap smoothly and evenly without letting the hair move from side to side. Insert more papers as necessary for a cushion wrap.

8. With the rod securely against the scalp, flick the band loose with your thumb. Move your other hand straight across the rod and fasten. Avoid reaching up and over the rod to grasp the end as this will rock the rod off your selected base (Figure 16.29).

9. Fasten the rod parallel to the base parting (Figure 16.30). You can check this from the side. If the rod is correctly fastened, the bands will form a line exactly parallel to the head form. Bands incorrectly placed will break the hair if too tight and result in weak or no curl if too loose.

10. Check the tension on the rod by gently pulling the rod with your thumb and middle finger at each end. A correctly wound rod will return to its original position when released. If the hair is too tight, breakage could result. If it is too loose, you will get uneven or no curl at all.

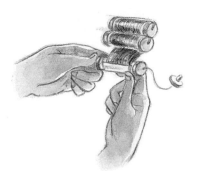

16.28 Direct rod with other hand

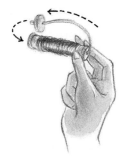

16.29 Loosen band

16.30 Fasten band

11. To establish the next base, slice the hair at the very bottom of the wrapped rod. This will provide a base exactly the size of the rod above. Wind as outlined and position so that the rod is almost touching the one above it.

Checklist for Winding

Remember that the quality of the wrap determines the quality of the finished perm. Spend the time necessary on your mannequin and fellow students to perfect your technique. Check each finished wrap for the following:

- ☐ Partings are clean and straight.
- ☐ Rod is consistently placed in relation to base chosen.
- ☐ Rods almost touch one another. There are no gaps between sections.
- ☐ The rod moves slightly within its base without being loose.
- ☐ Each subsection is the length of the rod selected and the depth of the rod diameter.
- ☐ The hair is wound smoothly around the rod without any crossed hairs or clumping. The hair wound around the rod looks much like thread wound around a spool.
- ☐ The hair is spread evenly from the outside edge of the rod to the other edge (within $\frac{1}{4}$ inch of the edge if you choose to use concave rods).
- ☐ The bands are straight across the rods and form a pattern parallel to the head form when checked from the side.
- ☐ The ends are smooth against the rods and completely covered with the end paper.

◆ **Key Point** ◆
The quality of the wrap determines the quality of the finished curl.

THE CHEMISTRY OF A PERMANENT WAVE

A chemical wave is permanent, therefore changes must occur to the bonding structure within the cortex layer of the hair. Refer to Chapter 2 for details of the structure of the hair and to Chapter 13 for a discussion of the chemical aspects of permanent waving. This section will cover practical issues involved in the chemical wave process.

Chemical waving is both a physical and a chemical process. It is called chemical, or permanent, waving to distinguish it from wet styling techniques that last only from shampoo to shampoo. Previous sections described the importance of the manual skills—sectioning, wrapping, and winding—to the success of the perm. This section will focus on the chemical activities of a permanent wave.

Processing

The permanent wave lotion is the first chemical applied during a permanent wave service that alters the structure of the cortex of the hair. **Processing** refers to the time between the application and the removal of the lotion.

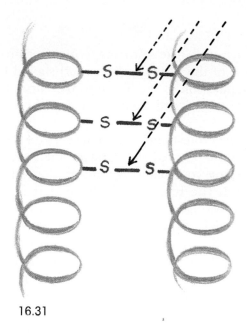

16.31

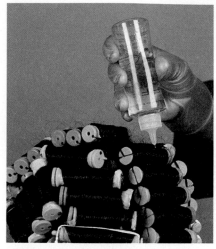

16.32   Lotion application

The active ingredient in the vast majority of chemical waves and in all cold waves is **ammonium thioglycolate** (uh **MO** ni uhm theye oh **GLEYE** co late). This reducing agent, which we will call thio, is formed by the combination of ammonia gas and thioglycolic acid. When the resulting alkaline (9.3 pH) solution is applied to the hair, it first penetrates the cuticle layer. The thio then begins the process of disassociating, or breaking, the disulfide bond in the cortex layer. This is the bond that is responsible for the natural curl pattern of the hair. If the natural bond is straight, so is the hair. If it is formed at an angle between polypeptide chains, the hair is wavy. And if the bonds are formed at a severe angle, the hair is curly to extra curly, depending on the sharpness of the angle.

The chemical effect of the processing lotion is to soften the cuticle layer of the hair by decreasing its protective function. The lotion also reduces the disulfide bond by adding hydrogen. When this happens, the hair can conform to the rod chosen and assume its shape. The amount of time that this takes depends upon the texture and the porosity of the hair. As the hair structure is altered, so too is the chemical composition of the permanent wave lotion. A chemical reaction occurs when thio comes into contact with the disulfide links in the amino acid cystine (sis **TEEN**) in the cortex (Figure 16.31). Check the illustrations to see what chemically happens.

The illustrations show how 2 hydrogen atoms are released from the thio and combine with 2 sulfur atoms to break bonds (Figure 16.32). This reduction breaks the disulfide linkage across 2 polypeptide chains and forms 2 molecules of cysteine (sis teh **UHN**) (Figure 16.33). The lotion is now di-thio, which cannot effectively break any more bonds. Of course what we are looking at is one tiny bond in the cortex, and there is much more free thio available to attack and break other bonds. Chemists formulate most alkaline perms so that they will be effective for 10–12 minutes.

CLIENT   T I P ◆◆◆◆◆◆◆

Blot lotion from the rod before taking a test curl. Do not stretch or push the hair as you examine progress.

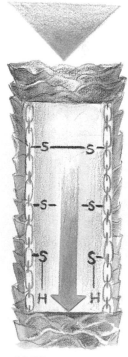

16.33

The Test Curl

During the processing, take test curls to monitor progress and check the effectiveness of the formula. A test curl should be taken as soon as you finish application of the lotion to the entire head. Test where you began application and then test every three to five minutes thereafter.

When checking a test curl (see Figures 16.34–16.36), first gently blot lotion from the selected rod. Unwind the hair one and one half turns while keeping your hands resting on the rod beneath. As you unwind the rod, the hair will arch up if it is not completely processed. If processing is complete, the hair will fall into a wave pattern equal to the size of the rod and the subsection of hair will break into separate strands.

If the test curl is incomplete, rewind and fasten the rod. Apply one or two drops of lotion to reactivate processing. When test curls indicate that the hair is processed, proceed to the removal of lotion as recommended by your instructor or the manufacturer.

Underprocessing is the term that refers to the removal of lotion from the rods before a satisfactory test curl is achieved. This typically occurs when you push a wave in during the test curl and a false wave shows. If the hair is not sufficiently processed the wave achieved, if any, will be very weak. The slight wave will relax very quickly. To correct, reperm the hair.

Overprocessing is the opposite condition. The hair is processed further after the bonds are already broken. This can happen if the hair is pulled so tightly during test curling that the wave does not show, or if the processing lotion is left on the hair too long. While the bonds themselves cannot be overprocessed, having only two sulfur atoms to donate, the hair can be severely damaged by processing further. Overprocessed hair is usually very dry and often loses its elasticity. The only correction is deep conditioning and removing the worst of the damage by cutting.

Self-timing perms are formulated with the correct balance of thio and di-thio to work for a specific amount of time. The manufacturer

> **CLIENT TIP ◆◆◆◆◆◆◆**
>
> If you do not have a successful test curl after 10–12 minutes, blot the rods gently with a damp towel. Apply drops of fresh lotion to reactivate processing.

> **CLIENT TIP ◆◆◆◆◆◆◆**
>
> Make sure that each rod is completely blotted, but be careful not to hurt your client by pressing too hard. Fold a paper towel to the width of the section and blot again by weaving the towel underneath each rod with the tail of your comb and applying gentle pressure.

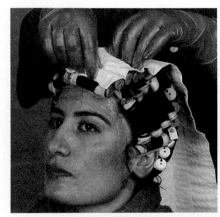

16.34   Blot test curl

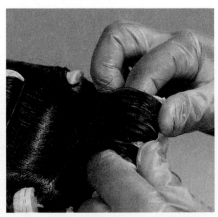

16.35   Unwind test curl

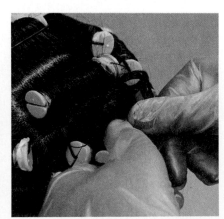

16.36   Check test curl

has estimated the strengths of these formulas for each hair type. It is always best to confirm correct processing by taking a test curl. Only you can determine what is right for your client in your situation.

Removing the Processing Lotion

The two commonly accepted methods for the removal of lotion are towel blotting and rinsing. To blot, saturate a terry towel in hot water and thoroughly ring it out. Place the towel (see Figure 16.37) carefully over the rods and press gently on each individual rod. Rinse the towel repeatedly.

The benefits of towel blotting are as follows:

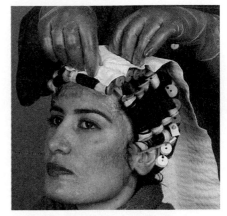

16.37   Towel blotting

☐ The wrap pattern is not disturbed by rinsing. This is especially important for short or fine hair.
☐ Hair made more porous by processing does not absorb excess water that could prevent complete neutralization.
☐ Sections or curls that process faster can be stopped while the rest of the hair continues to process.
☐ Specialty wraps such as stack or spiral perms can have the lotion removed without client discomfort at the shampoo bowl.
☐ Blotting allows ammonia to dissipate, or evaporate, preventing alkaline damage to the hair.

If you decide to rinse, seat your client at the shampoo bowl as comfortably as possible. Adjust the water so that the temperature is just warm enough for your client's comfort and the pressure will rinse the rods without moving them from their base (Figure 16.38). Take special care to protect the nape rods and avoid pressure that could cause breakage. Rinse thoroughly and towel-blot excess water. Blot the individual rods, rather than the entire head. Check each rod to see if it has been loosened during this process and carefully rewind as necessary.

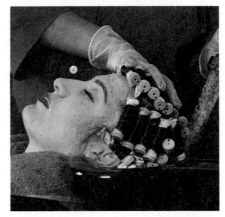

16.38   Rinsing

Process Conditioning

Once the lotion is removed from the hair, you may condition the hair and prevent damage during the neutralizing process. This should be done if you are using an alkaline perm or your analysis indicates the need. Use a liquid conditioner in a spray bottle. Hold it about 12 inches away from the client's head and *lightly* mist the back, each side, and the top. Only a light misting is necessary since the cuticle is lifted and the conditioner will penetrate instantly. Let your client relax a few minutes before you proceed to the next chemical step—neutralizing. Do not overcondition.

Neutralizing

The second phase of the chemical process of a perm is that of oxidation. The neutralizer is a diluted solution of hydrogen peroxide or sodium bromate mixed with buffers and conditioners. The application of this solution neutralizes the effect of the lotion by rebonding the disulfide structure in its new shape (see Figure 16.39).

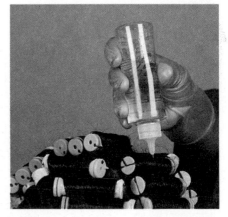

16.39

The disulfide links in the hair are reformed in their newly waved position. When the neutralizer releases its oxygen into the hair (Figure 16.40), the oxygen combines with the hydrogen deposited during reduction or processing. The disulfide bond is reformed, recreating cystine (Figure 16.41), and a molecule of water is formed as a byproduct. Since the hair is in its new position around the rods, the newly formed bond creates the curl that you desire.

The timing of the neutralizer is very important. Follow the manufacturer's suggested timing and avoid overneutralization. If the hair is overoxidized, it will lose color, become very dry and brittle, and the ends or even the entire hair shaft may break away. Overoxidation is very difficult, if not impossible to correct.

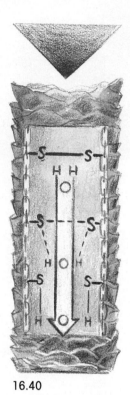

16.40

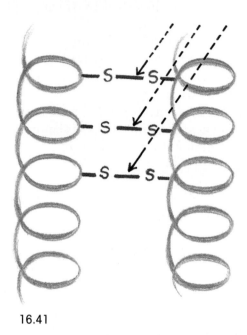

16.41

Remove the neutralizer when the suggested timing has passed and the hair on the rods feels cool. If the hair is less than six inches long, you will first remove the rods. Start at the hairline and gently remove each rod without stretching the hair. When all rods are carefully removed, work the neutralizer through to the ends with your fingers and then rinse thoroughly. Use low pressure and cooler water to protect the newly formed curl.

If the hair is longer than six inches, or you have used a specialty technique with a large number of rods, rinse before removing rods. Again, use low pressure and comfortably cool water to avoid distorting the new curl. Blot the rods and remove carefully from the hairline up toward the crown. Apply neutralizer to the ends and work through for one to two minutes, then rinse again.

Acid-Balanced Perms

These permanent waves are a derivative of traditional alkaline perming. The main active ingredient is **glyceryl monothioglycolate** (**GLY** ser ohl mo noh theye oh gleye **KOH** late). Acid-balanced perms operate at a lower pH in a range from 4.5 to 7.9. Typically, these perms take longer to process, require some form of heat, and can cause allergic reactions on the scalp. The curl is softer and usually does not last as long as traditional methods. Heat can be applied in two ways:

1. **Exothermically** (ex oh **THER** mick lee). The perm is activated by the heat produced when an additional chemical is mixed with the product. Once the chemicals are mixed, these perms act as alkaline waves. A cap is usually placed over the rods to retain the heat.
2. **Endothermically** (en doh **THER** mick lee). The perm is activated by an outside heat source, such as a dryer, when the heat is absorbed by the chemical.

GIVING A CHEMICAL WAVE

The following procedure is the most common method of giving a chemical wave. Follow manufacturer's directions for the products you use.

Material and Equipment

Cotton	Fan-tail or a styling comb	Moisturizer
Protective gloves	Selected rods	Plastic cap (optional)
Client record card	End papers	Plastic cape
Release form	Selected lotion and neutralizer	Plastic clips
Protective cream	Applicator bottles	Scissors or razor
Prepermanent shampoo	Neutralizing bib (optional)	Timer
Liquid conditioner	Towels (paper towels optional)	Picks (optional)
Wide-tooth comb	Acidifier	Spray bottle

Procedure for Giving a Chemical Wave

1. Sanitize your hands.
2. Seat client comfortably and drape for a chemical service (Figure 16.42). Have client remove ear and neck jewelry.
3. Analyze hair and scalp. Record results on client record card. Have client sign the release form.
4. Shampoo the hair gently. Do not scratch or irritate the scalp. If the hair is coated with conditioning or styling products, use a special shampoo designed for preperm services (Figure 16.43).
5. Clarify or chelate the hair if you live in a hard water area or your client is on medication. Follow manufacturer's directions.
6. Condition the hair as your analysis indicates and proceed with wrapping. You may place picks between the bands and the rods to prevent band marks.
7. Apply protective cream around hairline and over ears (Figure16.44).
8. Place cotton around hairline. Put on your protective gloves.
9. Apply perm lotion from an applicator bottle. Begin at the top of the center-back section. Slowly draw applicator across rod with-

CLIENT TIP ◆◆◆◆◆◆

Process conditioning corrects damage done during the perm and is ideal for tinted or frosted hair. Mist conditioner lightly to protect the hair without interfering with neutralizing activities.

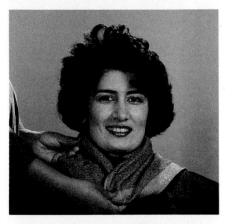

16.42   Chemical service drape

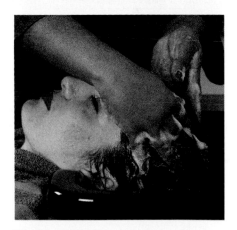

16.43   Shampoo

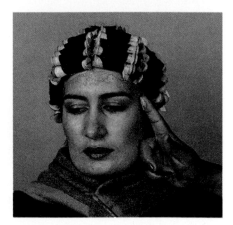

16.44   Apply protective cream

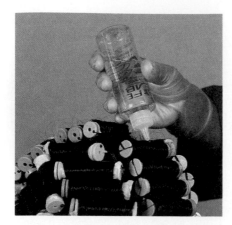

16.45   Apply perm lotion

out disturbing the hair. Roll the rod up and apply underneath in
the opposite direction. Proceed to each rod in a systematic fashion (Figure 16.45).

10. Remove saturated cotton.

11. Take a test curl at the first rod where you applied lotion. Check
that saturation is sufficient and note if the processor has penetrated the hair. (Smooth hair textures will appear more dull, and
curly hair textures will appear more shiny when the lotion has
penetrated.) Apply more lotion only if necessary.

12. Cover the rods with a plastic cap if directed. If the hair is resistant or you are using a heat-activated wave, place the client under
a preheated dryer (Figure 16.46).

13. Test-curl every three to five minutes, testing a different curl each
time. If you have not received satisfactory curl development after
12 minutes, blot the rods gently with a damp towel and apply
drops of fresh lotion to each rod.

14. When a satisfactory test curl is evident (Figure 16.47), test at
least two more curls in different areas of the head. If processing
is even, remove the lotion by rinsing or by blotting.

15. Blot the rods (Figure 16.48). Condition the hair if your preperm
analysis indicated this would be beneficial. Lightly mist the conditioner over the rods.

16. Let the hair rest slightly before neutralizing (Figure 16.49).

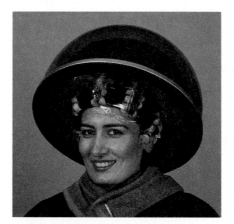

16.46   Place client under dryer

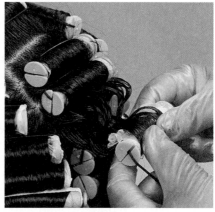

16.47   Check test curl

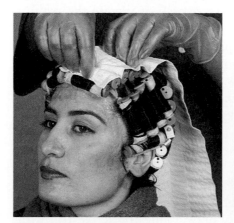

16.48   Towel blot rods

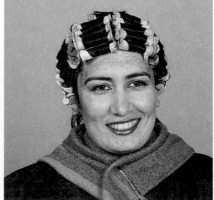

16.49

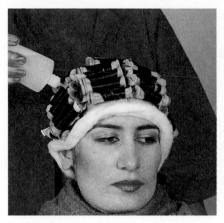

16.50 Apply neutralizer

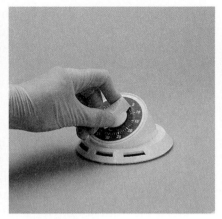

16.51 Set timer

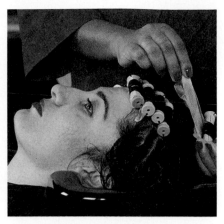

16.52 Carefully remove rods

17. Check protective cream and replace as needed. Apply cotton around hairline.
18. Apply neutralizer to the top and bottom of each rod in a systematic fashion (Figure 16.50). Start at the center back, work to each side of the back, then do the sides, top, and front. Have your client tilt the head back to avoid any dripping into the face.
19. Remove saturated cotton.
20. Time according to manufacturer's directions (Figure 16.51).
21. Carefully remove rods to avoid stretching (Figure 16.52). Work neutralizer through ends gently. Rinse thoroughly.
22. Towel blot and acidify the hair. Moisturize and rinse as needed (Figure 16.53).
23. Record all results on the client's card.
24. Proceed with styling. Avoid excessive heat or tension when styling (Figure 16.54).
25. Suggest client purchase quality products to protect perm at home.
26. Clean work station and prepare for your next service.

CUSTOM PERM TECHNIQUES

Once you have mastered the basics of classical chemical waving, you will be ready to customize your perm services. When you can customize techniques for your clients, you can offer them a unique service that no one else can. This spells good income, reputation, and creativity.

Waving Tinted, Bleached, or Damaged Hair

The secret to a successful perm on damaged hair lies in the analysis. Apply the appropriate conditioner for the hair type before wrapping the hair. Use less tension and slightly larger rods than you would for virgin hair. Carefully monitor progress with test curls as processing will be faster due to porosity. Blot, rather than rinse, the lotion from the hair.

CLIENT TIP ◆◆◆◆◆◆◆

Let the hair rest before you apply the neutralizer. A minimum of 10 minutes of air oxidation will produce visible results.

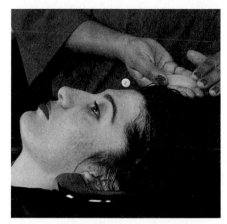

16.53 Moisturize hair

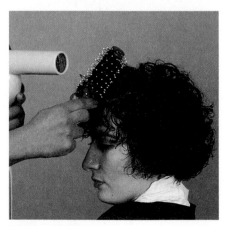

16.54 Style hair

Mist the hair lightly with conditioner and let it rest before neutralizing. Acidify the hair after the perm is complete and apply moisturizer. Use a wet setting technique for soft styling. Suggest your client purchase the proper products to maintain the terrific perm at home.

Air Oxidation

The terms **air perm** and **air oxidized** refer to a technique of neutralizing using the oxygen present in the atmosphere rather than oxygen supplied from a chemical neutralizer. It is by far the best perm technique, but there are some practical considerations.

In an ideal situation, you would process your client's hair, blot the solution from the rods, mist the hair lightly with a conditioner, and let the hair dry naturally on the rods. When the hair was completely dry, you would remove the rods, shampoo, moisturize the hair, and have a perfect perm. Depending upon the length and the density of the hair, however, it could take as long as twenty-four hours for the hair to dry. So you can see that this technique is not very convenient or comfortable for the client. In addition, the salon would have to have a huge supply of perm rods to service all the clients.

Some clients are willing to do this, especially those who have never before had successful perms. For most of your clients, however, you will find that a compromise can improve the quality of your perms and still be practical. With a minor adjustment to your scheduling, you can easily leave 30-minute air oxidation time between the processing and the neutralizing. This amount of time will let the hair adjust to the chemical changes occurring and improve results.

Style Perming

This technique attempts to permanently set a style into the hair with a chemical wave. Here again, the concept is terrific, but it has limitations. First, perms are not effective on rods large enough to produce a particular style. The polypeptide chains cannot shift enough; therefore the bonds are not broken. The hair can be softly permed, however, in a pattern that follows the style you have in mind.

Style or design perming is only effective on short hair that goes around the rod two times or less. Why? Once the hair begins the third turn, a wave results and the hair reverses direction. You also have to consider damage or breakage that can occur when you wrap against the natural growth direction of the hair. As the hair grows, it will grow in that natural growth direction, not in the style direction selected.

There will be times, however, when you decide to style-perm. For example, you may want to direct the hair back from the face or control an obvious cowlick. First, check the condition of the hair to make sure it can withstand the stress of the wrap. Second, mold or sculpt the style into damp hair. Place rods within the shapings, beginning at the closed end of each shaping. Use picks to support the rods in place and consider using bandless, interlocking rods. Process and neutralize as normal and style into the direction permed.

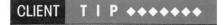

CLIENT **T I P** ◆◆◆◆◆◆◆

If you must rinse because of the perm selected, thoroughly blot afterward and let the hair rest for at least 10 minutes.

CLIENT **T I P** ◆◆◆◆◆◆◆

Baby fine or thin hair, which is often very difficult to perm, responds well to air oxidation. This type of hair will often dry completely in three to four hours.

Root Perms

This perm is designed to give lift and volume to the hair without adding curl to the ends. Special end wraps and heavy conditioner are used to prevent penetration of the lotion to the ends. Wrap the perm on base to create volume, as long as the hair is of good enough texture and condition. The effect is not long lasting, as the hair will continue to grow, but can be one that produces a fun, free style.

Transfer Perms

Very fine hair has traditionally been difficult to perm. The hair is limp, has a small cortex (and therefore fewer bonds that can be affected), and is often fragile. One method that addresses these problems is commonly called a transfer perm. The hair is permed on rods small enough to break down the bonding structure in the cortex. The lotion is then removed and conditioner misted over the rods. Next, two rods are removed, and the hair strands are combed gently together and rewrapped on a rod two sizes larger. Hair processed on pink rods, for example, would be rewrapped onto white rods. Two more rods are unwrapped, combed, rewrapped, and so forth until all the hair has been wound onto the larger rods. The hair is then neutralized on the larger rods. The smaller rod is needed to process the hair. The larger rod for neutralizing prevents frizzy, overly tight curls. This is a time consuming technique that requires advanced mechanical skills.

Partial Perms

Perms that do not affect the entire head of hair are called partial perms. Partial perms can be used to support a particular style, or to refresh a section of hair that has relaxed from a prior perm.

Part off the section to be permed; clip the rest of the hair out of the way. Wrap in the pattern you have selected and encircle the wrapped rods with cotton. Be very careful not to apply lotion to the unwrapped hair. You may wish to apply a cream conditioner to the unwrapped hair for extra protection. Process as usual and neutralize, but be careful not to contact the unwrapped hair.

Perm Techniques for Long Hair

There are a variety of perm methods available for your clients with long hair. Your instructor can keep you abreast of the latest methods in addition to those outlined here. The two general categories covered in this section are those that use traditional perm rods and those that use special rods designed for long hair.

Stack perms have the same effect, that of curling only the ends, but the placement of the curls creates a definite line of curl at a distance you choose from the scalp. For a stack perm, part the hair into even sections the length of the rods you will use. Begin at the hairline and wrap one to two rods down to the scalp. Insert sticks at the outside edges of the rods as shown in Figure 16.55 and move the sticks to the angle you want. Continue wrapping within the sticks and fastening the rods around them. Process as normal, sliding rods

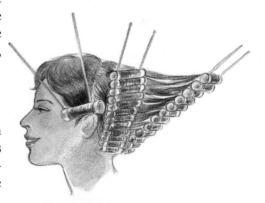

16.55 Stack perm

up the stick to give you room to take test curls. When the hair has processed, blot the lotion from the rods, again moving rods up and down the sticks to give you access. Neutralize, remove the sticks, rinse the hair and remove the rods.

The hair can be left to air dry for a dramatic effect, or can be blown smooth with volume at the ends.

The **end perm** was the first technique developed for longer hair. The hair is dropped from the crown, and wound only on the ends on concave rods (see Figure 16.56). Only the wrapped hair is processed and neutralized.

A **reverse stack** is wrapped closer to the head at the top and further away from the head at the bottom of each section. Begin the wrap in the top of the section and place sticks at an angle moving away from the head.

Piggyback perms are one option for the client who wants wave all the way to the scalp of her long hair. More than one rod is used on each subsection. The number of rods will be determined by the length of the hair as no more than 8 inches should be wrapped on any one rod. The rods selected can be one size, or larger rods can be used at the scalp.

Section the hair for control. Part off a subsection equal to the size of the rod placed nearest the scalp. Place the rod under the hair approximately 6–8 inches from the head (Figure 16.57). Roll the rod to the scalp while holding the rest of the strand to the side (Figure 16.58). Comb through the unwound part of the strand, use papers on the ends, and wrap the second rod to the base rod and fasten (Figures 16.59 and 16.60). You may wish to place a plastic pick under the bands to hold the two rods together for stability.

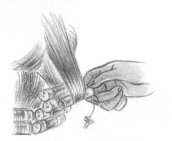

16.56   End perm

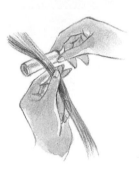

16.57

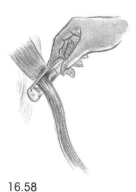

16.58

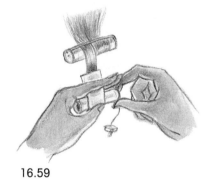

16.59   16.60

Process as directed and take test curls on both rods. To test curl near the scalp, unwind the hair by maneuvering under the end rod. You may need to blot the solution from the end rods before the scalp rods are processed. Or you may choose to wrap the porous ends with conditioner to slow processing.

An alternative to the piggyback wrap is the **double rod wrap**. This is an advanced technique that involves wrapping the hair from the ends. When approximately 6 inches of the hair have been wrapped, a second rod is inserted underneath the hair. Winding continues around both rods until the scalp is reached. Use special caution when applying and removing lotion to make sure all the hair is covered.

◆ **Key Point** ◆

Custom perm techniques provide you with excellent income as you produce one-of-a-kind results. Most custom techniques also create a style effect.

Ponytail wraps are a variation of end curls for very long hair. Pull the hair into several ponytails at the top of the head and fasten with elastic bands or locking clips (Figure 16.61). Separate the ends into strands and wrap around rods. Process, taking special care that the tails do not swing into the face or drip onto the scalp.

A **spiral perm** uses a custom-made rod or a straight rod that is wrapped vertically to the head. Very small subsections equal to the diameter of the rod are parted off, beginning at the hairline. The hair is wrapped around the rod in a spiraling fashion and secured at the scalp. The second row of rods should be "brick layered" over the first. The hair is then processed (see Figure 16.62). Spiral perms give a long-lasting defined curl pattern for long hair.

Custom rods can help you achieve special effects as well. Most, but not all, are designed for hair longer than 8 inches (see Table 16.1).

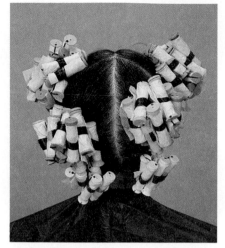

16.61   Ponytail wrap

Reconstruction Perm Waving

The process of permanently waving curly coarse hair to a larger wave pattern is known by several names. **Reconstruction perm**, **reverse perm**, and **soft curl perm** are but a few. Many manufacturers refer to the technique by a brand name they produce.

The "curl" was first introduced in the 70s when wet-look curls became stylish among black clients. While that fad has passed for the moment, the use of permanent wave techniques to expand the natural pattern of curly coarse hair has not disappeared. Today, chemical reconstruction is as viable a salon service for people with curly coarse hair as permanent waving is for the client with straight hair. The soft-curled hair can be blown dry, wet set, or left to air dry for a soft, curly look.

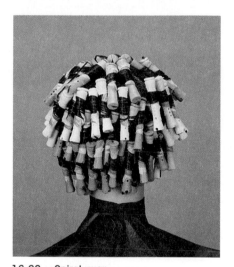

16.62   Spiral wrap

Preparing for a Reconstruction Perm

A reconstruction perm can be applied to virgin hair or to hair that has previously had a curl. Do NOT apply a soft curl over hair that has been relaxed. Sodium hydroxide-type relaxers permanently alter the bonding in the cortex so that the disulfide links necessary for permanent waving are not present. Applying a reconstruction curl to relaxed hair would not produce satisfactory results. It would, however, run a very large risk of extensively damaging the hair.

Analyze the hair as you would for any perm service. Check to see if there is any buildup of product on the hair that should be removed prior to the wave.

If the client has been having her hair pressed, wait about two weeks before attempting a reconstruction perm. In the interim, apply conditioning treatments and acidify the hair to see what natural curl will return. If you have any doubts, take precurl test curls at the side or back of the head. Pressing, especially hard pressing, can have the effect of permanently straightening the hair over time. You may need to cut the hair before you can successfully administer a soft curl.

> **◆SAFETY P R E C A U T I O N◆**
>
> DO NOT give a soft-curl perm to hair that has been processed with sodium hydroxide relaxer. You will not get good curl, and could seriously damage your client's hair.

CLIENT **T I P** ◆◆◆◆◆◆◆

Use rods at least twice the size of the natural curl. Make sure that the hair is long enough to wrap around the rod at least two and a half times.

Since the rod size determines the size of the curl, you will usually use rods with a large diameter. As a general guide, use rods that are at least $2\frac{1}{2}$ times larger than the natural curl for visible results. As with all perming, the hair should be long enough to encircle the rod at least $2\frac{1}{2}$ times for a complete wave effect.

The double flat wrap is usually the preferred method of wrapping extra curly hair. It provides more protection for the cuticle and the ends, and also gives you more control as you wind the hair smooth. Keep the papers damp by misting lightly with water to increase your wrap control and to ensure that the lotion is spread to the ends once applied.

Reconstructing Extra Curly Hair

Reconstruction, or soft curls, work on the same principle as permanent waves. Most soft curls are alkaline, having the main active ingredient of ammonium thioglycolate. The lotion is usually thick, often a creamy liquid or light gel.

The feature that distinguishes the soft curl process from the chemical wave is that the hair is first softened so that wrapping is possible. The prewrap solution, or gel, is a reduced-strength thio cream that penetrates the cuticle layers, begins the softening process of the hair, and also reduces the natural curl.

Materials

Client record card	Scissors or razor	Cotton
Release form	Acidifier	Plastic bag or
Plastic cape	Moisturizer	cap (optional)
Towels	Liquid protein	Plastic clips
Preperm shampoo	conditioner	Spray bottle
Wide tooth and tail or	Timer	Rod picks
styling combs	Applicator bottles	
Protective gloves	Selected rods	
Protective cream	End papers	
Selected	Prewrap solution	
reconstructor	(optional)	

Procedure for Reconstructing Extra Curly Hair

1. Cleanse your hands.
2. Seat your client comfortably and drape for a chemical service.
3. Analyze the hair and record all observations on the client record card. Have client sign the release form.
4. Shampoo the hair, being careful not to irritate the scalp (Figure 16.63). If there is a buildup on the hair from styling aids, use a special preperm shampoo. If the buildup is extreme, completely remove by deep shampoo and chelating treatments. Condition the hair, and wait a week before attempting to give a soft curl.
5. Section the hair into four or five sections. Secure with plastic clips.

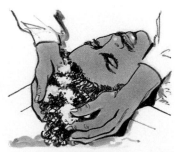

16.63   Shampoo hair

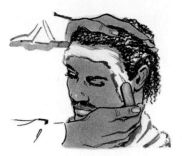

16.64   Apply protective cream

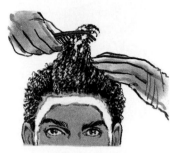

16.65   Apply prewrap gel

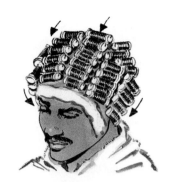

16.66   Off-base double flat wrap

6. Apply protective cream around the hairline and over the ears (Figure 16.64). (Some manufacturers recommend that you "base" the entire scalp with protective cream.) Put on your protective gloves.

7. Apply prewrap gel or cream to one section at a time, using the back of a comb, a relaxer brush, or your fingers. Begin in the most resistant or the curliest area. Keep the prewrap off the scalp itself (Figure 16.65).

8. Comb the gel gently with a wide-tooth comb. If the hair is very resistant, recomb with a finer-tooth comb. Be careful to avoid damage.

9. When the hair becomes controllable and the curl is relaxing, remove the gel as directed. Most reconstruction perms require that you rinse thoroughly with water just warm enough for your client's comfort. Towel blot gently.

10. Section the hair and begin the wrap. Most curls are done with the double-flat wrap. The condition of the hair will determine the base for the rod setting (see Selecting the Base). Insert picks under the rod bands if necessary to maintain tension (Figure 16.66).

11. Check protective cream around hairline and add more as needed. Place cotton under rods around hairline.

12. Apply processor carefully to each rod by drawing the applicator bottle across the top of the rod (Figure 16.67). Be careful that you do not drag the bottle tip on the hair. Roll the rod up and apply to the bottom of each rod.

13. Remove saturated cotton.

14. Place plastic cap or bag over rods if directed. Some reconstruction perms are speeded by placing the client under a preheated dryer.

15. Test-curl frequently. Check development on a different curl every few minutes. You will first note that the hair gets more sheen as the cuticle softens and the curl smooths. At that point, begin taking a test curl every three to five minutes. To test, blot the rod, unfasten it and unroll one to two turns, keeping your fingers anchored on the rod beneath. If the hair arches up from the rod, continue development. If the hair collapses into a wave the size of a rod (Figure 16.68), proceed to remove the processor.

16. Remove the lotion from the hair (Figure 16.69).

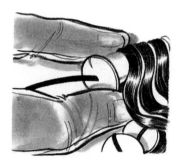

16.67   Apply processor

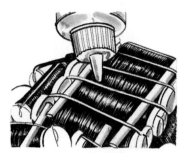

16.68   Test curl

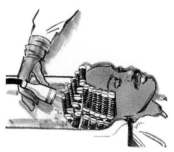

16.69   Rinse lotion

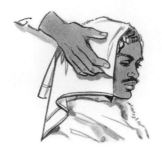

16.70   Blot each curl

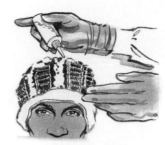

16.71   Apply neutralizer

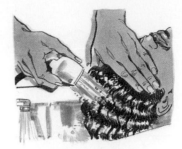

16.72   Rinse neutralizer

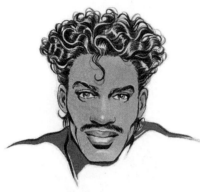

16.73   Finish style

CLIENT   TIP ◆◆◆◆◆◆

Most manufacturers recommend rinsing with water due to the thickness of the processor. Rinse thoroughly with warm water. Use low pressure so you do not disturb the rods.

◆ **Key Point** ◆

Reconstruction perms provide versatility of styling for over-curly hair. They can be air-dried, blown-dry, or wet-set to create any style desired.

17. Blot each curl individually to remove excess water (Figure 16.70).
18. Let the hair air oxidize for at least 10 minutes before applying neutralizer.
19. Check protective cream around hairline and reapply as necessary. Place cotton under rods around hairline.
20. Apply neutralizer, beginning at the crown (Figure 16.71). Slowly apply across top of rod with applicator, turn the rod up and return back across the bottom of the rod.
21. Remove any saturated cotton.
22. Time as manufacturer's directions require.
23. Carefully remove rods without stretching the hair and gently work the neutralizer through the ends.
24. Rinse thoroughly (Figure 16.72). Towel blot.
25. Apply a moisturizing conditioner that will normalize the pH of the hair. Avoid a strong acidifier as it will cause the curl to draw up.
26. Record all results on the client's card.
27. Proceed with styling as desired (Figure 16.73).
28. Suggest that your client purchase quality products to maintain the reconstruction perm at home.
29. Clean work areas and prepare for your next client.

SAFETY PRECAUTIONS FOR CHEMICAL WAVING

Safety for you and your client should be uppermost in your mind. During chemical services, there are several additional precautions that you should observe for everyone's benefit.

Be aware of the hazards associated with the chemicals used in the salon. Protect yourself by ensuring adequate ventilation. Post emergency numbers you can call if you accidentally spill or splash chemicals on yourself or your client. Know immediate steps you should take to remove chemicals from the skin or scalp, and what to do to counteract their harmful effects.

The following guidelines will get you comfortably and safely through your day.

1. Do not apply a perm if the scalp is irritated or has abrasions.
2. Analyze the condition of the hair and record results.

3. Do not brush or irritate the scalp immediately prior to a permanent wave.
4. Carefully drape your client to protect skin and clothing.
5. Use a protective cream around the client's hairline skin. Protect your hands by wearing gloves.
6. Remove and discard any cotton that is saturated with solutions.
7. Blot any lotion that contacts the scalp with cotton saturated in water. Blot the area and apply neutralizer with cotton. Blot with damp cotton again. Apply protective cream to sensitive area.
8. Test curl frequently to avoid overprocessing.
9. Follow manufacturer's directions.
10. Do NOT leave your client during the processing or neutralizing segments of the perm.
11. Observe all sanitation rules.
12. Never apply a perm to hair that has been treated with sodium hydroxide.
13. Never apply a perm to hair that is severely damaged.

> ◆ **Key Point** ◆
> Use chemicals safely for your protection and for that of your client.

SUMMARY

The mastery of chemical waving is an important addition to your menu of salon services. It is probably the chemical service that you will be most often asked to perform. Careful analysis is critical: you must be able to determine the scalp condition, the texture or diameter of the hair, and the porosity or ability to absorb liquids. You will test for elasticity, the ability of the hair to stretch and return; this is critical for a successful chemical wave. The density, or thickness of the hair, will help you determine the blocking pattern.

The rods you select determine the size and the shape of the curl. You will select the correct rod according to the length of the hair so that it will go around the rod at least two and one-half turns. The placement of that rod within the sectioning pattern will determine the final effect that you get. You must perfect your wrapping techniques in order to get successful results.

The chemical wave process involves processing (when the bonds are broken), and neutralizing (when the bonds are reformed). You will select the correct formula based upon your analysis and you will determine when that processing is complete by test-curling. You will then remove the lotion as directed and apply neutralizer to complete the chemical wave process.

Custom perm techniques offer advanced methods either to achieve a style result or to overcome a difficult hair type. Air oxidation and transfer perming give you the ability to chemically wave damaged or very fine hair. You will select style or root perm techniques when the effect you desire is a subtle one lasting only six to eight weeks. As a professional cosmetologist, you must be able to offer a variety of perm techniques for long and very long hair. You will select the one best suited to the style desired and the length of the client's hair.

Reconstruction, or soft curl chemical waves give you the ability to reduce curly coarse hair for more manageability and a looser curl pattern. You will perform this service by reducing the natural curl, wrapping the hair on larger rods, and then chemically creating the new curl. As with all chemical services, you will follow safety precautions to prevent injury to your clients or to yourself.

QUESTIONS

1. Why is hair analysis important to the success of the perm service? What information do you get during the analysis and how do you use it?
2. What different types of rods are available to the professional perm artist? What effect does each create on the hair?
3. Why do you section the hair before wrapping?
4. What are the two commonly accepted methods of sectioning?
5. What are the characteristics of a well-wrapped perm?
6. What chemical activity takes place during a permanent wave?
7. What is the procedure for giving a chemical wave?
8. What custom perm techniques are available to the progressive stylist?
9. What are several ways of wrapping long hair?
10. What is the difference between a soft or reconstruction perm wave and a regular permanent wave?
11. What safety precautions should be used to protect you and your client during perm processes?

PROJECTS

1. Perform an analysis service on at least three of your fellow students. Determine the correct rods and perm to give the results they describe. Fill out record cards and then have your instructor estimate the results you would get.
2. Research the types of rods that are available in your school and the benefits of each. Check what other rods are used in key salons in your area and why.
3. Section your mannequin for each sectioning pattern you have learned. Explain when each is preferred.
4. Perform the amount of practice wraps on mannequins required by your school. Check each wrap yourself against the "checklist for winding" and compare your rating to your instructor's.
5. Working with magazines, select six pictures of models with different styles and lengths of curled hair. For each, determine the wrap, custom wrap, and rod size for the look shown. Check your results in a discussion period with your fellow students and instructor.
6. Research the MSDS sheets for the perm products available in your school. Outline the hazards posed, how the perm can be safely used, and what to do in the event of a safety problem.

CHEMICAL RELAXING

CHAPTER • 17

CHAPTER GOAL

Chemical relaxing is the most common salon service to loosen natural curl for manageability. After reading this chapter and completing the projects, you should be able to

1. Explain the two primary types of relaxer available and briefly explain their effects on the hair.
2. Demonstrate the components of a complete hair analysis for a relaxer service.
3. Demonstrate the procedures of preparing for a relaxer including the strand test, sectioning, and applying protective cream.
4. Outline the procedure for relaxing virgin hair and for doing a retouch relaxing service.
5. Explain specialty relaxer service techniques and relate them to today's styles.
6. List at least eight safety precautions to protect you and your client during the relaxer service.

The history of chemical relaxing is primarily a story that developed in the United States. As slavery gradually caused the disintegration of African culture, it also eliminated the richness of tribal styling. Efforts to straighten the hair usually involved wrapping and twisting—a method that could result in hair loss. Attempts were also made to soften the hair with a mixture of mashed potatoes, lye, and oil.

The foundation of today's black styling services was laid by Madame C.J. Walker. The Walker creations, a hair softener and a straightening comb, were used in one of the first methods of relaxing. These innovations also began a road to success that made Madame Walker America's first self-made black female millionaire.

Relaxers progressed over the years and chemical improvements made them kinder to the hair and more effective in reducing the natural curl present. Today, relaxers are available in many formulations and strengths for different hair types. By mastering the art of chemical relaxing, you can follow in Madame Walker's footsteps and begin your journey to fortune.

To master chemical relaxing, you will examine the scalp and analyze hair qualities. You will section for control so your application will be fast and accurate. You will determine when processing is complete and will safely follow all removal techniques.

HAIR RELAXING PRODUCTS

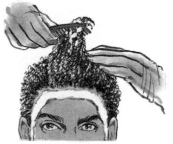

17.1

There are three general categories of relaxers available to you as a professional cosmetologist. There are **thioglycolate**, **acid**, and **hydroxide** (high **DROK** seyed) **relaxers**. Of these, the hydroxide types are used more frequently in the salon. Thio relaxers are closely related to the development of permanent waves. Let's take a look.

Thioglycolate Relaxers

These relaxers contain thio (the same ingredient used in permanent wave solutions) as the active ingredient. The relaxer is a thick cream or a gel; the weight of the product will help remove curl from the hair (Figure 17.1). When the relaxer is applied, usually to shampooed hair, the cuticle layer is softened. The hair is then combed or smoothed until the desired degree of curl is removed. Figure 17.2 shows that the disulfide bond in the cortex is broken as the curl is removed.

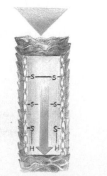

17.2   Breakdown of disulfide bonds

Once the curl has been removed as desired, the relaxer cream is rinsed from the hair and the hair is neutralized in its straighter position. The disulfide bonds are reformed in the straight position as shown in Figure 17.3. This is often done through a net, especially if the hair has been molded into a style shape or waves.

Thio relaxers are often not effective on coarse hair textures, or on hair that has extreme curl. Extra care has to be taken to keep the relaxer off the scalp, especially during the combing phase. Use protective cream to protect the hairline and blot any thio that contacts the scalp.

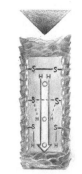

17.3   Reformed disulfide bonds

Acid Relaxers

These relaxers also work like permanent waves. The active ingredient is usually a **bisulfite**. These relaxers are very mild in their action and are more often used in a soft curl process than as a relaxer alone. You should always research the manufacturer's directions and consult with your instructor before you combine different chemical products in a service. If the chemicals are not compatible, your service will not be successful and you risk damaging your client's hair and scalp.

Hydroxide Relaxers

Relaxers based on **sodium hydroxide** work on an entirely different principle. They are most often used to remove curl from the hair. These relaxers are usually available in a cream formulation in varying strengths of mild, regular, and super. The difference between the strengths depends upon the percentage of active ingredient, which varies between 5 and 10 percent. These relaxers are alkaline in pH, ranging at 10.0 and above. The alkalinity forces the cuticle to soften so that the relaxer can penetrate into the cortex layer of the hair (Figure 17.4). Once there, the sodium hydroxide (NaOH) breaks the disulfide or sulfur bond (Figure 17.5). When this happens, the hair will smooth out to a straighter form due to the weight of the cream, the pressure of smoothing, or—in extremely curly hair—the gentle combing of the hair.

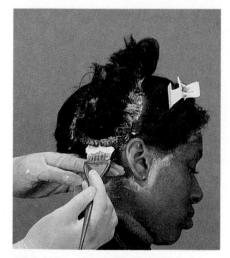

17.4   Theo relaxer removes curl

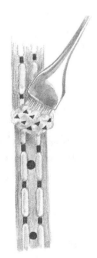

17.5   NaOH breaks disulfide bond

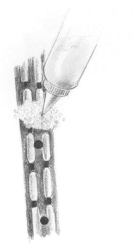

17.6   Shampoo forms lanthionine

Once the hair has relaxed to the desired degree of smoothness, take your client to the shampoo bowl and rinse very thoroughly. The rinsing is necessary to remove all traces of relaxer from the hair so that its action is stopped. You will speed this process by using warm water and gradually increasing your water pressure from a moderate setting. Rinse the hair from the scalp out to the ends, avoiding excessive pressure around the hairline. Lift the hair from the crown and separate layers in the back to ensure thorough rinsing. Lift the client's head gently so that you can remove all traces of relaxer in the nape. The temperature of water is important and should be comfortably warm. Hot water could damage the hair, cause scalp irritation, and be extremely uncomfortable for your client. Water that is too cool, on the other hand, will not remove the oil and wax bases that form the relaxer cream, thus leaving the relaxer to continue processing.

Next, and most important, shampoo the hair thoroughly (Figure 17.6). An acid-balanced (4.5 to 5.5) shampoo is recommended as the acid will neutralize any remaining alkali inside the hair shaft. You will know that this is happening when you smell sulfur (somewhat like the aroma of rotten eggs). Shampoo the hair until it rinses clear with warm water. This may take as many as three shampoos if the relaxer you choose has a heavy wax base. The hair should then be deep conditioned according to your analysis.

A **lanthionine** (lan **THEE** oh neen) bond is a permanent bond and cannot be broken or altered any further. It is for this reason that sodium relaxers were once referred to as *perms* (permanent) to separate them from temporary pressing methods. Today, with many clients choosing soft curl processes to reduce curl, the term *perm* is not used for relaxers in order to avoid confusion.

Potassium hydroxide is often an ingredient in sodium relaxers and occasionally is used as the primary active ingredient. These relaxers work in the same manner as sodium and are also referred to as "lye" relaxers.

Calcium hydroxide relaxers work on the same chemical principle as those outlined previously. Calcium hydroxide is slightly milder and works more slowly on the hair. Many professional technicians feel that calcium hydroxide relaxers are more damaging to the cuticle layer of the hair and leave it in a more roughened state. Calcium hydroxide relaxers are often mistakenly referred to as "no lye" relaxers.

Base Creams

A **base** is a petroleum cream designed to protect the scalp during a relaxing service. These creams have a lighter consistency than petroleum jelly and are designed to melt at body temperature. They cover the scalp with a thin, oily coating and prevent irritation or burning from the relaxer cream.

No-base relaxers are available. These relaxers are milder to the scalp and often have a protective base conditioner added into the cream. This type of relaxer does not require a base unless you determine that the client might be especially sensitive.

A protective cream should be used around the hairline and over the ears before beginning any relaxer application.

HAIR ANALYSIS

When offering a relaxing service, it is most important that you select the correct product and the correct application technique for your client's hair. In order to do this, you will need to increase your knowledge of the hair, the chemistry of relaxers, and the different types of relaxers available. Practice your skills of analyzing your client's scalp, hair, and natural curl so that you can provide a professional relaxing service.

Your hair analysis for a relaxing service should include checking for the same characteristics discussed in Chapter 15, Chemical Waving. In addition, you will need to analyze the natural curl present in the hair. Carefully record all of your data on the client's record card.

Choosing the Correct Formula

Sodium relaxers are available in regular, mild, and super formulas. Mild formulas are suggested for softer, finer hair and hair that has had a previous chemical treatment such as coloring. Super formulas are stronger and sometimes also more alkaline. They are designed for resistant, coarse hair that is extremely curly.

In order to determine the correct formula, first analyze the texture. To do this, estimate the diameter of the hair shaft. Is it thin, medium, or thick? Check the amount of natural curl present, especially in the area closest to the scalp. Next, analyze the porosity of the hair because this will affect the speed at which the relaxer penetrates the cuticle layer.

When you do your analysis, be certain to include hair from the hairline, the nape, and the crown. Consider the hair closest to the scalp and also the hair shaft and ends. You will often notice that the hair around the hairline has a different texture and is less thick. The hair in the nape is sometimes more curly and of a different texture from the rest of the hair. Even if the hair has not had prior chemical services, you may notice changes in the condition of the hair further from the scalp. This could be from thermal pressing, from harsh shampoos, or just normal wear and tear that is more obvious in hair that is naturally more dry.

Varying textures over the head may occasionally dictate use of more than one strength of relaxer. More often, however, you can equalize the results by your application method or by the use of conditioners on more fragile or damaged hair. The varying textures affect where you begin relaxer application. Start application in the most resistant area; either where the hair is curliest or where it is the most coarse.

Scalp Analysis

It is especially important that you examine the scalp for abrasions or irritations prior to giving a chemical relaxing service. Part the hair in

CLIENT TIP ◆◆◆◆◆◆◆

Include hair from the front, back hairline, crown, and side when you give an analysis. The differences in the condition and the varying textures will determine the correct formula and application method.

◆ **Key Point** ◆
A thorough analysis of the hair is critical to your success. The amount of curl and the hair texture will determine the strength of relaxer to use, the timing, and correctional treatments.

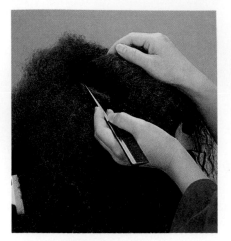

½-inch to 1-inch sections, being careful not to scratch the scalp. Use the tip of your finger, or the tail of a comb (Figure 17.7). Push the hair away from the parting so that you can clearly see the scalp. Check to make sure there are no abrasions or irritations. If you see redness or sores you should advise your client to postpone the relaxing service until the scalp is healed.

Keeping Client Records

Keep a record for each client to help you achieve consistent results and avoid problems. The card should include the client's hair history and notes concerning how the hair reacted to specific chemical products (Figure 17.8).

17.7   Examine scalp

Relaxer Record Card

Name .... Phone ( ) -
Address ....
City .... State .... Zip ....
Analysis of Scalp
Condition .... Base used Y .... N ....
Analysis of Hair
Porosity .... Elasticity ....
Texture .... Condition ....
Length .... Natural Curl ....
Previous Chemical Treatments ....
Relaxer Selection
Relaxer used ....
Strength ....
Strand Test Timing .... Results ....
Additives or special instructions ....
....
Processing Time .... Shampoo Used ....
Results ....
Conditioning ....
Date .... Stylist ....

Date	Relaxer Used	Results	Stylist

17.8

PREPARING FOR A RELAXER

The most important step in learning to give a relaxing service is hours of application practice. Speed and accuracy of application are important in all chemical services so that the results you achieve will be even. Precise application techniques will prevent scalp irritation and hair damage which can be caused by overexposure to chemicals. Your instructor will work with you to ensure that you develop a pattern of application that covers the most resistant, coarsest, and curliest, hair first. Try to develop a rhythm or application that is both fast and accurate.

◆ Key Point ◆

Establish a working rhythm for application of the relaxer. Your strand test will indicate the amount of time that you have for application. Section for control and work in a pattern for speed.

The Release Form

Inform your client of the results of your hair and scalp analysis. Explain how the condition of the hair and scalp affect the choices you make about the relaxer. Make sure the client understands the processes involved in the relaxer service, then ask him or her to sign a release form. This form indicates that the client is aware of the processes of the service; it does not release you from the responsibility of damage or accidents.

The Strand Test

Because every head of hair reacts differently to chemicals, you should perform a strand test before each relaxer service. A strand test *must* be done if you are at all unsure about results.

Follow the manufacturer's instructions for the product selected. The directions will include guidelines for timing, safety, and application.

Procedure for Strand Testing

1. Select a ½-inch square section at the back of the head.
2. Place the strand over a strip of foil or transparent plastic.
3. Apply the relaxer to the strand (Figure 17.9).
4. Fold the strip over the strand to protect the rest of the hair.
5. Process the strand until the desired degree of relaxation has been achieved. Note timings.
6. Rinse the strand thoroughly with a spray bottle. Towel-blot excess relaxer (Figure 17.10).
7. Apply shampoo to the strand only and massage through. Rinse with the spray bottle and reapply until the strand is completely clean.
8. Compare strand to virgin hair to determine if you have the results you want (Figure 17.11).
9. Analyze the condition of the hair. Make necessary adjustments to formula and techniques chosen for application to the entire head.
10. Cover the strand test liberally with protective cream to prevent reprocessing during the full service.

◆SAFETY **PRECAUTION**◆

If you cannot apply relaxer in the time indicated by the strand test, alter your method. Use a slower-acting formula or select a different service to remove excess curl without hair damage.

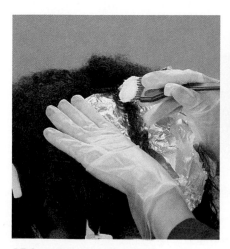

17.9 Apply relaxer to strand

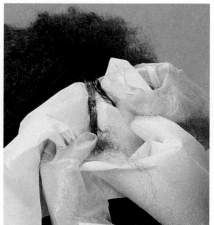

17.10 Towel blot strand

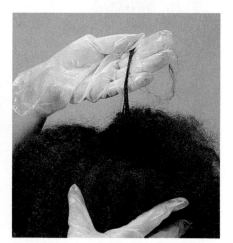

17.11

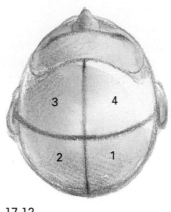

17.12

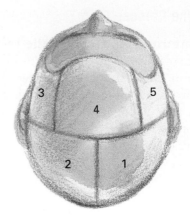

17.13

Sectioning the Hair

Part the hair into four or five sections for control. The most common sectioning is into four parts as shown in Figure 17.12 so that you can equally process the entire head. First, part the hair from the front hairline to the nape of the neck into two equal sections. Next, part the hair from ear to ear, across the crown of the head. Secure each section with a large plastic clip.

Some technicians prefer to use three sections in the front. First, part the hair from ear to ear over the top of the crown. Split the back section into two equal parts and clip securely. Next, section out a panel from the crown to the front hairline. Clip this and each of the two remaining side sections (Figure 17.13).

Applying the Base

Most of today's relaxers are "no base." However, you may select a relaxer that requires the use of a base to protect the scalp.

To apply, release one of the sections. Part the hair into a subsection $\frac{1}{2}$ to 1 inch in thickness and apply the base directly to the scalp. Continue through each section, applying base to the scalp only (Figure 17.14).

Apply protective cream around the hairline, over the ears, and at the base of the nape to all heads, whether a base is used or not (Figure 17.15).

RELAXER PROCEDURES

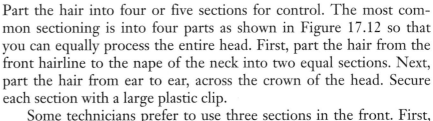

The following is the procedure for a sodium hydroxide, no-base relaxer on virgin hair. Before beginning any relaxing service, thoroughly read the manufacturer's instructions for the particular product you are using.

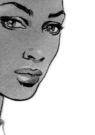

17.14 Apply base to scalp

17.15 Apply protective cream

Materials

Relaxer	Protective cream	Timer
Neutralizing shampoo	Conditioner	Plastic clips
Towels	Gloves	Record card
Neck strip (optional)	Wide-tooth comb	Applicator brush,
Plastic cape	Spatula	spatula, or comb

Procedure for Sodium Hydroxide Relaxer

1. Seat client comfortably at your station.
2. Sanitize your hands.
3. Drape client and ask him or her to remove neck and ear jewelry. Do NOT irritate the scalp by brushing or shampooing.
4. Analyze hair and scalp. Record results. Have client sign release form.
5. Perform a strand test. Make note of results and timing. The total timing will be your guide for application and processing of the entire head. For example, if the strand processed in 20 minutes, you must be able to apply relaxer to all four sections, cross-check, and begin final strand-testing in 20 minutes.
6. Section the hair and clip securely.
7. Apply base if needed or recommended by the manufacturer.
8. Apply protective cream around entire hairline and over ears. Put on your protective gloves.
9. Open relaxer container. Place the container on a terry towel to prevent slipping during application. Select applicator.
10. Release one back section of hair. Set the timer as directed by the manufacturer and the strand-test timing.
11. Outline the section, except the hairline, with relaxer. Begin application ½ inch from the scalp.
12. Part a ½-inch horizontal subsection, beginning at the top of the first quadrant. Hold subsection straight out from the head and apply relaxer to the top (Figure 17.16). Begin ½ inch from the scalp and apply out to, but not through, the ends. Apply relaxer to underside of the strand in the same manner (Figure 17.17). Lay the hair up, out of the way and quickly proceed to next subsection.
13. Quickly apply to the entire quadrant in this manner (Figure 17.18) until you reach the hairline. Lift the subsections away from the top of the head, turning them back down to the nape (Figure 17.19).
14. Proceed in the same manner in the second back section. Outline the section, part off a ½-inch subsection and quickly apply to the top and bottom of the subsection. Apply from ½-inch away from the scalp up to, but not through, the ends. Avoid application at the hairline (Figure 17.20).

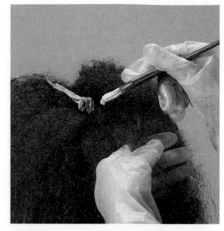

17.16　Apply to top of hair

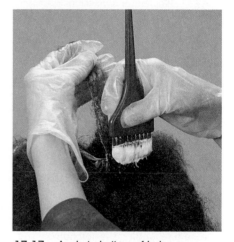

17.17　Apply to bottom of hair

CLIENT　TIP ◆◆◆◆◆◆◆

Your instructor may advise you to use a base if the client is sensitive, regardless of the relaxer chosen.

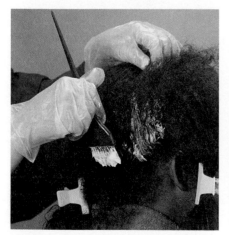

17.18　Complete to entire quadrant

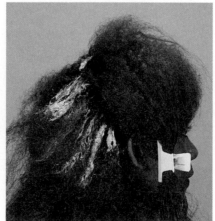

17.19　Turn hair back down

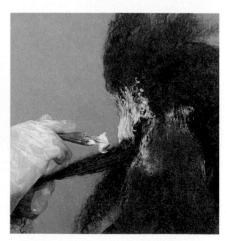

17.20　Apply to second quadrant

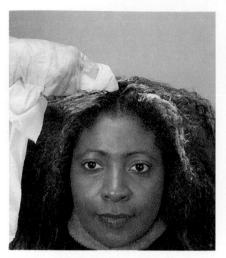

17.21   Blot relaxer from scalp

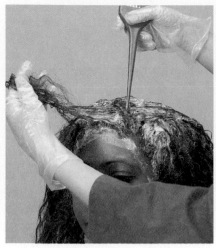

17.22   Cross check

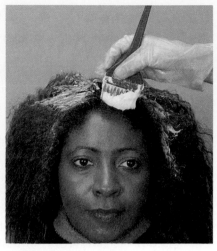

17.23   Apply to hairline

15. Continue around the head by applying to the adjoining front section (Figure 17.20). Outline the section and apply to each subsection as described in step 13. Avoid pressing the hair down to the scalp.

16. Apply relaxer to the last section. You should have used half, or less, of your total timing.

17. Immediately begin cross-checking your application in the last quadrant. Part the hair vertically. Apply relaxer to the area closest to the scalp, to the hairline, and to any areas that you may have missed. If any relaxer should touch the scalp, thoroughly blot it away with a damp towel (Figure 17.21). Cross check the entire fourth quadrant.

18. Move to the third quadrant and use vertical partings to cross-check (Figure 17.22). Apply relaxer to the hair near the scalp and the hairline (Figure 17.23). Add any additional relaxer as needed.

19. Cross-check the second quadrant (Figure 17.24) where you applied relaxer, then the first. Apply relaxer to the hair near the

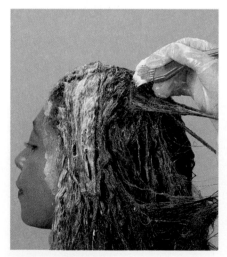

17.24   Cross check

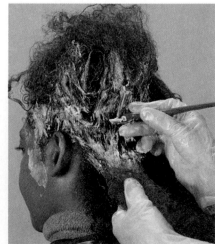

17.25   Apply to hair near scalp

scalp (Figure 17.25). You should have one quarter, or more, of your total time remaining.

20. Work the relaxer through the ends according to your analysis of the hair.

21. Test the action of the relaxer by slightly stretching a small subsection and seeing how fast the natural curl is being removed (Figure 17.26). Remove the relaxer from the strand with your gloved finger. Watch for the degree of relaxation and for the amount of curl that returns as you release the hair. You do not want to completely straighten the hair; this causes excess damage and gives you no styling options. Remove curl until the hair has a loose, controllable wave.

22. Smooth the hair only as necessary to even processing. Gently lift the hair from the scalp, stretching slightly and smoothing the relaxer into the subsection. Today's relaxers are formulated to need little, if any, smoothing.

23. When the timer indicates that processing should be finished, remove the relaxer from several strands. Select a strand from the front, the back, and the side hairline. Place the strand over a towel. Remove excess relaxer and mist with water if needed to assess relaxation. If processing is not complete, work relaxer back into the hair. When processing is complete, proceed with your client to the shampoo bowl.

24. Seat the client comfortably at the shampoo bowl, making certain that all of the nape hair is inside the bowl. Adjust the water so that the temperature is warm and pressure is medium. As you will still be wearing your gloves, check that the client is comfortable with the water temperature. Water that is too hot will burn the client and cause hair damage. Water that is too cool is also uncomfortable and will not stop the action of the relaxer.

25. Rinse the hair thoroughly. Use one hand as a shield around the hairline so water does not splash into the client's eyes. Lift the hair in sections out away from the head so that you can completely rinse the relaxer from the underneath layers. Lift the client's head gently and rinse the nape area. Pay attention that no chemical remains in this area.

26. Rinse the hair from the scalp out to the ends until all traces of the relaxer are removed and the hair no longer foams. This step stops the action of the relaxer and is extremely important.

27. Remove your gloves.

28. Shampoo the hair with an acid-balanced shampoo or the neutralizing (stabilizing or fixative) shampoo provided by the manufacturer. Apply the shampoo to the palms of your hands, work them together, and gently begin manipulations on the hair. Work underneath the hair to prevent tangling and to ensure that all the hair is shampooed. This step neutralizes the chemical action inside the hair and forms the new lanthionine bond. (Refer to the section, Hydroxide Relaxers, on page 361.)

29. Rinse and repeat as necessary until the hair lathers well and rinses clear. Frequently, three shampoos are necessary to ensure that this phase of the relaxing process is complete.

CLIENT **T I P** ◆◆◆◆◆◆◆

As you cross-check the hair, add gentle pressure that will speed the processing of the relaxer. Work backwards from your initial application, so the degree of relaxation will be uniform over the entire head.

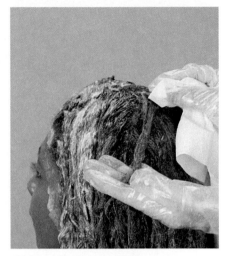

17.26 Observe progress

CLIENT **T I P** ◆◆◆◆◆◆◆

Protect your client's eyes. For extra client comfort, cover the eyes with cotton pads saturated with herbal tea.

30. Apply conditioner according to manufacturer's instructions, your analysis of the hair, and your instructor's directions. Time as necessary, rinse, and towel-blot.
31. Style the hair, using caution to avoid excess heat or stretching.
32. Complete and file the record card; clean your station and shampoo area.
33. Suggest your client purchase the products to maintain the hair and the style at home. Give any tips that would be helpful.

Sodium Hydroxide Retouch Application

As your client's hair grows, you will need to repeat the relaxing process on the new growth at the scalp. This usually happens anywhere from six weeks to two months after the initial relaxing service, depending upon the degree of natural curl, the rate of hair growth, and the style. Most hair grows $\frac{1}{4}$ to $\frac{1}{2}$ inch a month.

Materials

Relaxer	Conditioner	Plastic clips
Neutralizing shampoo	Gloves	Record card
Towels	Wide-tooth comb	Applicator brush,
Neck strip (optional)	Spatula	spatula, or comb
Plastic cape	Timer	Release form
Protective cream		

Procedure for a Sodium Hydroxide Retouch Application

1. Seat client comfortably and drape. Discuss the success of the previous relaxer and perform analysis of the hair and scalp. If you have not given your client a retouch before, give a strand test.
2. Apply deep conditioners to the hair if it is damaged. Apply protective cream around hairline. Section the hair. Put on your protective gloves.
3. Begin application in the opposite back section from initial application. If you applied initially in the right back and proceeded clockwise 1,2,3,4, your retouch application will be, counterclockwise, 2,1,4,3. (See Figure 17.27.) This ensures the most even results possible.

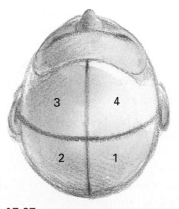

17.27

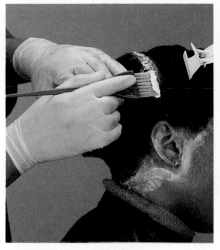

17.28 (a)   Outline quadrant

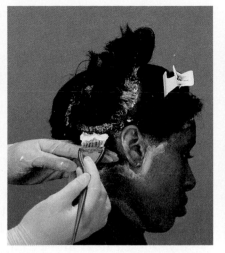

17.28 (b)   Apply in ½-inch sections

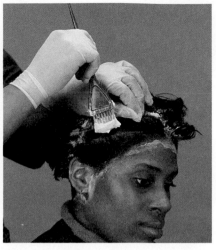

17.29   Apply to remaining hair

4. Set timer according to your record card or the strand test. Outline the quadrant with relaxer (Figure 17.28a). Make ½-inch horizontal partings and apply from the scalp up to the line of demarcation (Figure 17.28b). Use caution to avoid overlapping. Proceed through all quadrants (Figure 17.29).
5. Cross-check the last quadrant vertically, applying more relaxer as needed and to the hairline (Figure 17.30). When cross-checking, reverse the order of application in your quadrants so that processing is equalized (Figure 17.31).
6. Check progress by strand-testing and gently smooth the hair only if necessary.
7. Thoroughly rinse the hair with warm water.
8. Shampoo the hair until it lathers well and rinses clear.
9. Condition as needed and proceed with styling.

For damaged hair, your instructor may direct you to cleanse the hair with conditioner instead of shampooing as in step 8. Apply the conditioner and massage into the hair as you would shampoo. Rinse and repeat, leaving the conditioner on five or more minutes before rinsing.

Thio Relaxer Procedure

Consult the manufacturer's directions when using a thio relaxer. Some relaxer involve a two-step process, while others require three steps. Some relaxers require preshampooing and some do not. Thio relaxers are usually advised for finer-textured hair with less curl.

Materials

Relaxer	Protective cream	Plastic clips
Neutralizer	Conditioner	Record card
Shampoo	Gloves	Applicator brush,
Towels	Wide-tooth comb	spatula, or comb
Neck strip (optional)	Spatula	
Plastic cape	Timer	

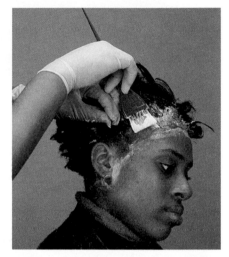

17.30   Cross check and apply to hairline

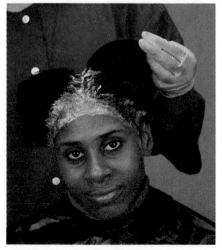

17.31   Finished application

Procedure for Thioglycolate Relaxer

1. Sanitize your hands.
2. Seat your client comfortably and drape.
3. Shampoo the hairs as directed, using caution not to irritate the scalp.
4. Apply protective cream around the entire hairline and over ears.
5. Section the hair for control. Put on protective gloves.
6. Apply relaxer with brush or comb as directed. Apply relaxer to ½-inch subsections from the hair at the scalp out to the ends. Apply relaxer section by section until all hair is covered.
7. Cross-check application and begin timing. Comb the relaxer through the hair as directed. Use caution to avoid hair breakage during this process. Avoid working the relaxer into the scalp. Blot any exposed areas with a damp towel.
8. Rinse the relaxer from the hair when the desire degree of relaxation has been achieved. Rinse thoroughly from scalp to ends, paying special attention to the nape area.
9. Towel blot and gently comb hair back into a smooth position. You may wish to cover the hair with a net if you are molding a style into the hair, such as waves, before you neutralize.
10. Apply neutralizer and time as directed. Rinse, towel-blot, and condition as your analysis indicates.
11. Style hair and recommend correct retail products.
12. Complete record card and file. Clean styling area and shampoo bowl.

Thio Retouch

Thio relaxers may require a retouch after the hair has grown. The line of demarcation will not always be clear because the curl is never completely removed and some curl returns over time. Follow your instructor's expert advice as to the procedure and method of application should you need to offer a thio retouch.

Specialty Reaxing Services

Chemical hair relaxing adds another texture-control method to your professional styling repertoire. In addition to the procedures outlined previously in this chapter, there are two custom techniques you will need to know: relaxing tinted or damaged hair and style relaxing.

Relaxing Tinted Hair

Consultation and analysis are two critical tools that will help you with a client who has tinted hair and wishes to relax it, or has relaxed hair and wishes to color it. There are may options available, but first determine how committed your client is to the upkeep of double-processed hair.

Confirm your analysis with a strand test. Choose either a tinted or mild relaxer formula. Apply conditioner as needed according to your analysis and proceed with relaxer application as detailed in this chapter. Pay special attention to the timing of the process and the condition of the hair as the curl is relaxed. Remove relaxer as directed and deep condition.

Darker tones will be pulled from the hair as a result of the relaxing process. Refresh those tones with a temporary or semipermanent color designed for use after a chemical service. Keep all color application at least $\frac{1}{4}$ inch off the scalp.

If the colored hair is lighter than the natural shade, suggest that your client switch to a highlighting technique. Perform that service within a week of the relaxer.

Style Relaxing

The concept of creating a style with the aid of a relaxer is not new, but it is certainly exciting. There are two methods that withstand fads and fashion trends. The first is to apply relaxer according to the style desired. Relax the nape and perimeter, for example, for whatever this year's version of the flattop is called. Or, just the opposite, leave the nape area natural and relax the top and sides to help you create this year's version of the timeless wedge shape.

The second method of style relaxing reduces curl all over the head. The key difference between this method and regular relaxing is the degree of curl removed. This technique removes a small amount of curl and leaves the hair in a more manageable and stylable condition while still appearing to be "natural."

> ◆ **Key Point** ◆
> Style, or design, relaxing is the service that can help you build a clientele. Study the hair, listen to your customer's requests; and then create a one-of-a-kind style.

SAFETY PRECAUTIONS FOR CHEMICAL RELAXING

1. Follow manufacturer's instructions and precautions carefully.
2. Conduct a hair analysis. Confirm your results with a strand test.
3. Do NOT perform a relaxing service if the scalp shows sign of abrasion, irritation, or redness.
4. Do not brush the hair and scalp before applying relaxer.
5. Apply base if directed or if the client's scalp is sensitive. Advise client to avoid drinking caffeinated beverages during the relaxer process.
6. Protect your hands with gloves and protect your client with cream around the hairline and over the ears.
7. Avoid contacting the scalp directly with the relaxer. If relaxer should accidentally touch the scalp, gently remove it with a damp towel and apply protective cream.
8. Carefully adhere to timing limits from the manufacturer and your strand-test results.
9. Rinse all relaxer from the hair and thoroughly shampoo to neutralize chemicals.

10. Never apply sodium hydroxide to hair treated with thioglycolate. Never apply a thio relaxer over a sodium hydroxide product. These two chemicals are not compatible and mixing them on hair can cause severe damage and failed services.

SUMMARY

Chemical relaxers help you obtain control of the texture of your client's hair for increased stylability. Sodium-type relaxers are by far the most often used; although thio type relaxers are still available. You will perform hair analysis and examine the scalp as a key to your success with relaxing. This will assist you in determining the strength relaxer to use and the amount of time that it will take to process. The timing from your strand test is critical as it tells you the maximum time the relaxer can stay on the hair without damage. You must be able to apply and cross-check the entire head in that amount of time. You will also strand test at the end of that time to determine if the hair is sufficiently processed for good results.

Relaxers can also be used alone to create a style in combination with a precision cut. The hair is partially relaxed to expand the curl to a wave and then the hair is cut. Relaxers should not be used to completely straighten hair, but to give you the stylability you need.

QUESTIONS

1. What are the two primary types of relaxers available?
2. What are the components of a complete hair analysis for a relaxer service?
3. What is the procedure for a relaxer strand test? How should you section the hair for a relaxing service? Where do you apply protective cream?
4. What is the procedure for relaxing virgin hair? How does this differ from a retouch application?
5. How can you alter basic relaxer techniques to obtain today's styles?
6. What are the safety precautions you should follow to protect you and your client during the relaxer service?

PROJECTS

1. Research the relaxers available at your school. Determine if they are sodium, potassium, or calcium hydroxide based. Check if each requires a base or is designated as "no-base."
2. Study the directions of all the relaxers available at your school and see what is the most common timing limit. Practice relaxer mock application to mannequins until you can apply, cross-check, and strand test relaxer within that amount of time.
3. Research the MSDS sheets for the relaxer products available in your school. Outline the hazards posed, how the product can be safely used, and what to do in the event of a safety problem.

SKIN CARE

CHAPTER 18

CHAPTER GOAL

Skin care is an additional service offered in a full-service salon. After reading this chapter and completing the projects, you should be able to

1. Describe the types of massage and explain the benefits of each.
2. Outline the preparation, cleansing, and analysis for a plain facial.
3. Demonstrate the basic manipulations for a facial.
4. Describe the skin treatments that are recommended for dry, oily, and combination skin types.
5. List 15 elements of infection control that are critical for the protection of the public and for the safety and welfare of the practitioner and the client.

As a specialty, esthetics (ess **THET** ix)—the science of massage, facials, and skin treatments—is relatively new to the United States. Until the 1960s, skin care in this country was restricted to simple pampering and makeup application without any scientific approaches to skin treatment in cosmetology salons.

This began to change, primarily due to the arrival in the United States of Christine Valmy from Romania. Upon her arrival, she quickly grasped the differences in the approach to esthetics and set out to bring European techniques and science to the American practice of skin care. In 1965, she opened the first school for skin care and in the 70s received official recognition from Congress for starting the field of esthetics in America.

Today the study of esthetics is very extensive, and specialty licenses are available in a majority of the states for those who wish to specialize without taking the entire cosmetology course. This chapter is intended to give you an overview of this dynamic field.

As a cosmetologist offering skin care, you will cleanse the face and analyze it. Your analysis will help you determine the correct treatment in the salon and the proper maintenance products for your client to use at home. You will apply and remove products according to the infection control guidelines for your state.

THEORY OF MASSAGE

The word **massage** comes from the Arabic word *masa*, meaning "to touch" or "to stroke." Massage is a scientific method of manipulating the body by rubbing, kneading, tapping, or stroking with the hands and fingers. The value of massage has long been known. It was used by the ancient Greeks as a cure for ailments even before Hippocrates, the Father of Medicine lived in the fifth century B.C..

In many states, cosmetologists are limited to massage of a client's head, face, neck, arms, hands, and feet. Full body massage is usually administered by licensed estheticians and massage therapists.

Benefits of Massage

For thousands of years, people have enjoyed the benefits of massage. Quick, gentle pressure in the correct direction provides the following benefits:

1. Relaxation of the nerves
2. Relief from body tension

3. Increase in blood circulation
4. Increase in lymph circulation
5. Contraction of muscles for toning
6. Stimulation of skin gland activity
7. Relief from muscle pain
8. Softening of the skin when lotions and creams are used
9. Calming and relaxation effects for the client

Types of Massage

Effleurage (ef **LOO** rahzh) is a stroking massage. It is used for relaxing and soothing effects and done with the pads of the fingers or the palms of the hands. Effleurage increases the circulation on the skin surface and is very soothing (Figures 18.1 and 18.2).

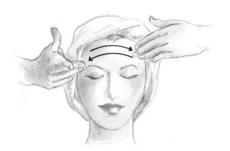

18.1   Effleurage on forehead

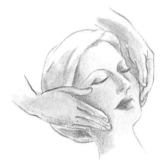

18.2   Effleurage on cheeks

Petrissage (PE tri sahzh) is the technical name for kneading movements. This rolling and gentle squeezing of the muscles under the skin increases circulation of blood and lymph and stimulates muscles for a toning effect (Figures 18.3 and 18.4).

CLIENT   T I P ◆◆◆◆◆◆◆

Warm your hands before you touch your client. Your first touch should be gentle, yet firm and on a large area, such as the jaw or forehead.

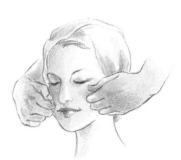

18.3   Petrissage on cheeks

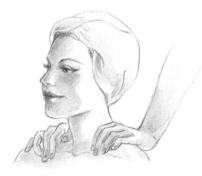

18.4   Petrissage on shoulders

Friction is a circular, deep rubbing movement. Friction greatly increases circulation and is used most commonly on the scalp, arms, and hands. Friction is used with less pressure in facial manipulations (Figures 18.5 and 18.6).

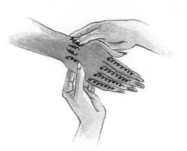

18.5   Friction massage on hands

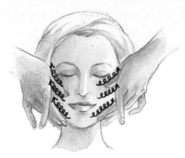

18.6   Friction massage on face

Tapotement (ta POHT ment) is a movement that consists of tapping or lightly slapping the skin. It is done in a rhythmic and springy fashion with the pads of the fingers or the sides of the palms. It increases blood circulation and promotes muscle contraction (Figures 18.7 and 18.8).

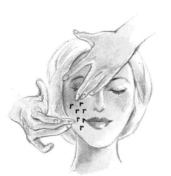

18.7   Tapotement on face

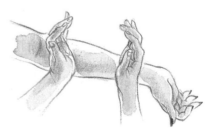

18.8   Tapotement on forearm

Massage Techniques

The beneficial effects of massage are ensured when proper techniques are used. Once you have begun massage movements, it is very important that you maintain a steady rhythm. Do not lift both hands from the client at the same time until the entire massage is completed. Breaking contact with your client will spoil the soothing and relaxing effects the massage would otherwise provide.

Use a slow, steady rhythm in your massage movements. Try thinking of the steady 1-2-3 count of a slow dance. Move from one area to another slowly and smoothly, without breaking contact.

Muscles should be massaged from their insertion to their origin. The origin is the fixed attachment of the muscle to a bone or other tissue. The insertion is the more movable and stretchable end. By massaging from insertion to the origin, you increase muscle tone and avoid any stretching that could cause premature aging. As a general rule, massage *up and out* on the face, and *up* on the neck. To begin a movement on the neck, lightly trace *down* the sides of the neck. Directly under the eye move from the *outside corner in* toward the nose (Figure 18.9).

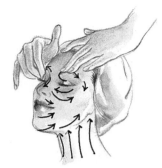

18.9   Direction of massage

Precautions and Reminders

1. Never massage over any area where redness, swelling, or pus is present. Examples of these conditions are **pustules** (pimples), **papules** (hardened red elevations), and acne.
2. Never massage when there are **abrasions** (cuts) on the skin.
3. Do not break contact with the client's skin until the massage is finished. Keep movements rhythmic and continuous.
4. Keep your fingernails filed short enough so that you will not scratch your client. Care for your hands so the skin is soft and there are no rough edges. Avoid using sculptured nails, tips, or any covering that could trap bacteria.
5. Massage toward the origin of the muscles.

Pressure Points

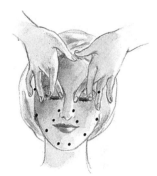

18.10   Key pressure points

Nerves control the muscles of the body. A muscle may be stimulated and its nerve relaxed by the correct manipulation of the **pressure point**. This point is where the nerve fibers enter the muscles that control the skeleton. The pressure points to the face are shown in Figure 18.10. The three nerves you as a cosmetologist affect most in massage are the 5th, 7th, and 11th cranial nerves. These and other points of anatomy are explained to you in Chapter 3. The nerves are listed in Table 3.4.

Whenever you are moving from one area of the face to another, end your massage movements over a pressure point. Pause for a few seconds and then gently "feather off" the area by decreasing pressure as you lift one hand at a time from the face. Place the first hand on the next area to be massaged before lifting the second hand from the skin.

> **◆ Key Point ◆**
> Use a slow, steady rhythm in your massage movements. Try thinking of the steady 1-2-3 count of a waltz. Move from one area to another slowly and smoothly so the client does not feel a break in contact. Finish each massage movement by pausing at a pressure point.

FACIALS

A facial service is one of the most pleasant treatments available in the salon. Unfortunately, it is one that is too often neglected. The area for facials should be removed from the noise and activity of the central salon. It should be quiet, immaculately clean, comfortably warm, and indirectly lit. The client cannot relax if these conditions are not met.

The facial chair, or lounge, should be comfortable and adjustable. Your stool should also be adjustable so that you can easily reach all treatment areas easily.

A thorough knowledge of the underlying structure of the skin is essential for anyone practicing massage or giving facial treatments. Chapter 2 covers this important topic for you.

Facials are not designed to treat skin diseases. If there are signs indicating disease or infection, refer your client to a dermatologist or a physician. However, there are a number of skin conditions that can be greatly improved with treatment and a number of aging symptoms that can be prevented or at the least slowed. The beneficial effects of facials are most evident when the client begins a professional regimen at a young age and follows it.

Preparing for a Plain Facial

You will begin most of your skin services with a plain facial. The following procedure outlines the steps. Your instructor may suggest slight alterations for a particular client.

Materials

70% alcohol or approved hospital-grade disinfectant	Spatulas	Linen facial towels
Cleansing cream or lotion	Two or three steam towels	Sheet
Massage cream	Body drape	Gloves (optional)
Cotton pads or sponges	Head drape	Analysis light(s)
Skin lotion or astringent	Booties for feet (optional)	Steamer (optional)
	Neck strips	

Procedure for Preparing for a Plain Facial

1. Clean the facial chair and table with a hospital grade disinfectant.
2. Arrange cosmetics and supplies on facial table. Place table to the left or right near the head of the chair for easy access. Place analysis light at the other side (Figure 18.11).
3. Place a clean towel over the back of the chair so that your client's bare shoulders will not directly touch it. Place a second towel, folded diagonally, across the head rest.

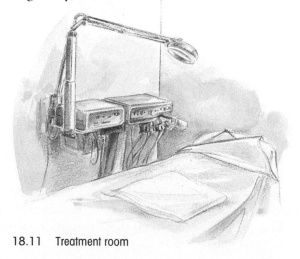

18.11   Treatment room

4. Cleanse your hands by washing carefully with an antibacterial scrub.

5. Direct your client to an area for changing from clothes to a body drape that exposes the shoulders. Ask client to remove jewelry and place it safely away.

6. Seat your client in the center of the facial chair. Remove their shoes and lift legs onto the chair. Cover the client's feet with a cloth or with booties.

7. Assist your client into a comfortable reclining position. Cover client loosely with the sheet and tuck the ends under the feet lightly. Fold the top edge back over the body drape. Place a linen towel across your client's chest and pull up to shoulders (Figure 18.12).

8. Smooth hair back from the face and secure under a neck strip if desired. Bring ends of towel on head rest up and join at center of client's head to create a protective turban. Fasten with a large bobby pin or with clips. Gently move fastened towel back until all of the face is exposed (Figure 18.13).

9. Re-cleanse your hands.

CLIENT TIP ◆◆◆◆◆◆◆

Ensure that your client is comfortable and warm before beginning the facial. Speak in a low, soothing tone of voice.

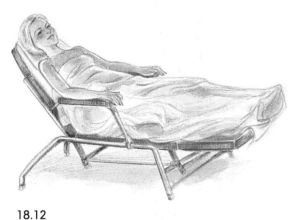

18.12

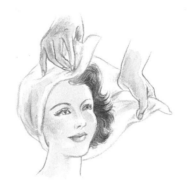

18.13 (a)

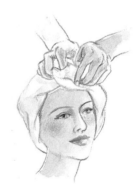

18.13 (b)

TABLE 18.1 Cosmetics Used with Facial Massage

Cosmetic	*Skin Condition*	*Recommended Product*
Cleanser		
Used to clean face before massage	Dry or normal	Liquefying cleanser
	Oily	Gel cleanser
Massage cream		
Lubricates skin	Dry or normal	Essential oils
Use so fingers glide		Aromatherapy balm
smoothly over face		Moisturizing cream
Avoid excessive oil	Oily	Cleansing cream
Skin Refiner		
Removes massage	Normal to dry	Skin fresheners
cream and cleanser		Toners
	Oily	Astringent

CLIENT TIP ◆◆◆◆◆◆◆

Freshener can be misted over the face for a cooling effect. Cover the eyes with pads and blot excess freshener after misting.

Cleansing the Face

A most important phase of any facial work is the proper cleansing of the skin. This prepares the skin for any treatments you may choose to give and begins relaxation of your client so that the facial can have maximum benefit. All of the materials you will need to cleanse the face were gathered during the preparation procedure. Check Table 18.1 to decide which cosmetic treatments to use for your facial procedure.

Procedure for Cleansing the Face

1. Cleanse your hands.
2. Place a small amount of the cleansing product into the palm of your hand (Figure 18.14). Remove all creams with spatulas.
3. Rub your fingers together to warm and distribute the cleansing product (Figure 18.15).
4. Apply the cleansing product with upward strokes, beginning on the neck (Figure 18.16). Work cleanser over the chin and lips. If your client is wearing lipstick, remove it first.
5. Continue applying cleanser with upward strokes over the jaw and cheeks (Figure 18.17). Add more cleansing product to your fingers as you need.
6. Apply the cleanser over the nose, using your fingertips to make circular movements at the nostrils (Figure 18.18).

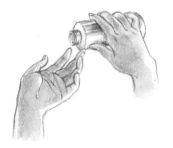

18.14   Pour cleanser into hand

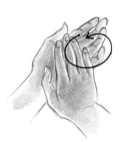

18.15   Distribute cleanser

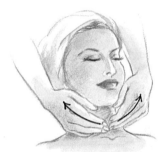

18.16   Apply cleanser to neck

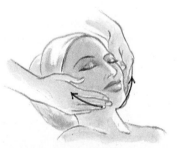

18.17   Apply cleanser to cheeks

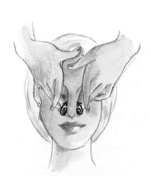

18.18   Cleanse nose

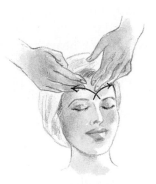

18.19 Cleanse forehead

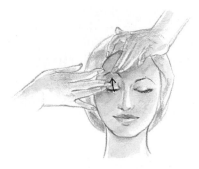

18.20 Cleanse eyelids

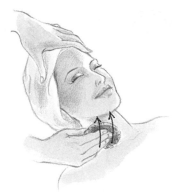

18.21 Remove cleanser

7. Apply the cleanser to the forehead. Move one hand upward, then the other, and follow with strokes across the forehead (Figure 18.19). Pause at the temple and repeat.

8. Lift the eyebrow with one hand. Apply cleanser with the other hand over the eyelid, gently working down and over the eyelashes (Figure 18.20). Be careful that product does not get in your client's eye. Cleanse the other eyelid in the same manner.

9. Remove cleanser with dampened cotton pads or with a moistened sponge (Figure 18.21). Begin removal at the neck and work up and out over the face until all cleanser is removed. Rinse sponges as necessary in warm water, and squeeze out excess water. Work carefully around the lips and over the eyelids. Finish by cleansing gently under the eyes with the cotton pad folded in half. Always work from outside corner of the eye toward the nose.

10. Apply skin freshener or astringent to clean cotton. Follow the movements outlined in steps 4–7 to ensure that all cleanser is removed. Do not apply freshener around the eyes.

Skin Analysis

A thorough analysis is key to any effective facial or skin treatment (Figure 18.22). This helps you determine the correct creams and lotions to use during the plain facial and also helps you suggest the appropriate products for your client to use at home. Record your observations and place the client card in a file so that you can keep track of the effectiveness of services given.

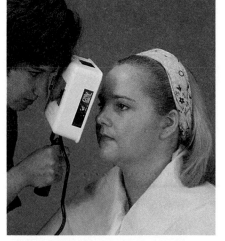

18.22 Skin lamp

Dip small cotton pads, the size of quarters, into cool water or witch hazel. Squeeze out excess moisture and place a pad over each eye. Then, turn on the magnifying analysis light and swing it over your client's face. Place one hand on the face, and with the other, bring the lamp down close so you can observe the quality of the skin (Figure 18.23).

Elasticity is observed by gently lifting the skin on the cheeks with the thumb and forefinger. Release the grasped skin to observe how quickly it springs back into place. Loose or aging skin will leave a ridge for a few seconds, while elastic skin will immediately return to its original position.

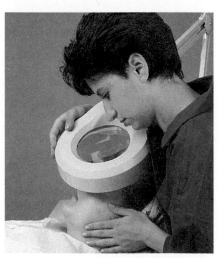

18.23 Magnifying analysis light

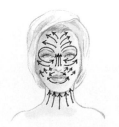

18.24 Apply massage cream

Pliability is determined by how resistant the skin is to movement. On the cheek, use gentle pressure to move the skin up and out. If the skin is very tight or dry, you will need to use a heavier massage cream.

Hydration (high **DRAY** shun) is the amount of moisture present in the skin. Dehydrated skin typically has lines and very small, tightly closed pores. In addition, milia are often seen on dehydrated skin. Sometimes these pores are so tight that they are not even visible under the magnifying lamp. Normal skin should have pores that are small in size, yet visible under the lamp. Check for flaking skin, especially in the forehead, the center cheek, and on the chin.

Excess oil creates a sheen that is easily visible. Under the lamp, the skin resembles an orange peel and may be yellow in color. The pores of this skin type are usually enlarged, especially across the forehead and down the nose (an area known as the **T-Zone**), and may be clogged. Comedones and pimples may also be present.

Cuperose (**KOO** per rose) are damaged capillaries that are visible under the lamp as tiny red lines. Cuperose indicate fragile, aging skin or an area where damage may have been done due to injury, pinching, smoking, drinking, sun exposure, etc. You should note these areas and avoid massage there to avoid further damage.

Record all data from your analysis on a client record card. This will help you keep track of progress as well as note the effectiveness of products recommended for home use.

FACIAL MANIPULATIONS

The massage movements are the most important, and the most pleasant, part of any facial. Practice the movements outlined in this section on your mannequin and your fellow students until you have established the correct rhythm and pressure. Be certain that your touch is not so light as to be ineffective, and not so heavy as to cause tissue damage. Massage from the insertion to the origin of facial muscles. Do not break contact once you have begun the massage process. Move from one area to another slowly and smoothly. Finish each massage movement by pausing at the pressure points and then moving smoothly to the next area.

First, apply massage cream. Remove approximately 1 teaspoonful from the jar with a spatula. If you use a liquid, squeeze it from the bottle onto your hand, using care that the bottle lip does not touch your skin. Warm the massage cream by working it between your fingers. Apply the cream to the face and neck as shown in Figure 18.24. You are now ready to begin the massage portion of the facial.

Movement 1: Up and Down on the Forehead (Figure 18.25)

1. Starting on the right side of the client's face, use the middle and ring fingers of both hands to stroke up and down on the forehead. Holding the left hand on the client's left temple, glide the right hand back across the forehead to the right temple. Pause and rotate with both hands.
2. Glide both hands to the cheek in front of the ear. Pause and rotate.
3. Glide to the lower jaw, below the earlobe. Pause and rotate.
4. Glide up to the front of the ear. Pause and rotate.
5. Glide up to the temples. Holding the right facial fingers on the right temple, glide the left hand across the forehead.
6. Repeat the entire movement two more times.

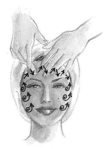

18.25

Movement 2: Lead and Rotate (Figure 18.26)

1. Glide your left hand across the forehead to the right temple. Lead with the left hand and rotate with the right hand across the forehead to the left temple.
2. Holding the left fingers on the left temple, glide the right hand across the forehead to the right temple. Pause and rotate with both hands. Glide both hands to the cheek in front of the ear. Pause and rotate.
3. Glide both hands to the lower jaw, below the earlobe. Pause and rotate.
4. Glide up to the cheek in front of the ear. Pause and rotate. Glide up to the temple and hold the right facial fingers on the right temple.
5. Glide the left hand across the forehead.
6. Repeat the entire movement two more times.

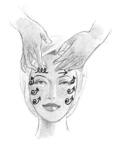

18.26

Movement 3: Rotate the Center of the Forehead (Figure 18.27)

1. Hold the skin at the center of the forehead taut with the index and the middle fingers of the left hand.
2. With the middle and ring fingers of the right hand, rotate upward on the muscle.
3. Glide the right hand down to the center of the brows.
4. Repeat two more times.

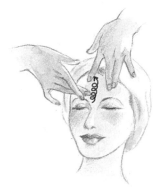

18.27

Movement 4: Stroke the Center of the Forehead (Figure 18.28)

1. Place the middle and ring fingers of the left hand on the bridge of the nose and stroke upward to the hairline.
2. With the right hand, repeat the same movement without breaking contact. Continue alternating hands and repeat three times.

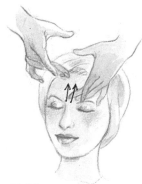

18.28

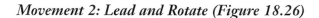

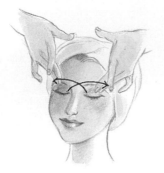

18.29

Movement 5: Crisscross at the Center of the Forehead (Figure18.29)

1. Place the middle and ring fingers of the right hand on the left eye.
2. Cross up and over to the corner of the eyebrow of the right eye. With the ring finger down, glide over the forehead to the temple. Repeat with the left hand, moving from the inner corner of the right eye to the eyebrow of the left eye until both eyes have been treated three times.

Movement 6: Outline the Eyes (Figure 18.30)

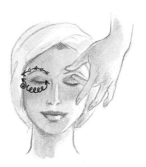

18.30

1. Place the middle fingers of both hands under the eyebrows. Place the thumbs on top. Glide the middle finger across the bone while pinching the eyebrows with the thumb to the count of one-two-three-four-five. Rotate on the temples.
2. Massage very lightly under the eyes with the middle finger.
3. At the sides of the bridge of the nose, turn the hand in and up so that the thumbs grasp the eyebrows.
4. Repeat the entire movement two more times.

Movement 7: The "Headache" Movement (Figure 18.31)

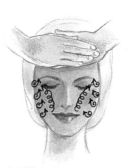

18.31

1. Glide the left hand to the forehead. Place the right hand on top of the left. Do not place the hands on top of the eyebrows.
2. Press while counting to three and then relax to the count of three. With both hands glide firmly out to the temples. Pause and rotate with the fingers.
3. Glide to the cheeks, in front of the ear. Pause and rotate.
4. Glide to the jaw, below the earlobe. Pause and rotate.
5. Glide to the middle of the lower jaws. Pause and rotate.
6. With both hands, use rotary massage up the cheeks to the temples. Pause at the pressure points.
7. Repeat the entire movement two more times.

Movement 8: Rotate the Nose (Figure 18.32)

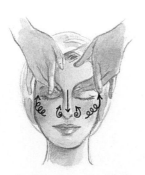

18.32

1. Glide the middle fingers of both hands across the forehead to the bridge of the nose. Slide down the center of the nose, being careful not to close the nostrils. Pause on the cheek at the side of the nostrils and rotate.
2. Rotate out and up on the cheeks to the temple.
3. Glide across the forehead very lightly to the bridge of the nose and repeat the entire movement two more times. After the last repetition, glide the fingers down to the jaw, just below the earlobes.

Movement 9: Circle the Lips (Figures 18.33 and 18.34)

1. Hold the fingers of the right hand on the jaw.
2. Place the index finger of the left hand in the middle of Cupid's bow, the thumb on one side, and the middle finger on the other side (Figure 18.34a). Make nine quick lifting strokes.
3. Glide the fingers of both hands under the lower lip. Using tapping movements with the fingertips, circle the lips at least three times (Figure 18.34b).

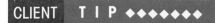
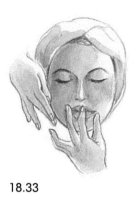

18.33

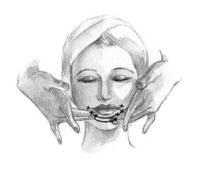

18.34

Movement 10: Rotate the Cheeks (Figure 18.35)

1. Glide the fingers of both hands to the tip of the chin.
2. Rotate out to the jaw, in front of and below the earlobe. Pause and rotate.
3. Glide the fingers lightly toward the corners of the mouth. Pause and rotate, one-two-three.
4. Rotate the cheeks up and out to the middle front of the ear. Pause and rotate.
5. Glide down to the earlobe. Pause and rotate. Glide to the chin.
6. Repeat the entire movement two more times.

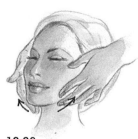

18.35

Movement 11: Scissor the Chin (Figure 18.36)

1. Glide the left hand to the earlobe. Spreading the index and middle fingers of the right hand like scissors, place the index finger on the chin and the other three fingers on the underside of the chin.
2. Draw the hand firmly across the jawline toward the ear.
3. Repeat with the left hand, being careful not to break contact. Repeat the movement two more times on each side of the face.

18.36

◆ **Key Point** ◆

Rhythmical movements following an organized pattern are essential to a successful service. Memorize these movements for best results.

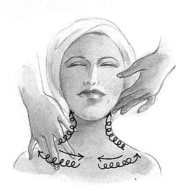

18.37 (a)

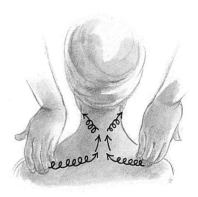

18.37 (b)

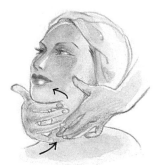

18.38

Movement 12: Massage down the Sides of the Neck (Figure 18.37)

1. Glide the fingertips of both hands to the sides of the neck under the ear. Massage down the muscle.
2. Glide to the center of the chest and massage out to the shoulder (Figure 18.37a).
3. Turn the hands and massage the back of the neck (Figure 18.37b).
4. Firmly glide the fingers up the muscle to the hairline at the back of the neck. Press while counting to three, then relax to the count of three.
5. Glide to the muscle below the ear and repeat the entire movement two more times.

Movement 13: Stroke the Neck (Figure 18.38)

1. Glide both hands to the left side of the neck, under the ear.
2. Cup the hands and stroke upward, one hand following the other. Be very gentle over the Adam's apple.
3. Move the hands from one side to the other and then back to the starting area. Repeat two more times. On the last movement across the neck, stroke very lightly. Remove one hand and then the other.

Completion of the Plain Facial

1. Remove massage cream with moist sponges, cotton pads, or a damp towel. Rinse the cotton pads or sponges in warm water as needed.
2. Apply astringent for oily skin or mild freshener for normal or dry skin, as indicated by your analysis. Pour the freshener onto clean cotton and gently sponge the face, excluding the eye area.
3. Apply moisturizer or protective lotion.
4. Remove the covering sheet, assist your client in getting up, and refresh their hairstyle. Direct your client to the dressing area to change.
5. Complete record card.
6. Clean and disinfect work area. Discard all disposable supplies and materials. Close product containers and return them to the dispensary.

Plain Facial at a Glance

1. Prepare facial area.
2. Cleanse your hands.
3. Seat client comfortably and drape.
4. Cleanse skin.
5. Analyze skin.
6. Perform massage movements.
7. Remove massage cream.
8. Refine skin and moisturize.
9. Remove client draping.
10. Clean facial area.

Skin Treatments

Minifacial

Today's client is often pressed for time—juggling the responsibilities of home, career, and social life. A minifacial is a treatment that offers the benefits of relaxation and skin stimulation to the client with pressing time restraints.

The minifacial consists of the cleansing procedure outlined on pages 382 and 383. Then a light massage lotion is applied, and each massage movement is performed once. The facial is completed by removing the lotion, applying freshener, moisturizer, and makeup if the client desires.

> **CLIENT TIP** ◆◆◆◆◆◆
>
> Practice your techniques so you can give a minifacial in 30 minutes without making your customer feel rushed.

Facial for Dry Skin

Facials for dehydrated (dry) skin incorporate steaming into the plain facial procedure. If you have a steamer in your school, warm it while you are preparing your client, cleansing the face, and performing the analysis. Then turn the steamer so that it makes a fine mist over the face. Move the steamer 12–20 inches away so your client does not feel moisture droplets. Client should feel a fine, warm mist that is soothing and moisturizing at the same time.

Apply a massage cream as outlined in the previous section. For dry skin, you may choose one that also contains natural oils that can be absorbed by the skin. Continue through the massage movements as outlined, turn the steamer away, and remove excess massage cream.

If you do not have a steamer available, saturate a towel with hot water. Cover the eyes with protective pads. Thoroughly wring excess water from the towel, and beginning at the chin, wrap the face in the steaming towel. Press gently at the forehead and on the cheeks. Let the towel remain on the face for a few moments while you prepare a second towel. Exchange it for the first and repeat several times.

> **CLIENT TIP** ◆◆◆◆◆◆
>
> Saturate eye pads in chamomile tea or witch hazel for extra soothing effects. Thoroughly squeeze excess moisture before placing on eyes.

Select a treatment mask that will add humectants. These natural ingredients attract and draw moisture into the deeper levels of the skin, especially when the pores are open due to steaming. Your instructor will assist you in selecting the correct product. Protect the eyes with cotton pads and apply the mask according to the manufacturer's directions. Cover the face with cotton strips to fit the face as your instructor recommends. Remove after the recommended time has gone by, cleanse any traces with a nonalcohol freshener, and finish the facial by applying a moisturizer.

Treatment for Oily Skin

Oily skin can effectively be treated by regular facials. In combination with correct nutrition, oily skin can be prevented from developing into more complex skin problems, such as acne or comedones.

First, cleanse the skin thoroughly with a water-based product. Use a hydrating massage cream that is not heavy in waxes or oils. After you have completed the massage movements, deep-cleanse the skin. If you have access to facial machines in your school, use the vacuum attachment to gently deep-cleanse pores.

If such a machine is not available, turn on the analysis light and then swing it over the face. Sanitize your hands. Gently apply pressure at the sides of comedones or pimples to remove clog. DO NOT puncture the skin and DO NOT mark the skin with your fingernails. DO NOT use an extractor. These metal implements can puncture the skin or cause bruising. Rather, wrap your fingertips with cotton or tissues to protect the client's skin.

Next, apply a pack designed for oily skin that will reduce pore size and pull impurities from the skin. Check the manufacturer's recommendations for product selection and use. Apply with a sanitized spatula, being careful not to contaminate the pack in the jar. Protect the eyes with pads, and leave the pack on the skin for the prescribed amount of time.

Treatment for Combination Skin

It is quite common to find a combination of skin types when you analyze your client's skin. This is especially true as the skin matures. It is not uncommon to find an oily T-zone across the forehead and down the nose. On the same client, the cheek area—especially directly under the eye—could be lacking in moisture. In addition, the areas around the eyes and mouth are the most likely to show evidence of dryness and the first signs of aging.

Treatment of combination skin should begin with a plain facial as outlined previously in this chapter. After the massage is completed, either treat the skin for the primary condition or apply the mask and/or pack in the appropriate areas. Use a separate spatula for each formula to remove the product to your hand. Discard the spatula. Use special care to avoid any contamination of the product in the jar. Cover the eyes with soothing pads and time the treatment as recommended by the manufacturer of the products chosen.

Exfoliation Treatment

Exfoliation (ex FOH lee **AYE** shun) is the process of sloughing off, or removing, dead skin cells. Some of the materials used to exfoliate dead skin cells are: gentle brushes attached to skin-care machines, specially designed cleansers, and custom-designed treatment masks containing enzymes.

Removal of dead skin cells is essential to maintenance. Exfoliation prevents clogged pores and helps to retard wrinkling, especially around the mouth and nose. These treatments are especially good for your clients who tend to neglect their skin or who work out-of-doors. The skin is constantly producing new cells in the deeper levels of the epidermis. These cells gradually dehydrate as they work their way toward the surface. Dead surface cells should be removed about every 10 days.

Treatment for Male Clients

Minifacials are excellent for your male clients. Many salons offer special services for men one evening a week. While some men are still reluctant to come to a salon, this is a stereotype that is rapidly disappearing. The minifacial shows results right away and the service is quick for those men who are hesitant to receive salon services.

When applying creams, lotions, and masks to a man's face, gently work in a downward direction on any areas that are covered by facial hair. To remove products from the face, gently wipe material from beard and sideburn stubble. Use linen towels rather than cotton to avoid fiber residue getting caught in facial hair. Male skin has a tendency to be oily, but only your analysis will determine what is the correct treatment for each and every client.

◆ **Key Point** ◆

Each skin treatment should be custom designed for your client. Record and review treatments to monitor progress. Adjust treatments as necessary.

INFECTION CONTROL FOR ESTHETICS

Disinfection, sanitation, and safety are always important considerations when you treat the public. In the case of skin care, there are several situations that deserve special attention. Make sure that the area of the salon where facial treatments are given is sufficiently wired for necessary electrical equipment. Use outlets that have GFIs (ground fault interrupters) to protect you from the possibility of electrical shock. These outlets will disrupt the flow of electricity if faulty wiring or moisture causes problems in an electrical circuit. (See Chapter 22, Electricity, for more information.) The list that follows offers guidelines to a safe and sanitary skin care environment.

CLIENT   T I P ◆◆◆◆◆◆◆

Practice sanitation in front of your client to demonstrate your professionalism.

1. Be certain that the floor, implements, equipment, and surfaces are dry so that a short circuit will not occur.
2. Disinfect the chair and table before and after each facial service with an approved hospital-grade product.
3. Sanitize your hands before seating and draping your client. Use an antibacterial scrub, and sanitize again after you drape your client and arrange equipment.
4. Remove products from jars with a sanitized spatula. Have several spatulas available so you do not mix various products.
5. Keep all jars and containers tightly closed when not in use.
6. Label all jars clearly and store in a cool place to avoid spoilage.
7. **Never** treat infected skin. Refer a client with skin that shows signs of redness, swelling, or pus to a physician or dermatologist.
8. Dip eyepads in cool water and squeeze to remove excess moisture. Use eyepads to protect and soothe the eyes when applying packs or masks, and when analyzing the skin.
9. Switch the analysis light on when it is turned away from your client, then swing it over the face. Curve your hand over the edge to ensure that the lamp does not touch the face and cause discomfort.

10. Wear gloves when treating acne. You may choose to wear gloves for all treatments.
11. Keep a record card on all clients and especially note any allergic reaction to a product.
12. Cotton pads that are discarded after use are more sanitary than reusable sponges. If you do select sponges, make sure you disinfect them according to state board guidelines.
13. All nonsanitizable implements should be discarded immediately after use. If you use disposable spatulas, break them in front of the client before disposing.
14. Wipe all spatulas to remove creams before immersing in a disinfectant solution.
15. Keep fingernails short and manicure often to avoid scratching your client. Keep your fingertips smooth and soft so the massage sensation will be a pleasant one.

Summary

Esthetics is a specialty field within cosmetology that deals with the care, treatment, and massage of the skin. Esthetics licenses are available in a majority of the states for those persons who wish to specialize without cosmetology training. Esthetician training focuses on various treatments for all skin conditions and is far more extensive than what is presented in this chapter. The basics of esthetics: cleansing, massage, applying treatment product, and toning are essential to healthy skin.

Skin care is a preventive measure to retard the aging effects of the environment on the skin. It is also a great stress reducer that aids in the elimination of toxins from the skin. Correct skin care, regularly applied, will normalize oily skin, moisturize dry skin, and prevent minor skin conditions from becoming more complex.

Esthetics is one of the largest areas of growth in today's cosmetology market. To offer skin care services, you must be able to analyze the skin and determine the most effective treatments. You will cleanse the skin, massage it in the correct direction for best results, and apply the chosen treatment product. You must follow infection control guidelines to protect yourself and prevent bacterial infection.

Questions

1. What are the types of massage? What is the benefit of each?
2. What are the steps for preparing for a facial? What is the procedure for cleansing? What are the steps for a plain facial?
3. Demonstrate the basic manipulations for a facial.
4. What skin treatments are recommended for dry, oily, and combination skin types?
5. List at least 15 procedures an esthetician should follow to ensure proper infection-control practices in the salon. What special safety precautions should you follow to protect yourself as well as your client?

1. Practice the basic massage movements until you have them memorized. For practice, sit in a chair, cross your legs, and imagine that your top kneecap is a face. Or you can take your mannequin and grasp the neck between your knees, again while seated. Rest the back of the mannequin head in your lap, apply massage cream, and practice until you are ready to work on your fellow students. Once you have all the manipulations memorized and your rhythm established, perform at least 12 facial services.

2. Research treatments available from different manufacturers. Outline the benefits and the key features of at least three for dry skin, three for oily skin, and three for exfoliating treatments.

3. Research the effects of ultraviolet light from the sun on skin. Report back to the class and cite at least three prevention measures listed by skin care experts, the American Cancer Society, or the American Medical Association.

4. Describe the daily regimen that is ideal for care and preservation of the skin.

5. Research the SPF (sun protection factor) ratings of competitive sun products. In conjunction with their ingredients, draw up a list of the top three you would recommend for each skin type.

6. Report to the class on the interaction between nutrition and the health of the skin.

7. Sketch the facial muscles onto a facial form. With a green pen, insert arrows to indicate the proper massage direction. With a red pen, indicate the primary pressure points.

8. Perform an analysis on at least 6 of your fellow students. Record recommendations for skin care treatments and products to be used. Check each with your instructor and discuss any suggestions for improvement made.

MAKEUP

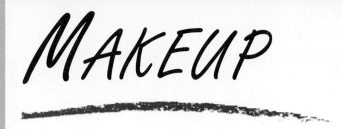

CHAPTER GOAL

In order to apply cosmetics properly, the cosmetologist analyzes and enhances the client's whole appearance. After reading this chapter and completing the projects, you should be able to

1. Explain the purpose of makeup and describe the primary cosmetics used.
2. Name three types of makeup application and describe how they differ.
3. Explain how corrective makeup uses dark and light colors to create optical illusions.
4. Demonstrate the application of strip and individual false eyelashes.
5. Explain the importance of the eyebrow to the facial balance and indicate the characteristics of the correct arch.
6. Demonstrate eyebrow and lash tinting.

CHAPTER·19

Applying color to the body, especially the face, has been a custom throughout recorded history. We know that both Neanderthal men and the men of the New Stone Age used body paint and tattoos for ornamentation. Makeup was used as a face and body camouflage against a hostile environment, to indicate status, as a tribal identification, and as a preparation for war and important religious ceremonies. History records the use of makeup changing. It was soon primarily used by women for adornment. Cleopatra's makeup made the dramatic Egyptian eye famous. Makeup was an advanced art form in ancient China, available only to nobility. Makeup was usually a combination of vegetable dyes, mineral salts, and ground alabaster or starch.

The cosmetics business blossomed into large, commercial companies in the 1930s when Elizabeth Arden introduced a line of makeup. Max Factor opened a salon devoted to beauty in London in 1936. Meanwhile, the cinema was creating superstars such as Greta Garbo and Jean Harlow. Consumers sought cosmetics to imitate the glamorous styles. The demand increased and products were soon available to customers of all economic means.

In recent years we've seen trends in makeup change from dramatic to more natural styles. You will enhance your client's appearance by properly shaping their facial features with color, contour, and highlights. You will add artificial lashes for special effects.

THE PURPOSE OF MAKEUP

The purpose of applying makeup is to enhance the beauty of the face by bringing out good features and minimizing less attractive ones. Makeup application is an art. It requires practice and a fundamental knowledge of (1) the structure of the face, (2) the action of colors and their relationships to one another, and (3) the principles of optical illusions. The makeup artist must realize that total beauty is an illusion that depends on how the following factors work together: (1) face makeup, (2) hairstyle, (3) harmony of color in the clothing, eyes, skin, and hair, (4) individuality of features, and (5) personality.

Cosmetics Used in Makeup

Makeup is available in liquid, cream, powder, and stick forms. Many of today's products are interchangeable and can be used wherever color is desired. The following list outlines the basic cosmetic categories:

1. **Foundation.** Used as a base for the makeup and as a concealer and highlighter. It is available in cream, liquid, semisolid, cake, and stick form. Foundations are available in water-based formulas for normal or oily skin and in oil-based formulas for dry skin.
2. **Cheek color.** Used to give the cheeks a soft, warm glow. Rouges come in cream and powder form.
3. **Lipstick, lip color, and lip gloss.** Used on the lips. Lip color is available in stick and cream form. **Lipliner pencils** are used to outline the lips.
4. **Eye shadow.** Used to add color to the eyelids. It is available in cream, pencil, powder, and crayon form.
5. **Eyeliner.** Used to outline the eye close to the eyelashes. Eyeliners are available in pencil, cake, and liquid form.
6. **Eyebrow color.** Used to draw in fine lines in the eyebrow area. Eyebrow color is available in pencil and compressed-powder form. Compressed powder is applied with a small brush.
7. **Mascara.** Used to add color to the eyelashes. It is available in cake, cream, and liquid form. The cake and cream types are applied with a brush. Liquid mascara comes in a tube. Disposable applicators should be used to protect the client from infection.
8. **Powder.** Used to help the makeup to set. It also gives the face a dull, matte finish. This cosmetic is available in the form of a very fine powder or a compressed cake. The powdered form is ideal for professional makeups. The compressed powder is usually available in compacts.
9. **Brushes.** Brushes are used to apply different cosmetics. They range from thin liner brushes to fat, fluffy powder brushes.
10. **Underbases.** Used to neutralize unwanted skin tones. They are available in lavender to offset yellow, and mint green to neutralize red tones. Underbases are applied as needed under foundation.

How to Choose the Correct Colors

Color selection presents a problem for most women when they are trying to choose lipstick, rouge, eye shadow, and foundation. Should the eye shadow match the eye color? Should cheek color be exactly the same as lip color? Should one use a dark foundation in the summer and a light foundation in the winter? All these questions can be answered very simply by using *The Color Key Program* system of color selection described in Chapter 1. All colors, including skin tones, have been classified into either the *Key 1* or *Key 2 Colors* palette. Every person belongs to one of the two palettes. *Key 1* people can use any shade in the *Key 1 Colors* chart. *Key 2* people can use any shade in the *Key 2 Colors* chart.

Lipstick and rouge do not have to be the same color, but they must be in the same *Color Key* palette. Eye shadow does not have to match the eyes. Simply select the eye shadow color from the correct *Color Key* palette.

Color coordination is the prime requisite. If you use *The Color Key Program* system of color selection, you can be sure that your hair color, makeup, and clothing colors will harmonize with your natural skin tones.

Selecting a Foundation Color

Foundation color is extremely important and should be chosen with great care. To select the proper color, dab some foundation on the jaw and blend it up onto the face and down on the neck. The shade of foundation you use should blend with this skin tone. Clients who have blotchy skin of different shades should match their foundation to the darkest areas.

As many as three colors of foundation may be used at the same time for corrective makeup. Highlights and shadows are created by using a lighter or darker foundation than the basic color. If all three foundation colors (basic, light, and dark) are selected from the correct *Color Key* palette, the makeup will blend together and will look natural.

How to Determine Facial Balance

Just as an artist divides his canvas into sections, so a cosmetologist divides the face into sections before applying corrective makeup. The face is divided into three horizontal sections (length) and three vertical sections (width). Figure 19.1 shows these divisions for an oval face.

Length (Figure 19.1, Pink Lines)

1. From the hairline to the bridge of the nose.
2. From the bridge of the nose to the tip of the nose.
3. From the tip of the nose to the tip of the chin.

Width (Figure 19.1, Blue Lines)

1. From the right hairline to the pupil of the right eye.
2. From the pupil of the right eye to the pupil of the left eye.
3. From the pupil of the left eye to the left hairline.

By dividing the face into these sections, you will be able to spot any areas that need corrective makeup.

Accepted Standards of Facial Harmony (Figure 19.2): A Perfect Oval Face

1. An oval face is usually five eyes wide across the cheekbones. It is slightly wider across the forehead than at the chin.
2. Eyes should be set one eye's width apart.
3. The distance between the eyebrow and eye socket should be one eye's height.
4. The eyebrows should extend approximately ½ inch beyond the outer corner of the eye.

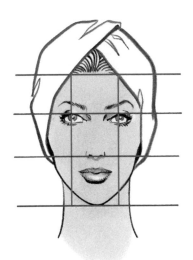

19.1   Divisions of an oval face

19.2

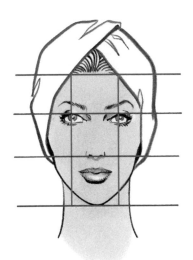 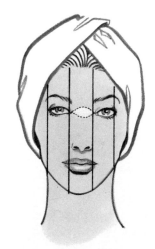

5. The highest part of the eyebrow should be above the outside edge of the iris of the eye.
6. The inner corner of the eyebrow should be directly above the inner corner of the eye.
7. The inner and outer ends of the brow should be at the same level.
8. The flare of the nose should be the width of one eye.
9. The mouth should be the width of two eyes.
10. The bottom of the ear and the end of the nose should be at the same level.
11. The length of the nose should be one-third the length of the face from the hairline to the chin (Figure 19.1).
12. The upper lip should be slightly thinner than the lower lip.
13. The corners of the mouth should be directly under the pupils of the eyes.

TYPES OF MAKEUP APPLICATIONS

Makeup application varies according to the time of day and the occasion. The following guidelines offer basic advice.

Daytime Makeup

A very soft, natural-looking effect is best for daytime. The makeup should enhance the natural beauty but should not appear artificial. For office settings, makeup tones should be slightly warm (pink) to offset the effects of fluorescent lighting.

Evening Makeup

The principles for evening makeup are the same as for daytime makeup. However, more color can be used on the cheeks and lips and around the eyes to counteract the effect of artificial lighting on the face. Frosted colors may be used on the cheeks and around the eyes. Gold and silver eye color may also be used on the eyelids. Artificial lashes may be longer for evening wear.

Glamour Makeup

This makeup is more elaborate and exotic than is the usual daytime or evening makeup. Eyebrows may be winged or arched in a dramatic fashion. Eyeliners may be wider and the eyelashes longer. Eyeliners tend to vary with the fashion trend. Colors, too, may be used in an unusual manner. A mixture of golds, silvers, mauves, bright blues, browns, pinks, greens, and whites may be applied to the eye area (Figure 19.3). The cheeks may be devoid of color or may be covered with intense color. Lip colors usually blend with the cheek color. To complete the high-fashion or trend look successfully, the hairstyle and wardrobe must be compatible. Trend makeup techniques change to keep up with new trends in fashion.

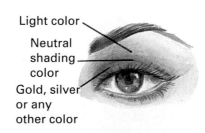

Light color

Neutral shading color

Gold, silver or any other color

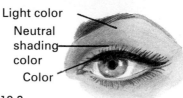

Light color

Neutral shading color

Color

19.3

Materials

Headband	Moisturizer	Eyeliner
Disposable neck strips (opt.)	Sponges	Eyebrow brush
Makeup drape	Skin lotion or astringent	Lipliner pencil, if desired
Spatula	Foundation	Mascara
Cotton	Cheek color	Orangewood stick
Wet sanitizer	Lipstick	Face powder
Towels	Eye shadow	Assorted brushes
Facial cleanser	Eyebrow pencil	

Procedure for Applying Daytime Makeup

1. Cleanse hands.
2. Drape the client. Use a neck strip around the hairline so that the head covering does not touch the client's skin. If using a short makeup drape, place a neck strip under the neckband of the drape.
3. Cleanse the face and neck thoroughly with cleansing cream or lotion. Warm the cleanser slightly by working it between your fingers. Apply the cleanser to the client's face and neck (Figure 19.4).
4. Remove the cleanser from the face and neck with cotton pads (Figure 19.5).
5. Moisten cotton pads and apply an astringent (for oily skin) or a skin lotion (for dry skin) to the face and neck. This will remove all traces of cleanser. Apply moisturizer.
6. Place a small amount of foundation in the palm of the hand. Apply a few dots to the cheeks, nose, forehead, and chin (Figure 19.6). Spread the foundation with a makeup sponge and blend carefully as shown in Figure 19.7. Make sure to select the foundation color according to the client's *Color Key* palette. If correc-

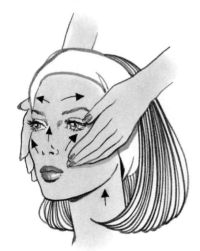

19.4   Apply cleanser

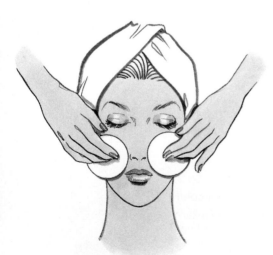

19.5   Remove cleanser

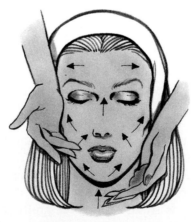

19.6   Apply foundation

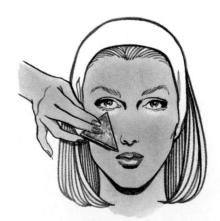

19.7   Blend foundation

tive shading is necessary, apply the correct shade of foundation as required (see the following section on corrective makeup).

7. Apply cheek color. With a cotton-tipped orangewood stick or cotton swab, remove either cream or liquid rouge from the container. Place dots of color along the lower ridge of the cheekbone. The cheek color should be placed in the "apple" of the cheek. (The "apple" is the pouch formed when you smile.) With the fingertips, blend the cheek color up and out along the cheekbones to the hairline (Figure 19.8).

   Select a complementary cheek color from the *Color Key* palette. Black women should use berry colors—a light tone for those with lighter skins and a dark berry for those with darker skins.

   a. Place cheek color as outlined above, beginning at least ½ inch away from the nose.

   b. Do not blend cheek color into the eye socket area.

   c. Cheek color should not extend on the cheeks below the top of the lips.

   d. If using a powdered blusher, apply face powder first (see step 9). Use a stiff brush to apply the blusher.

8. Apply eye shadow. With a cotton-tipped orangewood stick, remove a small amount of shadow from the container. Place it on the back of the hand. With the fingertip or a disposable applicator, apply the shadow to the upper eyelid. Blend it out to the corner of the eye (Figure 19.9). Or use a crayon and apply to the lid. Smudge the edges for a softer look.

9. Place face powder in the palm of one hand. With a dome brush, apply the powder to the client's face. Remove excess powder with clean cotton or a clean sable brush. Powder helps set creamy makeup and gives it a matte finish. If using powder blusher apply the face powder before step 7.

10. Apply eyeliner, if desired. With a sharp eyeliner pencil, or with a small brush and liquid eyeliner, draw a fine line as close to the eyelashes as possible (Figure 19.10). Sharpen the pencil before each use as a sanitary measure. When using eyeliner on the upper and lower lids, use a lighter shade on the lower lid. At the outer corner of the eye, the lines may be turned up slightly. Strip eyelashes can be applied at this point, if desired. The eyeliner helps hide the base of the lashes.

11. Measure the eyebrows.

   a. Place an eyebrow pencil diagonally from the flare of the nose and past the outside corner of the eye, and mark a light dot on the skin at the brow. This measurement determines the outside of the brow.

   b. Hold the pencil at the inner corner of the eye and mark the skin above this point. This determines the inside of the brow. The inner and outer edges of the brows should be at the same level.

   c. The highest part of the brow should be above the outside edge of the iris of the eye when the client is looking forward.

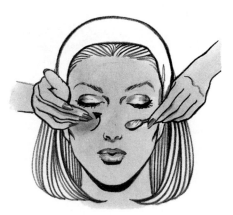

19.8   Blend cheek color

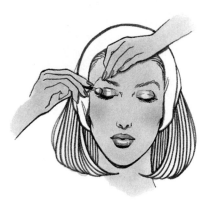

19.9   Apply eye shadow

CLIENT   T I P ◆◆◆◆◆◆◆

Brace the client's eye by placing your little finger against the client's temple. When applying makeup around the eye, hold the center of the eyelid to protect your client and make application more comfortable.

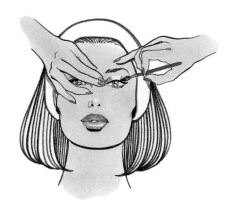

19.10   Apply eyeliner

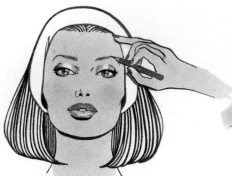

19.11   Apply eyebrow pencil

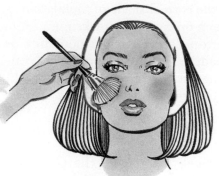

19.12   Apply face powder

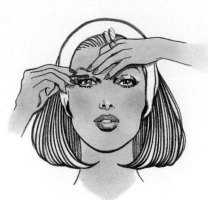

19.13   Apply mascara

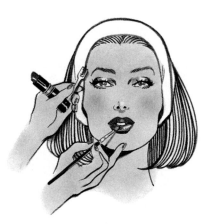

19.14a   Apply lipstick

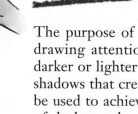

19.14b   Blot off lipstick

◆ Key Point ◆

Daytime makeup should look natural and blend the skin tones together. Accent the eyes and add cheek color. Finish the face and blend tones together with powder. Lip color should complement the facial tones and the clothing worn.

---

12. Apply eyebrow pencil. Lightly draw short, hairlike strokes with a sharp eyebrow pencil (Figure 19.11). Remember to sharpen pencils before each use as a safety precaution. Use several shades of pencil to achieve a natural-looking effect.

13. Reapply face powder over the entire face (Figure 19.12). Dust off the excess with a soft brush or a cotton ball. Brush down lightly on the face, because the facial hair grows down. Brush the brows with an eyebrow brush. Face powder helps set the makeup.

14. Apply mascara. Ask the client to look forward. Apply mascara with a disposable mascara brush to the upper lashes by stroking from underneath. To apply mascara to the bottom lashes, stroke down from the top (Figure 19.13). If artificial strip lashes were applied, brush mascara on them if desired. Hold the center of the eyebrow to protect your client.

15. Apply lipstick (see Figure 19.14). First outline the lips with a lipliner pencil or a lip brush. If using a lip brush, remove some lipstick from the container with the spatula. Draw a fine line of lip color to outline the lips. Add more lip color to the brush. Ask the client to open the mouth and hold the lips taut. Apply more color until the lips are completely filled in. Blot off the excess lipstick with a tissue. A cotton swab may be used to apply lip color if desired. Black women should outline the lips with a light brown pencil.

16. Optional: Lightly mist the face with water. This step helps set the makeup and gives the skin a dewy appearance.

CORRECTIVE MAKEUP USING OPTICAL ILLUSIONS

The purpose of corrective makeup is to minimize poor features by drawing attention away from them. By using a foundation that is darker or lighter than the skin color, you can produce highlights and shadows that create optical illusions. In the eye area, eye shadow can be used to achieve the same effects. **Shadows** are created by the use of darker colors. Darker colors make the facial features appear

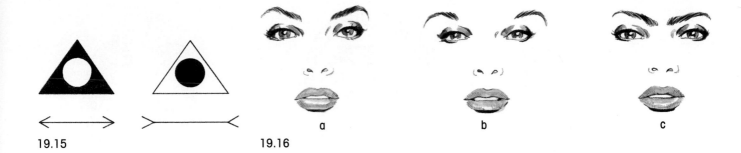

19.15   19.16

a   b   c

smaller. **Highlights** are created by the use of lighter color. Lighter colors make the features seem larger. You are probably familiar with these principles with regard to clothes. Black clothing makes a person look thinner; white clothing will make the same person look heavier. In Figure 19.15, the circles within the triangles are of equal size, but the white circle appears larger than the black circle. The dark area around the white circle recedes, and the white seems larger.

Lines are also used to achieve optical illusions, especially in the eye area. Lines drawn with an eyebrow pencil can be used to increase or decrease the length of the eyebrow in order to achieve facial balance. Eyeliner can also be used to make the eyes seem wider or narrower. In Figure 19.15, the lines are of equal length, but the line at the right seems longer. This is because of the direction of the arrows at the ends of the lines. Eyeliner that ends in an upward "wing" will lengthen the eye, while a line that goes into the outside corner will shorten the eye.

Corrective Eye Makeup

The eyes are the most important feature of the face. This means that proper eye makeup is very important. When necessary, lines, shadows, and highlights can be used to create optical illusions in order to achieve facial balance.

The eyes in Figure 19.16 are all the same size and the same distance apart. Yet they appear different. In part *b* the eyes seem farther apart than do the eyes in part *a*. This is because (1) there is a greater distance between the eyebrows in *b* than in *a*, and (2) the eye shadow is concentrated at the outer corners of the eyes in *b*. The eyes in part *c* look closer together than do those in part *a*. This is because (1) the eyebrows have been drawn closer together in *c* than in *a* and (2) the eye shadow is heavier at the inside corners of the eyes. This illustration shows how highlights, shadows, and lines can be used for correction in the eye area.

Corrective Nose Makeup

1. A wide nose can be made to appear narrower by using a darker foundation on the sides (Figure 19.17).
2. A thin nose can be made to appear fuller by using a lighter foundation on the sides (Figure 19.18).

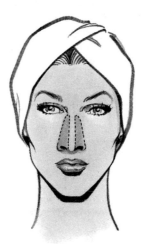

19.17

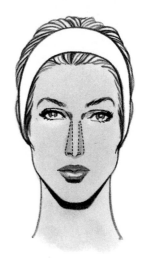

19.18

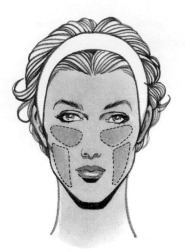

19.19   Hollows in the cheeks

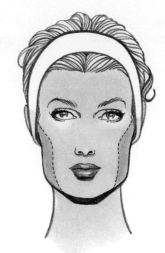

19.20   Heavy jaw

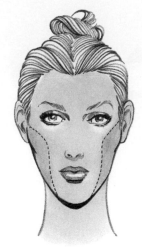

19.21   Narrow jaw

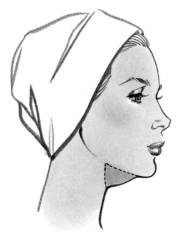

19.22   Double chin

Corrective Cheek, Jaw, and Chin Makeup

1. Large cheekbones can be subdued by using a darker foundation on them.
2. Hollows in the cheeks under the cheekbones can be filled out by using a lighter foundation (Figure 19.19).
3. Large, heavy jaws can be made less noticeable by using a darker foundation on them (Figure 19.20).
4. Very narrow jaws can be made to seem wider by using a lighter foundation on them (Figure 19.21).
5. A double chin can be reduced by applying a small amount of darker foundation to a triangular area directly under the chin (Figure 19.22).

Corrective Lip Line

Changing the natural line of the lips is very difficult, so correction of this type is not recommended. The natural outline of the lips is very definite, and the texture of the skin of the face and the skin of the lips is different. Adding color to the skin above the lips or below the lips for correction is too obvious. The length of the lip can be altered by the use of a heavier or lighter application of color in the corners of the mouth. The Cupid's bow can be rounded or altered slightly without causing it to look unnatural.

To accentuate the lips, try the following ideas:

1. Outline the rim of the lip with a darker shade of lipstick or lip color, using a very fine, stiff sable lip brush. Then fill in the inner part of the lip with a lighter shade or a lipliner pencil.
2. Outline the outer rim of the lip with a shade of brown. Then cover the same area with a shade of red and blend this color into the full part of the lip. Finally, add a lighter shade over the full part of the lip.

Be creative and experiment, but always try to please your client with a natural, pretty mouth.

Seven Basic Facial Shapes

There are seven basic facial shapes: oval, square, round, triangle (or pear), diamond, inverted triangle (or heart), and oblong. An oval face is considered to be ideal. Your facial shape is determined by your bone structure. If you face is not oval, you cannot change your bone structure to make it more oval. However, you can use makeup, hairstyling, and hair coloring to make your face seem more oval (see Chapters 10 and 15) by using the principles of optical illusion.

The measurements to determine facial shape are taken at three different places on the face:

1. Across the forehead, from hairline to hairline.
2. From cheekbone to cheekbone.
3. Across the chin line at the hinge of the jaws.

The faces of most people do not perfectly fit any one of these categories. However, a face will usually be "most like" one of the basic shapes even though it may have some of the characteristics of another shape. To determine your facial shape, read the description of the various shapes and look at the illustrations that follow. Then pull your hair away from your face and look into a mirror. You will discover your facial shape.

Oval

This face is considered to be classically proportioned (Figure 19.23). No corrective makeup is required.

Square

The forehead and chin line across the jaw are almost equal in width. Apply corrective makeup as follows (Figure 19.24):

1. To make the face seem longer, arch the eyebrows to a high, natural-looking curve.
2. Subdue the square jaw by using a darker foundation on the sides of the jaw. Make sure you blend well.
3. Use heavier eyeliner at the center of the upper eyelids.
4. Place eye shadow across the upper lid and blend out to the corner of the eye.

Round

The cheeks and jaw are wide and full (full-moon face). Apply corrective makeup as follows (Figure 19.25):

1. To make the face seem longer, arch the eyebrows to achieve a winged effect lifting up at the outside edges.
2. Reduce the roundness of the face by using a darker foundation from the temples to the jawline.
3. Keep the eyeliner as close to the upper lashes as possible. Extend the lines past the outer corners of the eyes, turning the lines up at the ends.
4. Place eye shadow across the upper lid. Use more color at the inner and outer corners of the eye. Blend the shadow from the outer corner of the eyelid to the brow.
5. Avoid all circular lines when working on this facial shape.

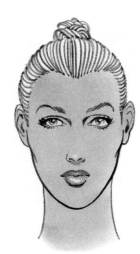

19.23   Oval

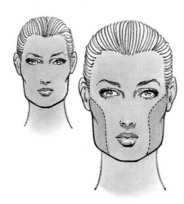

19.24   Square

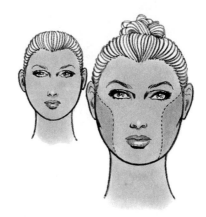

19.25   Round

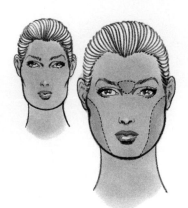

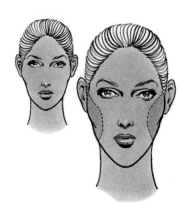

19.26 Triangle or pear

Triangle (or Pear)

The forehead is narrow and the jawline is wide. The eyes are usually close-set. Apply corrective makeup as follows (Figure 19.26):

1. To make the forehead seem wider, move the highest part of the eyebrow arch to the outer corners of the eyes.
2. Tweeze the brows slightly so that they do not extend to the inner corners of the eyes (see Chapter 20).
3. Use a lighter foundation between the eyes and on the bones under the eyebrows. Make sure you blend well.
4. Draw a very fine line with eyeliner from the center of the eyes to the outer corners.
5. Place eye shadow at the center of the eyelid and blend it to the outer corners of the eyes.
6. Shadow the broad jaw with a darker foundation.

19.27 Diamond

Diamond

The forehead and chin are narrow and the cheekbones are wide. The eyes are near the widest part of the face. Apply corrective makeup as follows (Figure 19.27):

1. Arch the eyebrows and gradually narrow them at the ends.
2. Subdue the wide cheekbones by shadowing them with a darker foundation.
3. Apply eye shadow to the upper lids and blend up to the brows.
4. If eyeliner is used, make a very thin line close to the lashes. Do not extend the line.

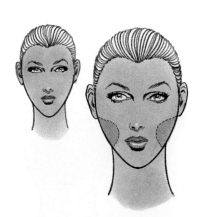

19.28 Inverted triangle

Inverted Triangle (or Heart)

The forehead is wide and the chin narrow. The eyes are often set far apart, and the cheekbones are large. Apply corrective makeup as follows (Figure 19.28):

1. To bring the eyes closer together, extend the eyebrows toward the bridge of the nose past the inner corner of the eye.
2. Eye shadow should be heaviest from the center of the eye to the inner corner of the eye.
3. The eyebrows should just barely arch.
4. Apply eyeliner close to the lashes. Do not extend it beyond the lash line.
5. Use a lighter shade of foundation at the center of the jaws. Blend well.

Oblong

This face is usually long and angular, with fairly straight lines. Apply corrective makeup as follows (Figure 19.29):

1. The brows should have a natural, rounded arch. Avoid turning the ends down.
2. Blend eye shadow across the eyelid.
3. Eyeliner should be heaviest in the center of the eyelid. Give the line an upward sweep at the outer corner.
4. Use a darker foundation at the tops of the cheekbones.
5. If the nose is long, apply a darker foundation along the center.
6. If the cheeks are hollow or sunken in, use a lighter foundation in the hollows of the cheeks. Blend the foundation well.

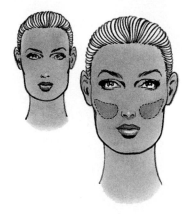

19.29 Oblong

Safety Tips and Client Protection

1. Do not get mascara in the eyes.
2. Sharpen eyebrow pencils, eyeliner pencils, and lipliner pencils after each use. Sharpen pencils with a sharpener made especially for them. Do not use an ordinary pencil sharpener.
3. Sanitize mascara, eyebrow, and lip brushes after each use.
4. Discard all sponges.
5. Wash all drapes that touch the client's skin.
6. Be sure that your fingernails are filed smoothly, so that you do not scratch the client.
7. Pour lotions from bottles.
8. Shake powder from a powder container similar to a salt shaker. Do not dip into the box.
9. Remove cleanser from the container with spatulas, not with the fingers.
10. Remove cream cosmetics from the container with a small spatula or an orangewood stick.
11. Do not touch a lipstick to a client's mouth. Remove a small quantity of lipstick with a spatula and apply it to the lips with a lip brush or a cotton swab.
12. Sanitize your hands before and after makeup application.

> **◆ Key Point ◆**
>
> All makeup should look *natural*. Makeup should be applied so skillfully that it is hardly noticeable. This takes practice. When using foundation for correction, always make sure that you blend it well. Corrected areas should not appear to be darker or lighter than the rest of the face. If you use a darker foundation on one area, blend it in so the tone changes very gradually.

FALSE EYELASHES

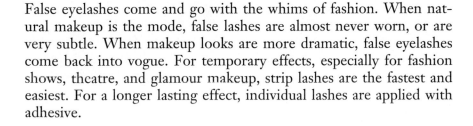

False eyelashes come and go with the whims of fashion. When natural makeup is the mode, false lashes are almost never worn, or are very subtle. When makeup looks are more dramatic, false eyelashes come back into vogue. For temporary effects, especially for fashion shows, theatre, and glamour makeup, strip lashes are the fastest and easiest. For a longer lasting effect, individual lashes are applied with adhesive.

Applying Strip Lashes

Materials

Eyelashes	70 percent alcohol	Aluminum foil
Adhesive	or any other	Toothpicks
Manicure scissors	approved germicide	Mascara brush
Tweezers	Adhesive applicator	Mascara (if desired)

Procedure for Applying Strip Lashes

1. Sanitize hands.
2. Read the manufacturer's directions enclosed with the eyelashes. Examine the lashes carefully and select the correct lash for each eye. They are different. One lash is designed for the left eye, the other for the right eye.
3. Remove one of the eyelash strips from the container. Handle gently. Place it against the eyelid and measure for length. If the base of the lash is too long, cut off a few hairs at a time (Figure 19.30). Trim from the outer edge where the lashes are the thickest. The lash should be cut so that it will rest about ¼ inch away from the corner of the eye.
4. If the hairs of the eyelash are too long near the corner of the eye, shorten one hair at a time. If the hairs are too long and lashes are placed too close to the corner of the eye, the eye may be irritated and the client may be uncomfortable.
5. Squeeze a little adhesive from the tube onto the lash strip (Figure 19.31).
6. Let the adhesive set for 30 to 60 seconds. Flex and bend the eyelash to help contour the base (Figure 19.32).
7. Have the client look down with eyes half open.
8. Place the eyelash down at the inner corner of the eye and gently press the base along the base of the natural eyelashes (Figure 19.33).
9. Secure the lash firmly by pressing with the finger along the full length of the base. The adhesive will dry in 3 to 5 minutes.
10. With a clean mascara brush, blend the natural lashes with the false lashes by brushing them from underneath.
11. If mascara is desired, apply it to the eyelashes from underneath.

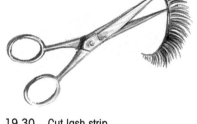

19.30   Cut lash strip

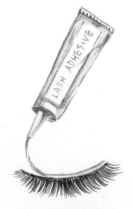

19.31   Apply adhesive

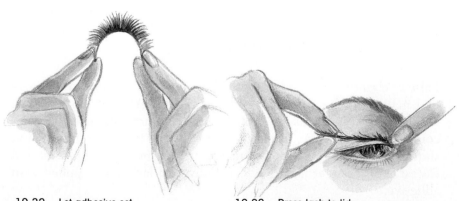

19.32   Let adhesive set   19.33   Press lash to lid

Removing Strip Eyelashes

1. Lift a corner of the base strip from the outer corner of the eye and gently peel off (Figure 19.34). Be careful not to pull the real lashes.
2. Lift the strip of adhesive off the base with tweezers (Figure 19.35) and store the eyelashes in the original container.

19.34 Lift lash from corner

Safety Tips

1. Always use a hypoallergenic adhesive, a surgical type of glue. An allergy test can be given by putting a dot of the adhesive near the eyelash at the outer corner of the eye. If there is no reaction within 24 hours, strip lashes may be worn safely.
2. Be careful not to point the tweezers into the client's eye.
3. Do not get mascara in the eye.
4. Do not place eyelashes under the natural lashes. This can cause irritation to the eye.
5. Place eyelashes as close to the base of the natural lashes as possible and not on the skin above the lashes.
6. When removing strip lashes, be careful not to pull the skin or the natural lashes.
7. Sanitize hands before applying false eyelashes.

19.35 Remove adhesive from lash

◆SAFETY PRECAUTION◆

Some people may be allergic to the adhesive used to apply artificial lashes. An allergy test can be given by putting a dot of adhesive behind the client's ear or by attaching a single lash to each eye. If there is no reaction within 24 hours, you can apply the lashes safely.

Applying Semipermanent Individual Eyelashes

Customized eyelash service is a technique of applying individual eyelashes one at a time to the client's own eyelashes. The eyelashes, when attached correctly, will stay on about six weeks. Generally two or three natural eyelashes fall out per week. When the natural eyelash falls out, the artificial lash falls with it. The operator then reapplies the required number of eyelashes each week.

Artificial lashes come in three lengths: short, medium, and long. Artistic and natural-looking effects can be accomplished by using a combination of long and medium or medium and short lashes. It is usually advisable to use short lengths at the inner corners of the eyes. For a heavier look, several artificial lashes can be glued to the base of an artificial lash after it has been glued to a natural lash. This gives a kind of feathered look (Figure 19.36). The same procedure can be used if there are gaps between the natural lashes.

Artificial lashes can be applied to both the upper and lower eyelids. Lashes for the lower lid are usually shorter than those for the upper lid. Lashes for both lids are applied in the same manner. Usually the bottom lashes do not stay on as well as the upper lashes because the natural bottom lashes are shorter and weaker. The operator works in front of the client when applying bottom lashes, behind the client when applying top lashes.

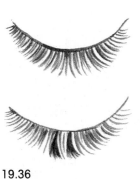

19.36

Materials

Tweezers	Aluminum foil	Adhesive
Eye-makeup remover	Eyelashes	Adhesive solvent
Cotton swabs	Adjustable light	Empty lash container
Wet sterilizer	Eyelash brush	or small dish
Tissues	Eyelid and lash cleaner	

Procedure for Applying Individual Lashes

1. Cleanse hands.
2. Have the client recline on a lounge-type chair. Work from behind the client.
3. With a cotton swab, apply eye cleanser over the lids and the lashes. Be careful that all makeup is removed. The adhesive will not stick if any oil or cream is left on the eyelash. Do not get cleanser in the eye.
4. Brush the upper eyelashes to separate them (Figure 19.37).
5. Place a small quantity of adhesive on an empty eyelash tray or in a small dish. The adhesive dries very quickly, so use only a small amount.
6. With the tweezers, remove a lash from the tray (Figure 19.38). Dip the end of the lash into the adhesive (Figure 19.39). Spread some of the adhesive onto the client's eyelash (Figure 19.40). The client should keep the eyes half open, while looking down.
7. Place the artificial eyelash on top of the client's lash, toward the base of the natural lash (Figure 19.41). Do not apply the lash to the eyelid. Start the application near the center of the eye, working carefully. Steady your hand by supporting it with your other hand.
8. Apply about four lashes to one eye and then go to the other eye. Continue moving from eye to eye, applying four lashes at a time.
9. Continue until all the lashes are applied.

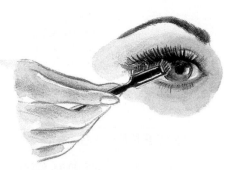

19.37   Brush upper lashes

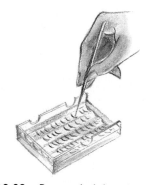

19.38   Remove lash from tray

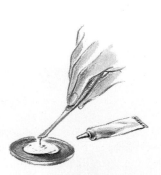

19.39   Dip lash in adhesive

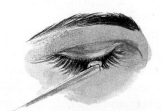

19.40   Spread adhersive to eyelash

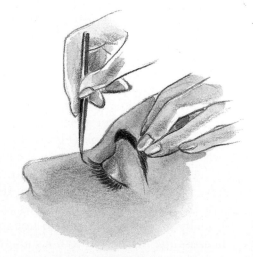

19.41   Place artificial lash

10. When you are finished, have the client sit up and look into a mirror. If a lash is out of line, remove it by putting some adhesive remover on a cotton swab and rubbing the swab over the eyelash. Protect the client's eye with a shield. Do not get adhesive remover in the eye.

Safety Tips

1. Do not get adhesive, adhesive remover or eyelid cleanser in the eyes.
2. Always have the client sit up when you are using adhesive remover.
3. Work in a quiet, well-lighted, well-ventilated room.
4. Do not glue an artificial eyelash to two natural lashes. This could cause discomfort to the client.
5. Always work with clean tweezers, and be careful when using the tweezers around the eyes.
6. If the glue dries on the tweezers, remove the glue with adhesive remover.

> **◆ Key Point ◆**
> The popularity of false eyelashes is determined by fashion trends. They are seldom used for daytime makeup, unless the client has very sparse natural lashes. Practice application on a mannequin so you will be comfortable when the occasion arises to apply lashes.

EYEBROW ARCHING

In Chapter 20, we will discuss how to remove unwanted hair from the face for a balanced look. This section describes the importance of the eyebrow to the overall balance of the face and what attention eyebrows should receive in makeup application.

The eyebrow should be in proportion with the facial structure, especially the bones surrounding the eye socket. Fads sometimes influence the shape of the eyebrow. Caution your client not to remove eyebrow hair in the interest of fashion. The eyebrows are secondary hair and grow back very slowly or not at all. Removal can be permanent over time.

The eyebrows are used to balance the eyes if they are too widely spaced or too close together. Refresh your memory in this area by reviewing the section on corrective makeup in this chapter. If the face is balanced, the eyebrow should begin at the end of an imaginary line drawn from the flare of the nostril past the inside corner of the eye (see Figure 19.42). The highest point of the eyebrow should be directly above the iris of the eye when your client is looking straight ahead. If you trace a line from the corner of the nose to the corner of the eye, you will see that the eyebrow ends about ½ inch outside the eye, completing that imaginary line.

In your makeup application, use pencil strokes to fill the eyebrow in as necessary. In general, eyebrows are heaviest from the nose to the arch. Brush the natural eyebrows into the lines you have created for a natural effect and brush lightly with mascara for a darker look.

Read the precautions at the end of this section before starting the procedure.

> **CLIENT TIP ◆◆◆◆◆◆◆**
> Brace your little finger against the temple area when drawing eyebrows. Add short strokes of color, much like hair, for a natural effect.

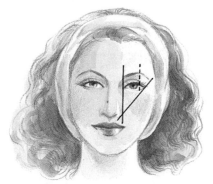
19.42

> **◆ Key Point ◆**
> The eyebrow determines the balance of the eye within the cheekbone. It serves to frame the eye and add expression to the face.

EYEBROW AND LASH TINTING

Some clients have very light eyelashes and eyebrows. Without some color to frame the eyes, the face has a blank look. This service is not a luxury but a great convenience to these people.

Materials

Cotton swabs or toothpicks with cotton	Towels	Package of brow and lash tint
Petroleum jelly	Two washcloths	(contains two
Cotton	Shampoo cape	different
Mild soap	Disposable neck strips	solutions)
	Eye shields	Stain remover

Procedure for Eyebrow and Lash Tinting

1. Sanitize hands.
2. Drape the client with a shampoo cape.
3. Have the client sit in an upright position with the eyes closed.
4. Using a soft washcloth and mild soap, wash the brows and lashes and rinse them well. Be certain that all eye makeup is removed.
5. Put petroleum jelly on the eye shields and place the shields under the eyelids (Figure 19.43).
6. Apply petroleum jelly to the skin below the eyebrows and over the upper lid but not on the eyelashes or the eyebrows themselves.
7. Use a cotton swab, or make a swab with a toothpick and cotton, and saturate it with solution 1. Carefully touch the brows and the upper and lower eyelashes with the solution and let it dry (Figure 19.44).
8. Saturate another swab with solution 2 and touch the brows and the lashes. Don't let the solution run or get in the eyes.

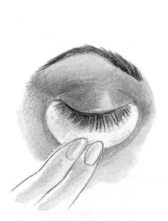

19.43   Place shield under eye

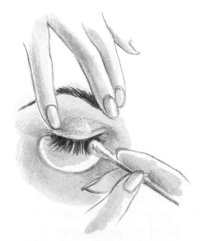

19.44   Apply solution 1 to lashes

9. After about a minute, wash the brows and lashes with mild soap and water, using a small, soft cloth (Figure 19.45).
10. If any color gets on the skin, remove it with soap and water or with stain remover.

Inform the client that this service lasts approximately 6 to 8 weeks. Arch the brow the week before or the week after the tint, if desired.

Safety Tips

1. Recap bottles tightly with original caps as soon as possible.
2. Do not mix solutions or interchange applicators.
3. Do not use applicators for more than one treatment. Swabs should be discarded after use.
4. Discard any unused solution. Do not pour it back into the bottle. Pour out only a little of each solution at a time.
5. Remove stains quickly with soap and water. Stubborn stains can be rcmoved with stain remover.
6. Delicate skin can be easily irritated if you rub too hard. Be gentle.
7. Follow manufacturer's directions.

Permanent Makeup

"Permanent makeup" is a modified tattooing process that can be used to create semipermanent to permanent eyebrows, eyeliner, lipliner, shadowing, etc. Originally designed for use as a finish to cosmetic surgery, permanent makeup is now a specialty area for many makeup artists. If you are interested in this service, ask your instructor where you can obtain the special training necessary. In some states, permanent makeup artists are licensed by the Board of Cosmetology; in other states, such licensing is done by the Board of Health or another state agency.

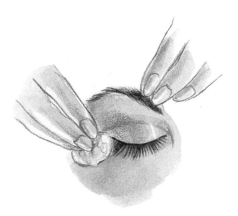

19.45 Wash lashes

> ◆ Key Point ◆
> Follow manufacturer's directions and safety tips closely when tinting brows and lashes.

Makeup is the art of enhancing the face with colored cosmetics. Both men and women use makeup today; however makeup for men is very subtle and is more restricted to those in the performance fields. As a makeup artist, you will choose from the liquids, creams, pencils, and powders available according to the skin tones and the eye and hair colors. You will select the foundation to nearly match the skin tones when compared at the jaw.

Daytime makeup is more subtle; evening and glamour makeup use brighter colors and more heavy application. You will determine the correct application for the occasion, and adjust it to the life style of your client and the colors he or she chooses to wear. False eyelashes are more for evening and gala makeup and are sometimes out of fashion totally. You should be able to apply both strip and semipermanent, or tab eyelashes, in a safe, quick manner.

Corrective makeup combines the artistry of color with the prin-

SUMMARY
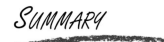

ciples of art and design. Light colors enlarge; dark colors diminish areas of the face for a total balanced look. Any color added around the eye will make it appear larger and more expressive. As a creative makeup artist, you will use color to enhance your client's features.

QUESTIONS

1. What is the purpose of makeup? What are the primary cosmetics used?
2. What are the three types of makeup application?
3. How do these makeup applications differ?
4. How does corrective makeup use dark and light colors to create optical illusions?
5. How are strip false eyelashes applied?
6. How are individual false eyelashes applied?
7. How is the eyebrow important to the facial balance?
8. What are the characteristics of the correct arch?
9. How is eyebrow and lash tinting accomplished?

PROJECTS

1. Analyze the facial bone structure of at least six of your fellow students. Pull their hair straight back from their faces and away from their necks. Secure the hair in place. Working with a headform on a piece of paper, redraw the outline of each face you are analyzing. Note the bone on each face that is the structure for the most prominent feature.
2. Using the drawings from your facial analysis (project 1), indicate where you would highlight and contrast each face for best effect. Recommend colors and placement.
3. Working with the drawings (project 1), shade in the eye, contour, cheek, and lip color.
4. Apply makeup to each person's face according to your drawings.

REMOVING UNWANTED HAIR

CHAPTER GOAL

Removing unwanted hair can enhance your client's appearance by strengthening individual facial features. After reading this chapter and completing the projects, you should be able to

1. Explain the two categories of hair removal.
2. Demonstrate the procedure for removal of the hair by tweezing.
3. Outline the procedure for using a depilatory.
4. List the methods of waxing and explain the procedures.
5. Describe the benefits of facial hair lighteners.

Unwanted hair has been a concern for centuries. Early methods of hair removal were either painful or damaging to the skin. Primitive peoples used knives made of stone or iron to shave hair. The Egyptians removed hair with a mixture of river muck and alum. This compound was very unpleasant and could pit the surface of the skin. Abrasives such as pumice stones have been used throughout history to remove hair, but always with the side effect of irritating the surface of the skin.

The most common method of removing hair—shaving—is done at home by the customer, not the cosmetologist. In the salon, epilation, or removal by pulling, is the most common professional method.

Unwanted hair is of great concern to the client. You will want to learn the best ways to remove the hair with the least discomfort and the longest lasting results. You will determine where hair should be removed and use the selected technique in a safe manner. You will analyze eye structure and remove hair accordingly, always following sanitary procedures.

METHODS OF HAIR REMOVAL

The presence of unwanted, superfluous hair can often detract from a person's appearance (see Chapter 2). There are many ways of removing unwanted hair, or it can be bleached so that it is less noticeable. Methods of hair removal fall into two categories: depilation and epilation.

Depilation (dep ih **LAYE** shun) means that the hair is removed at the skin line. **Shaving** and using **chemical depilatories** are methods of depilation.

Epilation (ep ih **LAYE** shun) means that the hair is removed below the skin. Both the hair shaft and the root are removed. Methods of epilation are **tweezing**, **waxing**, and **electrology**.

Permanent Hair Removal

Electrology is the only safe method of removing hair permanently. It is a specialty service that requires additional training, and in many states, an additional license. Electrology works by the insertion of a very fine filament (thread or fiber), called a probe, into the follicle. The goal is to insert the probe along the hair until the papilla of the hair is reached. Electricity is then applied so that the papilla is destroyed either by heat or by alkalinity, depending upon the method of electrology used. The hair is then removed by epilating (tweezing). A new hair will not grow from the follicle once the papilla has been destroyed. Electrology should only be performed by a qualified, licensed practitioner.

Choosing a Temporary Method

Most states permit cosmetologists only to remove hair by tweezing, by using chemical depilatories, or by waxing. In the salon, you may be called upon to remove hair from the face, the underarms, the arms, the legs, or anywhere on the torso. The method you choose will often depend upon where the hair is located, the amount of hair to be removed, and your client's particular preference. For example, unwanted hair on the upper lip can be removed with a depilatory, waxed, or bleached. Shaving, waxing, and depilatories work well on the legs, but you would not tweeze such a large area because it would take too much time and be too painful. You can also bleach the hair on the legs, but unless it is very fine, the hair will not be concealed.

TWEEZING

Tweezing is an excellent way of removing small amounts of individual hairs. Tweezers are most often used to shape the eyebrows, but they can be used elsewhere to remove scattered hairs. Tweezers come in a variety of styles (Figure 20.1). Experiment until you find the shape that is most suitable for you. Because the hair is removed below the skin line, tweezing can be uncomfortable if it is not done properly.

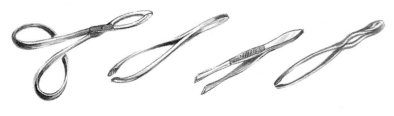

20.1

Materials

Wet sanitizer containing 70 percent alcohol or any approved germicide	Towels
	Eyebrow pencils
	Disposable neck strip
Tweezers	Astringent
Cotton	Boric acid solution
Eyebrow brush	

◆ **Key Point** ◆

Depilation, removing the hair at the skin surface, is seldom a professional service. Epilation, removing the hair from the follicle, is accomplished in the salon by tweezing, waxing, and electrology.

CLIENT   T I P ◆◆◆◆◆◆◆

Make sure that your client is comfortable. Tweezing the individual hairs in a quick motion and sponging the treated skin with astringent will ease discomfort.

◆SAFETY **P R E C A U T I O N**◆

1. Read the labels on the bottles.
2. Do not put alcohol or astringent on the eye pads.
3. Tweeze one hair at a time.
4. Do not catch the skin between the tweezers.
5. Do not allow tweezed hairs to fall into the client's eyes.

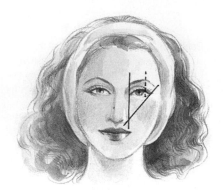

20.2

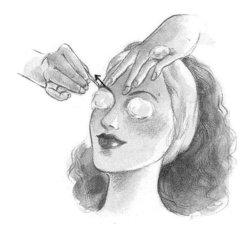

20.3

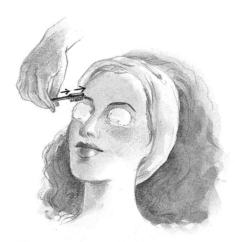

20.4

Procedure for Tweezing the Eyebrows

1. Place a towel over the headrest.
2. Cleanse your hands.
3. Fasten a disposable neck strip around the client's hair, if desired. (You may at this point steam the eyebrows with a hot, wet towel, to relax the skin. This step is optional.)
4. Measure the brow for the correct length and arch (Figure 20.2).
   a. Place an eyebrow pencil diagonally from the flare of the nose past the outside corner of the eye, and mark a light dot on the skin at the brow. This will establish the outside of the eyebrow about ½ inch past the corner of the eye.
   b. Hold the pencil at the inner corner of the eye and mark the skin above this point. This determines the inside of the brow.
   c. The highest part of the brow should be above the outside edge of the iris of the eye when the client is looking straight ahead.
5. Make eye pads from cotton by shaping them with the fingers. Moisten the eye pads with boric acid solution and place them over the eyes. The pads should fit securely into the eye socket (Figure 20.3). (This step is optional.)
6. Moisten a cotton pad with boric acid solution and place it on your index finger like a ring (Figure 20.3). Tweezed hairs are to be placed on the top of this cotton ring.
7. Begin tweezing the hairs between the marks you made at the inner corner of each eyebrow. Hold the skin taut with one hand by stretching it between the index and middle fingers. Tweeze the hairs with the other hand in the direction of the hair growth (Figure 20.3).
8. Remove excess hairs above the brows. The brows should gradually arch to the highest point marked on the skin (step 4). If any hairs extend beyond the outer corners of the eyes, remove these hairs in the direction of their growth.
9. Tweeze the hairs below the brow.
10. Brush the eyebrows against their growth (Figure 20.4). Look for any stray hairs.
11. Rebrush the brows in the direction of the growth.
12. Remove the eye pads.
13. Apply astringent to the skin and the eyebrows.

Electric Tweezers

One of the methods of hair removal employs electric tweezers. As the name implies, electrically charged tweezers are used to pull the hair. Because each hair must be removed individually, as with ordinary tweezers, this method is very slow. Some manufacturers claim that the hair is removed permanently, but this is not true.

♦ Key Point ♦

Tweezing is often the preferred method for arching eyebrows as individual hairs can be removed. Tweezing is not practical for large surface areas because it would be too painful.

DEPILATORIES

Depilatories are chemicals that dissolve the hair so that it can be wiped or washed away. Because they are applied to the skin, care must be taken so that they do not dissolve the skin as well. Depilatories can be used over large and small areas. Some products are made for use on the face and others for use elsewhere on the body. Be extremely careful when using a depilatory on the face. Never put a depilatory near the eyes. Be sure to read and follow the manufacturer's directions very carefully.

Materials

Cotton	Skin lotion
Spatula	Talc
Towel	Depilatory
Soap and water	

Procedure for Using Depilatories

1. Wash the area to be treated with mild soap and water. Pat dry. Do not rub.
2. Apply the depilatory with a spatula to the area where hair is to be removed.
3. Leave the depilatory on the skin for 5 to 15 minutes. Check every few minutes by removing a bit of cream with the spatula. If the hair has not been removed, reapply.
4. Remove the cream and hair with water-soaked cotton. Do not rub the area.
5. Blot dry.
6. Use a mild skin lotion or talc over the area to soothe the skin.

◆SAFETY P R E C A U T I O N◆

Always perform an allergy test at least 24 hours prior to applying the depilatory. Apply a small amount of depilatory cream behind the ear. Leave it on for 15 minutes and then remove. If there is no positive reaction (redness or swelling) after 24 hours, proceed with the treatment.

◆SAFETY P R E C A U T I O N◆

1. Do not use a depilatory if there are any abrasions, lesions, or pustules on the skin.
2. Do not use a depilatory if the client has a positive reaction to the skin test.
3. Take care not to let a depilatory get into the eyes or the mouth of the client.
4. Always read and follow the manufacturer's directions.

◆ Key Point ◆

Depilatories dissolve the hair. Their use in the salon is limited primarily to "mustaches."

WAXING

Waxing is an effective method for removing unwanted hair in large and small areas. There are three types of wax: **hot (hard) wax**, which is heated and applied when melted; **warm wax**, which comes in a semisolid form and is heated in a thermostatically controlled warmer; and **cold wax**, which comes ready to use in tubes, in jars, or on strips.

The three types of wax are applied and used in basically the same way. The main difference is that the warm and cold waxes are applied thinly and removed with strips of cotton or muslin fabric, called **epilating strips**, which are rubbed over the wax. Hot wax must be applied in thick layers so that there is enough to grasp when it is pulled off.

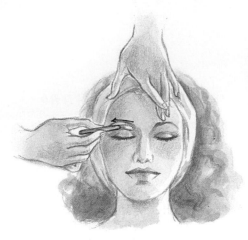

20.5

Following are procedures for shaping the eyebrows with hot wax and removing hair from the upper lip with warm wax. (These directions would also apply for cold wax.) Which type of wax you use will often depend upon your own preference and the equipment available at your salon. Become familiar with all three methods so that you can decide which you prefer. When using any wax, be sure to follow the manufacturer's directions carefully.

If not done properly, waxing can be quite painful. Practice to perfect your technique.

Materials for Hot Waxing

Hot plate	Skin lotion
Foil	Talc
Spatula	Special wax
Wet sanitizer	Towels
Cotton	Soap and water

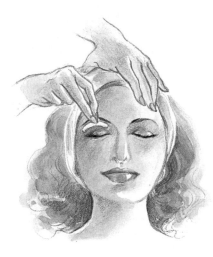

20.6

Procedure for Waxing the Eyebrows

1. To determine the proper shape for the eyebrows, see the Procedure for Tweezing the Eyebrows, step 4.
2. Cleanse the skin. Blot dry.
3. Before applying the wax to the client's skin, test a drop on your arm or hand to make sure it is warm enough but not too hot. Do not burn the client.
4. Start under the brows. With a spatula, apply the wax in the direction of the hair growth (Figure 20.5). Do not get wax on the eyelids.
5. Press the wax with the fingers until it is cool. The hairs will become lodged in the wax (Figure 20.6).
6. With a spatula, lift up an edge of the wax, hold it firmly between the thumb and index finger, and remove it quickly (as if it were an adhesive bandage) in the direction opposite that of the hair growth. Hold the skin taut with one hand as you remove the wax with the other hand (Figure 20.7).
7. Apply wax to the excess hair over the brows and follow steps 4, 5, and 6.
8. Apply wax between the brows and follow the same directions.
9. Apply skin lotion with cotton to soothe the skin from which hair has been removed.

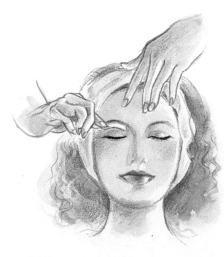

20.7

Warm Wax

Materials for Warm Wax

All materials for
 using hot wax
 except the hot plate

Thermostatically controlled warmer
Epilating strips

Procedure for Warm Waxing the Upper Lip

1. Use soap and water or a specially formulated lotion to cleanse the skin. Blot dry.
2. Divide the lip area into two equal sections from the center of the lip (the Cupid's bow) to the corner. Determine the direction in which the hair is growing (Figure 20.8).
3. Hold the spatula at a 45° angle to the skin, as shown in Figure 20.9 and apply the wax in a thin, transparent layer in the direction of the hair growth. Use short strokes. Take care not to allow the wax to touch the lips.
4. Apply two-thirds of an epilating strip over the wax and rub in the direction of the hair growth. Be sure that one-third of the strip is left free (Figure 20.10).

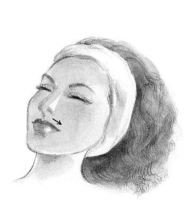

20.8

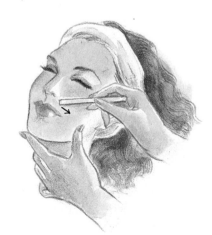

20.9

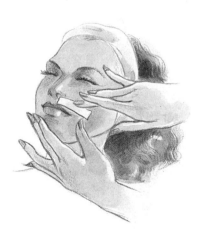

20.10

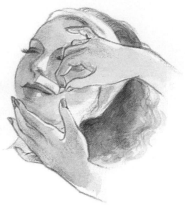

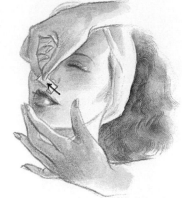

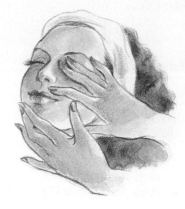

20.11   20.12   20.13

5. Hold the corner of the lip taut (Figure 20.11) and grasp the free end of the strip. Quickly peel off the strip in the direction opposite that of the hair growth. Be sure to peel the strip as close to the skin as possible (Figure 20.12).
6. Because this is a very sensitive area, apply firm pressure to the lip with the cushions of your fingers (Figure 20.13).
7. Apply an antiseptic cream followed by a skin lotion to soothe the skin.

> **◆ Key Point ◆**
> Waxing is the most common method of removing hair in the salon. Large or small areas can be treated with a minimum of discomfort.

LIGHTENING UNWANTED HAIR

Oil lightener mixed with two parts hydrogen peroxide, or specially formulated products, can be used to lighten unwanted hair. This works best on the soft, downy hair (lanugo hair) that grows on the face and arms, but it can be used anywhere. However, lightening can cause an allergic reaction, so a predisposition test should be performed before application (see Chapter 14). Read and follow the directions carefully.

> **◆ Key Point ◆**
> Lightening of facial hair is an alternative to removing it. Lightening is more effective on fine, sparse facial hair.

SUMMARY

As a cosmetologist, you will be asked to remove unwanted hair, especially the eyebrows, or to lighten facial hair. If you choose to specialize in esthetics you will add other services to your skills, if state laws permit. You will become experienced in waxing, the use of depilatories, and possibly even electrology.

Hair is removed by depilation, the dissolving of the hair beneath the surface; or by epilation, the physical pulling of the hair from the follicle. Epilation is more common and can be permanent (electrology) or temporary. You will perform the temporary methods of tweezing and waxing with either soft or hard wax. Hard wax is the least common and is a hot technique. Soft wax can be applied either warm or cold. You will determine the proper wax according to the amount and length of the hair and the sensitivity of your client's skin.

It is important to follow sanitary guidelines when removing unwanted hair. You will cleanse the skin prior to treatment and apply a cooling antiseptic afterwards. You must follow all safety precautions to protect your client from inflammation and infection.

1. What are the two categories of hair removal?
2. What temporary methods of hair removal are there?
3. What is the procedure for removal of the hair by tweezing?
4. What is the procedure for using a depilatory?
5. What methods of waxing are available? What are the steps for each method?
6. What is the difference between soft and hard waxes?
7. What are the benefits of facial hair lighteners?

1. Research the waxes that are available. Determine if each is hard or soft and whether it is to be applied hot, warm, or cold. Outline the features of each and report back to the class.
2. Analyze the facial features of at least six people and determine ideal placement of their eyebrows. Recommend the best method for removing unwanted hair on each person.
3. Perform at least six eyebrow archings. Follow all sanitary procedures.
4. Determine the natural growth pattern of excess hair on three clients. Demonstrate the direction in which you would apply wax, and how you would remove the epilating strips.
5. Research facial hair lighteners. List the directions for each and explain how they differ from lighteners used for hair on the scalp.

NAIL AND HAND CARE

21

CHAPTER GOAL

Nail and hand care are offered in today's full-service salon. After reading this chapter and completing the projects, you should be able to

1. List the implements, equipment, and supplies necessary for a basic manicure service.
2. Demonstrate the procedures for a basic manicure and a man's manicure.
3. Demonstrate the procedure for a hand and arm massage.
4. Outline the technique for applying nails using the sculptured, fiberglass, and tip techniques.
5. Explain repair techniques for acrylic and fragile natural nails.
6. List the procedure for a pedicure service.
7. Explain the importance of safety precautions for you and your client during nail care procedures.
8. Explain safety requirements for the nail salon and explain the importance of safety to the technician.

The ancient people of China and Egypt regarded long colored nails as a distinction separating the aristocracy from common workers. Nails were shaped with pumice stone and colored with vegetable dyes. In the late 1800s, painted fingernails were in vogue among the Parisian elite. American women began wearing nail polish in imitation of glamorous film stars. By the 1920s, the idea was so popular that barber shops began to offer services for the care and beautification of the nails for both men and women.

As styling salons became popular, the demand for qualified manicurists increased. By the late 1950s virtually every state offered a specialty license for manicurists. The nail industry expanded with the introduction of the first build-on nails in the 70s. Following the development of natural looking artificial nails in the 1980s, the nail industry became the largest growth area in the entire cosmetology market. The field of manicuring has changed so dramatically since the basic filing and polishing of years gone by, that those who earn specialty licenses in this area are now called nail technicians.

In many states, the basic cosmetology license covers manicuring; however, additional coursework and the specialty license is available for those individuals who wish to concentrate their studies. Nail technicians now work in full-service styling, manicuring, and esthetic salons. To begin nail care, you must select the correct implements for the effects you want to create. You will handle the tools safely and disinfect them according to the health guidelines in your state. You will shape the nails and treat the surrounding skin. You will add length to the nails by sculpting, tipping, or wrapping. You will then complete the service by adding color to the nails if your client wishes.

EQUIPMENT, IMPLEMENTS, AND COSMETICS

Equipment and implements for manicuring refer to those durable articles that are reused after sanitization. *Equipment* generally means large articles provided by the school or salon as well as electrical items such as the heater for reconditioners and drills, or the bath for hot paraffin. *Implements* refers to your own tools that you will disinfect after each use and sanitize before and during the manicure. Any implements that you use to cut the skin must be sterilized. Refer to

Chapter 4 for approved methods of infection control. *Supplies* are disposable items that cannot be sanitized and cosmetics that are used during the nail service.

Equipment for Manicuring

1. **Manicure table** with lamp
2. **Chair** for the client
3. **Stool** for the manicurist
4. **Cosmetic tray**, including a container with clean cotton and a wet sanitizer
5. **Finger bowl** for soaking client's fingers
6. **Appliances** for treatment manicures

Implements for Manicuring

1. **Nail file** and/or **emery board** for shaping the nail (Figure 21.1). Files are available in various grits. The higher the grit number, the finer the file.
2. **Cuticle pusher**.
3. **Orangewood stick** (Figure 21.2).
4. **Swabs** for applying cosmetics. (You can use an orangewood stick wrapped in cotton.)
5. **Cuticle scissors** or **nippers** for removing dead skin.
6. **Acrylic nippers** for clipping loose or lifted product.
7. **Emery disks** and **blocks** for buffing and shaping nails (Figure 21.3).
8. **Nail brush** to cleanse the nails (Figure 21.4).
9. **Nail buffer** (optional) for polishing the surface of the natural nail.
10. **Spatulas** to remove any cosmetics from jars or containers.
11. **Tweezers**.

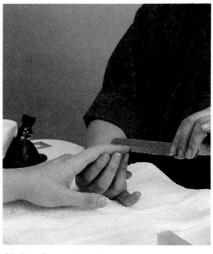

21.1　Emery board

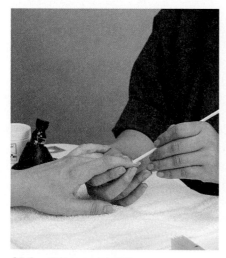

21.2　Orangewood stick

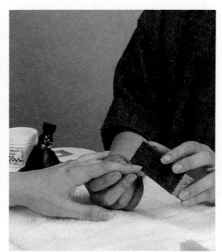

21.3　Emery block

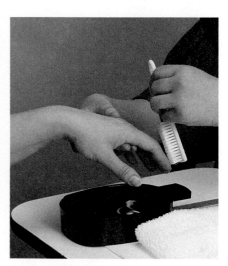

21.4　Nail brush

Cosmetics for Manicuring

1. **Acrylic Liquid.** Monomer (single unit molecule) with or without oil. It is mixed with a powder to form a sculptured nail.
2. **Acrylic Powder.** Polymer (long chain of repeating single units) mixed with liquid to form a sculptured nail.
3. **Alcohol.** A 70% solution is approved as a disinfectant when imple-ments are completely immersed for at least 20 minutes. You may also use alcohol to sanitize the table. Alcohol may be used to sanitize your hands and your client's hands, however, it is considered to be drying because it removes the skin's natural oils.
4. **Alum Solution.** Used to stop bleeding. For sanitary reasons it must be in a liquid or powder form.
5. **Base Coat.** Colorless liquid polish that is brushed on the nail before colored polish is applied. It provides a base for adhesion of the colored polish and helps prevent staining of the nail.
6. **Cleanser.** Liquid or cream that is added to the finger bath to help soften the skin, remove dirt and debris from under the nail, and remove oils prior to polish application.
7. **Cuticle Cream.** Creamy emulsion to soften the cuticle. Cuticle creams or oils have an emollient base and are used to treat dry cuticles and brittle nails. Cuticle cream is optional during the manicure and is an excellent at-home treatment.
8. **Cuticle Oil.** Vegetable oils are often used to soften dry, brittle cuticles. Heated oil is often used in a reconditioning manicure.
9. **Cuticle Softener.** Solution, usually of potassium hydroxide and glycerine, that softens the skin around the nail. Can be harsh and drying and should be avoided on thin, brittle nails or dry cuticles.
10. **Disinfectant.** A hospital-grade disinfectant for preparing the manicure table and for the wet sanitizer. A hospital-grade disin-fectant is preferable to alcohol.
11. **Primer.** Any liquid that will remove moisture from the nail plate so that artificial nails will adhere.
12. **Hand Lotion.** Used to soften the skin and to replace natural oils. These lotions contain emollients and humectants to moisturize the skin.
13. **Liquid Nail Dryer.** Product sprayed or brushed on following the final coat of polish. They are oily to the touch and add a pro-tective film to the nail while enamel dries.
14. **Nail Enamel.** Liquid polish with heavy color pigment, available in a wide range of colors.
15. **Nail Polish Remover.** Liquid solution, either using acetone or a substitute (non-acetone), that dissolves nail enamel. Non-acetone polish remover should be used on artificial nails.
16. **Nail Strengthener.** Liquid or cream that is applied to the nail for its strengthening action. Liquid strengtheners may contain formalde-hyde, which can cause allergic reactions, dryness to the cuticle, and may be carcinogenic.
17. **Paraffin Wax.** Used as a specialty treatment in a reconditioning manicure. Mitts are placed over hands dipped in heated wax for maximum benefits.

18. **Paste or Powder Polish.** Used to give gloss to the nail, especially in conjunction with buffing. Mild abrasives are sometimes used, which can be damaging to the nail.
19. **Reconditioner.** Any cosmetic used as a treatment during the manicure for dry cuticles, split nails, etc. Most reconditioners are hydrating, meaning they carry moisture into the skin and cuticle. Many also contain hydrolyzed protein and plant extracts to strengthen the nail.
20. **Ridge Filler.** Polish used when the surface of the nail needs a base coat that is thicker. Used to fill in minor depressions and imperfections in the natural nail. Also used with tips and wraps.
21. **Top Coat.** Liquid polish that dries quickly on the surface of the nail, leaving a tough film. Protects the colored polish, helps prevent chipping, gives a hard glossy finish, and strengthens the nail.

> **◆ Key Point ◆**
> As a professional nail technician, it is most important that you use implements in a professional manner and follow all infection control regulations.

Basic Manicuring Techniques

The word manicuring comes from the Latin *manus* meaning "hand," and *cura*, meaning "care." The purpose of basic manicuring techniques is to maintain the health and beauty of the hands and nails. The procedures that follow are those that you will incorporate as your basic menu of preservative and corrective treatments for the hands and nails.

Preparation for a Manicure

The following list includes the basic materials needed for a plain manicure. Your instructor may add to the list for a specific manicure treatment.

Materials

70% alcohol or approved hospital-grade disinfectant	Cuticle pusher
	Emery boards or disks
Wet sanitizer	Metal nail file (optional)
Cotton	Cuticle nippers (optional)
Polish remover	Cuticle softener
Cosmetic tray	Cuticle cream or oil
Hand lotion	Nail buffer (optional)
Two towels	Waste basket or bag
Finger bowl	Base and top coat
Nail brush	Colored enamel

Procedure for Setting Up Manicure Table

1. Move the manicure table in front of the chair where you will seat your client.
2. Sponge the table with an approved disinfectant.
3. Arrange supplies with labels facing you for your convenience.

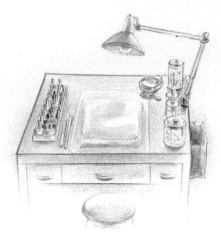

21.5

4. Tape a small plastic bag to the table for soiled, disposable materials.
5. Place clean metal implements in container for wet sanitizer. Fill sanitizer with an approved disinfectant until implements are covered.
6. Fold a towel to make a cushion. Then cover it with a second towel, leaving one end free. Place cushion in the middle of the table with free end toward you.
7. Arrange the lamp over center of cushion, 12–16" above it.
8. Place a few drops of cleanser in the finger bowl. Fill with warm water. Place on the opposite right-hand side of the table. See Figure 21.5 for the recommended setup as explained in steps 3–7.

Plain or Water Manicure

The following procedure is for a basic manicure. Your instructor may recommend a procedure that is slightly different, or may suggest that you alter a few steps if your customer is also receiving an advanced nail service.

Procedure for a Plain or Water Manicure

1. Seat your client in a comfortable chair. Sit opposite your customer with both feet on the floor. Turn your knees to the left or to the right to allow room for your client's comfort.
2. Cleanse your hands and then those of your client with 70% alcohol or an approved antiseptic. Pour a few drops into the palm of your hand and then rub your hands together. Take a piece of cotton, moisten it with alcohol, and rub it over your client's hands thoroughly (Figure 21.6).
3. Remove polish. Start with the little finger and work toward the thumb. Roll cotton between the palms of your hands to remove fuzz, saturate the cotton with nail polish remover, and press firmly against each nail. If your own nails are polished, hold cotton between your fingers rather than with your fingertips. Hold the cotton against the nail for a few seconds, then wipe the nail clean from cuticle to free edge (Figure 21.7).

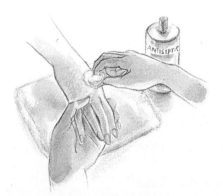

21.6   Sanitize client's hand

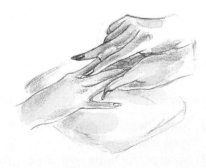

21.7   Remove polish

Use a fresh surface of the cotton for each nail, discarding and using new cotton as necessary. Cleanse around the cuticle gently with a swab dipped in polish remover.

4. Shape nails. Starting with the first hand, hold your client's little finger between your thumb and first two fingers. Gently roll the side wall away from the nail. Place the file straight across the end of the free edge and shape the nail, working from the outside edge in, toward the center (Figure 21.8). Do not file into the corners of the nail as this could cause chipping and splits. Never file on the surface of the natural nail.

5. Soften cuticle. After filing the client's first hand, place the fingers in the water bath to soften the cuticle (Figure 21.9).

6. Shape the nails of the other hand.

7. Remove the first hand from the bowl. Carefully dry the fingertips, gently pushing the cuticle back with the towel (Figure 21.10).

8. Apply cuticle softener around the base of the nails. Push back the cuticle gently, using a pusher or a cotton-tipped orangewood stick. Brace your little finger against the cushion and gently push the cuticle in a small circular motion, starting at the sides and working toward the center (Figure 21.11). Keep the cuticle moist while pushing and only use slight pressure so that you do not cause discomfort to your client or damage the nails. Injury to the root area will cause permanent nail irregularities. Remove any cuticle fragments from the pusher by wiping with the towel end before placing back in the wet sanitizer.
Note: Wrap the corner of your towel around your index finger and wipe away excess cuticle and solvent.

9. Immerse the second hand in the water bath.

10. Clean under the free edge of the nails on the first hand with an orangewood stick wrapped in cotton. Dip the swab into the finger bath and gently work debris out from under the nail.

11. Remove dead cuticle very gently with tweezers or pusher. Clip only if absolutely necessary. Use extreme caution not to cut your client or cause further hangnails by improper technique. Your instructor will advise you about regulations for nipping cuticles in your state.

12. Apply cuticle cream or oil to the first hand. Using a cotton-

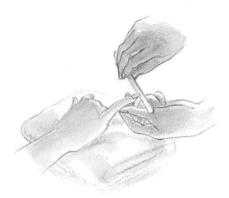

21.8   File nails

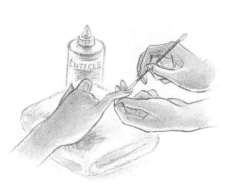

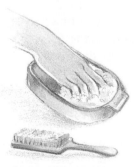

21.9   Soften cuticles

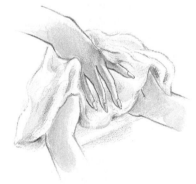

21.10   Dry hand

21.11   Push back cuticles

tipped orangewood stick, apply the oil or cream around the base and sides of the nail. Massage into the cuticle with the pad of your thumb.

13. Remove the client's other hand from the water. Repeat steps 7 through 10 and 12 on the other hand.
14. Brush the nails. Place the fingers in the finger bowl one hand at a time. Remove excess cream or oil by brushing with a downward motion from the base to the fingertips.
15. Thoroughly dry the nails.

Nail Polish Techniques

Application of nail polish is most often the final step of the manicure service. Assist your client in selecting the best color. Choose a color that will complement the wardrobe and also the season of the year. Usually, darker colors are worn in the cool months and lighter tones are selected in the warm months. Nail polish colors are also affected by fashion trends and fabric colors.

Procedure for Applying Polish

1. Thoroughly blend base coat by tapping bottom of bottle against the heel of your hand or rolling the bottle between your fingers.
2. Dip applicator all the way into the bottle. Make sure that enough polish is on the brush.
3. Wipe the brush on the bottle lip to remove excess polish. Wipe back side of brush gently.
4. Let polish collect into a small ball on the tip of the brush.
5. Brace your hand when applying polish so your stroke is smooth. Rest your forearm on the table for stability.
6. Stroke the center of the first pinky nail, starting near the cuticle and extending to the tip. Begin application $\frac{1}{16}$ of an inch from the cuticle. Hold the brush at a 45 degree angle to the nail plate with the drop of polish against the nail. Place brush on the nail. Gently push to almost touch the cuticle, then brush in one smooth move to free edge. Do NOT lift brush from the nail.
7. For second stroke, apply to right side of nail from barely above cuticle to tip. Hold side wall away from nail while applying polish. Avoid getting polish on the cuticles.
8. The third stroke covers the left side of the nail from cuticle to free edge. Hold the sidewall as outlined in step 7.
9. Examine nail and apply more polish only if needed.
10. Clean cuticle of any excess polish with a brush or swab dipped in acetone or polish remover. Discard soiled cotton.
11. Clean free edge with swab held straight up and down against free edge.
12. Continue to polish nails from ring finger to thumb. Continue to second hand from little finger to thumb.
13. Test if polish surface is dry by lightly touching the nail plate with the pad of your finger. If surface is not tacky, apply one or two coats of colored polish, then top coat. Blend each polish thoroughly prior to application.

CLIENT **TIP** ◆◆◆◆◆◆◆

Have a large selection of nail enamel on hand. Be prepared to sell the polish to your client for touch-ups at home.

CLIENT **TIP** ◆◆◆◆◆◆◆

To avoid smudges, suggest that your client arrange for payment, has car keys readily available, etc., before you begin polish application. Encourage your client to relax a few minutes before leaving the salon. Arrange for assistance with coat, accessories, or anything else that could distort the manicure while the polish is still damp.

The shape of the nail should always be considered before applying polish (Figures 21.12 and 21.13). The shape of the nail should complement the shape of the finger tip. You can best enhance your female clients' nails by making them appear longer and more slender. If the nails are already in the ideal shape and length, polish the nail from the cuticle to the free edge, and from outside edge to outside edge. If, however, the nail is short or wide, apply the polish so that a hairline edge remains free at both sides. As fashion dictates, you may choose to leave the lunula free of colored polish (or create the appearance by leaving a half moon free at the base).

"French" manicure polish techniques apply a white polish to the free edge, tapering toward the center (Figure 21.14). Clear, neutral, soft pink, or peach polish is then applied over the entire nail.

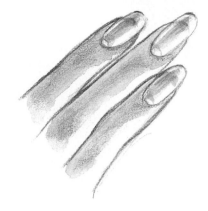

21.12

Reconditioning Manicure Techniques

Many of your clients will seek your advice and services because they have dry skin, brittle cuticles, or damaged nails. Reconditioning manicures are a treat as well as a treatment and should be a part of your basic menu of hand and nail services.

Hot Oil Manicure

A hot oil manicure differs from a plain manicure in that the hands are soaked in warm oil or cream rather than the water bath. An appliance is used to maintain the temperature of the oil or reconditioning cream at a comfortable level (Figure 21.15). This manicure is especially beneficial for clients whose hands are often in water, or those who suffer from dry skin and brittle cuticles. Definite improvement will be noticed after just a few reconditioning manicures.

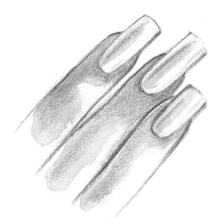

21.13

The procedure for a hot oil manicure follows that of a water manicure, steps 1 to 4. Then you will place the hand in the heated oil, replacing the water bath. As you remove the hand from the conditioner, give a minimassage. Work the cream or oil into the cuticle and fingers, finishing off by massaging the hand.

Repeat steps 1–4 on the right hand. Push back the cuticle and remove only jagged edges with the cuticle nipper. If possible, avoid any cutting of the cuticle and discourage your client from picking or trimming the cuticles at home.

Wipe each nail carefully with polish remover to clean traces of oil before applying polish.

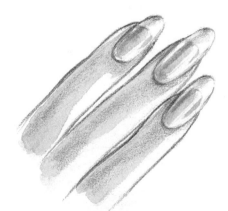

21.14   French manicure

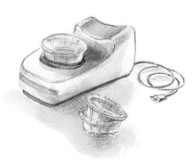

21.15   Hot oil heater

Paraffin Treatment

A paraffin treatment is a special luxury for the hands because it forces moisturizing agents into the deeper layers of the skin. It is beneficial for all skin types, but particularly effective for dry skin.

Complete the basic water manicure, apply hand lotion, and give a hand and arm massage. Test the wax temperature, then dip each hand three times in the paraffin bath. Cover each hand with a plastic bag, being careful not to disturb the wax. Wrap each hand in a towel mitt. Let the wax cool for a few minutes. Using the plastic bag, gently peel the paraffin mitt from the hands, working from wrists to fingertips. Complete the process by massaging the hands. If polish is desired, cleanse the nails by gently swabbing with alcohol or nail polish remover.

Manicures for Male Clients

Manicures have always been popular for men in barber shops. The basic water manicure procedure most often fills the needs of the male clientele. Pay special attention to smoothing the tips of the finger and removing any dead tissue with pumice stone. Nails should be kept short and filed to conform to the shape of the fingertips. Colorless polish or the use of a high-grit buffer block will add sheen to the nail plate.

Buffing should only be done if the nails are strong. The buffer must have disposable or washable cover. Buff nails in one direction, using a downward stroke from the base to the free edge of the nail. Lift buffer after each stroke.

> ◆ **Key Point** ◆
>
> The basic water manicure is the foundation for advanced nail services. Mastery of these techniques is essential.

MASSAGE FOR MANICURING

See Chapter 18 for a detail discussion of massage and massage techniques.

Hand Massage

Hand massage is an important part of every manicure. It not only relaxes the client, but also stimulates blood circulation to help keep the hands flexible and the skin smooth.

Procedure for Hand Massage

1. Apply hand lotion. Holding the client's hand in the palm of your hand, apply the lotion to the back of the client's hand. Gently distribute the lotion to the wrist and the fingers.
2. Place the client's elbow on the manicuring pillow. Hold the hand in an upright position, supporting it with your hand. With your right hand, slowly bend the client's hand back and forth (Figure 21.16). This helps to limber the wrist and relax the hand. All manipulations are repeated three times.

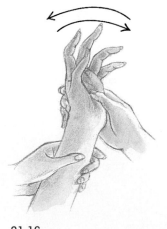

21.16

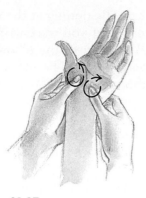

21.17

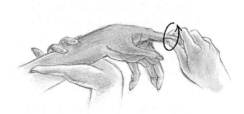

21.18

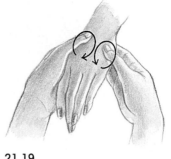

21.19

3. While the hand is in this position, place the cushions of your thumbs in the palm of the hand and massage in a circular movement from wrist to fingers (Figure 21.17).

4. Rest the client's arm on the manicuring table and put the hand in your own. Grasp each finger between your thumb and index finger and rotate it in a circular motion (Figure 21.18).

5. Hold the client's hand with both of your thumbs on the back of his or her hand at the wrist. Massage in a circular sliding movement down the back of the hand, following the line between the bones from the wrist to the knuckles (Figure 21.19). Slide back to wrist and give it a wringing motion.

6. Rotate each finger in a circular motion, beginning at the base and working up to the fingertip (Figure 21.20). Slide back and, with your thumb and fingers, pull down toward the fingertips in a tapering motion.

7. Repeat steps 1 through 6 on the other hand.

Arm Massage

When you give an arm massage that includes the upper arm, drape the client before beginning. Take a manicure towel, hold it lengthwise, and fold it around the arm. Pin the ends together at the shoulder. This will protect the clothing during massage.

Procedure for Arm Massage

1. Turn the client's palm downward and place the arm on the manicuring table. Apply lotion.

2. With your thumbs on the top of the wrist and your fingers on the inside, massage to the elbow in a circular motion, rotating your thumbs in alternate directions (Figure 21.21).

3. Turn the client's arm so that the palm faces up and repeat the first massage.

> **◆ Key Point ◆**
> Develop your touch until your massage movements are firm and rhythmical. The hand and arm massage is an especially pleasant part of hand care services.

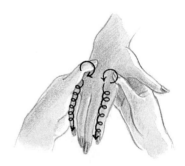

21.20

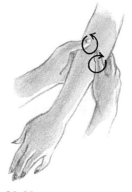

21.21

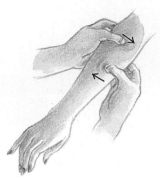

21.22

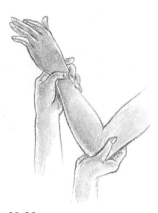

21.23

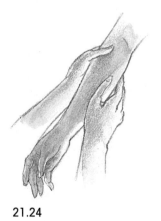

21.24

4. Place your hands around the client's arm. Beginning at the wrist, move your hands in opposite directions as if you were wringing out a piece of cloth (Figure 21.22). Work up to the elbow and then slide hands back to the wrist and repeat. The elbows are often neglected in beauty care, even though this is where dryness and scales show up first. Give extra attention to the elbows when giving an arm massage.
5. Support the client's arm with your left hand. Cup the right hand around the elbow and massage in a circular motion (Figure 21.23).
6. Work from the elbow up the arm, repeating steps 1 through 4 of the massage.
7. With your hands placed around the arm above the elbow, massage the arm in opposite directions, continuing to the wrist (Figure 21.24). Give extra massage when you reach the elbow.
8. Slide back to the shoulder and repeat, finishing with a gentle squeezing and tapering of the hand and fingers.

TECHNIQUES FOR ARTIFICIAL NAILS

Artificial nails have become more popular with the development of better materials. Artificial nails can be used to protect the natural nail, or to add length (an extension). Artificial nails are generally stronger than natural nails; they are less prone to splitting, cracking, or breaking.

The correct maintenance prevents the growth of mold or fungus between natural and artificial nails. As a technician, you will detect indications of allergic reactions to the nail product.

In this section, we will discuss the basic artificial nail applications: sculptured, fiberglass, tips, and extensions.

Sculptured Nails

Sculptured nails are built on a form, using an acrylic powder and an activating liquid. Acrylics can be used in many nail techniques that we will discuss, but first let's learn the basics of sculptured nails.

Materials

In addition to the materials for a plain manicure you will need:

Nail forms	Emery files in	Antiseptic
Acrylic powder(s)	various grits	Brush cleaner
Acrylic liquid	Buffer disks	Oil
Dappen dishes	Manicure brush and	Antimicrobial soap
Paper towels	finger bowl	
Sable brush	Primer	

Procedure

1. Sanitize work area and set up table for manicure.
2. Seat client comfortably.
3. Sanitize your hands, then your client's.
4. Give plain water manicure, if requested.
5. Lightly roughen the nail plate. File from the cuticle to the free edge (Figure 21.25). Be careful not to file the skin or cuticle — it could be painful for your client.
6. Dust each nail with the manicure brush. Brush down and away from the cuticle (Figure 21.26).
7. Work in a well-ventilated area. Apply primer as directed by your instructor and the manufacturer (Figure 21.27). Do not allow the primer to come into contact with the cuticle or skin. Let dry. If you are using an etching primer use extreme caution. This primer etches microscopic grooves in the nail plate to which the acrylic will adhere. The primer will also etch holes in the skin or eye.
8. Peel a nail form from its paper backing. Using the thumb and index finger of each hand, bend the tip to the desired nail shape. To apply the nail form, position it so that it rests under the free edge and extends past the natural nail. Press the adhesive tabs at the sides of the fingers with your thumb and index finger. Check that the form is snug under the free edge of the nail (Figure 21.28).
9. Lightly apply a second coat of primer if required by the manufacturer.
10. Pour acrylic liquid into a small (dappen) dish. Dip the brush into the liquid mixture, wipe excess material from one side of the brush against the side of the bowl. Immediately dip the tip of brush into the powder. Rotate the brush slightly and draw it toward yourself to form a smooth ball of acrylic at the tip of brush.

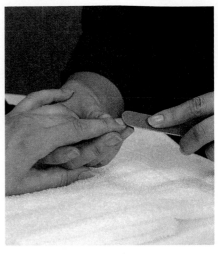

21.25   Roughen nail plate

CLIENT   T I P ◆◆◆◆◆◆◆

Use nail forms to correct nail problems. If your client has a nail that grows to one side, place the form extending straight out. If the free edge flips up, curves down, flairs out, or grows into the sides, file it or clip straight across and adjust the form to create the shape of extension desired. The pressure of the acrylic nail will encourage the nail to grow straight.

◆SAFETY P R E C A U T I O N◆

Prepare the nail file by smoothing the edges with another file. This removes sharp edges that could injure your client.

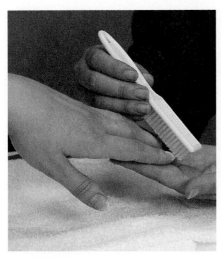

21.26   Dust nails

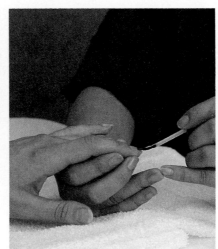

21.27

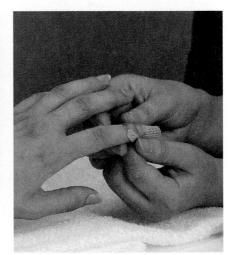

21.28

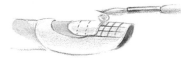

21.29   Place ball on free edge

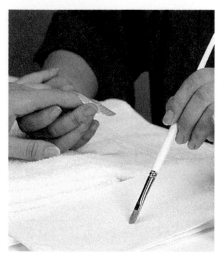

21.30

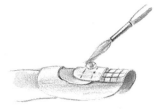

21.31   Place ball on center of nail

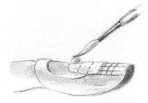

21.32   Place ball at base of nail

11. With the brush almost flat against the nail, place the ball of acrylic on the tip of the free edge of the nail (Figure 21.29). Lift brush and pat the ball into a square or rectangle shape. Work from the stress line (the free edge) out to the length desired. Make sure that the nail extension is not wider than the natural nail at the side.

12. Wipe brush on manicure mat or paper towel to remove excess product (Figure 21.30).

13. Start to form the second ball by immersing the brush in the liquid and stroking away excess on side of dappen dish. Dip brush in powder, making ball of desired size on tip of brush.

14. Clean brush against mat.

15. Apply ball to the center of the nail (Figure 21.31). Press ball down and lift brush quickly, patting the product into shape. Hold brush at a 45 degree angle so you are using the tip. Begin light strokes forward, toward and across the free edge. Clean nail groove as necessary with the tip of brush.

16. The third ball you form should be extremely wet. Apply to the area at the base of the nail, avoiding the cuticle (Figure 21.32). Press down quickly and stroke product from cuticle to free edge.

17. Reinforce stress area between the second and the third balls with a small wet product ball.

18. Use the sides of the thumbs to apply pressure to the stress area of the nail, creating a C curve. Apply this pressure right before product is set or when it becomes cloudy and is no longer sticky. (Some manufacturers do not recommend this step. Follow directions for best results.)

19. Tap nail surfaces gently with brush handle to see if product is set. Nails should sound hollow. Remove nail forms.

20. File the nail. Use a coarse grit file to form the nail straight out from the side wall (Figure 21.33).

21. File the free edge. Create the shape desired by your client (Figure 21.34).

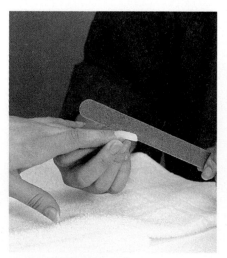

21.33   File sides of nails

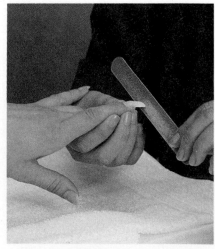

21.34   File free edge

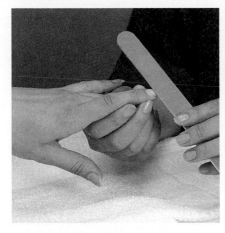

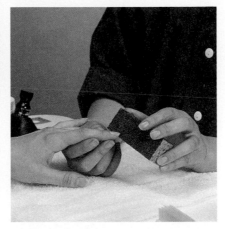

21.35   Shape base of nail   21.36   Buff nails

22. Use a medium-grit file to form the area at the base of the nail and across the contour of the nail bed (Figure 21.35).
23. Buff all nails. Apply cuticle oil to the surface of the nails and cuticles. Use block buffer to shine (Figure 21.36).
24. Cleanse fingers. Dip fingers in the water bath and brush nails firmly with a downward motion.
25. Polish nails as desired.
26. Sanitize work area and disinfect all implements. Break disposable files and discard all used materials.

Gel Nails

Acrylic nails can also be formed using gel systems that are either cured by light or sprayed with a catalyst. Consult manufacturer's directions and discuss the features and benefits of these systems with your instructor.

Fiberglass Nails

Fiberglass nails are formed by combining an acrylic system with a catalyst (often in the form of a spray). Most fiberglass systems offer the benefit of being odor free. Consult manufacturer's directions and discuss the features and benefits of these systems with your instructor.

Tips and Extensions

The length of the natural nail can also be extended by the use of tips. This method is sometimes preferred because it is faster than sculptured nails. The tips themselves are prefabricated nails used as extensions. They are available in many shapes and sizes.

Materials

In addition to the materials for a plain manicure you will need:

Non-acetone polish remover	Block buffer
Acetone or glue remover	Large clippers
Glue	Ridge filler
Tips (in various sizes)	Primer

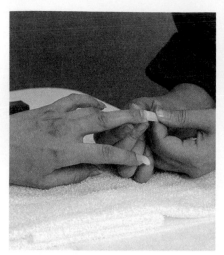

21.37 Select tip

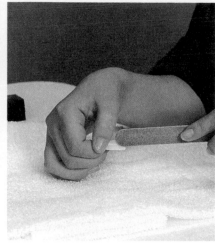

21.38 Etch tip

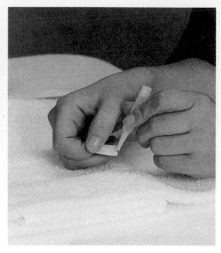

21.39 Apply glue to tip

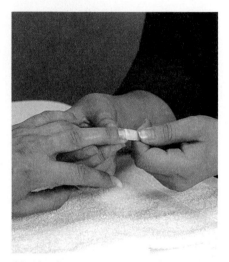

21.40 Press tip on nail

Procedure for Applying Tips

1. Select tip to match the width of the natural nail at the free edge (Figure 21.37).
2. Etch the underside of the nail tip with the nail file so it will adhere well (Figure 21.38).
3. Prime and etch the nail as manufacturer directs.
4. Apply glue to base of nail tip (Figure 21.39). Grip nail tip at free edge. Press the tip to natural nail (Figure 21.40), covering no more than one-third of the nail plate. The ridge of the tip must seal to the free edge of the natural nail.
5. Cut tip to desired length with large clippers.
6. Shape free edge.
7. Smooth the seam between the tip and natural nail with a medium-grit file.
8. Dust acrylic debris from nail with brush.
9. Apply glue as directed to strengthen the nail.
10. Apply oil and buff with block buffer.

> **CLIENT TIP ◆◆◆◆◆◆◆**
>
> After tip application, proceed with a wrap or acrylic overlap if you wish.

> **CLIENT TIP ◆◆◆◆◆◆◆**
>
> Many nail problems can be avoided with good care. Advise your customer to have professional manicures on a regular basis and avoid filing into the corners of the nails (this practice can cause splits below the free edge). Encourage your clients to allow the sides of their nails to grow or only file the free edge to a gentle oval.

Repair Techniques

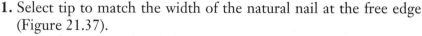

In spite of the best of care, nails will occasionally split, crack, or break. There are a variety of repair techniques available to you. Here we will discuss the basic repair techniques.

Nail Wrap Techniques

A manicure incorporating wrapping the natural nail with paper, fiberglass, silk, or linen can be preventive, strengthening, or corrective. The procedures vary slightly according to the product selected.

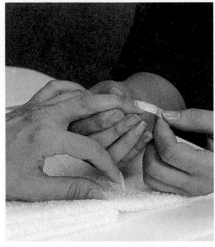

21.41 Place material on nail

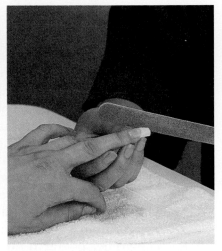

21.42 File off excess material

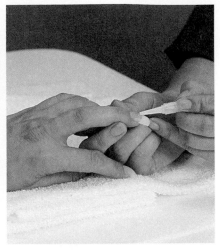

21.43 Reinforce nail with glue

Materials

In addition to the materials for a plain manicure you will need:

Non-acetone polish remover
Wrap material (silk, linen, paper, fiberglass)
Ridge filler
Glue

Accelerator spray or liquid
Primer
Block buffer

Procedure for Nail Wrapping

1. Perform plain water manicure. Dip nails in the bath to remove any film, but do not soak the nails.
2. Remove oil shine from natural nails by etching.
3. Apply antiseptic to natural nail.
4. Select mending material; cut and glue in place over natural nail (Figure 21.41).
5. Bevel off excess material by filing (Figure 21.42).
6. Reinforce with glue or acrylic as directed (Figure 21.43).
7. Apply accelerator if suggested by manufacturer (Figure 21.44).
8. Shape and buff nail using a medium-grit file.
9. Apply oil and buff with block buffer.

21.44 Apply accelerator

Fill-ins

When your client opts for extensions or sculptured nails, you should immediately schedule a series of fill-in appointments. A fill-in is the application of nail-extension products to the new growth area. It is very important that the client receive fill-ins on a regular basis to avoid lifting of the artificial nail. Lifting can lead to nail damage and the growth of mold and fungus. The following is a maintenance procedure for acrylic or sculptured nails.

Materials

Nail forms
Acrylic powder(s)
Acrylic liquid
Dappen dishes
Paper towels

Sable brush
Emery files in
      various grits
Buffer disks
Primer

Antiseptic
Brush cleaner
Oil

◆SAFETY **P R E C A U T I O N**◆

Do not stick the point of the nippers under the nail product. This will cause it to become loose. Prying off the artificial nail will make the natural nail thin and sensitive. Nip only where necessary. Remove the artificial nail if it is too loose.

CLIENT T I P ◆◆◆◆◆◆◆

Schedule the next appointment before your nail client leaves the salon. Send reminder notices to any client who misses an appointment.

Procedure for Fill-ins

1. Sanitize your hands and those of your client.
2. Remove polish.
3. Nip any loose product at the base of the nail.
4. Etch the artificial nail for adherence. Smooth the ridge of the extension where it meets the natural nail.
5. Prepare any cracks or breaks in the artificial nail by using a file to create a V in the product. File flush with the natural nail at the point of the break.
6. Gently push back cuticle and etch natural nail near base.
7. Dust with the brush to remove debris.
8. Apply primer to new growth area of natural nail. Slightly overlap acrylic onto extension. Let primer dry.
9. Reapply primer lightly, if directed, and then immediately apply acrylic ball at the growth area. Use an additional ball if necessary to reinforce stress point. Apply a thin layer of acrylic along the length of the nail.
10. File and buff nail.

TABLE 21.1 Trouble - Shooter Guide for Nail Problems	
Problem	*Treatment*
Dry Cuticles	Give reconditioning manicure.
Split Nails	Give reconditioning manicure. Etch edges of splits and apply acrylic product.
Peeling Nails	Gently buff peeling nail. Apply wrap to strengthen natural nail.
Lifted Sculptured Nail	Clip lifted area. Proceed with fill-in procedure.
Mold (Pseudomonas Aeruginosa)	Remove any artificial nail product. Thoroughly sanitize natural nail and refer client to a physician.
Fungus (Tinea Ungium)	Remove any artificial nail product. Thoroughly sanitize natural nail and refer client to a physician.
Hangnails	Give reconditioning manicure.
Bitten Nails	Schedule regular manicures. Keep natural nails short and treat rough areas on fingertips. Suggest nail extensions.
Crooked Nails	File natural nails to camouflage distortion. Apply nail forms for acrylic nails to create straight nails. Adjust polish technique to create illusion of a straight nail.
Allergic Reaction	Immediately refer client to a physician. Soak fingertips in baking soda solution. Remove artificial nails and polish as physician directs.

Removing Sculptured Nails

You may choose to remove sculptured nail product for many reasons. Sculptured nails need to be removed if they are very loose. You may also want to remove sculptured nails from clients who have had extensions applied and feel that their natural nails are grown out. Sculptured nails should be removed if you or your client suspect allergic reaction. The client should first be referred to a physician or a dermatologist. Of course your client may simply choose to discontinue wearing sculptured nails.

Procedure to Remove Sculptured Nails

1. Sanitize your hands and those of your client.
2. Pour acetone or recommended nail remover into a glass bowl.
3. Place fingers into bowl. Soak according to manufacturer's directions.
4. Remove fingers from the bowl and gently file away softened product.
5. Wash hands of all traces of nail remover. Resanitize your hands and those of your client.
6. Proceed with manicure or other nail technique.

> **◆ Key Point ◆**
> Proper maintenance will help your clients grow long healthy nails without danger of mold or fungus.

Pedicure Techniques

The word pedicuring comes from the Latin *ped, pedis* meaning "foot," and *cura*, meaning "care." Basic pedicuring techniques cleanse and relax the feet while smoothing rough skin and long nails.

Plain Pedicure

A pedicure may be considered a luxury treatment. It makes the feet feel more comfortable and helps to eliminate rough scales. It also beautifies the feet and toenails and is therefore an important part of the total grooming effort.

Materials

Pan with warm water	Manicure towel	Neck strip
Disinfectant solution	Cuticle softener	Hand lotion or foot cream
Orangewood sticks	Cuticle cream	70% alcohol
Toenail nippers	Polish remover	Two terry towels
Cuticle nippers	Sterile cotton	Antiseptic
Emery board	Nail polish	Antimicrobial soap

Arrange materials needed on a manicure table or a commercial pedicure machine. Seat the client comfortably. Place one terry towel on the floor near the client's right foot and the other near the left. Have the client remove the shoes and hose or socks. Fill the pan with the required amount of antiseptic solution (according to state

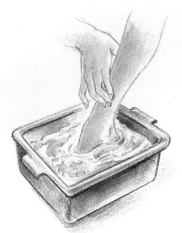

21.45 Foot bath

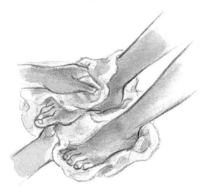

21.46 Dry foot

requirements) and warm water. Place a towel over your lap to protect your clothing. Cleanse your hands and your client's feet before beginning the pedicure. Most pedicurists begin work on the left foot and continue on the right.

Procedure for a Pedicure

1. Soak the client's first foot in the disinfectant solution for 3 or 4 minutes (Figure 21.45). The other foot remains on a towel placed on the floor or on the leg rest of the pedicure chair.
2. Dry the first foot, holding it in your lap while drying or place it on the leg rest of the pedicure chair (Figure 21.46).
3. Remove nail polish from the first foot (Figure 21.47).
4. Shape the nails by filing them straight across (Figure 21.48). If the nails are long, shorten them with the toenail clippers and then file to smooth the edges.
5. Place the second foot in the disinfectant solution.
6. Use cuticle softener around the nails of the first foot. Work gently to remove excess cuticle, using a cotton-tipped orangewood stick (Figure 21.49). Do not use a steel cuticle lifter, because the toe could easily be injured.
7. Apply cuticle cream and massage it into the cuticle around the nail.
8. Clean under the free edge of the nail with the cotton-tipped orangewood stick.
9. Apply hand lotion or foot cream and massage the foot, paying special attention to rough areas such as the heels (see foot massage).
10. Dry the second foot.
11. Repeat steps 2 through 9 on the second foot.
12. Hold the first foot at the edge of the pan, using the nail brush to remove the cuticle cream.
13. Trim the cuticle with cuticle nippers if necessary.

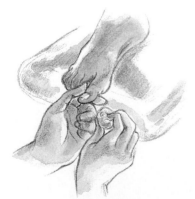

21.47 Remove polish

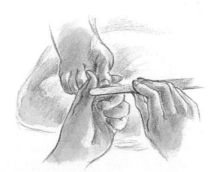

21.48 Shape nails

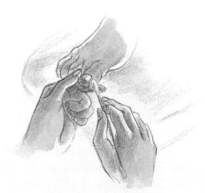

21.49 Apply cuticle softener

14. Space the toes, using folded neck strip or cotton strips between them (Figure 21.50).
15. Use alcohol to clean the surface of the toenails.
16. Apply base coat.
17. Repeat steps 12 through 16 on the second foot.
18. Apply nail polish to the toes of both feet.
19. Allow polish to dry thoroughly. Wait 15 or 20 minutes before allowing the client to put shoes on.
20. Clean up: Wash tools with soap and water and then disinfect them. Discard all materials that cannot be disinfected.

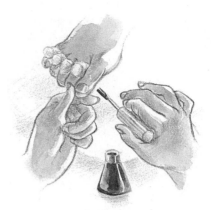

21.50   Apply polish

Foot Massage

Procedure for Foot Massage

1. Apply lotion or cream to the foot.
2. Start by placing both thumbs on the top of the foot, bracing the instep with the fingers on the bottom of the foot. Using a firm rotating movement, work down to the center of the toes (Figure 21.51).
3. Slide back to the instep and repeat the same movement.
4. Continue to massage until you have covered the top of the foot completely.
5. Holding the client's foot with your left hand, rotate each toe three times (Figure 21.52).
6. With the foot in an upward position, massage the sole of the foot from the heel to the toes by rotating in small circles with your thumbs.
7. Slide your right hand to the ankle and rotate the foot (Figure 21.53).
8. Repeat steps 1 through 7 on the other foot.

> ◆ **Key Point** ◆
>
> Pedicures are especially enjoyed by clients who are athletes or who work on their feet. Offer services to a local team to begin your client base.

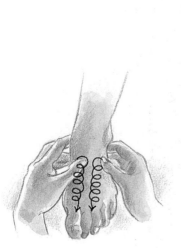

21.51

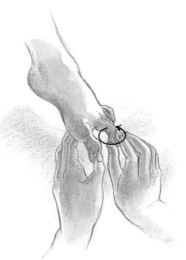

21.52

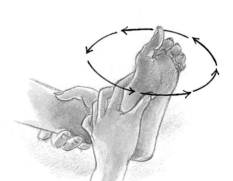

21.53

INFECTION CONTROL FOR THE NAIL SPECIALIST

1. Sanitize the work area before and after each client.
2. Sanitize your hands, then those of your client.
3. Never work on an area that shows signs of infection (is red, swollen, or has pus).
4. Remove all cosmetics from jars and bottles with a sanitized spatula.
5. Keep all sanitized implements submerged in an approved disinfectant. Wipe any debris from an implement before returning it to the disinfectant solution.
6. Use a primer before the application of an artificial nail.
7. Encourage your client to have frequent fill-in services to avoid lifting, breaking, or peeling.
8. Etch the nail before the application of acrylic to avoid lifting and remove shine.
9. Sanitize the natural nail with an approved antiseptic.
10. Discard all disposable materials after each manicure. Break paper emery boards in front of your client or give them to client for use at home.
11. Use files that can be cleaned and disinfected for artificial nails.
12. Remove all artificial products if there are any signs of mold, fungus, or allergic reaction. White patches on the nail, yellow streaks under the nail, and a thickening of the nail itself can indicate fungus. Dark streaks or green spots often indicate mold.
13. Do not cut cuticle unless absolutely necessary. Follow guidelines established by your state board if a cut occurs.

SAFETY FOR THE NAIL TECHNICIAN

The Occupational Safety and Health Administration (OSHA) protects both you and your client. As a professional nail technician, you should keep abreast of the latest information from the Food and Drug Administration regarding approved ingredients for nail care products.

Air quality is of critical concern to the nail specialist. Offer your services in a well-ventilated area of the salon or school. Ventilation must remove fumes and infuse fresh air. Research the latest products to find those with lower odor, fewer fumes, and safer ingredients. Protect yourself from dust with a mask and offer one to your client.

Schedule time between appointments to get outside and to enjoy the fresh air. Offering nail services can be enjoyable, profitable, and safe if you follow basic guidelines of infection control and product awareness.

Keep all products off the skin. Keep bottles capped when not in use to avoid spills. Do not use liquids directly from the bottle. Pour into a secondary dispenser to avoid contaminating the product.

SUMMARY

Nail services are presently the fastest-growing cosmetology services. To become an active manicurist, you must be able to select the proper implement and use it correctly to obtain the result your client wishes.

The basis of all nail techniques is the plain, or water, manicure. You should be proficient in the procedure and be able to adapt your techniques for reconditioning manicures. Hand and arm massage will be used to complete any nail service.

Artificial nail techniques are expanding. Your ability to provide sculpturing, gel, fiberglass, and tip and extension services will increase customer satisfaction. You must be able to provide nail repair services such as fill-ins, wraps, and the removal of artificial nails.

Infection control is critical for the nail and pedicure technician. You will identify disorders, mold, and fungus, determining what you can service and what must be referred to a physician for treatment.

QUESTIONS

1. Describe the implements, equipment, and cosmetics you would set up at your station before performing a basic manicure service. What have you included that is not mentioned at the beginning of this chapter. Why?
2. What are the procedures for a basic manicure and a man's manicure?
3. When is it appropriate to offer a client a full hand-and-arm massage?
4. What are the common procedures for all nail applications, including the sculptured, fiberglass, and tip techniques?
5. How do repair techniques differ for acrylic and for fragile nails?
6. How would you perform a pedicure?
7. What is the importance of safety precautions for you and your client during nail care procedures?
8. What are the safety requirements for the nail salon? How are they important to your safety?

PROJECTS

1. Research products for basic manicure services from at least three manufacturers. Compare the ingredients and discuss the effects of the ingredients on hands and nails.
2. Perform at least 6 men's and 6 reconditioning manicures. Give at least 12 plain water manicures.
3. Perform hand-and-arm massages on at least 6 clients.
4. Compare various artificial nail techniques. On a sheet of paper, list the features and benefits of each. For each technique, list the products available in the school and any special instructions.
5. Prepare procedure sheets for each repair technique for both natural and artificial nails.
6. Obtain Material Safety Data Sheets for the products used in your school. Compile them in a safety manual for use after you graduate. Complete the safety information by listing all emergency procedures and numbers.

ELECTRICITY AND THE COSMETOLOGY SALON

22

CHAPTER GOAL

The modern salon cannot function without electricity. As a cosmetologist, you must know how electricity works in order to maintain a safe environment for yourself and your clients. After reading this chapter and completing the projects, you should be able to

1. Explain how electricity is produced by the two steady currents.
2. Outline how electricity is measured for safe operation of a particular piece of equipment. How is that measurement reflected on a utility bill?
3. List the three major uses of electricity in the salon and how they are applied.
4. List the three most common electrical hazards in the salon. Explain how each situation can happen.
5. Explain the steps to take in case of an electrical outage in the salon.

Energy. It's needed for everything. It is really what makes the world function. And it is critical in your life and in the salon in which you will work. Electricity is the principal form of energy that is used to control the environment of the school and the salon. It is also the energy source for equipment that you will use from blow dryers to lights to air purifiers to temperature control. Electricity even works overtime to protect the salon from break-ins and to advertise around the clock.

As a cosmetologist, you don't have to be an electrical wizard. But you should know how to operate the equipment and safety precautions related to electricity. Electricity should be treated with the matter-of-fact respect that comes from understanding. By knowing the full capabilities and limitations of the equipment you use, you strengthen your professional skills and your career.

ELECTRICITY AND ELECTRIC CURRENT

Electricity is a form of energy. It is sent through wires by means of a flow of tiny particles called electrons. (Refresh your understanding of electrons by referring again to Chapter 13.) The flow of electrons is known as **electric current**. The unique thing about electricity is that it is a directed movement of electrons creating a current. By *directed*, we mean that all the electrons move in the same direction at a given moment. The more electrons that are in motion, the stronger the current. Electron currents can be momentary or steady. We are interested only in steady currents for cosmetology. (Radios, televisions, and stereos use momentary currents.) There are two types of steady current: **direct current** and **alternating current**.

In direct current (DC), the electrons move only in one direction all the time. The electron flow is something like water flowing through a garden hose, in one end and out the other. DC current is most commonly provided by batteries, and is used in some specialized facial and hair removal equipment.

In alternating current (AC), the electrons move in one direction for a short period of time, then reverse their direction and move the opposite way for an equal amount of time. This change of direction occurs many times each second. Picture these electrons as tennis balls played side by side at the same time in many games. All would serve from the left at the same time, and return from the right together. Now, speed the game to fast forward until the serves and returns happen several times per second! AC current is the common household current in the United States. It is what you use whenever you plug a blow dryer or a curling iron into an outlet.

Current can be changed from DC to AC, or vice versa, by special devices. An **inverter**, for example, changes DC to AC. A **rectifier**, on the other hand, changes AC to DC. You will use these more often when you are on vacation in foreign countries and want to style your hair than you will in the professional salon. Most salon equipment that uses DC current is designed to be used in a regular outlet. The current is converted as needed inside the equipment to perform the function desired.

Producing Electric Current

Remember that an electric current is a movement of electrons. How is this movement produced? For an electric current to exist, two conditions must be met:

1. There must be a closed path for the electrons to move upon.
2. Somewhere in that path, a device must give the electrons a push.

In some ways, electric current is like water. To get water to go where we want, we have to provide a pipe or a channel, and then some sort of pump to push it through.

A **circuit** (**SIR** kut) is the closed path that electric current follows. The "pump" in the circuit is the **source**. The device to be operated, that needs the current, is the **load**. Figure 22.1 is a simple diagram of an electric circuit.

The arrows around the outside of the diagram show the movement of the electrons. Notice that the path is closed. The electrons leave the source, travel through one wire to the load, pass through the load, and return to the source through the other wire. If there is a break anywhere in the path, the current will stop immediately. It will start again, and continue, when the break is mended. That is why the word *closed* is so important. This is also why there are two wires in every electric cord and two prongs on the plug. One wire brings the electrons into the device, and the other provides a path back to the source. (The third prong, a safety device on larger and new equipment is a safety device discussed later in this chapter.)

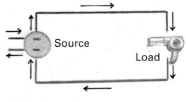

22.1 A circuit

Conductors and Insulators

What makes a good "pipe" for the flow of electric current? The most important factor is the material the pipe is made from. A material that allows current to flow easily is called a **conductor** (kun **DUCK** tor). All metals make good conductors. Silver is the best, and is used for critical parts in some electrical equipment. Copper is a close second, and is commonly used for most electric wiring. Carbon and water solutions containing ions (see Chapter 13) are weak conductors.

The human body is mostly composed of water and dissolved salts. Your skin can conduct a weak electric current.

A material that will not permit electric current to flow is called an **insulator** (inn **SUH** lay tor). Wood, glass, paper, brick, plastic, cloth, and rubber are common examples. Rubber and plastic are commonly used as insulators and cover the conducting wires of electrical appliances. The insulating material keeps the two wires from touching each other, and gives you the ability to handle the equipment safely.

Electrical Sources

As we said, every electrical circuit needs a "pump" to give the electrons a push to start the flow of current. This pump is called the source. Every source must have at least one pair of terminals where the wires connect. Although there are many kinds of electrical sources, as a professional cosmetologist you will only be concerned with two: batteries and wall sockets.

A **battery** is a DC source of electricity. This means that one of its terminals is always positive and the other is always negative. You will notice when you insert batteries into your Walkman® or camera a diagram directing you to place the positive pole in the correct position. If you do not, your flash won't operate. The charges at the terminals are created by a chemical reaction going on inside the battery. When these chemicals are used up, no more charge is produced and the battery is pronounced "dead."

A generator is actually the source of AC power, even though we think of the source as the electrical outlet. A generator is a rotating machine that produces electricity from mechanical energy. You have a little brother to the generators creating salon power in the battery of your car. Generators also have two terminals. At any given moment, one is positive and one is negative. When you insert the prongs of a plug into an outlet, you connect to these terminals. These charges are not permanent, however, and constantly alternate from positive to negative and back to positive. This chain of happenings is called a **cycle**. The number of cycles that occur in one second is called the **frequency** of the generator. In the United States, all commercial AC generators are designed to produce exactly 60 cycles in one second. The nameplate of an American appliance will usually say "60-cycle" or "60 Hz (Hertz)" on it to indicate the frequency. If an AC appliance is used on a current of the wrong frequency, it will not work properly and may even be damaged.

MEASURING ELECTRICITY

For most professional salon services, accurately measuring the amount of a chemical or solution is important. You will learn how much color is needed, for example, to mix with a certain amount of activator to cover gray hair. You will need to know how much conditioner is needed for long hair. Electricity, too, has its measurements. The name of one of those measurements is already familiar: **cycle**. A

◆ Key Point ◆

To produce an electric current, we must have a circuit. This circuit includes a source, a load, and two connecting wires. If the source is a wall outlet, alternating current is used. If the source is a battery, direct current is used.

cycle (per second) is the unit for measuring the frequency of alternating current. We will be using five more units of measurement: amps, volts, ohms, watts and kilowatt-hours. You may already be familiar with some of these measures from your utility bills. Let's take a look and see what they mean. And even more important, let's see what they mean to the operation of a salon.

The most basic measurement of an electric circuit is the amount of current flowing. An **ampere** (**AM** peer), or amp, is the unit that tells how much current is passing through the circuit.

How much current flows through a given circuit depends upon the strength of the source, or its ability to push electrons. How much push or pressure the source can give to each electron is measured in **volts.**

Batteries produce low voltage. This is because they depend on the energy from the chemical reactions taking place inside them. For example, your Walkman® batteries produce only 1.5 volts each. A basic flashlight uses larger, C, batteries that can produce current longer but still only provide 1.5 volts. A car battery only produces 12 volts. The wall socket that provides energy to your salon, on the other hand, provides 110 to 120 volts. This is why you use your electric sockets when at home, and only use the batteries when you are away from a regular power source. Very large equipment, such as heating and air conditioning units use 240-volt outlets for safety and to reduce cost.

Ohms are a unit of resistance, or friction. This naturally occurs because of the difficulty of the electrons to travel along the conductor. Ohm's law states

$$ohms = \frac{volts}{amperes}$$

By the same method, you can determine the amount of current by using the formula

$$amperes = \frac{volts}{ohms}$$

This is important if you want to be an electrical engineer, or design the wiring for your future salon. As a cosmetologist, you should know the basics of electricity and apply that knowledge to assure safety for yourself, your client, and the salon.

The next important quantity to talk about is power. Electrical power is measured in **watts**. This tells you how fast energy is being used. One watt represents a small amount of energy. A basic curling iron uses electric energy at 20 times that rate. Most blow dryers are 1500 watt. The implements in the salon use power so fast that it makes no sense to measure usage in watts. You will see a reading on the salon electric bill of the term **kilowatt** (1,000 watts). Your bill will compute your expense by how many kilowatts are used per hour. If you use, for example, a 1500-watt blow dryer for 8 hours a day, you would be billed for 12 kilowatts of energy.

To understand power, ask yourself two questions. How much power (electrical source) do you have and how much (load) do you need? Figure 22.2 shows the information found on the nameplate of an appliance. First, the manufacturer's name and address are given. Next, the power drawn (wattage) and operating voltage are listed. The appliance in Figure 22.2 draws about 650 watts of power and is designed to operate on 120-volt AC current. The frequency, 60-cycle, is often given. When you are purchasing equipment, look for the Underwriters Laboratories symbol (UL) . This group, supported by the underwriters of fire insurance, has examined the design and construction of the unit to be sure that reasonable care has been taken to make it safe from fire and shock hazards.

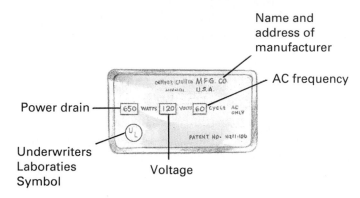

22.2   Appliance nameplate

ELECTRICITY AND SALON SERVICES

Electric current is used to produce a number of different effects for salon services. In the salon, you will be most concerned with **heating** effects, **mechanical** effects, and **chemical** effects.

Heating Effects with Electricity

If you rub your hands together, they get warm. This shows how mechanical energy is changed by friction (rubbing) into heat energy. In a similar way, the rubbing of electrons in the electrical current against the conductor produces heat energy. When an electrical load is connected to a source, current flows. The greater the friction, the more heat is produced. Electrical appliances such as curling irons and heat lamps use this energy to heat an element. Other appliances, such as clippers, do not need the heat to operate and are designed to cool off the heat as soon as possible.

Mechanical Effects with Electricity

Magnetic fields are generated around conductors. Properly arranged magnetic fields create a push-pull effect between positive and negative poles. When this happens, mechanical motion is produced.

◆ Key Point ◆

Electric current is measured in amps, which represent how many electrons per second move through the circuit. The electric energy that you pay for is measured in kilowatt-hours.

Motors in your blow dryers, clippers, fans, and massage equipment produce motion with magnetic fields.

Chemical Effects with Electricity

Chemical effects involve the human body and its ionic solutions. The chemical effect of atoms moving toward or away from the point of contact is known as **phoresis** (for **EEZ** ees). In the salon, phoresis occurs when specialized electrical equipment for facial treatment or hair removal is used. These specialties require specialized training. We will discuss only the basics.

Anaphoresis (**ANN** uh FOR eez ees) is the process of forcing liquids into the skin from the negative toward the positive pole. Galvanic current can be used to stimulate the skin. When used for deep cleansing the skin and for electrolysis, a negative electric current creates a chemical effect. In the first, ingrained dirt is dissolved and in the second, the papilla of the hair follicle is destroyed for permanent hair removal.

Cataphoresis (**CAT** uh FOR eez ees) is the forcing of solutions into the skin from the positive toward the negative pole. This is used in specialized skin care services to force an astringent, or acid solution into the skin.

> ### ◆ Key Point ◆
> Electricity in the salon is used to create heat, mechanical, and chemical effects. Heat effects are commonly used in thermal styling. Mechanical effects are applied with fans and clippers. Chemical effects are restricted to specialized treatments for skin and for the permanent removal of unwanted hair.

ELECTRICAL HAZARDS

Electricity is a form of energy. It is not one that you should fear, nor is it a force that you should take lightly. A matter-of-fact respect is the healthiest approach to electricity.

Overloading

The most common cause of electrical problems is that of overloading. As cosmetologists, we use many electrical appliances and often have several in use at the same time. If the salon is not equipped to handle the load of appliances we use, an overload results. Let's see what we can do to prevent such a common electrical problem.

You will recall that an electrical circuit is a closed path for current to travel from a source to a load and back again to the source. The amount of current flowing through the circuit is measured in amperes. Overloading occurs when more current is drawn from the circuit than it was designed for. If, for example, all the appliances plugged into one circuit drain 25 amps, and the circuit was designed to only handle 20 amps, the circuit will overload. If there are no safety devices to break the circuit, the wires in the walls and the electrical equipment will become very hot. If the circuit still does not break, fire will occur, the equipment will be destroyed, the salon damaged, and your safety will be endangered.

> ### ◆SAFETY PRECAUTION◆
> Avoid an overload by spreading large appliances over several circuits. Avoid using extension cords or plugging too many high-wattage appliances into the same circuit.

> ### ◆SAFETY PRECAUTION◆
> Never use implements that have exposed wiring or plastic cording that is cracked. Select equipment for purchase that has a protective cushion where the cord enters the appliance. Never wrap the cord tightly around the base; leave a loop where the cord leaves the housing.

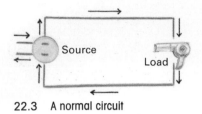

22.3   A normal circuit

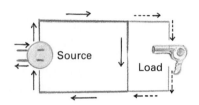

22.4   An overloaded circuit

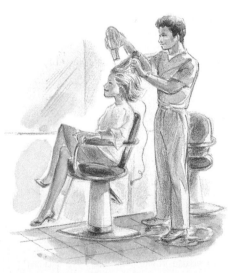

22.5   Do not stand in water

Short Circuits

Figure 22.3 shows a typical appliance operating normally. The current is flowing in a normal fashion from the source to the load and back again.

But, what happens if the insulation of your blow dryer cord is wearing? What if the stress area of the cord, right at the bottom of the handle is cracked? If this happens, the wires can work loose, even if the outside of the cord is not completely broken. The return wire touches the supply wire. This bypasses the load. Watch what happens in Figure 22.4.

The power leaves the source, traveling to the load. Where the wires touch, however, the power is short-circuited, meaning that it jumps past the load and begins the return to the source. But since the power has not been drained by the load, the amount returning is too strong for the wiring and overheats it. The dryer will smoke and begin to burn, and you or your client could very well get a nasty shock.

Grounding

Another hazard of concern to the stylist is one in which the power leaves its source, but is grounded out. What does that mean? How could it happen?

In the salon, we work around water all the time. Sometimes, water even gets on the floor. If we do not follow safe and sanitary procedures to remove it, we run the risk of electric shock. In Figure 22.5, the power will leave the source just as always. But, if the appliance is wet, or if the stylist is standing in water, power can be pulled from the circuit through the stylist's body. This usually does no harm to the equipment, but can give the stylist a nasty jolt.

Any of these electrical hazards can be easily avoided with sound safety habits and a good dose of common sense. There are also protective devices that should be in place in every salon to prevent fire, shock, and equipment damage.

SAFETY DEVICES FOR ELECTRICITY

We've talked about what could happen in unsafe situations or with a careless operator. But again, do not be fearful of the power that gives you the ability to make a living. Instead, familiarize yourself with the safety devices that should be built into the school and the salon. We'll also describe simple things that you can do to protect yourself and your customers in the salon.

Because of the potential danger of electricity, protection should be built right into the permanent wiring of buildings. This is part of the code that every building must meet before the owner can get a certificate of occupancy. Automatic devices designed to prevent fire or shock are described in the section that follows.

Fuses

A **fuse** is a wire link inside a plastic cap that will melt when it gets too warm. When this happens, the circuit is broken at the source and power is stopped from going along the path to the load. A fuse is a one-shot safety device and cannot be reused once it has blown. For that reason, wiring installed in recent years uses another safety device that is longer lasting. If your salon is in an older building, you may need to know about fuses in your day-to-day work.

When a fuse shuts off power to a circuit, it is actually a blessing in disguise. If the fuse had not blown, a fire would have occurred. To restore power safely, unplug or switch off as many items as possible on the failed circuit. Then, go to the electrical service panel—the metal box that houses the fuses. Your hands and the floor must be dry to avoid shock from faulty electrical components. As an added precaution, stand on a dry board or a rubber mat.

Open the panel door with one hand while keeping the rest of your body away from all other objects. To keep from touching another metal item while working, keep your other hand behind your back or in a pocket. Best yet, use it to hold the plastic flashlight that will help you see what you are doing.

The blown fuse will have a blackened window, or else a tiny metal strip visible through the window will be melted (Figure 22.6).

If the fuse is for a large appliance, it will be a cylinder. Before removing the fuse, shut off the main power switch, usually on the side of the box. Pull the blackened fuse with plastic pliers or tongs, and replace with one of identical rating with the pullers. Do not insert a higher rated fuse. That will only increase the fire hazard. Instead, change the appliances creating the overload to a different circuit.

Circuit Breakers

Most modern buildings are equipped with **circuit breakers**. These safety devices trip, or shut themselves off, when the load is excessive, yet can be reset for continued use. They are safer than fuses because they cannot be altered to temporarily restore power in a manner that is unsafe. Circuit breakers function much like a light switch. When the load does not exceed the source, the breaker remains in the ON position. When electrical demand is unsafe, the breaker will trip, breaking the circuit and shutting off the power. After you have unplugged the appliance that caused the problem, reset most circuit breakers by moving the switch to the OFF position, then back to ON.

The breaker that is tripped will be out of alignment with the others on the electrical panel (Figure 22.7).

Many times a red dot or other indication will also help you locate which breaker is tripped. Read the identifying chart next to the switch to determine where the problem lies and unplug appliances. If the circuit failed the instant an appliance was plugged in or a switch was turned on, the problem is probably a short circuit in that appliance. Unplug the appliance before power is returned and take it to a repair shop for inspection.

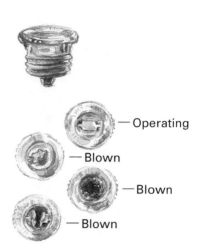

22.6   Electrical fuses

— Operating

— Blown

— Blown

— Blown

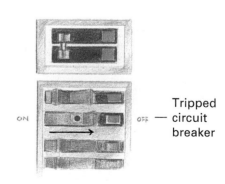

Tripped circuit breaker

22.7   Circuit breakers

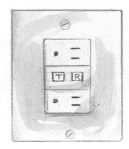

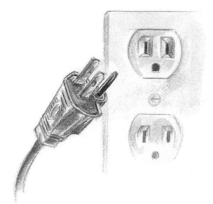

22.8　Ground fault interceptor

22.9　Grounding outlet

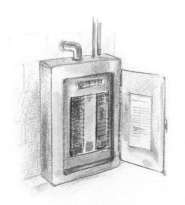

22.10

If the items on the circuit were working for at least a few minutes before the power failed, the problem is probably that too many appliances are plugged into the same circuit. To prevent the breaker from tripping again, move some of the equipment to another circuit. At the breaker box, move the switch of the thrown switch first to the OFF position, then to ON.

Any time that a fuse or a breaker switch continues to blow after the load has been reduced, call an electrician to inspect your system.

Ground Fault Interceptors

All new construction must provide GFIs or **Ground Fault Interceptors** in areas designed for heavy equipment, that have concrete floors, or that provide water. These safety devices are designed to protect you from electrical shock. You can identify a GFI outlet by the press switch in the center (see Figure 22.8).

If at any time, the amount of power returning to the source does not equal the amount going out, the GFI will recognize that electricity is being grounded (pulled from the path). At that point, the outlet itself will cut off before a circuit breaker trips. Grounding can easily be caused if you are standing on a wet floor, if the appliance is wet or dropped in water, or if there is a fault in the interior wiring. If the GFI pops, wrap your hand in a dry towel and unplug the appliance. Wait one to two minutes, then reset the outlet for use by pressing the reset button in the center. Take the appliance to a repair shop before attempting to use it again.

Grounding

Another safety device, called **grounding**, is the third prong on the plugs of larger and newer equipment (Figure 22.9).

This third prong is designed to run any misdirected electrical current to ground where it is absorbed, thereby preventing overheating of the wires and appliances. You should know, however, that the three-wire system has nothing to do with overloading, and will not prevent you from overusing a circuit. The purpose of the grounding safety device is to protect you from shock.

TROUBLE-SHOOTING

First let's see what we can do to avoid trouble. Locate the wall outlets in the school or salon and find out how much power they can provide. Determine how many blow dryers, curling irons, clippers, analysis lights, etc., can run off a particular circuit at one time. Know where the breaker box or fuse box is in case of emergency. It helps, in a dark stairway, to have a flashlight to guide you.

Another great timesaver is to have your electrical service box marked. On the door of most boxes, a blank chart is available (Figure 22.10). Fill it in with the outlets that run off each circuit. You can figure this by turning on all lights and running an appliance from each outlet. Then go to the box, flip one switch to the OFF position and make a notation of what outlets went without power. Turn that switch back on, and go to the next. Mark each breaker carefully, and make special note of the breakers that control the power to major equipment such as the furnace, air conditioner, or washing machine.

When a Breaker Trips

If you have just turned on an appliance, disconnect it. The problem is likely to stem from the use of that appliance. If you have been running equipment for a while without power interruption, the problem is likely to be an overload. Disconnect or turn off several appliances on the problem circuit.

1. Go to the breaker box and locate the breaker switch that is out of alignment. On some boxes, the flipped breaker will be marked in red (Figure 22.11).
2. Be sure that you are standing on dry flooring and that your hands are dry.
3. Push the breaker to ensure it is in the OFF position. If the switch feels warm, wait for it to cool.
4. Flip the switch to the ON position.
5. If power is restored, note the equipment that is not running and plug that equipment into an alternate circuit before using it. If the power immediately goes off again, disconnect more appliances, let the switch cool, and try again.
6. If power continues to be disrupted, call an electrician or the utility company.

When a Fuse Blows

Follow the steps outlined for basic safety.

1. Turn the main power switch at the box to the OFF position.
2. Locate the fuse that is blown by its blackened window or the broken filament.
3. Remove the blown fuse.
4. Replace it with a fuse of the same rating.
5. Turn the main switch back on and monitor the results.

Electric Shock

Electric shock is very rare in today's salon, thanks to the safety features of modern wiring and appliances. In the unlikely event that you or a client should suffer from electric shock, follow these guidelines:

1. Remove the source of electricity. Use an insulating material such as a wooden brush or a dry towel.
2. Disconnect the appliance, or turn the breaker switch for that circuit to the OFF position.
3. Call 911 or the Emergency Medical Service if your client is

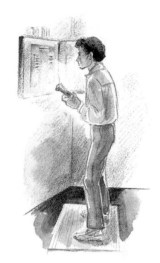

22.11

burned, unconscious, or in shock. If your client is in shock, do not move him or her.

4. Stay on the line with 911 for assistance while an ambulance is dispatched.

5. Remain calm and be prepared to give any information requested by the telephone operator. Follow instructions until help arrives.

Electrical Fire

Know the location of the fire extinguisher and how to operate it, even though the chances of you ever using it are slim. Be aware of the type of fire it is designed for. For electrical fires, the extinguisher should be marked ABC or BC. Never throw water on an electrical fire; the fire could spread and you could be electrocuted. Have the number of the fire department readily at hand for any emergency situation.

> **◆ Key Point ◆**
>
> Be prepared for any emergency in your salon. Have telephone numbers for help posted by the phone. Remain calm so you can give information while help is on the way. The odds of an emergency in your salon are slim, but precaution always pays.

Summary

Electricity is the energy source used to run the salon. It helps you create the environment you want with light, power, cooling, ventilation, and heat. Your key concern with electricity as a cosmetologist is one of safety. You want to be sure that you provide the salon atmosphere needed, and that you have the power to create styling effects without risking fire, damage to equipment, or electrical shock to either you or your client. Do not be afraid of electricity; but use it wisely.

Electricity moves from a supply source, along a circuit to the load, or demand point, and back again to the source. Electricity moves by means of conductors and is held within its circuit by insulators. Electricity is measured in kilowatts by the thousands of units per hour.

As a cosmetologist, you will establish safety procedures to prevent overloading the circuits. You will calculate the amount of electricity you need, and you will ensure that the circuit breaker or fuse can accommodate that amount. You will replace fuses or reset breakers when they blow due to overload after you have identified or removed the source of the problem.

You will have a listing of emergency numbers and established safety procedures to handle electrical problems in the salon.

Questions

1. How is electricity produced?
2. How is electricity measured for safe operation of a particular piece of equipment? How is the measurement reflected on a utility bill?
3. What effect does electrically generated heat have in salon services?
4. What are two major uses of electricity in the salon besides heat? Which effects do they have?

5. How does a circuit become overloaded?
6. How would you correct a circuit that has shorted?
7. What steps should you take in case of electrical outage in the salon?

PROJECTS

1. Identify the load that a particular breaker or fuse can handle in your school. Calculate the load that is placed on the breaker by the equipment that is running through it.
2. Describe the situation that could produce a short circuit in the school. Explain how that problem could be avoided and describe what you would do to correct the problem.
3. List the electrical equipment you have available. Indicate the effects each piece of equipment produces. Are they heating, mechanical, or chemical?
4. Develop a safe use procedure sheet for each piece of equipment available. Develop emergency procedures that should be followed in the event of an accident.

HEAT AND LIGHT

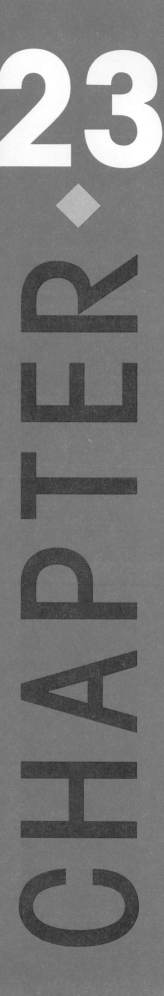

CHAPTER GOAL

Heat and light play important roles in the cosmetology salon. After reading this chapter and completing the projects, you should be able to

1. List the three different ways heat energy can be transmitted. Give an example of each.
2. Explain the electromagnetic spectrum, listing the bands and their functions.
3. List at least four devices that produce light, and describe the type of light generated.
4. Outline steps to protect yourself and your client when giving light treatments.
5. Explain the two main considerations when planning the lighting for your salon.

CAREER FOCUS

Heat and light have always been crucial to survival. In prehistoric times, heat and light from the sun meant life. The night, with its dangers and darkness, meant death. Virtually every early religion had some form of sun worship, celebrating the importance of heat and light for survival.

While we are certainly much more sophisticated and enjoy advanced technology, we are just as dependent on heat and light as our forebears. Can you imagine how your life would be without lighting, central heat, stoves, and microwaves? The modern salon uses heat and light extensively to establish a comfortable atmosphere, style and process hair, and treat nails and skin. Here we will explore various options for the safe and most efficient means of heating and lighting in the salon.

As a cosmetologist, you will work with both heat and light. You will describe to your clients the effect light from different sources has on the salon services you offer. You will be able to compensate for the effects of light on makeup and hair color. You will explain to your clients different ways to deal with the effects of heat and light in the salon, out of doors, at the office, or at home.

HEAT

Heat is a form of energy, just as electricity is a form of energy. *Heat energy is due to the motion of molecules.* A molecule is two or more atoms joined together by a chemical bond (see Chapter 13). In Chapter 22 we showed that electricity was due to the movement of electrons. Here, we are interested in energy that is related to the movement of whole molecules—that energy is heat.

Like any other form of energy, heat energy can be measured. In fact, you are probably already familiar with the unit of heat energy, the **calorie**, because this term comes up all the time in connection with diets. When we say that 1 tablespoon of butter contains 100 calories, what we really mean is that when this amount of butter is burned by the body, it can release 100 calories of heat energy. One calorie is the amount of heat required to raise the temperature of 1 gram of water by 1°C. So the 100 calories available from the tablespoon of butter would be enough to bring a gram of water from freezing to the boiling point.

Heat energy always flows from a hotter body to a cooler body. That's almost obvious, isn't it? If you place a hot object in contact with a cold one, you know that the hot one will get colder and the cold one hotter. The hot object will always give up heat to the colder one.

How Heat Energy Moves from One Object to Another

There are three different ways heat energy can get from a hot object to a cooler one: (a) conduction, (b) convection, and (c) radiation (Figure 23.1).

Conduction

Conduction refers to the transfer of heat by direct contact between hot and cool objects. This happens when you touch the hair with a curling iron. Conduction of heat is in many ways like the conduction of electricity. In fact, the materials that are good conductors of electricity—the metals—are also good conductors of heat; likewise, good electrical insulators are generally also good heat insulators.

Convection

Convection refers to the transfer of heat by means of a moving gas or liquid between a hot object and a cool one—for example, a stream of water or a current of air. Suppose you taste something you are cooking. You touch the hot food in the spoon with your tongue (conduction), and you burn your tongue. So what do you do to cool the food in the spoon quickly? You blow on it (convection), and the stream of cool air takes away the heat. A good example of heat transfer by convection is the hair dryer, and the cool object is the client's wet hair. The stream of air pushed by the dryer's fan takes heat from the hot coil by convection and then loses part of it, also by convection, to the wet hair.

Radiation

Radiation, the third means of transferring heat between two objects, occurs even when there is still air or empty space (such as a vacuum) between the objects. Some of the heat energy in the hot object is changed to **radiant energy**, which streams through space like light rays and then is changed back to heat energy when it strikes the cooler object. Radiation is most important when the hot object is much, much hotter than the cool object. If you hold your hand near (but not touching) a hot iron or a glowing light bulb, the sensation of warmth you feel is due to heat transferred to your hand by radiation. We will talk more about radiant energy later in this chapter.

How Heat Affects the Body

Scattered over the surface of the skin are special nerves that can sense the flow of heat. When heat flows out of the skin tissues, we get the sensation of coolness, and when heat flows in we get the sensation of warmth.

The human body operates within a very limited range of temperatures. Your body cannot stand to gain or lose very much heat. One of its main defenses is perspiration. If your body senses too much heat coming in, it slows down the rate at which it burns stored food, the pores open, and little drops of perspiration are released by the sweat glands in the skin. As the perspiration dries, it absorbs heat

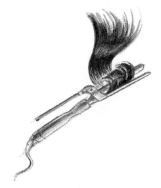

(a)   Conduction

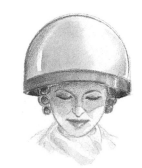

(b)   Convection

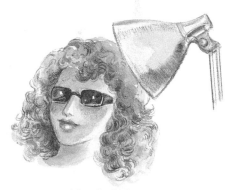

(c)   Radiation

23.1

◆ Key Point ◆

Heat is a form of energy used in the salon for drying, styling, and for speeding chemical processes.

---

from the skin and so cools your body. If the body senses too much heat being lost, the pores shut, perspiration stops, and the body steps up the rate at which it burns stored food, all of which warm you.

So far we have been talking about how heat affects the body generally. What happens when heat is applied locally to a particular part of the body? Mild heat can be very useful. It relaxes tissues, especially muscle tissue, and dilates (opens) blood vessels to increase the supply of blood to the tissue. It causes strands of hair to take a more or less permanent set, thus permitting waving and curling. Finally, heat always speeds up any chemical reaction, and so heat can be used to increase the effect of chemical solutions or shorten treatment times.

Intense heating of tissues can destroy them. The first effect of intense heat on the skin is to drive out water and oils—**desiccation**. Too much heat makes the skin dry and flaky and the hair brittle. Still greater heat causes **pyrolysis**—actual chemical breakdown under heat—which burns the skin and chars the hair. It does not take much heat for it to be considered "intense," so you must be extremely careful whenever you apply heat to the hair and body.

How Heat Is Produced

Heat is commonly produced in one of two ways: **electrically** or **chemically**. Chapter 22 explained how the flow of electric current in a conductor would produce heat. Where heat is required inside an electrical machine, a heating element is used. The metal wire or ribbon is wound on a material that is both an electric insulator and a heat insulator and that can also stand the high operating temperature.

Chemical heat sources are also used frequently. Many chemical reactions give off heat, the most obvious being the burning of a fuel with air. A chemical reaction between two liquids can sometimes release a lot of heat. Because this heat could harm hair or tender skin, you should always be very careful when mixing and applying solutions. Read the instructions thoroughly and be sure to follow any warnings or cautions noted in the manufacturer's directions.

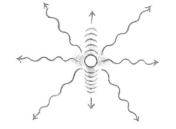

23.2   Electromagnetic radiation

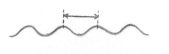

23.3   Wavelength

Light and Radiant Energy

Visible light is a very small part of something much broader called **radiant energy**. Radiant energy, like electricity, has to do with electrons. Whenever electrons vibrate (move rapidly back and forth over some path), they create ripply waves in the surrounding space which spread out at fantastic speed in all directions (Figure 23.2). The effect is similar to what happens when you drop a pebble into a still pond. The waves are called **electromagnetic radiation**, or **EMR** for short, and it is these waves that carry the radiant energy.

Each kind of wave has a particular **wavelength**, the distance between the top of one crest or peak and the next (Figure 23.3). The shorter the wavelength, the more radiant energy the wave can carry.

Electrons can be forced to move back and forth at almost any speed, and so the waves produced can have almost any wavelength. A collection of all the possible wavelengths is called the *spectrum of EMR*, or the **electromagnetic spectrum** (Figure 23.4).

In Figure 23.4, the longest waves are at the right, among the radio signals, and can actually be hundreds of miles long. As we move across the diagram to the left, the wavelengths become shorter and shorter. From radio signals, we pass into TV and FM signals and then into the waves used for radar. Next comes the group of wavelengths we call "light." As you can see, there are two kinds of invisible light in addition to the visible light that we see with our eyes. Passing beyond the "light" portion, we meet the X rays (like those the doctor uses to photograph the inside of your body) and finally the cosmic rays (high-energy waves coming from outer space). The wavelengths of cosmic rays are very short, unbelievably tiny fractions of an inch.

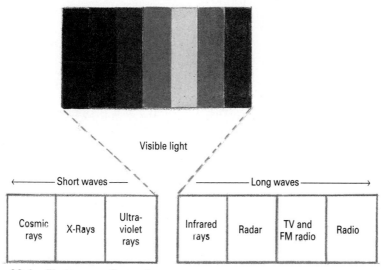

23.4   Electromagnetic spectrum

Having taken a quick trip through the whole electromagnetic spectrum, we can now fix our attention on the "light" portion. Here, the "light" means all those wavelengths that the human body can sense either by seeing or by feeling. The wavelengths of light waves are so short that using feet or inches to measure them would be like trying to measure a pinhead with a huge ruler marked off in miles. So scientists use a tiny unit of length called a **nanometer**, or just **nm** for short. If you can imagine cutting up an inch into 25 million equal pieces, the width of one of those pieces would be just about 1 nm.

Visible and Invisible Light

The portion of the light that we can see with our eyes is called **visible light**. It falls right in the middle of the "light" group and includes all the wavelengths from 390 to 770 nm. To the left and right of the visible light are two other bands of waves, which we can sense by the way our skin reacts to them but which we cannot see. These are the two bands of **invisible light**.

Within the band of visible light, the different wavelengths are seen as different colors. When all these wavelengths are mixed together in the right proportions, as in sunlight, what we call **white light** results. An object with color absorbs some of the wavelengths and reflects others. The ones it reflects produce the color that we say the object is. Black objects reflect almost none of the light hitting them.

Infrared and Ultraviolet

The band of invisible light to the right of the visible band in Figure 23.4 is called the **infrared**, or **IR**, because those wavelengths are below red (*infra-* means "below") in the energy they carry. The band of invisible light to the left of the visible band is called the **ultraviolet**, or **UV**, because its wavelengths are beyond violet (*ultra* means "beyond") in the energy they carry.

A Little More About Color

A lot has already been said in this book about color. Now we will discuss the way we *see* color.

When we see an object, we assume that it "has" a color. For instance, we think that a tomato *is* red or that a leaf *is* green or that hair *is* brown. This is not true. Color is *not* a property of an object, but a human sensation. As shown in Figure 23.5, the color we see is the result of five factors:

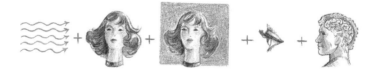

23.5

1. The type of light that falls on the object (what mixture of wavelengths it contains).
2. The nature of the object itself (which wavelengths it reflects).
3. The background against which the object is seen.
4. The eye of the person viewing the object.
5. The interpretation made by the brain of the person viewing the object.

Of course, people in general agree that a tomato is red. But that is because very similar tomatoes are *usually* seen by people with similar eyes and similar experiences, in *essentially white* (mixed) light, against fairly neutral backgrounds. But if you look at a tomato in the light of a sodium-vapor lamp (whose light contains a very narrow band of wavelengths with *no* reds), the tomato will appear almost black. Put the tomato back in sunlight, but in front of a very intense, deep red background, and the tomato will look yellowish orange.

And how does a tomato look to a color-blind person? To be sure, these are unusual ways of looking for color and are not of direct importance in the salon. They do point out, however, that the quality of light and background, even in ordinary circumstances, can vary enough to make subtle changes in the color an object seems to be at different places and times.

Our brains are wonderfully adaptable devices. They will accept many different softly colored kinds of light as "white" and shift our whole mental scale of color balance to correct for them. It is very important to understand this fact: **There is no single standard for what is white light.** Daylight is many kinds of white. It is always a mixture of all the colors in a rainbow, but on dull or cloudy days it is more bluish than it is on bright sunny days. The light from an ordinary 100-watt bulb is another kind of white. It is also a mixture of all the colors, but has far less blue and more red than does daylight. The "white" light from fluorescent tubes is still different. This light does *not* contain a mixture of all colors. Some colors are missing completely. But the balance of the colors that are present is good enough for the brain to accept the light as "white." The main point, in any case, is this: Anything that gives off, or reflects, even a reasonably good mixture of colors is usually called "white."

The importance of this discussion is that the operator must make some allowances for lighting in the selection of hair and makeup colors. What type of lighting is there likely to be in the place where the client works or lives? What correction must be made to compensate for the difference between the salon lighting and lighting where the client wishes to look the best? What will be the dominant color of clothing (background) the client will wear then, compared with the color worn to the salon? You should be able to advise your clients of the colors best suited to their skin tones.

Light

Light, as we now understand it, is made up of the band of wavelengths we can see plus the two bands we can't see, the IR (infrared) and UV (ultraviolet). Its effects upon the human body are of two kinds, **physical** and **psychological** (mental).

Physical Effects of Light

The body tissues absorb (soak up) at least part of the energy carried by all of the wavelengths of light. Much of this radiant energy is then changed back into heat. Remember that earlier we said that radiation was one of the ways heat gets from a warmer object to a cooler object? This ability to radiate heat is particularly true of the longer wavelengths of the IR and red-to-yellowish visible light. As a matter of fact, the only way our bodies know that IR waves are hitting them is by the feeling of warmth those IR waves produce. In mild doses, the warmth from IR relaxes the muscles and lets more blood flow to the exposed skin. Too strong a light of any kind, but particularly too much IR, can cause burns and can dry out skin and hair.

As the wavelengths of light get shorter—for example, in the bluish range of visible light and especially in the UV—the heating effect becomes smaller and smaller. However, these shorter waves produce strong *chemical* effects. Because of the greater energy they carry, short wavelengths not only make molecules vibrate (producing heat), but they can actually shake the molecules apart, thus causing the chemical effects. Light of wavelengths that cause chemical effects is called **actinic**, and UV is very actinic. *In small doses*, UV is good for the skin. It causes changes in the pigment in the skin (tanning) and aids the production of vitamin D. It also is able to destroy some of the bacteria on the skin or on equipment. For this reason, UV lamps are used in sanitizers. But too much UV can destroy tissues, and the result is much like the sun poisoning you get from an extremely bad sunburn. The eyes are particularly sensitive to UV and should always be protected from it. Too much UV can also destroy hair pigment and lighten the hair. You probably have often observed this effect in the hair of people who spend a lot of time in the sun (a UV source).

Psychological Effects of Light

We turn next to the psychological effects of light, which are not always easy to predict. Most people find the sensation of warmth from IR or UV light very pleasant, especially if the temperature in the salon is reasonably cool. Occasionally, however, you will have a client who finds this warmth disagreeable. As to visible light, psychologists have found that the "average" person finds reddish light mildly stimulating, possibly even a bit exciting, and bluish light quieting or relaxing. When we say the "average" person, we mean that if you asked 100 people how they reacted to these colors, 90 of them might agree that reddish light is exciting and bluish light relaxing. The point is that we must never forget the last factor in "seeing" of color—the mind of the person doing the seeing. The mind of each person contains a different set of life experiences. In the case of visible-light treatments, as with any other cosmetic treatment, you should understand that what is true for the "average" client may not be true for all.

Devices That Produce Light

There are many ways to produce light. We will talk only about the most important ones. Heat produces most of our visible light. When a material that doesn't burn is heated to higher and higher temperatures, it begins to glow. If you have an electric stove or hot plate, you've probably noticed that the element glows cherry red when it gets hot. If it got still hotter, the glow would become brighter and more yellowish, and finally almost white. Perhaps you've seen photographs of white-hot iron in a steel mill or a blacksmith's shop. This process of giving off light at high temperatures is called **incandescence**, and devices that use this principle are therefore called incandescent sources (Figure 23.6). Our sun is an incandescent source, and so are the flames of candles and kerosene lamps. Ordinary light bulbs are also incandescent sources. They contain a special metal wire that

> ◆ **Key Point** ◆
> Lighting in the salon should imitate natural light as much as possible. For best color analysis, work with incandescent light around the mirror and fluorescent light behind you. This combines warm and cool lighting for best color analysis.

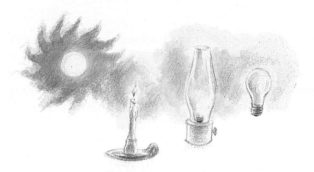

23.6   Incandescent light

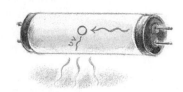

23.7   Flourescent light

becomes very hot. Although the light from all of these incandescent sources is different (some is redder and some bluer), they are all considered "white" light.

Another important source of visible light is the **fluorescent** tube, and it is worth a little discussion to understand how it works. The light is produced by a two-step process as shown in Figure 23.7. First, an electric current is passed through mercury vapor contained in the tube. This excites the electrons of the mercury atoms, and they give off mostly invisible UV wavelengths. The inside of the fluorescent tube is coated with a special mixture of powders called **phosphors**. In the second step, this powder absorbs the UV, is itself excited, and releases visible light. Each kind of phosphor gives off light of only few wavelengths, which would appear as some definite color if only that one phosphor were used. The mixture of phosphors is selected so that the overall effect is some acceptably "white" light. None of the UV gets out of the fluorescent tube because it is absorbed by the phosphors and the glass. One word of warning though: *Phosphors and mercury vapor are very poisonous. If a fluorescent tube should be accidentally broken, do not breathe the dust, and place the broken pieces in a closed bag as quickly as possible.*

IR Sources

Two kinds of incandescent sources produce IR light. One is a **heat lamp**, a special kind of glass bulb shaped like a floodlight with a reddish brown coating on the front. This bulb also produces some reddish visible light in addition to IR wavelengths. A more intense source of IR is an **infrared generator**. This is an electric heating coil inside a metal can that is fitted with a porcelain screw-in base like that of a light bulb. An infrared generator gives off almost no visible light, but it takes longer to heat up than does a heat lamp.

UV Sources

UV light is almost always produced by some kind of mercury-vapor lamp, also called a "sun lamp." Such a lamp is basically like a fluorescent tube without the phosphor coating. The UV lamp draws much more power than does an ordinary fluorescent tube. Sometimes UV lamps have cooling fans to get rid of excess heat.

Lamp Stands

Lamp stands are special floor lamps, designed to accept the different kinds of lamps or bulbs the operator may select for treatments that use light. They have reflectors to concentrate the light rays in a chosen direction and ceramic sockets that can stand the heat produced by the high-powered lights. They will accept either white or colored bulbs, for visible-light treatments, and IR lamps.

PROTECTING THE CLIENT AND THE STYLIST

From what has already been said in the previous sections, you should be pretty well aware of the dangers to the body from the different kinds of light. Here we will mention only a few specific do's and don't's.

Of all the organs of the body, the eye is by far the most sensitive to light. Eyes should always be protected. For IR or visible-light treatments, pads of damp cotton placed on the client's eyes are usually sufficient. Dark glasses may be used instead, but only for visible-light treatments. For UV treatments, the client should always wear special goggles that are usually provided with the UV unit. These goggles are not just dark glass; they are scientifically designed to filter out UV wavelengths.

Visible lights and IR bulbs should be placed 24 to 30 inches from the part of the body to be exposed. Visible-light and IR-treatment sessions may be as long as is necessary, provided the client does not become uncomfortable. When using these types of light, overexposure is difficult because the client will feel uncomfortably warm long before any physical harm could be done. A 15-minute exposure is usually sufficient. It goes without saying, of course, that no one should ever touch a heat lamp or light bulb while it is operating or just after shutting it off. If someone should do so accidentally, the resulting burn should be treated like any common burn: a gentle stream of cool water (or compresses), followed by a bland ointment. The burn should not be covered. You should not give an IR treatment if there is an infected sore on the skin.

When giving UV treatments, you should be especially careful. Because you have to see what you are doing, you cannot wear the special goggles that the client must wear. Wear regular dark glasses and be careful not to look into the UV lamp for long. The mucous membranes that line the eyes can be easily sunburned, resulting in a painful condition that doctors call **actinic conjunctivitis**. For general treatments, the UV lamp should be placed 24 to 30 inches from the client's body. The first exposure should not be longer than one minute. The exposure time can be increased by 30 seconds each time the treatment is repeated, up to a maximum limit of 10 minutes (seven minutes for very fair-skinned persons). For germicidal treatments of skin areas far away from the eyes, the UV lamp may be placed six to 12 inches from the skin, but only for periods of 30 to 60 seconds at a time. Exposure

◆SAFETY **PRECAUTION**◆

Follow all directions for timing and distance carefully. Overexposure can result in skin damage.

to UV first produces a reddening of the skin (medically called **ery-thema**), and overexposure results in the blistering typical of a bad sunburn. Treat overexposure to UV as you would treat sunburn.

In giving any type of light therapy, be alert for the albino client. You should never give any kind of treatment with lights, especially UV, to an albino without a physician's approval.

◆ **Key Point** ◆
Protective measures should be taken when using IR or UV lights. Many salons use visible lights for safety.

Lighting the Salon

In choosing the salon lighting, the things that must be considered are *visual effect* and *economics*. In other words, you should be aware of how the selected lighting affects colors in the salon, and how much it costs. There are really only two choices: incandescent lighting or fluorescent lighting.

It goes without saying that there must be enough light to work by, whichever type you choose. Lighting contractors and suppliers have helpful charts that show the number of light fixtures needed and how they should be placed in a salon of any particular size. They will usually provide this kind of assistance free of charge.

In selecting the type of lighting, keep in mind what we have said about the difference in color quality between the two. Incandescent light is generally redder than fluorescent light. Furthermore, the lower the wattage of an incandescent bulb, the redder it is. Also, incandescent bulbs of low wattage are less efficient; that is, they give less light per watt than a bulb of higher wattage. For example, you could get 300 watts of lighting in a particular area with either five 60-watt bulbs, three 100-watt bulbs, or two 150-watt bulbs. Yet, while all of these combinations eat up 300 watts of electricity (which is what shows up on the monthly bill), you get *more* and *whiter* light from the 150-watt bulbs than from either of the other two combinations. Of course, the question of where the bulbs are placed is also important, and this is where the suppliers' charts come in handy.

If fluorescent lights are chosen, they should be a neutral white, not pinkish (as in certain supermarkets, where they are used to make the meat look fresher) or bluish. Here again, the supplier can make helpful recommendations. Fluorescent lamps burn cooler than incandescent lights, since their light is not produced by high temperature. They are also about eight times as efficient, which means that one 40-watt fluorescent tube gives as much visible light as about eight 40-watt incandescent bulbs.

Fluorescent lighting fixtures cost more to install than incandescent fixtures, but this is a one-time-only cost. Fluorescent tubes cost more than incandescent bulbs to replace, but they also last much longer. The major advantage of fluorescent lighting is its greater efficiency. It provides more light per watt, which means more light per dollar on the monthly electric bill. When averaged over years of salon operation, fluorescent lighting usually comes out ahead, both in convenience and in dollars saved.

CLIENT **TIP** ◆◆◆◆◆◆◆

Always inquire as to the type of lighting your client has in the home or office. You may need to adjust your color work so they are equally happy with results in your salon and out of it.

◆ **Key Point** ◆
Lighting in the salon should consider both the effect of the light chosen and the cost of power needed.

SUMMARY

Heat is a form of energy that is measured in calories. In the salon, you will use heat to provide a comfortable environment, to accomplish styles, and to provide relaxing treatments for the face, hands and feet. You must determine the amount of heat to properly execute your treatments and apply heat in a safe manner.

Light, also a form of energy, has many effects in the salon. First, it provides lighting to enhance your decor and to enable you to see what you are doing. You will consider the type and placement of bulbs so that the light in your salon reproduces natural lighting as closely as possible. If the lighting in your salon is already established, you will use your knowledge to compensate for any bad lighting. You will evaluate the true effects of hair coloring or makeup services that you offer.

Light can be used as a therapeutic treatment in the salon, although a physician should recommend these treatments. You will apply the correct treatment and follow all guidelines for your own protection as well as to ensure that your client receives the full benefit.

QUESTIONS

1. What are the three different ways heat energy is transmitted? How do you use each in the salon?
2. What is the electromagnetic spectrum? Which bands in the spectrum affect your work as a cosmetologist? What are their functions?
3. What are four devices that produce light? Describe a service in the salon that would benefit from the use of each device.
4. How might the lighting in your school salon be improved? Which services have you performed that require better lighting than what you had available at the time?
5. What are the steps to protect you and your client when giving light treatments?
6. What are the two main considerations when planning lighting for your salon?

PROJECTS

1. Select sheets of colored paper that represent the primary and the secondary colors. Select color swatches that show an intense red, blonde and brown hair colors. Describe the color tones you see in each swatch and how the tones alter when you place each of the swatches on each of the sheets of colored paper.
2. Using the same color swatches, work with sheets of colored paper until you find the color backgrounds that most closely show true tones in the swatches. Design a salon decor using those background colors. Indicate how you would compensate for the colors you would like to use.
3. Construct a salon lighting system using a box with a slot cut in the top. Wire a light socket through the slot. Place a blond mannequin inside. Screw in a fluorescent bulb and note the hair color. Replace the bulb with an incandescent bulb and note the color change. Work with the two bulbs together until your mannequin has the same color tones inside the box as in natural light. Make your recommendations for ideal light placement in your "salon."
4. Research the regulations in your state to see what restrictions apply for heat or light therapy in the salon. Outline safety precautions for those treatments and report back to the class

BUILDING YOUR SALON SUCCESS

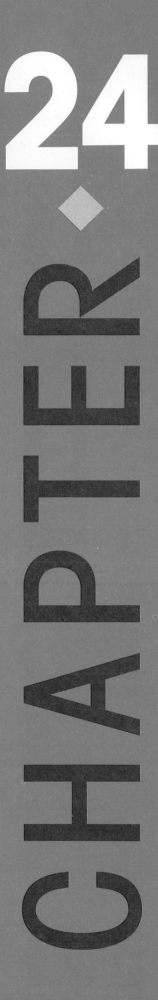

CHAPTER GOAL

Now, as you complete your studies, it's time to analyze the workplace you will be entering and study how you can best find a place in it. After reading this chapter and completing the projects, you should be able to

1. Explain the nature of personal service work and describe what this means in your chosen profession.
2. Demonstrate your preparation for the state board examination.
3. Outline the steps you should take to get your first job.
4. Describe how professional ethics are important to the operations of the salon and outline the benefits of ethics to you as a stylist.
5. List at least five ways of building a clientele.
6. Explain the different methods of compensation for cosmetologists. What employee benefits will you look for during your job search?
7. List the tax responsibilities of a regular employee and those of an employer.
8. List the important factors you should consider during the planning stage of opening your own salon.

Cosmetology got its start in this country in the 1930s, when legislation creating licensure was enacted. This radical development established standards for education, infection control, and the safety and welfare of the consuming public. Legislation made cosmetology in the United States very different from Europe, where apprenticeship was the method of training. The American model of education and licensing has been adapted by Asian countries and is being introduced in Europe. As you leave the school, find a mentor so you can hone your book skills to artistic standards so that you will have the best of both systems.

The salon industry today responds to the sophistication of its consumers and offers the most competitive marketplace in the world. The United States marketplace offers everything from budget shops to specialty salons and full-service establishments. Cosmetology has evolved from a guild craft passed down from generation to generation to a science.

While cosmetology is indeed a science, the art aspect of it provides room for creativity as a service-oriented industry. To build your salon success, you will develop a résumé and create advertising coupons for self-promotion. You will need to evaluate your paycheck and fulfill your tax liabilities either quarterly or annually. You will determine the type of salon best suited to you and the employee benefits that are essential for you. Are you ready for the challenge?

PERSONAL SERVICE WORK

Cosmetologists are listed by the federal government as **personal service workers**, meaning that they are in direct contact with the public. As a cosmetology student, you have learned the importance of your interpersonal skills; you will continue to develop these when you enter the professional world. One aspect that sets cosmetology apart from other career areas is the opportunity to develop a one-on-one relationship with each client. This fusion of interpersonal and artistic skills is what makes cosmetology unique and so much fun.

As a personal service worker, you must take special precautions to protect the health, safety, and welfare of the public. You are entering one of the few licensed professions that actually touch people. This means that you must follow infection control and OSHA standards as outlined in Chapter 4 to protect both you and your client.

Your personality and professional outlook will be very important in developing a clientele who recognize and appreciate your special skills. Technical as well as artistic skills are needed to be a success in this exciting business.

Personal Development

Your people skills will determine whether you become successful in this profession. Regularly conducted surveys indicate that while artistic skills are important, it is the stylist's personality that makes a customer select one stylist over another. To be most competitive in the job market, you should have equally developed technical, artistic, and interpersonal skills.

Appearance is one of the most important aspects of personal development. You are becoming a part of the fashion world, so make sure that your appearance fits. As a student you are probably on a limited budget, but you can begin now to develop a fashionable look you will present to your future clientele. To be well groomed, you must be perfectly neat at all times. Use accessories to update your wardrobe and style your hair in the latest trend. Women should wear makeup and men should be sure that facial hair is well tended. Jewelry is acceptable, but keep in mind that it must be functional in the salon. Long, dangling necklaces and earrings, bangle bracelets, and rings often pose an inconvenience. They make noise, dangle in your client's face, and sometimes cause dry skin problems on your hands. Fingernails should be shorter for the active stylist. If you are a nail technician or choose to wear longer nails, make sure that the free edge and cuticle area are smooth to avoid scratching your customer. Figures 24.1 and 24.2 show a classic stylist look that is easy on your beginning wardrobe budget, yet professional.

Hygiene is of great importance in the professional salon. You will be working very close to your clients, so make sure you have no offensive body or breath odor. Use a deodorant or an antiperspirant after your daily shower. Be prepared to brush your teeth during the day after meals, and keep breath fresheners or mouth mints on hand. Along the same vein, be aware of your perfume, cologne, or after shave lotion. Avoid heavy scents or too many scents from the combination of soap, body lotion and hair spray. Do not apply fragrance to the wrist area. You work with your hands close to your client, and often wet your wrists. This releases scent and could be offensive to your client.

Uniforms are seldom worn in today's professional salon, but you may be asked to adhere to a **dress code**. Some salons project a particular image through the colors and clothing worn by the employees. Keep comfort and style in mind when selecting a wardrobe. Washable clothing is more economical and practical in the salon setting than clothes that must be dry-cleaned. It is much easier to be cheerful and friendly when your feet don't hurt, so find comfortable shoes that are also stylish. Almost no salons permit the wearing of athletic shoes; however, you will find a large array of stylish shoes with cushioned soles.

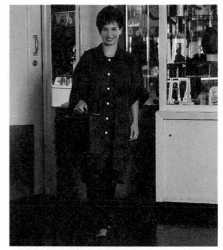

24.1

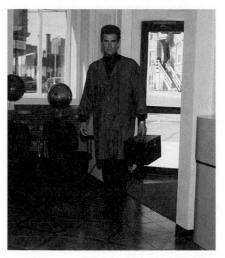

24.2

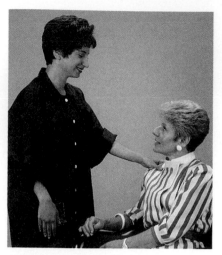

24.3

CLIENT TIP ◆◆◆◆◆◆

Make sure your new customer feels welcome and comfortable. Imagine how you would feel walking into your salon for the first time. Welcome your client as Mr., Ms., or Mrs., and be sure to introduce yourself by your first name.

CLIENT TIP ◆◆◆◆◆◆

Educate your clients while you perform services. You can make them look good on a long-term basis instead of just when they leave the salon.

CLIENT TIP ◆◆◆◆◆◆

Use the mirror to demonstrate how you will customize the look for your client. Look for a nod of the head or a smile in the eyes that says, "Yes, I want that," before you proceed.

◆SAFETY PRECAUTION◆

Do not perform a chemical service on hair that is damaged—even if the client insists. You will be liable in a malpractice proceeding, and could face fines from your state board as well.

Nutrition and **exercise** may be things you didn't think would be important to a cosmetologist. It is always important to take care of yourself. As a cosmetologist, you will be putting in long hours on your feet. Be sure to get adequate sleep so that you do not become overly tired on the job.

Nutritional experts recommend that you avoid fatty foods. Choose foods that give energy such as grains, fruits, vegetables, fish, and poultry. Be sure to drink at least eight glasses of water or more a day. Add nutritional supplements as recommended by your doctor.

A great way to work out stress and increase your resistance to common illnesses is to exercise. Strange as it may sound, exercise can give you renewed energy after working all day. Stretching exercises will help you relieve tension through the day. Use good posture to look your best and avoid fatigue. Work with your back straight but not tense. Try to keep your arms below shoulder level at all times. Learn the best settings for your chair, the facial lounge, and so on, so that you are comfortable and do not strain muscles.

Communication

Good communication skills are essential in order to develop a rapport with your employer, co-workers, and clients. A perfectly executed service will be considered a failure if it isn't what your client expected. Ask your client specific questions about what he or she wants. Listen carefully and then repeat the information to be sure you understand.

Greeting is the first communication skill you will use in the salon (Figure 24.3). Your greeting welcomes the client and helps him or her feel more comfortable. Meet and greet your client by name. Make sure they know your first name. A first-time client should be shown the basics of the salon: where to hang a coat, the location of the rest rooms, where to change into a smock for a service, the location of coffee, water, and so on. During the greeting, make note of client's height, weight, clothing, and overall appearance. These observations will help you later as you design a custom look for the client. Seat your client comfortably and proceed to the next step.

Assessment, the next step to effective communication, began when you greeted your client. Now you will follow through with the consultation phase. Discuss the desired result and analyze the aspects of the hair, face, and nails necessary to best perform the service. Ask what your client wants. Find out about the client's life style and how much time he or she has to maintain a particular style. Listen to what your client thinks the problems are and offer your suggestions to solve them.

If you are performing a chemical service, or if this is a new client, you may wish to record the consultation on a **record card**. Talk with your client about the analysis as you proceed. Explain what can be done at home to follow through on the service you are about to provide.

Agreement should always be reached before you proceed with the salon service. Paint pictures with words to make sure your client understands what you are about to do and believes it will improve his or her appearance. Be sure that both of you think, "over the ears," for example, means that you are going to cut up over the ears so they completely show. If your client thinks you're going to leave the hair long and over the ears, more talk is necessary! (See Figure 24.4.) Use pictures to help you communicate more effectively. Be certain that your client is looking at the hair, makeup, or nails rather than the glamour of the photograph or the beauty of the model.

Delivery, the next step, involves whatever steps are necessary to do what you have promised. This is the phase where technical and artistic skills will pay off. During the delivery phase, make sure that your client is comfortable. Drape client for protection of clothing and for comfort. Offer a beverage and a magazine during timing phases of services, or when you may not be nearby. If you are called away, reassure your client by gently resting your hands on the shoulders before you leave. Offer an additional service such as a paraffin treatment to the hands while a facial mask or permanent wave is processing.

Completion is the last phase of communication and of every salon service. Take a few moments to explain how your client should apply blusher and suggest the purchase of a new shade. Show your customer how to finish a blow-dry style to look its best and explain the products that will help re-create the style at home. Each and every service that you give should have this completion phase. Be sure that the customer

1. Is satisfied.
2. Has the products to duplicate the look.
3. Understands the upkeep necessary.
4. Is scheduled for the next appointment.
5. Knows how to contact you between appointments for assistance.

STATE BOARDS

You're almost there. You've completed you studies and now it is time to graduate and take your licensure examination. Scared? Why? This section will discuss those exams and the role the regulatory boards will play in your future.

Purpose of State Exams

As we've said, regulatory boards were created in the 1930s in this country. Their purpose and the purpose of licensing exams is to protect the health, safety, and welfare of the consuming public. As such, the exams operate as a screen to ensure that those people who claim to be cosmetologists have attained a prescribed level of skill. The regulatory boards require cosmetologists and the salons they work in to be licensed. One thing you should know is that the board is there for your benefit. The regulations ensure that cosmetologists in your state are providing good services.

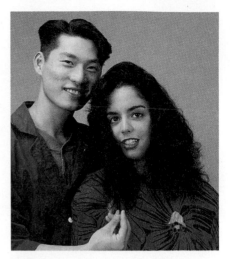

24.4

Preparing for Your Examination

Your school will certify your education when you apply for your licensure exam. You will apply to the board and pay a fee for the exam, which often includes the cost of your license. Licenses are good for one to three years, depending upon your state.

As an exam applicant, you are entitled to information regarding the content of the exam. This is called a **BOI**, a **Bulletin of Information**. It tells you the categories of the exam, what you must bring with you, and what you are expected to do. In many states, further information is available—sometimes in video—regarding the exam site, parking, models, and so on.

The vast majority of states require a written and a practical examination. You will take a written test, usually 100 questions, that covers all phases of cosmetology. The core of the practical examination accepted nationally includes haircutting, the chemical services (permanent waving, coloring, lightening, relaxing), and wet styling techniques. Your state may also choose to test you in additional areas of manicuring, facials, shampooing, thermal styling, and so on. You should know what is expected and be prepared to demonstrate all services required.

Be prepared for your license exam. Have all required supplies and a model who is willing to have the necessary services performed. Choose a model whose hair is easy to manage, and practice the skills outlined in the BOI. Make sure that you are on time for the exam; you can be disqualified for being late. Relax. You have practiced these skills in school and can do any of the basic skills they require. You will be allowed time to ask questions about any demonstration. Remember, the examiners are not the enemy; they are the people who will certify you to enter your chosen field.

In some states, you will be granted a temporary work permit on the day of your exam. This will allow you to be employed under the supervision of a licensed stylist until you learn the results of your test. If you should fail, ask for a **weakness report**, which outlines the areas of the examination you failed. Depending upon your state, you will be asked to repeat the entire exam, or just the particular phases where your scores were below minimum. But of course that will not be the case—you will pass your exam. If you are thoroughly prepared, you will be on your way to an exciting career in the cosmetology industry. Good luck!

GETTING A JOB

You've worked hard at school and practiced the skills you will need as a professional cosmetologist. Now it's time to think about where you will work when you have your license. Before you choose a work environment, make a list of things you want to accomplish in one year, three years, five years. Then select the salon that will best get you started on your career path.

◆ **Key Point** ◆

State board examinations are designed to ensure the health, safety, and welfare of the public you will serve. Request information from the school and the board so you will be totally prepared.

Developing a Resumé

A resumé describes you on paper. It outlines your employment experience and special achievements. As you progress through your career, you will update your resumé whenever you have added significantly to any of these categories. Not all salon employers will expect a resumé, but presenting one will give you an advantage.

Sample Basic Resumé

Resume	Gloria S. Jones 23 Morris Street Rochester, MI 55901 Telephone 000-111-2222
Career Objective	I am seeking full-time employment in a salon that will provide an opportunity to progress as a professional cosmetologist.
Education	Universal School of Cosmetology–18 Elm Street, Rochester, MN. Graduated June 2, 19XX. Northside High School–Rochester, MN. Graduated (with honors) June 12, 19XX. Majored in business and vocational cosmetology.
Experience	Universal School of Cosmetology–part-time office assistant; January 20, 19XX–November 19, 19XX. Elm Playhouse–19 Circle Pine Road, Elm, MO. Make-up assistant during summer season; May 1, 19XX-August 28, 19XX.
Job-Related Activities	Produced holiday makeup and hair fashion shows for ACE Department Store, and local salons; December 1, 19XX-January 3, 19XX. Directed and participated in fund-raising "Cut-A-Thon" for charitable organizations; sponsored by Chamber of Commerce, various events were held. Attended makeup seminar in New York City, sponsored by Universal School of Cosmetology; April 23, 19XX.
References	Available upon request.

24.5

To organize your own resumé, fill out the worksheet in Figure 24.6. Ask your instructor what you should include on your résumé. It is not necessary to offer information regarding age, race, religion, or health. You should include your education, special skills, and your career goal. Prepare a portfolio of your work as a senior students and don't forget to include those special projects that you completed during school. They may not seem important, but may be just the key for a prospective employer.

Your Resumé

Use this basic form to practice wiring your resumé. Then write your finished resumé on a separate piece of paper.

Name _____

Address _____

City _____State _____ZIP _____

Telephone _____

Career Objective:

_____
_____
_____

Qualifications:

_____
_____
_____

Education:

_____
_____
_____

Achievements:

_____
_____
_____

Work Experience:

_____
_____
_____

Personal Information is Optional:

_____
_____
_____

References:

_____
_____
_____

24.6

Types of Salons

As you go through the last phase of your cosmetology schooling, spend time researching the jobs available in your area. Think about the type of salon you would prefer to work in and check out the top salons in your area for opportunities. There are three different types of salons available for the entry-level cosmetologist.

Budget Salons

These low-cost salons came into being in the 1970s and serve an important need for today's consumer. They are also a good opportunity for entry-level employment. Most have a flat fee for a haircut; all other services such as styling and conditioning are additional. Some budget salons specialize in the type of services they offer, for example, haircut only, or children only. Most budget salons are chain operations, which will be discussed later in the chapter.

Specialty Salons

These salons are usually operated by an individual. Specialty salons are ideal for those licensed for just one service (nail technician, esthetician, haircutter, etc.). Some salons in large cities offer advanced services in a particular field such as specialty haircutting, long-hair styling, or cosmetic aids for medical patients. There are salons that only deal with toupees and wigs for men. Some salons add artificial hair by weaving; others are spas for full-body skin care. Others offer permanent or camouflage makeup. These advanced salons may not have employment openings for new stylists, but they can present excellent internship opportunities.

Full-Service Establishments

The full-service salon is usually independently operated, but can also be a chain operation. A full-service salon is one that offers services in many different areas. For example, a client can receive a haircut, style, permanent wave, or a hair coloring service. Facials, manicures, artificial nails, makeup services, and retail products are also available. Working in a full-service establishment will give you the broadest experience, and offer excellent internship opportunities. Most full-service salons are free-standing, meaning they are independently operated businesses. They can also be a salon operating as a contractor within a department store.

Choosing the Salon Experience for You

Your first job in a salon provides key experience. It is here that you will bring your school skills to salon level. This is also where you will learn from the masters to develop your own particular methods of styling, makeup application, or hair coloring. Choose your first salon carefully and learn as much as you can. You may very well spend years of your career, or all of it, with your first employer.

Your job search should begin with visits to several salons in your area. You may wish to visit as a customer and make special notations for future employment, or you may wish to identify yourself as a student interested in joining the industry. Talk to your instructor before you arrange these outings. Ask what particular features of the salon operation you should observe based upon your career plans.

Interview with the salons you are most interested in and be prepared to cut or style a model or mannequin. Discuss your career goals with the owner to see if the salon offers suitable learning opportunities. Express your willingness to be an intern, a junior stylist, until your skills reach expert level. Discuss salary options (detailed later in this chapter).

PROFESSIONAL ETHICS

The relationships that you build with your co-workers and your clients will help you be successful and enjoy your career to the fullest. As a licensed cosmetologist, you should be guided by a code of ethics. That means that you should conduct yourself in a way that does honor to you and to your profession. As an employee in the salon, you will find yourself developing three different types of relationships—with your clients, your co-workers, and your employer. All of these relationships should be governed by a standard of ethical behavior. Professionalism, competence, and courtesy should guide you in all of your actions. Treat others with the same consideration and respect you would like them to extend to you.

Your Relationship with Your Clients

Today's clients are sophisticated and will expect you to conduct yourself in a professional manner. They will appreciate your respect and will return it. Treat your clients as you would like to be treated yourself. Be proud of your profession and let your clients see that pride.

Be on time. As a professional cosmetologist you must pay very close attention to time. Start your day on time. Clients have a right to receive services shortly after they arrive. If you do encounter scheduling difficulties, make sure that waiting clients are comfortable, and have a realistic estimate of how long their wait will be. Statistics show that a client left three times during an appointment will probably not return.

Be clean. As simple as it may sound, your clients will be impressed by a clean workstation. Sanitize your station, sweep hair from the floor, and discard disposable implements between clients. Disinfect all other instruments before and after use. Be spotless in your own appearance.

Be competent. Your clients trust you to do your very best. Challenge yourself, but be certain that you can deliver what you promise. Do not be afraid to ask your co-workers for help and advice. Upgrade your skills through continuing-education workshops in the salon, and from seminars offered by manufacturers and at trade shows. Practice new skills on mannequins, models, or other salon stylists to whom you offer complimentary services. Give them your business card so they can advertise your skills to their friends.

Be safe. Infection control standards are developed for your safety as well as that of your client. Be aware of state regulations and follow them carefully. Check your electrical equipment for faults and have it serviced regularly.

Be caring. Customers will welcome an environment where their needs are put first. Don't try to sell them services they don't want, but be prepared to offer advice and salon treatments that would be of benefit. Treat your customers with respect and warmth. Avoid any ethnic or sexual slurs. Give your clients your full attention and let them know you appreciate their business. Address your customer as Mr., Mrs., or Ms. until you are asked to use the first name.

Be aware. Discuss current affairs with your clients, especially trends in fashion, hair, makeup, and nails. Avoid inflammatory topics or those that could be "hot buttons" for your client. Topics of religion, politics, personal or financial problems, or gossip about other clients or co-workers could offend your clients and send them to another stylist.

Be professional. Don't criticize a colleague's work, even if you are correcting it. Instead, offer your suggestions for a special look. Don't argue with your client. Handle each situation tactfully and offer what is expected. Eat, drink, and (if you must) smoke only in designated areas of the salon—never in front of a customer. Keep your salon environment alcohol and drug free.

Be fair. Ask fair payment for services rendered; offer fair value for the prices you charge. Some salons will have set prices; others have a scale according to the expertise of the individual stylist. Limit free services to charity, learning experiences, or promotional activities. Work in a licensed establishment.

Be sincere and truthful. Be honest about your abilities and ask assistance when you need it. Don't jeopardize your career by misrepresenting your experience.

Your Relationship with Your Co-Workers

Many of the same concepts you apply to your clients work with your colleagues as well. The stylists in any salon have much in common. All work for the same employer and try to do the best they can to make a living. Do your part to make the salon environment one that is very caring and sharing of knowledge.

Be honest. Be honest with your colleagues about your level of skill. Your co-workers can help where you need it and can learn from your expertise. Be willing to share and be equally willing to learn. Don't try to grab clients from your co-workers. Instead, help them out whenever you can, and they will do the same for you. Avoid gossip and don't "borrow" equipment or supplies from your fellow workers.

Your Relationship with Your Employer

Your initial impression of your employer may change once you experience the pressures of the job. Be loyal to your boss and always give a full day's work for a day's pay. If you can't be loyal, it may be time to look elsewhere for a job.

◆ **Key Point** ◆

Professionalism, competence, and courtesy should guide your behavior in the salon. Be loyal, dependable, and willing to learn. Treat others with the same consideration and respect you would like extended to you.

Discuss your goals with your employer to see if the two of you can work together to accomplish them.

There are many additional opportunities in the salon through retailing, outreach for clientele, and public relations that can offer you opportunities to increase your income and professional knowledge. Be cooperative and pitch in wherever you can. Remember that these are the masters that can give you the competitive skills you will need to excel in your cosmetology career.

BUILDING A CLIENTELE

The customer base, or **clientele**, that you build will directly affect your income. Your first salon can help you get started by giving you the customers left by a departing stylist as well as walk-in business.

Make an appointment with your employer to discuss ways to bring business into the salon to build your client list. Ask if the salon will absorb part of the expense of a promotion that would offer your introductory services at reduced cost. The section that follows offers several suggestions for you to build up your clientele. As your list of customers grows, work to develop your artistic and interpersonal skills. They will make the difference that starts you on your road to fame and fortune.

Business Cards

One of the first things you should do when you are established in a salon is to create a business card (Figure 24.7). Talk to your employer. It is possible that there is a standard design for the entire salon. If that is the case, simply go to the printer and have your name inserted. If there is not a salon design, draft your own. It should be simple, yet attractive.

The business card should give your name and identify what it is that you do. The name of the business should be clearly defined as well as the address and phone number, including the area code. A simple graphic will make your card eye-catching and finish the design.

The Look studio

210 N. Main
West Lansing, Michigan

701-555-4400   George, Stylist

24.7

Give your business cards to clients, with the day, time, and date of their next appointment. Have business cards available at your station; encourage clients to distribute them to their friends. Visit the other businesses in the area of your salon to see if they will display your cards at the check-out area. In return, you will display their cards in the salon. This is especially beneficial for fashion and personal-image-related businesses. Network with other young professionals and be prepared to exchange business cards. You never know when an opportunity may present itself!

Flyers

Speak with your employer about a simple flyer announcing your availability. The cost of flyers is minimal and they can be very effective. The printed information should include your name, business name and location, phone number, and the pricing information and expiration dates of the specials you are offering.

Advertising

Advertisements are slightly more expensive, especially if you choose a newspaper with a large circulation. Local or neighborhood papers can be very effective. Don't ignore the free press papers available at very low advertising cost. The advertisement should contain the same information as a flyer: your name, business name and location, phone number, and the expiration dates of the specials (see Figure 24.8).

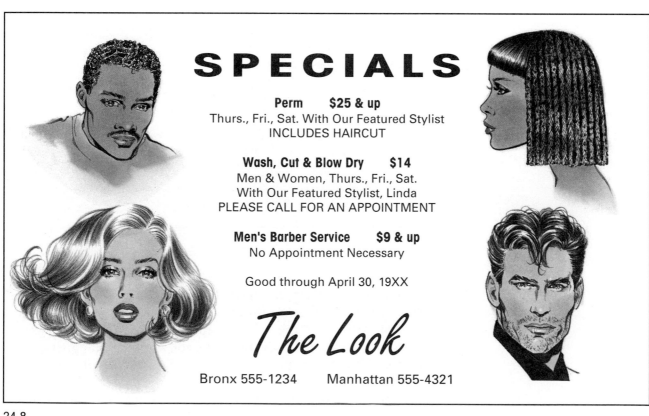

24.8

Gift Certificate

This promotional tool can be used in several different ways to get new customers into the salon. Gift certificates can be available for purchase, or included in packages for new residents distributed through local chambers of commerce (Figure 24.9). Many welcoming certificates offer a free or discounted service, such as a free manicure with the purchase of a cut and style, a free cut with a purchase of a permanent wave, or a discount on makeup with the purchase of a facial.

Gift Certificate
this certificate is good for
One Free Manicure
when you receive a cut and style

The Look   836 Smithtown Plaza
Anyplace USA 01234
(000) 111-2222

Welcome To The Community
This Entitles You To:
ONE FREE HAIRCUT
(One Coupon Per Person • Not To Be Combined With Any Other Offer)

The Look

Hair Designers For The Entire Family
170 North First St., Store #6
(Riverside Shopping Mall)
New Paltz • 555-1234
Full Service Hair Salon • Designer Fragrances • Cosmetics
Baby Sitting Service Available

24.9

You can also issue gift certificates to your existing clients. Let them know you will give a free service for every three new customers they send you. Give the same certificates to the new customers to keep your customer list growing. Do not worry about "giving away the store." Plan your promotions carefully so that you perform at least three full-price services to every free or discounted one. Many clients will send you one or two referrals, but only a few will get you three new customers. Make sure that all coupons and specials have a printed expiration date.

Client Reminder Cards

A variation of a gift coupon can be used to remind a client to schedule an appointment (see Figure 24.10). Computer programs store client records and can even print and address reminder cards for you. Offer an incentive to return, such as a free paraffin treatment, or a 10 percent discount on retail products. Take advantage of "down time" to send client reminder cards.

You can also program the computer to send cards for birthdays, anniversaries, and holidays. The key is to enter client data on a regular basis so the job is not huge when you decide to promote.

Dear Mr Jones,
It has been 8 weeks since your last cut & style. We value your business. Use this card for a 10% discount on retail products when you get your cut and style.
Yours truly,
363 Main st.
Freeport, TX 63297
offer good for 7 days from post mark

George Jones
2367 Allyn
Freeport, TX
63297

24.10

Self-Promotion

In order to build a clientele, you need to let the community know you are available and can provide excellent services. Check with local theatre groups to see if you can provide makeup or hair services for a performance. Explain that you will provide basic services in the salon for a fee, but will work backstage either for a reduced fee or for free. In return, receive credit in the program and the entire cast and backstage crew become potential clients. Besides those benefits, the experience you gain is terrific and it can be a whole lot of fun.

Check with your chamber of commerce to find out what organizations may be looking for someone to speak on personal-image-related topics. Make an appointment with the high school guidance counselor to see if you can make a similar presentation to the students. Teenagers are very anxious to learn how to look better and spend a great deal of their money on hair and other beauty items. They make excellent customers who can tell their friends about you.

Fashion shows, local television, charity fund-raisers offering cutathons, and other public events are all good opportunities to build your client list. These situations provide necessary public exposure, an opportunity to learn new skills, and free publicity. Be sure to distribute your business cards so you can maximize the benefits of your charity work.

> ### ◆ Key Point ◆
> Use all methods available to you to build a clientele. Network as much as possible in other professional organizations and be sure to join the cosmetology associations in your area.

CLIENT **TIP** ◆◆◆◆◆◆◆

Listen attentively to your client. Ask questions to be sure that you understand the client's particular needs before suggesting a service.

CLIENT **TIP** ◆◆◆◆◆◆◆

Work with the receptionist in the salon when you expand a client's service beyond what is booked. Learn how to work additional services in and how to keep all customers satisfied while offering additional services.

Selling Services and Products

Your success will depend on your technical and interpersonal skills and your ability to sell. You will sell yourself, your services, and your products.

You offer unique personal-image services to your clients. Every time you identify a client's need and match it with the correct service, you make a sale. When you teach your client how to duplicate your styling results at home with the correct retail products, you make a sale. When you explain to a client with an appointment for a haircut that only a perm will produce the desired results, you are selling. When a client worries about competing in the job market and you suggest subtle highlights for a youthful look, you are selling.

Building your book means that you fill the time slots you have available during the day and that you also increase the amount of services each client receives. How do you do this? Every client you have is a potential source of new clients: the father who can't understand his son's desire to establish his identity with a radical haircut, the teenager trying to look like the most popular kid in school, or the mother with business and social contacts trying to juggle the whole scene. As a cosmetologist, you must relate to all of these people. If you do it well, each will send you additional clients. The most effective means of marketing yourself is word-of-mouth.

Expand your book by offering additional services such as a perm to complement the desired volume of a cut, or highlights for a youthful look. Don't miss an opportunity to sell polish to touch up your nail artistry, or eye shadow to enhance your client's facial features. Suggest a relaxer for the ease of styling desired by your customer with extra curly hair.

Do everything you can to ensure that every customer who sits in your chair returns and sends other clients your way. Find out about family members and friends who might also have need of your services. Use the promotional tools outlined previously to remind customers when it is time to make an appointment. Offer free or discounted services to clients who refer new customers to you. Carefully study the methods of the successful stylists in your salon and ask their advice for selling. Your attention and admiration will encourage them to share their "secrets" with you.

Try to schedule the next appointment before your client leaves the salon. Haircuts should be scheduled in six-to-eight-week intervals. A hair coloring service will need attention in four to six weeks. If the client has received a perm, he or she should return in two weeks for a deep conditioning treatment. Hair removal must be followed up in four to six weeks. A fill-in is necessary for artificial nails in about four weeks.

Selling retail products is a method to increase your income and further fill your clients' needs. To sell successfully, you must be able to apply the following principles:

1. Know *who* you are selling to and what their needs are. Don't sell unwanted products; fill a need.
2. Know *what* the benefits of the product are.

3. Tell the client where and when to apply the products you suggest for best results.
4. Tell your clients why your products will fill their needs.
5. Emphasize the benefits of the product. Don't just sell! Suggest products and services that the client wants and needs.

You will have a unique advantage in selling cosmetics and salon services because of your relationship with your clients. Use retail sales to increase dollar volume during a slow week, or to cover your overhead costs.

Employee Compensation and Benefits

In years past, cosmetology was an industry that had few, if any, employee benefits. Most stylists were paid a commission, a percentage, of what they brought into the salon and that was it. Each stylist was responsible for his or her own insurance. Holidays and vacations were not paid, but simply time off from the salon. Pension plans did not exist and any continuing education was up to the individual to get. Times have changed.

There are appreciable differences in the way salons pay and offer benefits to employees. Discuss compensation and benefits during interviews and use the information to compare salons before making a decision.

Compensation

Compensation is the amount of money you get paid. In cosmetology, there are several ways that employers figure what that amount will be. A summary of basic compensation plans follows.

Straight salary means that you are paid the same amount, regardless of what you bring into the salon as income. This is usually figured as an hourly wage. This type of compensation is typically paid to cosmetologists who work for manufacturers as lab technicians or sales representatives. Flat salary is also paid to shampoo persons and some beginning stylists in budget salons.

Salary plus commission is a method of guaranteeing a certain amount per week, for example, but allowing for additional payment if you bring in more income than expected to the salon. Salary plus commission is a way that entry-level stylists are often paid. It guarantees that you will have a steady paycheck and rewards you for the efforts you make to build a clientele.

Straight commission means you are paid a percentage of the income you bring into the salon. This is a good method for the experienced stylist with a clientele because it directly rewards you for the amount of business you bring into the salon. Percentages vary according to the location of the salon: what part of the country it is in and whether the setting is urban, suburban, or rural.

The amount you make in commission is dependent upon two things: the amount charged for each service, and the number of clients coming into the salon. Consider the examples in Table 24.1

TABLE 24.1 Comparing Commission and Volume

Salon A		Salon B	
Commission paid:	40%	Commission paid:	60%
Haircut price:	$20.00	Haircut price:	$10.00
	x 40%		x 60%
	$8.00		$6.00
Average number of customers per day:	15	Average number of customers per day:	10
Total income:	$120.00	Total income:	$60.00

You can see that as the volume of customers changes so does the income, at either commission rate. Typically, lower commissions are paid in larger salons, those in high population areas, and those in more affluent communities. This is because the cost of operating the salon, the **overhead**, is high. However, it is in these areas that the price of a service is usually higher, there is a larger clientele base, and there are more advertising dollars to bring in customers.

There are benefits in both of the salons outlined in Table 24.1. Consider all the factors when choosing a salon; don't be fooled by looking at the percentage of commission alone.

Sliding Scale Commission is even more complicated. This is almost like getting a bonus for bringing in more customers than average. You might start at 40 percent, for example, but earn 45 percent of revenue over a certain dollar amount.

Retail commission is added to your paycheck, or is a separate monthly payment. It gives you a percentage of the purchase price of the retail items that you sell. Retail commission is not always separate income. An employer paying you a 65 percent commission, for example, may just expect you to sell retail products without additional compensation.

Benefits

Benefits refer to those things you receive as an employee for which you do not pay. Benefits are not available in all salons, and they vary greatly. Benefits count for a great deal. A one-week paid vacation equals a 2 percent increase in commission. Insurance paid by the salon amounts to a 3-5 percent increase in commission. As you interview potential employers, ask questions about profit sharing, savings plans, educational opportunities, company discounts, professional memberships, and insurance (health, life, and disability).

◆ **Key Point** ◆
Compare the methods of compensation and the benefit packages of the salons you consider as potential employers.

Taxes

Now that you are becoming a wage earner, you need to think about taxes. The way you pay taxes depends entirely on what type of employment you select.

Types of Employment

As a **regular employee,** either full or part time, your employer is responsible for deducting the correct taxes from your paycheck. You simply fill out a **W-4 form**, indicating your Social Security number and the number of dependents you wish to claim, and payroll will do the rest. When you claim more dependents, each paycheck will have less removed from income for taxes. You will receive more during the year, but may have a greater tax burden at the end of the year. If you are an independent contractor or a booth renter, however, your tax responsibilities are quite different.

The definition of an **independent contractor**, or **booth renter**, varies between companies. Typically an independent contractor rents space and equipment from an existing salon. Overhead for supplies is deducted from your earnings, and you determine your hours of business, provide your own phone, and booking. In this instance, you definitely need the assistance of a tax consultant to let you know what your tax obligations are and what expenses you have that can be deducted from the amount that you owe. In a booth rental situation you have no employee benefits at all. Booth rental is coming under increasing scrutiny by the Internal Revenue Service (IRS), and legislation is being passed in many states restricting it. Be sure you understand the situation before you agree to become an independent contractor, and that you know what your tax responsibilities are.

In most instances, an independent contractor is somewhere between an employee and a one-person salon. You will be your own boss; but you probably won't be around other stylists that can help you hone your skills and build your business. You will typically be paid a percentage of the business that you do. You are responsible for paying your own taxes (city, state, federal, Social Security, and unemployment) on a quarterly basis. And of course you are solely responsible for all promotional efforts to build a clientele.

Social Security

This tax, in effect since 1935, is deducted from your paycheck and placed in a trust fund in your name. In any given year, you will pay a fixed percentage of every dollar you earn until you reach a cutoff point beyond which you are not taxed. Your employer must contribute a matching amount to your fund. If you are self-employed, you make both contributions.

During your working years, you will continue to pay Social Security taxes. Then, when your earnings stop due to disability, retirement, or death, cash payments will be made from the fund on a regular basis to you or your dependents. You may ask the Social Security Administration (SSA) for an accounting of your fund by sending a postcard you can get from the local SSA office. The information you receive will tell you what to do if you disagree with the information provided.

Income Taxes

Your employer will deduct the correct amount from your earnings to meet your federal income tax requirements, according to the W-4 form you complete. In most states, you will have deductions for state taxes, and often for city taxes as well. If you are self-employed, this is also your responsibility.

At the end of every year, your employer will compute all the tax obligations that have been met. By the end of January, you will receive a **W-2 form** that indicates the amount you have earned, and the amounts contributed for federal and other taxes. This is not a tax return, but a receipt you must have in order to prepare your return. If you work for more than one employer, you will have as many receipts to compute.

Your income from salary, tips, fees, bonuses, commissions, pensions, vacation allowances, dismissal, severance, and retirement is subject to withholding taxes. Keep informed of changes in the tax laws by consulting an accountant or obtaining information such as *Your Federal Income Tax* and other guides available at local offices of the Internal Revenue Service.

Reporting Tips

Tips are considered part of your income and are subject to the same taxes as your salary. Keep a daily record of tips to help you make a written report for your employer. **Form 4070A, Daily Record of Tips,** may be used for record keeping and may be obtained free from the IRS.

The amount you must report depends on whether tip income is more than twenty dollars per month. If you make more than that in tips, you must report it to your employer by the tenth day of the next month. Your employer will then make the proper deductions for you. If you would like more information on reporting tips, ask for **Reporting Income from Tips, Publication 531,** available from the IRS.

Opening Your Own Salon

Owning your own salon may be an immediate or a long-range goal for you. Most students plan to work in a salon after leaving school in order to gain experience. When you are ready to open your own salon, you will need professional advice. The **Small Business Administration (SBA)** will be one source of excellent information. You will also want to research associations for entrepreneurs, people who run their own businesses, as they can offer advice and professional support. In many cities, retired executives are also available to offer free advice on own-

---

◆ Key Point ◆

Your employer is responsible for deducting tax amounts from your paycheck. If you are independently employed, or intend to hire your own employees, you are responsible for deducting the correct tax amount.

ing and running your own business. Check with your municipal government to see if this service is available to you.

Types of Ownership

When you do decide to open your salon, you have several options available to you. The first choice is whether you want to be the sole owner. You will want financial and legal advice before you decide the type of ownership for your salon.

An **individual proprietorship** is a form of business in which one person furnishes all of the capital (money needed to start the business). As sole owner of the salon, you would make the rules and regulations for your employees and receive all of the profits. On the other hand, you would bear all losses and be personally liable for any debts.

A **partnership** is a form of business in which two or more people contribute a share of the capital. To create a partnership, you need to draw up an agreement that clearly states how profits and responsibilities are to be shared. Partnerships have two main advantages: (1) There is more money to invest, and (2) your combined experience gives you a better chance for success. The key to a successful partnership is selecting the right people and drawing up a detailed agreement. On the other hand, so many partnerships fail because of personality and contract problems that some banks are hesitant to finance them.

A **corporation** is a form of business in which capital is raised from the sale of stock. A group wishing to incorporate must receive a charter from the state. As part owner of a corporation, your personal liability is limited to the amount of your investment. Stockholders select a board of directors to run the salon.

A **franchise** is a form of business in which you operate under a parent company name. As a franchised salon you typically pay a fee for the use of the franchise name and follow regulations established by the parent company. You are entitled to use the company logo and advertising campaign, and often get assistance in finding a good location. Other benefits of a franchise are better lease rates and financial assistance for equipment and decorating. Franchised salons are usually budget-type operations.

Salon Planning

Planning your salon is one of the most important steps in opening a successful business. Again, professionals are available to help you. Select a planner who has experience in the type of salon that you want to open. *Location* is vital to the success of the salon. You will want to consider these items:

1. Is it in a good neighborhood?
2. Is it easy to get to by car or by walking? Is there mass transit close by?
3. Is parking available? Is it free?
4. Does the area match the type of salon you want? Will the people who live or work there be able to afford your prices?
5. Does the rent fit into your business plan? Can you get a long-term lease?

6. Will you have to redecorate?

7. Is the space big enough? Will you have room for retail products?

8. Is there room for expansion?

Space is an important consideration when you select the location. You will need an average of 125 square feet for each stylist. This amount includes the reception area, workstations, dispensary, and storage. Plan enough room for efficient operations, but avoid excess space that will drive your rent up and your profits down. If the space is too large, consider subletting it to a related business such as a boutique. Make sure this is permitted by your lease agreement and follow city and state regulations. When figuring the size of your salon also consider

☐ **Equipment.** Will the space permit the equipment you need and want? For example, if you want a day spa, will you have room for shower facilities?

☐ **Shape of the salon.** Plan the workstations for efficiency. A long, narrow space requires totally different planning from a square one. Will the shape work?

Manufacturers of equipment frequently offer consultation and decorating services and can tell you the minimum space required for stations, chairs, manicure tables, shampoo bowls, etc. They can also provide layouts designed to increase efficiency or create the atmosphere you have in mind. Figure 24.11 represents a sample floor plan.

Cost must be considered in all of your planning. Figure all of the start-up costs as well as the amount of working capital you will have to have to sustain your business until it turns a profit. Experts suggest $100,000 as a minimum amount to open a salon. Many new salons fail

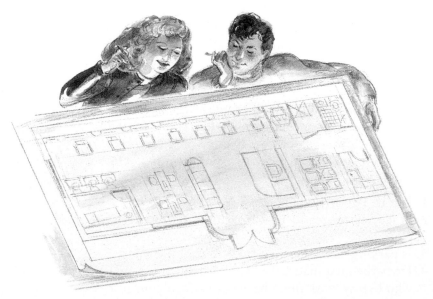

24.11

only because there is not enough capital to keep the salon open until the money generated can support the operation and the owner. Table 24.2 shows the accepted norms for a typical salon budget.

TABLE 24.2 Salon Expenses as a Percentage of Income	
Expense	*Percent of Income*
Salaries	53–55%
Rent	10–13%
Supplies	6–8%
Advertising	1–3%
Depreciation	1–3%
Laundry	1–2%
Utilities	1–3%
Maintenance	1–2%
Insurance	1–2%
Telephone	1–2%
Licenses and taxes	4–6%
Legal and professional fees	1–2%
Miscellaneous	4–5%

You can see that the salon that operates in the lower percentages has a total expense of 85%, leaving 15% for profit. The salon in the right column, however, is in big trouble. Total expenses add up to 104%, making the salon operate at a 4% loss. How could you correct the problems of this salon?

You must be sure that the prices you charge for your services cover all of your costs and give you a profit as well. Imagine that all the supplies you need to give a haircoloring cost $2.00. If you charge a customer $4.00 for a haircoloring service, will you make a $2.00 profit? *No*, because you have to pay salaries, rent, insurance, and many other things. All the general expenses a salon incurs as the cost of doing business are called **overhead**. It is important that the income you receive from your customers covers the costs of giving the services, your overhead, and your profit as well.

Cost of service refers to what it actually costs for every service you offer. The **break even price** is the price you must charge for a service to cover both your cost of services and your overhead. How do you figure out the least you can charge for a service to break even? You divide the cost of supplies by the percent of salon income that you spend on supplies. For example, if a perm wave costs $1.00 per application and you spend 6% of salon income on supplies (see Table 24.2), you make this calculation:

$$\frac{\text{Cost of supplies}}{\text{\% of salon income spent on supplies}} \quad \text{or} \quad \frac{\$1.00}{6\%} = \$16.66$$

So you need to charge at least $16.66 for a perm to met your costs or break even. Anything you charge above your break even price will be profit. This example is for the perm lotion and neutralizer only. Now add in the cost of cotton, shampoo, and conditioners. Add the cutting and styling costs to arrive at what you must charge for the total service. If you wish to charge a la carte, you will have separate service fees for the permanent wave, for the cut, and for the final style.

Services that have a very low product cost, such as cutting and styling, are the ones that will cover your other overhead costs and increase your profit. Retail products can also fill the gaps created when an expensive service must be discounted in order to be competitive (when you are offering specials, etc.). To price a retail product, you typically double the cost of the item. For example, a shampoo that costs you $2.00 will retail for $4.00. The typical commission on retail products is 10%. The following example illustrates the benefits of selling retail products.

Retail Price	4.00
Supply	-2.00
Commission	-.40
Overhead	-.33
Profit	1.28

While the profit might seem small in dollars and cents, the percentage of profit is 32%! The average salon nets 8% of its income from the sale of retail products. If you increase that by just 2%, you pay your rent.

Record Keeping

Keeping accurate records is essential. You need to be able to track your inventory to keep costs down. You must maintain accurate records to show that you have met your tax liabilities every quarter. Records are essential to ensure that your staff members are paid accurately and that you have withheld the taxes required.

Many salons today are relying on computers to maintain these records. Software programs are available that can operate your computer as a cash register, maintain client lists, keep salon service records, record inventory and flag when you are low on stock, etc. These programs can also be used for the promotional activities discussed earlier in this chapter. You have three methods of record keeping available to you: an accountant, a computer with selected software, or the traditional methods described in this section.

Cash receipts detail the monies collected on a monthly basis (see Figure 24.12). At the end of the month, you simply add the columns. The total of these columns should equal that of column 1, Net Deposit.

Cash disbursements is a monthly record of the money paid out. See Figure 24.13 as an example. Notice the difference in bookkeeping entries for check 303 (for supplies) and check 304 (payroll for John Smith). Such accurate record keeping is critical for proper preparation of your quarterly taxes and maintaining employee tax records.

The **book balance** is the amount of money you have available. To find it, add the net deposits to the balance from your previous month. Then subtract your disbursements. Here is the formula for finding the book balance:

CASH RECEIPTS – JULY

Date	Net Deposit ①	Services ②	Sales ③	Sales Tax ④	General ⑤
1	154.00	154.00			
8	57.78		54.00	3.78	
12					45.00
19	162.50	149.66	12.00	.84	
21	181.30	181.30			
30	259.60	206.10	50.00	3.50	
	860.18	691.06	116.00	8.12	45.00

24.12

CASH DISBURSEMENTS — JULY

#	Date	Payee	① Net Disbursements	② Social Security	③ Federal Tax	④ State Tax	⑤ Local Tax	⑥ Other Deductions	⑦ Pay Roll	⑧ Expences
303	1	The Apple Co.	27.68							27.68-Supplies
304	3	John Smith	109.90	10.05	17.50	4.50	2.00	6.05	150.00	
305	3	Mary Brown	90.23	7.37	9.80	2.60			110.00	
306	5	Telephone Co.	83.51							83.51- tele.
307	8	USA Towel Co.	54.15							54.15-towels
308	9	Bixby's	20.10							20.10-floor cleaner
309	10	John Smith	109.90	10.05	17.50	4.50	2.00	6.05	150.00	
			495.47	27.47	44.80	11.60	4.00	12.10	410.00	185.44

24.13

Book Balance = Total Net Deposits + Previous Book Balance
        – Total Net Disbursements

The **bank balance** is the amount of money remaining in your bank account according to your bank statement. Here is how you find it:

Bank Balance = Book Balance + Outstanding Checks

Insurance for the Cosmetology Salon

The purpose of insurance is to reduce your risk of loss from the operation of your salon. When you purchase insurance, you trade a large but uncertain loss for a small but certain loss—your premium. Some types of insurance are required by city, state, or federal regulation; make sure you meet all requirements before you open your business. The following are types of insurance you should consider:

- **Malpractice.** Covers injury to a client due to poor performance of a salon service.
- **Premise liability.** Protects against claims made by the public due to accidents inside or outside your salon.
- **Fire.** Protects the salon, equipment, etc., in the event of fire.
- **Workers' compensation.** Required insurance that covers any

injury or disease suffered by an employee as a result of performing his or her duties on the job.

- ☐ **Personal Illness, Hospitalization,** and **Accident.** These may be desired for yourself, or as a package of benefits for your employees.
- ☐ **Unemployment.** Required payroll deduction for your employees and one that you must match, dollar for dollar. If you are the sole employee, you will make both contributions.

Your Tax Obligations as an Employer

We talked about the types of taxes earlier in this chapter. As an employer, you are responsible for withholding the correct amount from each person's paycheck. The employee will complete a W-4 form so you know the number of dependents claimed. Then, using charts available from the city, state, and federal governments, you will withhold the correct amount from each paycheck and pay it into the employee's fund. At the end of the year, you must prepare a W-2 statement for each employee who is paid more than $600 during the year. As an employer, you must also be in compliance with any state labor laws regarding minimum wage.

> ◆ **Key Point** ◆
> With careful planning and advice from responsible business professionals, you can open a successful and profitable salon of your own.

Summary

There is much involved in building your career success, whether you choose to be an employee or to open your own salon. In either case, you have chosen to enter personal service work, which means that you must build your personal skills to deal with people effectively. Your image is your first means of communicating with your clients. The next impression is how well you greet your client and begin your consultation for a successful service. Good communication is as important as the work you do.

Establish realistic goals and a timetable for achieving them. Select the type of salon that suits your personality and your career goals. Strong promotion to the potential customers in your area will help you achieve your goals. You will determine the method of promotion that is most effective for your area. Be sure to use client follow-up methods that will help you retain the customers that you have and develop new ones.

Ethics are important in your business. Ethics involve good personal and business practices and will help you develop your professional relationships with clients, co-workers and employers. You must treat clients with honesty and integrity to build a solid foundation for your future.

If you decide to open your own salon, seek out the professionals that can help you determine the ideal form of ownership, location, and staffing for your new business. You will adhere to local codes and follow city, state, and federal requirements for taxes and licensure. Accounting methods will be essential to your success, whether you choose to track by computer or by hand. The world of cosmetology offers you many options, and you will build your own pathway to success.

1. What does it mean to be a personal service worker?
2. How will you benefit from the state examinations?
3. What steps should you take to get your first job?
4. Why are professional ethics important in the salon?
5. What are five methods you can use to build a clientele? Which methods will you employ and why?
6. Describe the methods of compensation for cosmetologists. What benefit packages are available to you as a cosmetologist from each?
7. What tax responsibilities do you have as a regular employee?
8. What important factors should you consider in the planning stage of opening your own salon?

1. Using the worksheet in this chapter, develop your own resumé. Ask a fellow student to comment on it and then refine it further. When you are satisfied, ask your instructor to critique your resumé. Which elements make it the most effective?
2. Research the salons in your locality. Determine whether they are full-service, a chain operation, franchise, or free-standing. Select the type of organization you would most like to work in. Explain why you made that selection.
3. At two of the salons in project 2, ask for information regarding the pay structure and the benefits available to employees. Compare the information and determine which offers the best potential income package.
4. Develop a business card, a flyer, and a client follow-up card. Why have you chosen the most effective advertising? Make notes of the features that worked best and refine your samples accordingly.
5. Obtain a Bulletin of Information (BOI) from your state exam administrators listing the expectations for the state exam. How will you prepare to meet those expectations?

APPENDIX A

EMERGENCY PROCEDURES

WHAT AN EMERGENCY IS

Emergencies are situations that call for immediate action. **First aid** is the action taken to assist people who suffer injuries or sudden illnesses until more complete help arrives.

Every agency has an emergency procedure. This includes telephone numbers of fire, police, and rescue squads. It also includes a plan of who to call during what emergency. It is your responsibility to be familiar with this plan and these telephone numbers.

If you need to call 911 be prepared to offer the following information:

☐ your name
☐ your exact location
☐ the situation or problem

If you are calling for medical assistance, it is helpful if you can specify symptoms. "The individual was having chest pains and has now collapsed," or "The individual is bleeding." Ask that an ambulance be dispatched immediately and stay on the line to offer further information.

Steps to be Taken in an Emergency

Before you take any action, you must know the following:

- What is the problem or emergency?
- What must be done?
- What *you* are capable of doing.
- Can the person be moved?

Get the person to safe, firm ground away from danger of electrical shock, fire, or explosion. Do not move the person unless there is danger of further injury. Remember, you should do this without causing serious injury to yourself.

Do not leave a person who needs help. Have someone else call for additional help. If the person does not need immediate help to maintain life, your responsibility is to prevent additional injury and to provide comfort and security until medical help arrives. Keep the person warm, comfortable, and safe. If the person is on the floor leave him or her there until medical help arrives.

RESTORING BREATHING

Choking

A person's airway can be blocked by

- Foreign matter in the mouth, throat, or windpipe
- Unconsciousness, leading to relaxed muscles and the tongue falling back

Children and infants are treated differently than adults when they have difficulty breathing. *If the child or infant is having difficulty speaking, or coughing, do not help, but call for assistance immediately.*

If the child or infant has had an infection, a high fever, or has taken medication and is having difficulty breathing, call for help immediately.

If the child or infant is unable to speak or cry and is conscious, use back blows and chest thrusts. Back blows are quick forceful blows between the shoulder blades used to dislodge objects when the person is an infant or young child. This causes waves of air to be forced out of the lungs and may dislodge the foreign matter. Talk to the child as you are doing this. Tell the child that you are going to smack their back to help them breathe easier.

1. Call for help
2. Support the child with one arm and the child's face down toward the floor.
3. Use less force than on an adult; hit quickly four times.
4. Keep the head supported and turn the infant over and place two fingers below the sternum and push down slightly four times (Figure A.1).
5. Repeat the entire process until the foreign object has been spit out.

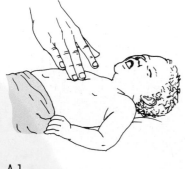

A.1

If the child or infant is unconscious, call for help.

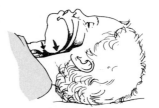

A.2

1. Open the child's mouth and remove the foreign object if you can see it.
2. Use the head-tilt/chin-lift and breathe for the child (Figures A.2 and A.3).
3. If the rescue breathing is not successful, perform one series of back blows and chest thrusts.
4. Perform rescue breathing again until help arrives.

Abdominal Thrust

Manual thrusts are a series of quick movements to the upper abdominal area or chest area to force the obstruction to move. **Abdominal thrust,** also called the **Heimlich maneuver,** is used when the person cannot breathe, cough, or speak. Talk to the person as you are doing this. Tell the person you are going to do the Heimlich maneuver to help them breathe easier. Do not use the Heimlich maneuver on pregnant women, infants, or small children.

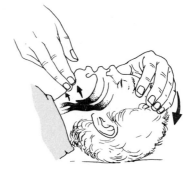

A.3

When the person is sitting or standing and is conscious:

☐ Stand behind the person and wrap your arms around his or her waist.
☐ Put the thumb side of one hand on the abdomen between the navel and the end of the breastbone. Do not actually touch the chest.
☐ Grasp this hand with the other hand and press it into the abdomen with a quick upward movement (Figure A.4).
☐ Repeat this six to times rapidly to dislodge the obstruction.

CONTROL EXTERNAL BLEEDING

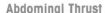

If a cut occurs during a salon procedure, immediately follow these steps:

1. Apply direct pressure to the wound to control bleeding and blot blood from the cut.
2. Dispose of soiled material in a sealed container used specifically for that purpose.
3. Clean and sterilize instruments.
4. Sanitize your hands. Put on a new pair of protective gloves.
5. Sanitize client's hands.
6. Apply sterile bandage to the injured area.

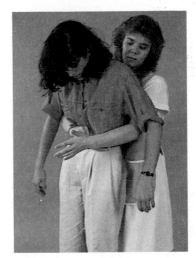

A.4

POISONING

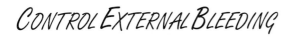

1. Look for a container that might have held the poison. (Remember, antidotes on the bottle can be incorrect.)
2. Check the mouth for chemical burns.
3. Check the breath for odors.

4. Gather as much information as possible about this incident before you act. A person can be poisoned by:

a. inhaling a poison through the mouth and nose.

b. swallowing it.

c. injecting himself or herself with it.

d. absorbing it through his or her skin.

No matter how a person is poisoned or how the poison acts, you must act quickly and correctly.

Swallowed Poisons

If the person is conscious and does not have convulsions:

- ☐ Dilute the poison with a glass of milk.
- ☐ Do not give oil.
- ☐ Call the poison control center with as much information as you have.
- ☐ Save any vomitus.

If the person is unconscious:

- ☐ Do not give anything by mouth.
- ☐ Position the person on his or her back with their head facing you.
- ☐ Maintain a clear airway. If the person stops breathing, give mouth-to-mouth resuscitation. There are times when you should not perform mouth-to-mouth resuscitation due to the type of poison involved. If poison remains on the person's mouth, or you could be poisoned by fumes. do *not* give mouth-to-mouth resuscitation. Check with your agency to see what the policy is in such situations.
- ☐ Call for help and remain with the person until someone arrives.

SHOCK

Signs and Symptoms of Shock

- ☐ Eyes are dull and pupils wide.
- ☐ Face is pale; may be bluish in color.
- ☐ Person may be nauseated.
- ☐ Respirations are shallow, irregular, and labored.
- ☐ Pulse is rapid and weak.
- ☐ Skin is cold and clammy.
- ☐ Person is restless.
- ☐ Person is very weak and may collapse.

Emergency Procedure

- ☐ Send someone for help.
- ☐ Position the person with the head lower than the legs. Keep him or her warm (Figure A.5).
- ☐ If a broken bone is suspected, keep the person flat.

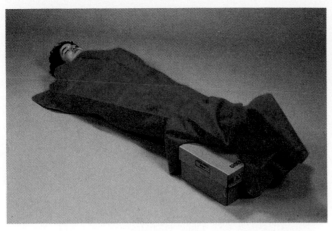

A.5

- ☐ Control bleeding.
- ☐ Do not give any fluids.
- ☐ Talk to the person and make him or her comfortable until help arrives.

Burns

Emergency Procedure

- ☐ Do not remove clothing stuck to the burned area.
- ☐ Put the body part in cool water, if possible. Let remain for two to five minutes. Do not put ice on the burn.
- ☐ Cover the area with a sterile or clean cloth.
- ☐ Continue to put cool water over the dressing.
- ☐ Get medical help. Stay with the person until someone arrives.

APPENDIX B

METRIC MEASUREMENTS

LIQUID

You are probably most familiar with measuring liquid in ounces. When you measure chemicals, you will be asked to record it in cubic centimeters (cc). This is a metric measure. A chart helps you determine how many cc are in a serving.

If you need to change ounces to cc, use this formula:

$$30 \times (\text{no. of ounces}) = \text{no. of cc's}$$

Example:

$$30 \times 8 \text{ ounces} = 240cc$$

1 gallon	— 4000 cc
1 quart	— 1000 cc
1 pint	— 500 cc
10 oz.	— 300 cc
9 oz.	— 270 cc
8 oz.	— 240 cc
7 oz.	— 210 cc
6 oz.	— 180 cc
5 oz.	— 150 cc
4 oz.	— 120 cc
3 oz.	— 90 cc
2 oz.	— 60 cc
1 oz.	— 30 cc
(2 tablespoons, 30 ml)	
1 teaspoon	— 4 cc
(15ml)	
1/4 teaspoon	— 1 cc
(1ml)	

cc = cubic centimeter   ml = milliliter   oz. = ounce

HEIGHT

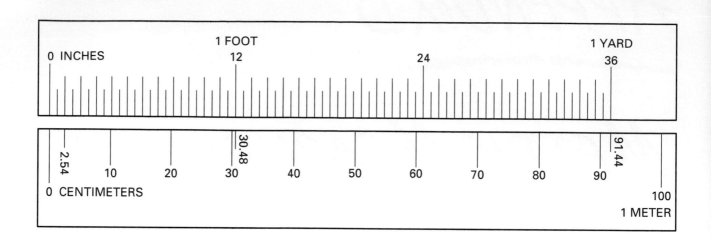

0 INCHES		1 FOOT 12		24		1 YARD 36

2.54	10	20	30.48 30	40	50	60	70	80	91.44 90	100

0 CENTIMETERS

1 METER

TEMPERATURE

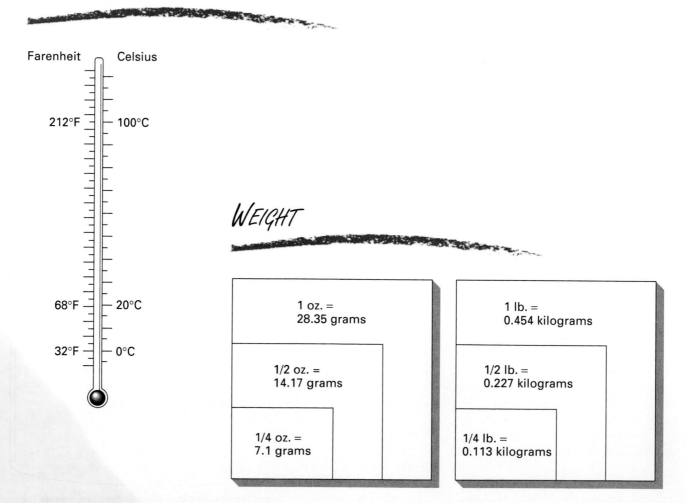

Farenheit   Celsius

212°F — 100°C

68°F — 20°C

32°F — 0°C

WEIGHT

1 oz. =
28.35 grams

1/2 oz. =
14.17 grams

1/4 oz. =
7.1 grams

1 lb. =
0.454 kilograms

1/2 lb. =
0.227 kilograms

1/4 lb. =
0.113 kilograms

GLOSSARY

abduction The action of the muscles that separate the fingers.

abductor Muscle located at base of fingers and thumb; separates fingers.

abrasion Scraping of the skin; excoriation.

abscess A hollow cavity containing pus surrounded by inflamed tissue.

absorb To take in or suck up (like a sponge).

accelerating machine A machine that can help some hair conditioners to work more quickly. The hair is not covered when using this method.

accelerator An additive to speed the hair lightening process. Also called a protinator, booster, or activator.

accent A concentrated formula that can be added to a color formula to intensify or tone down the color.

accessory A division of, and the name for, the 11th cranial nerve, acts on internal muscles; also, any attachment for a machine or device.

acetic acid (a SEE tik AS id) The chief acid vinegar.

acetone (AS e tohn) A volatile liquid used for removing nail polish.

acid A sour tasting substance that has hydrogen as one of its elements and that releases hydrogen ions when it is dissolved in water.

acid-balanced shampoo A low pH, conditioning shampoo for tinted, dry, damaged, or chemically relaxed hair.

acidic (a SID ik) The condition of a water solution with hydrogen ions in it and having a pH below 7.

acidification (a SID i fi KAY shun) Application of a low pH product to the hair.

acid rinse A mixture of water and vinegar or lemon juice.

acne A chronic inflammation of the sebaceous glands that results in pimples.

acne simplex A mild temporary variety of acne.

acne vulgaris (vul GAR is) A serious case of acne that requires a dermatologist's care.

acquired immunity An immunity that occurs once a person has had a particular disease or has been inoculated against it. Such immunity may be permanent or temporary.

actinic (ak TIN ik) Describing a kind of light that has a chemical effect.

actinic conjunctivitis (kon junk tih VEYE tis) A condition that results when the mucous membranes lining the eyes are burned by the sun.

active ingredient The substance in a cosmetic that gives special properties to the cosmetic and makes it do what it is supposed to do.

active stage The period during which bacteria are growing and reproducing.

adaptibility The quality that makes a hair design suitable to the client.

adduction The action of the muscles that draw the fingers together.

adductor Muscle located in base of fingers and thumb; draws fingers together.

adrenal gland (ad REE nal GLAND) An endocrine gland that secretes hormones into the bloodstream; increases energy.

adrenaline (a DREN a lyn) A hormone secreted by the adrenal glands in time of stress.

aerosol The name used for the fine spray that comes from an aerosol can; the fine drops of liquid or powder propelled from the can by means of gas pressure.

afferent nerves (AF fer ent NERVZ) Nerves that convey messages to the brain from the external organs.

agnails (AG naylz) Torn cuticle around the nail place.

air waver A device used to style hair as it dries; primarily used for platform and completion work.

AIDS Acquired Immune Deficiency Syndrome; an incurable disease, caused by the HIV virus, that destroys the immune system.

albino (al BEYE noh) A person born with little or no pigment in the hair, eyes, or skin.

alcohol A quickly evaporating, colorless liquid used to cleanse or sanitize the skin or implements.

alkali (AL kah lye) A corrosive compound having a pH of over 7 and marked basic properties; a hydroxide of an alkali metal.

alkaline (AL kah lyn) Term used to

describe a solution that contains hydroxide ions and has a pH above 7.

allergen (AL er gin) A chemical agent that causes an allergic reaction (especially skin problems) only in certain people.

allergy (AL er gee) Extreme sensitivity to specific foods, chemicals, and other substances that causes an abnormal condition.

alopecia (al oh PEE shee ah) Loss of hair.

alopecia adnata (ad NAYT a) The complete or partial loss of hair shortly after birth.

alopecia areata (air ee AH tah) A condition in which hari falls out in patches.

alopecia follicularis (foh lik yoo LAR is) Loss of hair caused by inflammation of hair follicles, usually in a small area.

alopecia prematura (pree ma CHUR ah) Loss of hair early in life.

alopecia senilis (se NIL is) Loss of hair in old age.

alopecia totalis (toh TAL is) Loss of hair from the entire scalp.

alopecia universalis (yoo ni VUR sal is) Loss of hair from the entire body.

alternating current Electric current in which electrons move first in one direction and then reverse their direction and move the opposite way; abbreviated AC.

alum solution An astringent used to stop bleeding; potassium aluminum sulfate.

amine (AYE mine) A reducing agent; alkalizer.

amino acid A special kind of organic compound that can form long chains called proteins; keratin is one such protein.

amitosis (ami i TOH sis) The process by which a cell splits in half; also called *direct division*.

ammonium hydroxide (uh MOH ni uhm hy DRAHK syd) A compound that is formed when ammonia dissolves in water.

ammonium thioglycolate (theye oh GLEYE coh late) A chemical used in permanent waving and hair relaxing; commonly referred to as "thio."

ampere (AM peer) The unit of strength of electric current (many electrons per second); called "amp" for short.

anabolism (ah NAB oh lizm) The building up of the body's cells; constructive metabolism.

anagen phase (AN uh jen FAYZ) The phase during which a hair is growing; lasts 2 to 6 years.

analysis The procedure by which hair is examined before a service in order to determine its condition.

analysis machine A device that tests the elasticity, strength, and moisture content of hair.

anaphoresis (ANN uh FOR eez ees) The use of a negative pole to introduce a negative charged solution into the skin.

anemia A condition in which the blood is deficient in red blood cells, in hemoglobin, or in total volume.

angiology (an jee OHL oh jee) The science of the blood vessels and lymphatics.

anhidrosis (an heye DROH sis) A condition that occurs when the sweat glands stop functioning and the body is no longer able to regulate its temperature.

aniline derivative tint (ANN i lynn dee RIV a tive TINT) A compound derived from coal-tar byproducts offering almost endless options in coloring services.

animal hair One of the types of hair used in the construction of wigs and hairpieces. Some manufacturers blend animal hair with human hair to made it more manageable.

animal parasites Small organisms or insects that live on or in another living organism; head and body lice are examples.

anions Negatively charged atoms.

anterior Before or in front of.

anterior dilator naris (dye LAY tohr NAIR is) Muscle located in the skin of the nostrils; opens the nostrils.

antibiotics Drugs used to kill bacteria and other disease-producing organisms.

antibodies Proteins in the blood that fight disease germs.

antigen (AN tih jin) A substance that, when introduced into the body, stimulates the production of an antibody.

antimicrobal soap (ant eye mih CROH bal SOHP) An antiseptic used to cleanse the hands.

antiperspirant A cosmetic used to restrict the flow of perspiration by swelling the openings of sweat glands on the surface of the skin.

antiseptic A chemical substance that retards the growth of bacteria.

antitoxin (an ti TAHK sin) A substance in serum that neutralizes poison (toxin).

aorta (ay OR tah) The largest artery of the body; starts blood circulation from the heart.

aponeurosis (ap oh noo ROH sis) Connective tissue that connects muscle to muscle or to bone. Differs from a tendon only in being flat or thin.

approximate symmetry Equal attractions on either side of the central axis.

arrector pili muscles (a REK tohr PEYE leye MUS els) Tiny muscles of the skin that can make the hair stand on end and cause gooseflesh when a person is chilled or frightened.

arteries Tubelike vessels transporting blood away from the heart.

asepsis (ah SEP sis) The methods of making or keeping free of pathogenic bacteria (aseptic).

aseptic (ah SEP tik) Free from pathogenic bacteria or microorganisms.

asteatosis (AYE stee ah TOH sis) A condition that occurs when the sebaceous glands do not secrete enough sebum and the skin becomes very dry and scaly.

astringent A substance or medicine that causes contraction of the tissues, arrest of secretion, or control of bleeding.

asymmetric (ay sim EH trik) Not having balanced proportions; not symmetrical.

asymmetry (ay sim EH trik kal BAHL ans) Unequal weights or attractions that must be balancd at various distances from the central axis. The larger attraction must be placed closer to the central axis and the smaller one farther away.

athlete's foot Tinea pedis; ringworm of the feet.

atom The smallest particle of an element that can exist by itself and still retain the characteristics of the element.

atrium (AY tree um) The main chamber of an auricle of the heart.

atrophied nails See **onychatrophia**.

atrophy A wasting away of the tissue.

auricles (OR ik kel) The two chambers on each side of the heart that receive blood from the veins.

autoclave (AW toh klayv) A device that uses hot steam under pressure to sterilize implements.

autonomic nervous system (aw toh NAHM ik NER vus SIS tem) The system of nerves that controls automatic bodily functions, such as respiration, digestion, and circulation.

axillary (AK si ler ee) The main artery that supplies blood to the armpit, upper art, and chest.

axons (AK sahnz) The long nerve fibers that carry impluses away from the cell body.

bacilli (ba SIL eye) Plural of bacillus.

bacillus (ba SIL us) A rod-shaped bacterium.

backbrushing Brushing the short hair toward the scalp while holding the hair strand in a vertical position.

backcombing Combing the short hair toward the scalp while holding the hair strand in a vertical position.

bacteria One-celled vegetable microorganisms, sometimes called germs or microbes.

bactericide (bak TEER ih syd) An agent that destroys bacteria.

bacteriology (bak teer ee OL oh jee) The science that deals with bacteria.**bacterium** (bak TEER ee um) Singular of bacteria.

balance A pleasing harmony of weight or visual attractions.

bangs Hair that is cut to fall on the forehead.

barber comb A flexible comb used to taper a short neckline haircut.

barrel curl A curl shaped like a barrel; used on short to medium-length hair; also called a *styling curl*.

basal cell layer (BAY zal SEL LAY er) The deepest layer of the epidermal division of the skin.

base A compound that will produce hydroxide ions in solution. Also a protective cream applied to prevent soap irritation or the combination of colors that make up the total foundation of a specific hair color.

base cream An oil designed to protect the scalp during a straightening service.

basic Describing a solution that contains hydroxide ions; alkaline.

basilic (ba SIL ik) The main vein that draws blood from the back of the forearm.

battery A cell used to generate electricity.

bile (BYL) Secretion from the liver to aid the digestive process.

birthmark An unusual mark or blemish on the skin at birth; usually a pigmentation defect.

blackhead See **comedone**.

bleach See **lightener**.

blocking Fitting a wig on a proper canvas head; following the customer's measurements. Also, sectioning for a perm.

blond, blonde A person of fair hair and complexion.

blond-on-blond effects Multiple shade of blond tones on one head.

blood vessel A vein artery, or capillary.

blow dryer A device used to dry hair by means of a stream of hot or cool air that permits the operator to brush or comb the hair while the dryer is on.

blowout See **chemical blowout**.

blue nail See **onychocyanosis**.

blunt cutting Cutting the ends of the hair straight across without thinning or slithering.

bobby pins Pins that have either a smooth or crimped pattern, used for pinning rollers and curls and controlling hairpieces.

bob curl A curl that is used with very short hair.

body odor See **bromidrosis**.

body wave A permanent that gives the hair structure without curl; also called a *support perm*.

bonding A joining together of amino acids to form the unique structure of the hair.

book wrap Wrapping the hair ends for a perm by folding the endpapers over the ends of each strand of hair.

boric acid An acid solution derived from boric oxide, used to cleanse the eyes.

brachial (BRAY kee al) The main artery that supplies blood to the upper arm.

bromidrosis (broh mi DROH sis) Body odor caused by bacterial deposits on the skin.

buccal (BUK ahl) A division of the 7th cranial nerve; acts on muscles of the upper lip and the sides of the mouth.

buccinator (BUK si nay tor) Muscle located at the sides of the mouth between the upper and lower jaws; compresses cheeks, aids in chewing.

buffering agent An agent that helps to maintain a given pH.

callus A thickening of the skin due to friction.

calorie The unit of measure for heat energy.

camphor A medicated ingredient often used in cosmetics.

caninus (kay NEYE nus) Muscle located above and at the edge of the mouth; drawn the mouth up and out.

canities (ka NIT eez) Loss of the pigment melanin, resulting in white or gray hair, a natural part of the aging process.

canvas head (KAN vas HED) A canvas-covered, cork- or sawdust-filled head used for setting, sizing, and blocking wigs.

cape The covering draped over a patron to protect clothing during a salon service.

capillaries (KAP ih lar eez) Very small blood vessels that connect the arteries with the veins.

capitis (KAP ih tis) Pertaining to the head or scalp.

carbohydrate Any substance made of carbon, hydrogen, and oxygen; a food that gives energy, such as a sugar or a starch.

carbon A chemical element found in hair and in all organic compounds.

carbon dioxide A colorless gas formed especially by the decomposition of organic substances; often used in fire extinguishers.

cardiovascular system The heart and various blood vessels.

carotid (kah ROT id) The main artery of the neck that supplies blood to the brain, eye socket, eyelids, and forehead.

carpal (KAHR pul) The two rows of bones that form the wrist and join the arm bones to the hand.

cartilage A tough connective tissue capable of withstanding pressure.

catabolism (kah TAB o liz em) The destruction of the body's cells.

catagen (CAT uh jen) The phase during which hair growth slows as the follicle shrinks and the hair bulb thickens and slightly lifts from the papilla.

cataphoresis (CAT uh FOR eez ees) The use of a positive pole to introduce a positively charged solution into the skin.

cations Positively charged atoms.

caustic A strong alkali capable of destroying or burning tissue by chemical action.

CDC Abbreviation for the Center for Disease Control.

cell A small mass of protoplasm that is the basic building block of all plant and animal life.

cell body The central part of a neuron.

central axis A point of reference that works like the point of balance on a scale.

central nervous system The portion of the nervous system composed of the brain and the spinal cord.

cerebellum (sair eh BEL um) One of three parts of the brain; controls the functions of the muscles.

cerebrum (se REE brum) One of three parts of the brain; controls thinking, remembering, speaking, moving, and the activities of the senses.

certified color A vegetable coloring product that is used to coat the hair shaft temporarily.

cervical (SUR vi kal) A division of the 7th cranial nerve; acts on muscles at the sides of the neck.

cervical bones Seven bones that form the top of the spine; the top seven vertebrae.

chemical blowout A hair relaxing service that removes a small amount of curl and leaves the hair more manageable. It is used to achieve natural styles.

chemical bond A force that holds atoms together.

chemical change A process by which new substances are formed through the rearrangement of atoms.

chemical hair relaxer A chemical used to straighten curly hair.

chemical tint remover A tint (dye) remover containing a chemical solvent.

chemistry The study of matter and the changes it may undergo.

chemosurgery (kee moh SER je ree) Removing layers of skin with chemicals.

chignon (SHEEN yahn) A knot or coil of hair worn at the crown or nape.

chloasma (kloh AZ mah) Large brown pigmentation spots on the skin.

cholesterol A fat from animal tissues, used as an emulsifier.

cilia (SIL ee ah) *See* **flagella**.

circuit The closed path via which electric current follows.

circuit breaker An automatic switch that trips, or shuts itself off, when current passing through the breaker is greater than it was designed for.

citric acid A weak acid, found in fruits such as oranges, lemons, and grapefruits, that is used in preparing an acid rinse.

clavicle (KLAV ih kul) A bone forming the front part of the shoulder.

cleansing cream A soothing cleansing cream; usually a perfumed emulsion of vegetable oil or mineral oil.

clicking The rapid opening and closing of a curling iron as the hair is rolled around it.

clip A single- or double-pronged clip used to hold a curl or the hair in place, but not for decoration.

clippers Electric and manual implements used for shaping hair, especially at the neckline.

clockwise In the direction of the hands of a clock.

coating tints Tints that deposit color only on the outside of the hair shaft, affecting only the cuticle layer.

cocci (KAHK seye) Plural of coccus

coccus (KAHK sus) A round- or berry-shaped bacterium.

coccyx (KAHK siks) The tail bone; consists of four fused bones.

cold waving lotion A chemical solution used to break the bonds in the hair so that they can be reformed on a rod; ammonium thioglycolate.

color additive A surfactant used in lighteners to add color tones to the hair to offset the harsher tones that appear as the hair loses color.

colorfast shampoo A shampoo

formulated to protect the color of hair that has been tinted or bleached.

color modifier A substance that changes the color of a dye.

color remover A product that removes artificial pigment from the hair. Also known as a *stripper*.

color rinse A rinse that gives a temporary color (highlight) to the hair.

color shampoo A preparation formulated to cleanse the hair and add color at the same time.

color spray A gold or silver spray that is applied for special effects.

color stain A hair-coloring technique involving the use of a permanent color without developer.

color test A method of determining the action of a selected tint by testing it on a small strand of hair.

comb-out brush A small brush to cushion hair, smooth out a style, or lock hair in place.

comb-out comb A large comb used for teasing and locking hair in place.

comedone (KOM ee dohn) Blackhead; a constricted mass or plug of sebum with a darkened top.

communicable disease A disease spread by direct contact when blood or other body fluids are passed from one person to another.

composition In hairshaping, the amount of hair to be cut short and the amount to be left long in order to achieve the desired style.

compound A substance that contains atoms of two or more different elements.

compound dye A combination of vegetable dyes and metallic salts.

compound henna Egyptian henna to which has been added one or more metallic substances.

concentration The quality of depth, or darkness.

conditioning Any application of an oil, protein, or other substance to the hair or scalp to counteract the effects of strong chemicals or

exposure to the sun and to protect the hair against breakage.

conduction The transfer of heat by direct contact between hot and cool objects.

conductor A material through which a current will flow easily.

cone curl A curl that has a lifted, sculptured, curved stem that is shaped like a cone.

consistency Degree of firmness or viscosity of a cosmetic.

contagion The transmission of disease from person to person by direct or indirect contact.

convection The transfer of heat by means of a moving fluid (gas or liquid) between a hot object and a cool one.

corium (KAW ree um) The derma.

cornified layer *See* **stratum corneum**.

corn-row Small braids created all over the head, often in a pre-planned design; also the basis for a hair-weave extension.

corpuscles Red and white blood cells. The red cells carry oxygen to the body cells; the white cells help to fight disease germs.

corrective makeup Makeup designed to minimize poor facial features by drawing attention away from them.

corrugations (kor oo GAY shunz) Wavy ridges on the nail.

corrugator (KOR oo gay tohr) Muscle located in the eyebrow; pulls eyebrow down.

cortex (KOR teks) The most important part of the hair shaft, located between the cuticle and the medulla.

cosmetic dermatitis Allergic reactions caused by the application of cosmetics.

counterclockwise Movement in a direction opposite to that of the hands of a clock.

covalent bond The kind of chemical bond that is formed when atoms share each other's electrons.

cowlick A tuft of hair that stands up and is difficult to manage; usually in the crown area.

cream lightener An easy-to-control lightener containing thickeners, conditioners, and emulsifiers. It is most often used for application at the hair closest to the scalp.

cream press A solid, waxy product that leaves the hair soft and pliable.

crepe wool (KRAYP WUHL) Strands of wool sued to control hair ends in winding.

cresol (KREE sohl) A liquid obtained from coal tar and used for germicides; has pungent odor.

croquignole (KROH keen yohl) A figure-eight curl.

crown The top part of the head.

cuperose (KOO per rose) Damaged capillaries, visible as tiny red lines, that indicate fragile, aging skin or an area of skin that has been damaged.

cupid's bow The center portion of the upper lip below the center of the nose.

curl Hair that has been molded or wound into a circular spiral-like wave or coil.

curler A roller on which hair is wound.

curl foundation The base on which a curl is formed.

curl parting *See* **parting**.

curling iron A heated instrument used for curling hair.

curved parting A C-shaped section used as the base for a sculpture or cone curl.

cuticle The outer layer or covering of a hair; also, the tough fold of skin that forms at the base and sides of the nail plate.

cuticle cream A cream with a lanolin or petroleum base that is used to treat dry cuticles and brittle nails.

cuticle softeners Substances used to soften the skin so that it is easier to remove the cuticle adhering to the nail.

cyst (SIST) A closed sac covered by a membrane that develops abnormally in a body cavity or structure.

cystine (sis TEEN) An amino acid.

cytoplasm (SEYE toh plaz em) A

semifluid that lies outside the nucleus of a cell.

damaged hair Hair characterized by split ends, dryness, lack of elasticity, and brittleness.

dandruff A flaking of the skin, usually in the region of the scalp.

dandruff shampoo A shampoo formulated to aid in the elimination or control of dandruff and flaking.

dart A flat seam used in altering wig caps.

daughter cells The two new cells produced when a cell splits in half.

daytime makeup Soft, natural-looking makeup for everyday use.

debris Waste; dead skin cells, dirt.

decolorize To remove color.

deionized water Water without an electrical charge.

deltoid Muscle located in the upper arm and shoulder; lifts, extends, and rotates the arm.

dendrites (DEN dreyets) The shorter nerve fibers that carry impulses toward the cell body.

density The number of hairs per square inch on the scalp.

deodorant A product that hides or conceals odors.

depilation (dep il LAY shun) Removing hair at the skin line by means of depilatories or shaving.

deposit The addition of color to the hair to make it darker.

depressor septi nasi (di PRES or SEP tee NAY see) Muscles located in the membrane dividing the nostrils; closes nostrils.

derma (DER mah) The sensitive second layer of the skin; located beneath the epidermis.

dermabrasion (der mah BRAYE zhun) The smoothing of the skin by rubbing a rotating brush over scars or acne pits.

dermatologist (der ma TAHL oh jist) A medical doctor who specializes in the diagnosis and treatment of skin disorders.

dermatology (der mah TAHL oh jee) The study of the structure, function, and diseases of the skin.

dermis (DER mis) *See* **derma**.

detangler A conditioner that acidifies or coats the hair cuticle to prevent or remove snarls.

detergent A special kind of organic compound that has one end that is attracted to water and one end that is attracted to hydrocarbons (oils and greases); a good cleansing agent.

developer The substance that develops or oxidizes tint, usually hydrogen peroxide.

diagnosis Determination of the nature of a condition by its symptoms.

diamond Describing a face with a narrow forehead and a narrow chin.

diaphragm (DYE a fram) The midriff area; muscular partition that separates the chest cavity from the abdomen.

diathermy (DYE ah ther mee) A treatment designed to produce warmth deep in the muscles by means of electric current.

diffuser An blow-dryer attachment used in drying curly hair. The air is directed over a wide area as the hair dries "naturally" without loss of curl.

digestion The process whereby food is broken down and utilized by the body.

diplococci (dip lo KOK seye) Cocci that divide and grow in pairs. They can cause disease themselves, but often they invade the body following other diseases.

direct current Electric current in which electrons move in only one direction all the time; abbreviated DC.

direct division The process by which a cell splits in half; also called *amitosis*.

directional rollers Rollers used to create a definite style, ranging from fullness to closeness, by directing the hair either backward or forward.

disease carrier An apparently healthy person who carries disease germs and can transmit them to others.

disease vector An organism (for example, a tick) that carries or transmits disease from person to person.

disinfectant A chemical solution that will destroy most pathogenic and nonpathogenic organisms.

disc buffer An emery disc used to shape the nails.

disulfide bond (die SUHL fide BAHND) A special kind of covalent bond between two sulfur atoms; often forms a cross-link between two protein molecules in hair.

double-application tint A two-process penetrating tint.

double bond A chemical bond, usually between carbon atoms, that consists of two pairs of shared electrons; an unsaturated bond.

double flat wrap A procedure in which one endpaper is placed underneath the hair strand and the other paper on top of the strand before wrapping a permanent.

double-prong clips Devices used to pin flat curls, moldings, and shapings.

drabber A preparation that is added to tints and lighteners to tone down red and gold highlights; the drabber is usually blue.

dry cell A battery; a direct current (DC) source.

dry sanitizer An airtight cabinet that contains a disinfectant, usually formalin, used to keep tools sanitary.

duct A tube by which fluids or other substances are conducted to the surface of the skin.

duct glands Glands that produce substances that travel through tubelike ducts; examples are the sweat glands and the glands concerned with digestion.

ductless glands Glands without ducts that secrete hormones directly into the blood.

eccrine glands *See* **duct glands**.

eczema (EK semah) An inflammatory condition of the skin characterized by redness, itching, and scaly lesions.

edema (eh DEE mah) A swelling.

efferent nerves (EF e rent NERVZ) *See* **motor nerves**.

effleurage (ef LOO rahzh) A smoothing, gentle movement in massage.

eggshell nails Thin, flexible nails that separate from the nail bed.

Egyptian henna A pure vegetable hair dye.

elasticity The ability of hair to stretch beyond its normal length and then spring back.

electric curling iron An electrically heated instrument used for curling the hair.

electric current A directed movement of electrons in more or less the same direction at a given moment.

electric heater A device used to heat straightening combs and curling irons.

electricity Energy provided by an electric current.

electric pressing comb An instrument used for straightening the hair.

electric sanitizer A dry sanitizer that contains an ultraviolet lamp designed to keep tools sanitary. (Tools must first be immersed in a wet sanitizer before being placed in the dry one.)

electric shock The reaction of the nervous system to the passage of an electric current through the body.

electrode An implement that is used to apply electrical current to some part of the body.

electrology A method of removing undersirable hair with an electric needle,using electric current.

electron A tiny particle of an atom that has negative electrical charge.

electrotherapy Cosmetic or medical treatment involving use of electric current.

element A simple substance that cannot be broken down by ordinary means; an element contains atoms that are all of the same kind.

elevation In hairshaping, how high or low you hold a strand of hair in relation to where it grown on the scalp.

emollient (i MOL yent) A compound that will make two other substances mix together; soap is an emulsifier for oil and water.

emulsion (ee MUHL shun) A solution produced by using an emulsifier to mix two substances.

endocrine glands (EN doh krin GLANDZ) *See* **ductless glands**.

endothermic perm (en doh THERM mick PERM) A perm activated by an outside heat source, such as a dryer, when the heat is absorbed by the chemical.

endpapers Special papers that are used to control the hair ends as they are being wrapped on a permanent rod or roller.

enzyme (EN zym) A protein that can speed up or slow down chemical reactions.

EPA A number that indicates that a product meets the claims on its label. Abbreviation for the Environmental Protection Agency.

epidermis (ep ih DUR mis) The outer layer of the skin, visible to the eye.

epilating strips Pieces of muslin or cotton fabric used to remove warm and cold wax.

epilation (ep ih LAY shun) Removal of the shaft and the root of the hair by tweezing or waxing.

eponychium (ep oh NIK ee um) The cuticle around the nail plate.

erythema (er ih THEE mah) The reddening of the skin through the use of an ultraviolet lamp or from inflammation.

erythrocyte (i RITH roh syt) A red blood cell.

esophagus (ih SOF ah gus) The tube that guides food from the mouth to the stomach.

estrogen A hormone that promotes development of the secondary sex characteristics in the female.

ethmoid (ETH moid) Bone that forms the root of the nose between the eyes.

eucalyptus (yoo kah LIP tus) A mild painkiller often added to cosmetics to soothe tender skin.

eumelanin (yoo MEL ah nin) A type of natural melanin pigment found in black, brown, and blond hair.

European hair Hair from European countries used in the manufacture of human-hair goods; considered to be the finest-quality human hair.

evaporate To dry up as moisture passes into the air as vapor.

evening makeup Similar to daytime makeup, but more color, especially frosted color, is used to counteract the effect of artificial lighting.

excoriation (eks koh ree AY shun) A wearing off of the skin; an abrasion.

excretion (eks KREE shun) The discharge of waste products from the body.

excretory system (EX skre tohr ee SIS tem) The system that eliminates solid, liquid, and gaseous wastes from the body.

exfoliation (ex FOH lee AY shun) The process of sloughing off, or removing, dead skin cells.

exocrine glands (EX o krin GLANDZ) *See* **duct glands**.

exothermic perm (ex oh THER mik PERM) A perm activated by the heat produced when an additional chemical is mixed with the product.

extensor Muscle located in the forearm; straightens the wrist to the hand points forward.

external jugular The main vein that draws blood from the surface of the cranium and face.

eyebrow color Pencil or compressed powder used to draw fine lines in the eyebrow area.

eyeliner Cosmetic used to outline the eye close to the eyelashes; available in pencil, cake, and liquid form.

eye shadow A cream or powder cosmetic; used on the eyelids to add color.

facelifting A surgical procedure

performed by a plastic surgeon to tighten loose or wrinkled skin.

face powder A cosmetic used to help set makeup; available in powder or compressed-cake form.

facial A procedure designed to relax, tone, and condition the skin of the face.

facial chaise A reclining chair or bed in a room or a stall where facials are given.

facial nerve The 7th cranial nerve.

fall A long hairpiece.

fan-tail comb A short comb with evenly spaced teeth and a tapered tail at one end.

faradic current A rapidly interrupted current of a safe level produced by a special machine.

fascia A fibrous membrane that covers, supports, and separates muscles.

feather Taper.

fibrinogen (fy BRIN o jin) A protein in the blood essential for clotting.

filler A product used to build color on damaged porous hair so that all the hair has an even color.

fill-in curl A curl used in the areas between shapings that frame the face and run around the crown.

finger wave The use of the fingers, lotion, and a comb to fashion waves into wet hair.

finger-waving comb A 7-inch styling comb with well-tapered teeth used to move scalp hair.

fishhook ends Hair ends curved like fishhooks; the result of improper winding in permanent waving.

flagella (flah JEL ah) Hairlike appendages to a cell; sometimes called *cilia*.

flare curl A curl that has a long, narrow stem, with the curl at the end of the stem.

flat base Preshaped hair that forms a foundation for a curl to lie on.

flexor Muscle located in the forearm; bends wrist and clenched fist backward.

fluorescent source A light source in which visible light comes from phosphors that have been "excited" by ultraviolet waves.

fly-away hair Hair with static electricity.

formaldehyde A gas with a pungent odor that is used for preparing a germicide.

formalin A chemical solution made from formaldehyde gas; usually 37 to 40 percent formaldehyde. Used to clean implements.

formula The symbolic expression of the chemical makeup of a molecule; also, any standard procedure for preparing a product; recipe.

foundation A cream, liquid, cake, or stick product used as the base for other makeup.

fragilitas crinium (frah JIL ih tas KRI nee um) Split hair, a disorder of the hair shaft.

franchised salon A salon that is operated by an individual and regulated by a parent company; such salons are usually "budget type" operations with faster customer turnover and a larger dollar volume than the average new salon.

freckles Reddish brown or yellow spots on the skin; usually caused by locally excessive pigment.

free edge The part of the nail plate that is not attached to the nail bed and extends beyond the fingertips.

frequency The number of times per second an AC current changes direction.

friction Resistance to the relative motion of two objects in contact.

fringe Hair on the forehead.

frontal Bone that forms the forehead.

frontalis (frun TAL is) Muscle located at the scalp, forehead, and root of nose; raises eyebrow, draws scalp back, and wrinkles brow.

frosting The lightening or darkening of a number of individual strands of hair in various areas of the head to give an overall high-fashion look.

full-base roller *See* **on-base roller**.

full-stem curl A curl that is place completely off its base, giving the hair the greatest mobility.

fungi (fun JEYE) Plant organisms, some of which can cause serious infections; many others are harmless and even beneficial.

furrows Depressions in the nail caused by injury.

fuse A special device designed to prevent an overload in an electric circuit; usually contains a wire that melts when the current passing through it exceeds the limit for which it was designed.

galvanic current Direct current of a safe level that can be used in electrotherapy.

gauze A very thin meshlike material used in preparing facial masks; sometimes called cheesecloth.

general infection An infection in which bacteria are carried in the bloodstream to all parts of the body.

general shock A condition that results when electric current passes through part of the central nervous system.

generator A machine that acts as a source of AC power.

gene The basic unit of heredity.

germ *See* **bacteria**.

germicide A chemical solution used to destroy most pathogenic and nonpathogenic bacteria.

germinative layer (jer me NAY tiv LAY er) *See* **stratum germinativum**.

glycerine (GLIS ih rin) A common humectant used in many cosmetics.

glyceryl monothioglycolate (GLY ser ohl mo noh theye oh gleye KOH late) The main active ingredient in chemical waves.

gonads (GOH nadz) The reproductive glands.

grabbing The tendency of the porous ends of the hair to absorb more of a tint than the rest of the hair and consequently become too dark.

granular layer *See* **stratum granulosum**.

groove The bowl part of a curling iron that is curved to fit around the prong when the iron is closed.

ground An object designed to prevent shock by conducting electrical current into the earth.

Ground Fault Interceptor Abbreviated GFI; a safety device designed to protect from electrical shock, identified by the press switch in the center.

hacking In massage, a chopping movement made with the edge of the hand.

hackle A device used for combing and intermingling hair; looks like a board with several rows of nails sticking out of it.

hackling A process by which tangled hair may be disentangled.

hairbrush A brush used for brushing out a set, for removing tangles, or in giving a scalp treatment.

hair bulb A hair structure that lies just above the papilla and fits over it tightly; the bulb, nourished by the papilla, gradually narrows as it approaches the surface of the skin.

haircolor A product used to tint the hair.

hair crayons Crayons used to retouch the new hair growth between tint retouches.

hair follicle A tiny, tubelike pit in the skin from which a hair grows.

hair goods A general term applied to all wigs, hairpieces, and falls.

hairpiece A partial headcovering made of human hair or synthetic fiber, such as a fall, cascade, or wiglet.

hairpins Double-prong pins, available in many lengths, used for control in dressing wet or dry hair.

hair pressing A procedure for straightening curly or kinky hair by means of a heated comb or iron.

hair relaxer *See* **straightener**.

hair root The portion of the hair below the skin and within the hair follicle.

hair sample A swatch of hair taken from the patron's head in order to match hair goods with the patron's natural hair.

hairshaping Cutting or thinning the hair to achieve the proper style or look desired by the patron.

hair shaft The portion of the hair that projects from the skin.

hair spray A product that acts as a light net to hold hair in place or to add body to the hair; usually comes in aerosol cans or pump containers.

hair tinting The act of adding color pigment to either virgin or tinted hair.

half-base roller A roller that sits halfway on and halfway off the section of hair used for the roller.

half-stem curl A curl in which the circle is place half off its base, giving more movement but less firmness to the curl.

hand dryer A hand-held device used for blow drying by means of a stream of hot or cool air.

hand lotion A preparation used to soften the skin and to replace natural oils.

hand-tied wig A wig or hairpiece made by hand.

hangnails *See* **agnails**.

hard press A hairpressing treatment that removes all curl from the hair.

hard water Water that contains calcium and magnesium and does not lather easily with soap.

harmony Unity; a condition in which all elements of a hair design complement the facial features.

Haversian canals (hah VER shun kah NALZ) The small channels through which the blood vessels spread through bone.

health hazard A chemical that may affect health by exposure to it.

heavy side The side of the part where the most hair falls.

heating cap A thermal cap.

heat lamp A glass bulb with a reddish brown coating that produces infrared light used in heat treatments

helix (HEE liks) A spiral shap with a straight backbone.

hematoma nail (hee mah TOH mah NAYL) A bruised nail with a blood clot under the nail place.

hemoglobin (HEE mo glob in) An iron-containing protein occurring in the red blood cells.

henna shampoo A shampoo containing Egyptian henna; gives hair an auburn-red tone.

herpes (HER peez) An inflammatory disease of the skin caused by a virus.

herpes simplex (SIM pleks) Cold sores.

high-frequency current High-frequency alternating current of a safe level produced by a special machine; also called *Telsa current*.

high-frequency unit A small machine to produce high-frequency (Telsa) current; it plugs into a standard outlet.

highlighting shampoo A combination rinse and shampoo that gives highlights and slight color tone to the hair.

hirsute (HER soot) Hairy

horizontal Running or moving from side to side.

hormone A substance produced in one part of the body that is transported to other parts of the body by the blood.

hot comb An electrically heated comb used to style the hair; may have a hairbrush attachment.

hot dye *See* **fabric dye**.

hot-iron curling An instant curling method that uses electric irons or irons heated in an electric or gas stove.

hot oil An oil used in giving a hot-oil manicure; formulated to eliminate the need for soapy water, cuticle softener, cuticle oil, and lotion.

hot rollers Electrically heated rollers used to set the hair.

human disease carriers People who have a natural or acquired immunity to certain diseases yet who still carry the disease germs in their bodies and can infect others.

human hair One of the types of hair used in the construction of wigs and hairpieces.

humectant (hyoo MECK tant) A compound that will collect water out of the air and hold on to it by means of hydrogen bonds; a moisturizer.

humerus (HYOO mo rus) Bone located in the upper arm.

hydration The amount of moisture present in the skin.

hydrocarbon An organic compound that contains only hydrogen and carbon atoms.

hydrogen One of the elements contained in hair; usually occurs as a colorless, odorless, highly flammable gas.

hydrogen bond A special kind of chemical bond formed between molecules.

hydrogen peroxide A chemical used as a bleaching agent (20-volume strength) or as an antiseptic (10-volume strength).

hydrolized protein (HEYE droh lyzed PRO teen) A protein that is broken down into a small molecular weight so it can penetrate the hair or skin.

hydrometer (heye DRO mi ter) A device for measuring the volume of liquids.

hydronium (heye DROH nee um) Acid H_3O^+ ions in water.

hygiene The science of establishing and maintaining health.

hyoid (HY oid) Bone located at the front of the throat between the root of the tongue and the Adam's apple.

hyperhidrosis (heye per heye DROH sis) Abnormal sweating in cool weather or when at rest.

hypertrichosis (heye per tri KOH sis) Excessive growth of hair.

hypertrophy (heye per troh fee) A thickening of the nail.

hypoallergenic (heye poh al er GEN ik) Describing cosmetics that are especially designed for use by persons who tend to have allergic reactions to normal cosmetics.

hyponychium (heye poh NIK ee um) The cuticle under the free edge of the nail.

imaginary balance line A line drawn by the eye through the two fullest points of a form. These points will be dominant weights in a design and assist in determining balance.

imbrication (im brah KAYE shun) Scale-like cells that overlap one another.

immune Free from the possibility of harmful effects from a pathogenic agent; not able to contract a given disease.

immunity The condition of being able to resist disease.

immunity, acquired Resistance to specific disease germs as a result of once having had the disease or having been inoculated or vaccinated against it.

immunity, natural Inborn power to resist disease.

impedance (im PEED ans) The resistance in an electric current to the flow of alternating current.

incandescence The ability of an object to produce visible light when it is heated.

incandescent lamp An electric lamp that produces light by means of incandescence.

infection The invasion of the tissues of the body by disease germs. *See also* **general infection; local infection.**

infection control Efforts to prevent the spread of disease, including sanitary habits such as general cleanliness, chemical disinfection, and sterilization.

infectious Capable of causing or spreading infection.

inferior vena cava (in FIR ee er VEE nah KAY vah) A large vein that carries blood to the heart from the abdomen, legs, and feet.

inflammation A response of the body tissues to irritation or infection, with accompanying reddening, pain, heat, or swelling.

infrared (in fra RED) A portion of the spectrum lying outside the visible portion and below the red rays; abbreviated IR.

infrared generator An electric heating coil that gives off almost no visible light but is an intense source of infrared radiation.

ingrown hair A hair that grows beneath the surface of the skin and can cause infection.

ingrown nails *See* **onychocryptosis.**

inoculation Introduction of a disease-causing organism into the body to stimulate the production of antibodies

in-process test curl A permanent-wave rod that is unwound during the chemical-wave process to determine if the wave formation is complete.

insertion The attachment of the end of a muscle to a movable bone or other muscle.

insulator A material through which an electric current cannot flow.

insulin A hormone secreted from the pancreas that regulates sugar in the blood.

insurance, fire Insurance that would provide cash to replace salon equipment of furnishings were the salon to be damaged by fire.

insurance, liability Insurance that protects a person against being sued for damage for which that person is responsible

insurance, malpractice Liability insurance that protects the salon from damage claims made on the grounds of negligence.

insurance, premises Protection against claims made by the public with regard to accidents that occur inside or outside your salon.

insurance, product Liability coverage that protects the salon when a patron is injured due to the fault of a product.

insurance, workmen's compensation Insurance that covers any injury or disease suffered by an employee as a result of occupational duties.

internal jugular The main vein that draws blood from the internal region of the cranium, face, and neck.

international color ring A ring of color samples used to match the patron's hair with hair goods; standardizes all colors of the major hair-goods manufacturers; also known as the *J & L Color Ring.*

intestine The digestive tube that runs from the stomach to the anus.

inverted triangle Describing a face with a broad forehead and a narrow chin.

inverter A device that can change DC current to AC.

invisible light Light that cannot be seen with the eyes but that can be felt on the skin; includes infrared and ultra-violet light.

involuntary muscle A muscle that is not controlled by the will.

iodine A nonmetallic element used as an antiseptic, especially in treating cuts and bruises.

ion A particle with an electrical charge.

ionic bond A chemical bond between charged particles (ions).

iris The colored part of the eye.

irritant *See* **primary irritant; secondary irritant.**

isopropyl alcohol (eye so PRO pil AL co hohl) A chemical used to cleanse hands, skin, and minute cuts.

joint The point at which bones are connected or joined.

keratin (CARE ah tin) A hard chemical substance that is the principle constituent of hair and nails.

kidneys Two bean-shaped organs whose job it is to filter out wastes as the blood passes through them.

kilowatt A unit consisting of 1,000 watts.

kilowatt-hours The number of kilowatts used per hour.

kneading A movement used in massage that involves squeezing the muscles between the thumb and fingers or pressing the palm of the hand firmly over the muscle and then squeezing with the heel of the hand and the fingers.

knotting In wig making, the process by which hair is attached to a foundation.

lacing Light teasing of the entire length of hair to give it a soft, delicate appearance.

lacquer Any of a special group or organic compounds often used in the manufacture of nail polishes.

lacrimals (LAK ri malz) Two bones located in the side walls of the nasal cavity.

lactic acid Sour milk, often used as a mild bleaching agent.

lanolin A fatlike substance derived from animals; used in conditioning cosmetics.

lanthionine (lan THEE oh neen) A monsulfide bond with only one sulfur atom that cannot be reduced or oxidized.

lanugo hairs (lah NOO goh HAIRZ) Fine body hairs that contain no medulla.

large intestine The region of the digestive system into which food passes after it has been digested.

larynx (LAIR inks) The voice box.

ledger A written record of all salon income and expenses.

lemon rinse Lemon juice diluted with water used after shampooing in order to remove soap curds.

lentigo (len TEE goh) A pigmentation defect characterized by dark spots similar to freckles.

lesion (LEE zhun) An abnormal change in structure of an organ or part due to injury or disease.

leucoderma (loo koh DER mah) White patches on the skin caused by lack of pigment.

leuconychia (loo koh NIK ee ah) White spots on the nail place.

leukocyte (LOO koh syt) A white blood cell.

lift The action of a hair lightening product on the natural pigment of the hair.

ligaments Tough bands of tissue that hold the bones together.

light Radiant energy that can be seen or felt by the human body.

lightener A compound that will break down or react to produce free oxygen atoms that can remove color from other substances; to lighten the hair.

lightening mixture A mixture of hydrogen peroxide and either a commercial lightener or white henna and soap flakes.

lipstick A lip color available in stick and cream form.

liquid dry shampoo Shampoo made from a dry cleaning product; no water is needed in giving a dry shampoo.

liquid nail polish A polish applied to the nail to give it color.

liver spots Dark blotches on the face (chloasma).

lubricity (loo BRI sit ee) Smoothness; slipperiness.

load The device in an electric circuit that does the useful work.

local infection An infection that is confined to one area of the body.

local shock The passage of electric current only through a small region of the body.

lotion-wrapped perm A conventional permanent wave during which the waving lotion is applied to each rod as it is wound and reapplied after the entire head is wrapped.

louse A parasite that lays eggs on the hair shaft.

lumbars The five vertebrae located beneath the thoracics

lunula (lu NOO lah) The white semicircular area at the base of the fingernail.

lymph (LIMF) A colorless fluid filtered out of blood plasma.

lymphatics (lim FAT ics) Lymph vessels collecting fluids that have separated from the blood.

lymphatic system A secondary circulation that is closely connected with blood circulation; the collection of vessels, spaces, nodes, and so on through which lymph flows.

lymphocyte (LIMF oh cyte) A type of white blood cell.

lymph nodes (LIMF NOHDZ) The parts of the lymphatic system that trap bacteria and foreign particles; also called lymph glands.

machine-wefted Machine-woven said of wigs and hairpieces.

mandible Bone that forms the lower jaw.

mandibular (man DIB yoo lar) A division of the 5th cranial nerve; transmits sensations from the lower teeth and gums, lower lip and jaw, and sides of the head; also acts on muscles connected with chewing. Also, a division of the 7th cranial nerve; acts on muscles of the chin and lower lip.

manicure The care of hands and nails.

manicure table A table used to give manicures.

manicurist A person who specializes in the care of the hands and nails.

manipulation Any of the various hand movements used by the operator to achieve the beneficial effects of massage.

marcel iron A curling iron.

marcel wave A wave produced through the use of heated irons.

mascara A cosmetic preparation used to impart temporary color to the eyelashes.

mask A product applied directly to the skin to deep cleanse, tighten the skin, firm of the skin, moisturize, or reduce wrinkles or pore size.

massage Scientific manipulation of the body by rubbing, pinching, kneading, tapping, or stroking with the hands, fingers, or an instrument.

masseter (ma SEE ter) Muscle located at the back of the jaw; closes jaw.

match test The burning of fiber or hair to determine whether it is human hair or a synthetic.

matrix The region of the nail where new cells are forming.

maxilla (MAX ila) Bone that forms the upper jaw.

maxillary (MAK si lair ee) A division of the 5th cranial nerve; transmits sensations from the middle of the face, the lower eyelids, and the upper lip.

maxillary artery The main artery of the skin and muscles of the lower region of the face that supplies blood to the mouth and nose.

maxillary bones The bones that form the upper jaw.

medial (MEE dee al) Midway, middle.

medicated ingredient A substance added to a cosmetic because it promotes healing or is a good germicide.

medulla (mih DUHL ah) The innermost part of the hair shaft.

medulla oblongata (ahb lawng GAH tah) One of the three parts of the brain; the part that joins with the spinal cord.

melanin (MEL ah nin) A brownish pigment that determines skin color.

melanocytes (MEL uh no seytes) Cells throughout the body that manufacture pigment.

membrane A thin layer of tissue that covers parts of the body.

mentalis (men TAY lis) Muscle located at the tip of the chin; raises lower lip, wrinkles chin.

Merthiolate (mer THY oh layt) A commercial product used to cleanse cuts, and wounds.

metabolism The chemical changes in living cells that involve the building up and destruction of protoplasm.

metacarpals (met a KAR pulz) The bones that form metallic salts containing, for example, silver, lead, or copper.

microbes *See* **bacteria**.

microorganism A very small organism

mildew A parasitic fungus.

milia (MIL ee uh) Whiteheads; an accumulation of sebum beneath the surface of the skin, resulting in a small, whitish pimple.

miliaria rubra (mil ee AYE ree ah ROOB rah) Prickly heat; a condition caused by inflammation of the skin around sweat pores; usually occurs in hot weather.

minifacial A treatment that offers the benefits of relaxation and skin stimulation to the client who has pressing time restraints.

mirror-image symmetry An exact duplication of form and design on either side of the central axis.

mixture Two or more substances combined physically.

modacrylic (moh da KRIL ik) A general term applied to synthetic fibers, designating a single, nonporous fiber that can be varied in thickness.

moisturizer *See* **humectant**.

mold A fungus growth.

mole A small, brownish spot or blemish on the skin; usually slightly elevated.

molecule Two or more atoms joined together by a chemical bond.

monilethrix (moh NIL eh thriks) Beaded hair, a disorder of the hair shaft.

motor nerves Nerves that carry outgoing messages from the brain and spinal cord to the muscles or other organs.

motor units The muscle fibers that are controlled by nerve fibers.

mucous membrane A membrane that lines body passages and cavities that have openings on the surface of the body.

mucus A slippery secretion produced by the mucous membranes.

muscle A tissue that can contract and cause bodily movement

myology (meye OL oh jee) The study of muscles and their functions.

nail bed The underlying flesh on which the nail plate rests.

nail brushes Small, round brushes used to clean the nail and wash away the lifted cuticle.

nail enamel dryer An oily product that is applied to the nails to prevent stickiness and to produce a tough protective film.

nail lacquer Liquid nail polish.

nail mender A product similar to a nail strengthener, often containing flecks of nylon.

nail plate The visible part of the fingernail.

nail-polish remover A solution, often containing acetone, that is used to remove nail polish from the nails.

nail root The part of the nail between the matrix and the nail plate.

nail strengthener A product that is brushed on the nails to strengthen them.

nail white A cream or paste used to bleach and whiten the free edge of the nail.

nasalis (na ZAY lis) Muscle located at the bridge of the nose; opens and closes nostrils.

nasals Two bones that form the upper part of the bridge of the nose.

natural bristle brush A brush made from animal hair, usually boar's hair.

natural immunity An inborn power to resist certain diseases, possible due to an inherited characteristic.

NDC A number that ensures that a product is registered and meets guides established by the Food & Drug Administration (FDA); abbreviation for National Drug Code.

nerve A band of fine fibers that connect part of the nervous system with other organs and conduct impulses and messages.

neurology (nuh ROLOH jee) The study of the structure and functions of the nervous system.

neuron (NOOR on) A nerve cell with its related structures.

neutralization The process by which an aid and a base react with each other to leave only a salt and water; the process by which hair is rehardened after waving or straightening.

neutralizer An oxidizing substance that stops the action of chemical-waving, straightening, or coloring products.

neutron A small, electrically neutral particle in the center of an atom.

NF Abbreviation for National Formulary; on a label NF means that the product meets the standards of the *National Formulary*, published by the American Pharmaceutical Association.

nit The egg laid by a louse.

nitrogen A colorless orderless, tasteless gaseous element that makes up 80 percent of the atmosphere and occurs in all living tissues.

no-base relaxer A relaxer that does not require the application of a base cream.

nonconductor A material through which electric current cannot pass.

nonpathogenic Not producing disease; not harmful.

no-stem curl A curl in which the circle is placed directly on the center of the base, producing a firm curl with little movement.

nucleus The center of the functional activity of the cell; the center of an atom.

nutrition The nourishment body cells receive from food eaten.

obesity The condition of having excessive body fat.

objective symptom Any visible irregularity of the skin that helps a dermatologist to diagnose skin disorders.

oblong Describing a face that is long, narrow, and usually angular.

oblong parting A long and narrow section used as the base for a flare curl or stand-up curl.

occipital artery (ok SIP i tal) The main artery that supplies blood to the skin and muscles of the scalp, back of head, and neck.

occipital bone Bone that forms the back of the skull.

occipitalis (ok sip i TA lis) Muscle located at the back of the scalp; draws scalp back.

off-base roller A roller that lies completely off the section of hair used for the roller.

ohm The unit used to measure resistance in an electrical device or system.

Ohm's Law A principle of physics that accounts for the resistance that materials offer to the flow of electricity.

oil An organic compound that has some unsaturated bonds in it; a liquid fat.

oil lightener A lightener that is seldom used alone because it is slow and very messy. It can be used for special-effects lightening or as an additive to other formulas.

oleic acid (oh LEE ik AS id) As acid derived from natural oils and fats.

on-base roller A roller that lies directly atop the section of hair used for the roller.

onychatrophia (on ih kah TROH fee ah) Atrophied, thin fragile nails.

onychauxis (on ih KOH sis) A thickening of the nail; also called hypertrophy.

onchia (on NIK ee ah) Inflammation of the matrix of the nail.

onychocryptosis (on ih koh krip TOH sis) Ingrown nails; a condition that occurs when the corners of the nail press into the skin, causing inflammation.

onychocyanosis (on ik koh sy a NOH sis) Blue nail.

onychogryposis (on ih koh greye POH sis) Excessive nail growth with an inward curvature.

onychology (on ih KOH loh jee) The study of the nails.

onychomycosis (on ih KOH meye koh sis) *See* **Tinea unguium.**

onychophosis (on ih KOH foh sis) Accumulation of horny layers of epidermis under the nail.

onychophagy (on ih KOH fah jee) Biting of the nails.

onychorrhexis (on ih koh REK sis) Split nails.

onychosis (on ir KOH sis) Nail disease.

onyx (ON iks) A fingernail.

ophthalmic (ahf THAL mik) A division of the 5th cranial nerve; transmits sensations from the forehead, eyelids, eyebrow, and nose.

optical illusion An effect, usually created with makeup, that causes the eye to see something as different than it really is; can be created with haircolor and hairstyling as well.

orangewood stick A small stick made of orangewood; used in manicuring.

orbicularis oculi (or BIK yoo lar is OHK yoo leye) Muscle that encircles the eye; closes eyelid.

orbicularis oris (OR is) Muscle

that circles the mouth; contracts and puckers lips.

orbit Eye socket; also, the path followed by electrons as they move around an atom.

organ A part of the body having a special function.

organic Any compound that contains carbon atoms; also, relating to an organ.

organism Any living thing, whether plant or animal.

Oriental hair Hair from Asian countries, such as China or Korea, used in the manufacture of hair goods.

origin The fixed attachment of a muscle to a bone or other muscle.

OSHA Abbreviation for Occupational Safety and Health Administration.

osteology (oh tee OL oh jee) The study of the bones or the skeletal system.

ovaries The female reproductive glands.

overcutting technique Rolling the fingers of the left hand up before cutting.

overload To draw more current through a circuit than it was designed for.

overprocessed hair Hair that has been left too long in the processing stage; has been incompletely neutralized, or has been subject to too strong a waving lotion; the hair is dry, frizzy, dull, and brittle.

oxidizer A special kind of compound that supplies oxygen and removes hydrogen; bleaches are oxidizers. *See* **developer**.

oxidation A chemical reaction that forces a compound to lose electrons. This process is used in the salon to reform bond, join together artifical pigment molecules in color, or lighten natural color pigment in the hair.

oxygen A tasteless, odorless, gaseous element that makes up 20 percent of the atmosphere; essential animal and plant life.

oxygenated (AHK si jin ay ted) Containing oxygen.

pack A cosmetic preparation that is spread on the face and allowed to dry before it is removed; stimulates and conditions the skin.

palate (PAL at) The roof of the mouth.

palatines (PAL i teyens) Two bones located at the back of the nasal cavity that form the roof of the mouth.

pancreas A gland that secretes fluid to aid in digestion; it acts primarily as a duct gland.

pancreatic juices Fluids that flow from the pancreas into the small intestine to help the digestive process.

papilla (pa PIL ah) A structure that lies at the base of the hair follicle, deep in the dermal layer; it is well supplied with blood vessels and nerves.

papillary layer A layer of the dermis that contains tiny fingerlike projections (papillae) that anchor the dermis to the epidermis.

papule (PAP yool) A hardened red elevation on the skin.

paraphenylenediamine A color molecule made from coal tar.

parasite An organism that must live in or on another organism in order to survive.

parathyroid gland A gland attached to the back of the thyroid that regulates the calcium and phosphorus in the blood.

parietals (pah RYE i tals) Two bones that form the sides and upper part of the skull.

paronychia (pare oh NIK ee ah) An accute infection of the structures around the nail.

parting The area of the hair sectioned off for a curl. *See* **curved, oblong, square,** and **wedged parting**.

paste polish *See* **powder polish**.

patch test The application of small amount of tint or toner to the patron's skin 24 hours prior to a color application to determine a possible allergy to the preparation.

pathogenic (path o JEN ik) Causing disease.

pattern baldness Baldness in which hair recedes from the hairline toward the back of the head and also becomes very thin and recedes in the crown area.

pectoralis major (pek tohr AL is MAY jor) Muscle that runs across the chest from the breastbone to the upper arms; draws arm across chest, elevates ribs.

pectoralis minor Muscle located underneath and below pectoralis major; draws shoulders forward and down.

pediculosis captitis (pe dik yoo LOH sis KAP tis) Head lice.

pedicure Care of the feet and toenails.

pelvic region The region of the body that contains the reproductive organs and some of the digestive organs.

penetrating tint A tint that penetrates the cuticle layer of the hair and deposits color in the cortex.

pepsin An enzyme that breaks down proteins in food that is eaten.

peptide bond A special kind of covalent bond that is formed between two amino acids.

pericardium (per ih KAHR dee um) The tough membrane that surrounds the heart.

perimeter The circumference (outer edge) of a haircut.

periosteum (per ih OS tee um) The membrane that covers the exterior of the bone.

peripheral nervous system All the sensory and motor nerves that carry messages to and from the central nervous system.

permanent haircolor An aniline-derivative tint that is mixed with peroxide to make a penetrating, permanent color.

permanent wave The procedure using chemicals or heat to change the structure of hair so that it is permanently wavy or curly.

peroxometer *See* **hydrometer**.

perspiration The excretion of water and minerals through the sweat glands.

petrissage (PE tri sahzh) A light or heavy kneading of the muscles.

petrolatum (pet roh LAY tum) Petroleum jelly; a mixture of hydrocarbons used as a lubricant and as an ingredient in many cosmetics.

phalanges (fa LAN jeez) Long bones that form the fingers and toes.

phenol (FEE nohl) A good disinfectant for sanitizing and cleaning.

pheomelanin (FEO mel ah nin) A type of natural melanin pigment found in red hair.

phoresis (for EEZ ees) The chemical effect of atoms moving toward or away from the point of contact; used to introduce solutions into the tissues through the skin.

phosphor A substance that gives off visible light when it is struck by ultraviolet waves; used in fluorescent lamps.

pH scale A scale for rating the acidity or alkalinity of a solution; a measure of the hydrogen ion concentration of a solutions.

physical hazard A chemical that is combustible, flammable, or explosive.

physiology (fiz ee AHL oh jee) The science that deals with the functions of living things.

pigmentation A general term to describe the coloring of the skin and hair.

pigment granules The matter that gives hair its color.

pin curl A small section of hair that is wound around the index finger to make a curl and then pinned with hairpins or clippies.

pituitary gland (pi TOO i tair ee) A small gland located near the brain; involved in the regulation of most body functions.

pityriasis (pit i REYE ah sis) Dandruff.

pivot curl See **pin curl**.

plasma The fluid part of the blood and lymph.

plastic surgeon A medical doctor who specializes in facial surgery.

platelet A very tiny, flattened particle found in blood that aids in the clotting process.

platysma (pla TIZ mah) Muscle that runs from the chin to the shoulders and chest; draws down lower jaw.

pledget (PLEJ et) A square of cotton used to apply lotions or other liquids to the skin.

polarity The condition of having two opposite poles; for example, a positive pole and a negative pole.

polyethylene glycols (pol ee ETH i leen GLEYE calls) A complex family of large molecules that form chain polymers.

polypeptide A long molecule containing two or more peptide bonds.

pomade A cosmetic preparation used for the hair and scalp.

pore A small opening on the skin through which sweat is secreted.

porosity The ability of hair to absorb moisture.

posterior Located behind or toward the back.

posterior auricular (aw RIK yoo lar) A division of the 7th cranial nerve; acts on muscles behind the ears.

posterior auricular artery The main artery that supplies blood to the scalp behind and above the ears.

posterior auricularis (aw rik yoo LAR is) Muscle located behind the ear; draws ear backward.

posterior dilator naris (dye LAY ter NAIR is) Muscle located in the skin of the nostrils; opens nostrils.

postiche (poh STEESH) An artificial hairpiece, especially curls, braids, or any other extra hairpiece, used in creating a particular hairstyle.

powdered lighteners A lightener that is usually faster in its activity and slightly more alkaline than other lighteners. It can also be drying to the hair.

powder polish Used to give gloss to the nail, specially in conjuction with buffing.

precision haircutting A system of hairshaping.

predisposition test See **patch test**.

prelightening A lightening service that must be given before application of a tint when a patron choses a tint that is much lighter than her natural hair color.

preliminary test curl Advance application of waving solution to a small strand of hair to determine processing time and the hair's reaction to the chemical solution.

presoftening A service designed to soften and lift the cuticle of resistant hair so that tint can reach the cortex; given before a coloring service.

pressing See **hair pressing**.

pressing oil A preparation applied to the hair before pressing; deposits an oily film on the hair; lets the hot comb glide through the hair and gives it a sheen or gloss.

prickly heat See **miliaria rubra**.

primary colors Red, blue, and yellow.

primary irritant A mild cosmetic that has a minor irritating effect on the skin only at the point of contact.

procerus (pro SEER us) Muscle located between the eyebrows; pulls forehead down.

processes The short, threadlike fibers in a nerve cell.

processing The complete waving procedure—wrapping, testing, and rinsing.

profile proportion The standard proportion of three parts hair to two parts face from a profile view.

progesterone (proh JES ti rohn) A female hormone.

progressive rhythm Repeating patterns that gradually become larger or smaller.

progressive tint A tint that oxidizes slowly, so that the color develops gradually.

pronator (PROH nay tohr) Muscle located in the forearm; turns hand so that palm faces back or down.

prong The solid, perfectly round part of the curling iron that fits into the groove when the iron is closed.

prophylaxis (proh fi LAK sis) Prevention of the spread of disease.

protective base *See* **base cream.**

protein A special kind of organic compound made of many subunits of amino acids held together by peptide bonds; proteins are found in all living tissues, including skin, hair, and nails.

protein conditioner A conditioner that adds amino acids to hair that has been weakened by chemical services or exposure to the environment.

proton (PROH tahn) A small particle in the center of an atom that has a positive electrical charge.

protoplasm (PROH toh plax em) A substance present in all living matter.

psoriasis (soh REYE ah sis) A skin disease characterized by red patches covered with white scales.

pterygium (te RIJ ee um) An overgrowth of cuticle on the nail plate.

pulmonary Relating to the lungs.

pulmonary artery The artery that carries blood poor in oxygen from the right ventricle to the lungs.

pumice (PUM is) A very light mineral used for polishing and buffing.

pus The fluid that oozes from an infected wound.

pustule (PUS tyool) An inflamed or infected pimple containing pus.

pyrolysis (peye ROHL i sis) Chemical breakdown under heat.

quadratus labii inferioris (kwah DRAY tus LAY bee y in feer ee OR is) A muscle located below the lower lip; that acts to pull down lower lip.

quadratus labii superioris (soo peer ee OR is) Muscle located above the upper lip; lifts upper lip.

quat (KWAHT) The short name for a quaternary ammonium compound.

quaternary ammonium compound (kwah TER ne ree ah MOH nee um KAHM pownd) A compound used as a germicide.

radial The main artery that supplies blood to the front of the forearm and hand.

radial rhythm Regualar and even patterns emerging from a center point.

radiation The process by which an object gives off heat or light.

radius Long bone forming the thumb side of the forearm.

rash Skin inflammation or eruption having little elevation.

razor A useful hairshaping tool for certain textures of hair.

receptors Nerves that are sensitive to cold, heat, or pain.

reconditioning The process of improving the condition of damaged hair through the application of conditioners.

reconstruction perm A two-part permanent-wave procedure during which the hair is first chemically straightened and then chemically waved.

record card A card that contains all pertinent information about each patron, including name, address, and telephone number, a record of all services and products used, hair condition at the time of each service, and so on.

rectifier A mechanism that can change AC current to DC.

relaxer *See* **straightener.**

reduction A chemical reaction that forces a compund to gain an electron.

resilient Springy, flexible, and strong.

resistance The force that limits the flow of current in an electric circuit.

resistant hair Hair that is not easily penetrated by coloring, waving, and straightening products.

respiration The act of taking air into the lungs; breathing.

respiratory system The body system that takes in needed oxygen and eliminates carbon dioxide and moisture. The lungs, windpipe, and bronchial tubes are the key organs of respiration.

resume (REZ uh may) A typed summary of vital statistics and past experience that is given to a prospective employer.

retail department A section of the salon in which cosmetics, hairpieces, jewelry, and other products are available for purchase.

reticular layer (re TIK u lar) The second layer of the derma, beneath the papillary layer, that contains sensory nerves, oil glands, sweat glands, hair follicles, and blood vessels.

retouch A touch-up; applying a lightener, tint, or hair straightener to the new growth of hair.

rhinoplasty (RYE noh plas tee) Surgery designed to reshape the nose.

ribs Twelve pairs of bones located in the thorax.

ridge filler Polish used when the surface of the nail needs a base coat that is thicker. Used to fill in minor depressions and imperfections in the natural nail. Also used with tips and wraps.

ringworm A highly contagious skin disease caused by a fungus; takes the form of circular lesions

rinse To cleanse hair with water after shampooing, permanent waving, coloring, or other services.

risorius (ri SOR ee us) Muscle from the corner of the mouth to the masseter; draws mouth out and back.

roller A cylindrical object on which hair is rolled in order to curl it

roller base The section of hair at the scalp that is parted off for a sculpture curl or a roller.

rouge Cheek color, available in cream, dry, liquid, brush-on, and moisturized form.

round Describing a moonshaped face.

rubbing alcohol An isopropyl alcohol that can be rubbed on the skin to stimulate the tissues.

sacral (SAC ral) Five fused bones beneath the lumbar vertebrae.

saliva The fluid secreted by the salivary glands; spittle.

salivary gland (SAL i vair ee GLAND) The gland in the mouth that secretes saliva.

salt bond *See* **ionic bond.**

sanitizing The physical or chemical means used to keep the salon and its equipment as clean and free of germs as possible.

scabies (SKAY beez) A contagious disease caused by a mite.

scalp The thick layer of skin covering the top of the head.

scalp-and-hair conditioner A cosmetic applied to the hair and scalp to prevent dryness and brittleness.

scapula (SKAP yoo lah) The back of the shoulder, forming a part of the socket for the arm; the shoulder blade.

scissor An instrument used for cutting and shaping the hair.

sculpture curl A curl made by circling the hair around like a spring, with each circle slightly smaller than the one before and with the ends of the hair in the center of the circle.

sculptured nails Artificial nails, either brush-on or applied by means of a special mold.

sebaceous glands (si BAY shus) Glands that secrete oils vital to the skin.

seborrhea (seb or REE ah) A condition cause by overactivity of the sebaceous glands.

seborrhea oleosa (oh lee OH sa) Oily dandruff.

sebum (SEE bum) The fatty matter secreted by the sebaceous glands.

secondary colors Orange, purple, and green.

secondary irritant Alkaline chemical agents that cause serious skin eruptions.

secretory nerve The nerve that affects the activity of the sweat and oil glands.

secretion (se KREE shun) The discharge of hormones or other vital products by the glands.

sectioning Dividing the hair into separate parts in preparation for hairshaping or hairstyling.

semipermanent hair color A non-permanent hair color that coats and stains the hair, imparting color without peroxide.

sensitivity The quality of skin that causes it to be easily affected by cosmetic products, chemicals, or heat.

sensory nerve receptors Nerve endings that convey messages to the brain and spinal cord and react to heat, cold, pain, and pressure.

sepsis A poisoned state caused by the spread of pathogenic bacteria from a region of infection to the bloodstream.

septic Relating to, or characteristic of, sepsis.

setting lotion Lotion used to help provide better hair control and manageability; it is available in either liquid or gel form.

shade The gradation of difference between one hair color and another.

shampoo To cleanse the hair and scalp with soap and water

shampoo basin A basin, usually mounted to a wall, used in giving a shampoo.

shampoo-in color A type of glamour shampoo.

shaping In hairstyling, hair that has been molded in a straight line vertically, horizontally, or on the bias.

shears An instrument used for cutting or shaping.

sheen Brightness or luster.

shell The path electrons take around the center of an atom; orbit.

shock The condition that results when an electric current passes through the body. *See also* **local shock** and **general shock**.

short circuit An accidental direct contact between a supply wire and a return wire in an electric circuit; generates heat and can cause fire.

single-application tint A one-process penetrating tint.

single flat wrap The process of using a single endpaper placed lengthwise on top of the hair strand when wrapping a permanent.

single-prong clips Used to pin small curls or stand-up curls on thin hair.

sinusoidal current (SEYE nus OI dal) Alternating current of a safe level.

sizing Fitting or altering a wig to fit a person's head.

skeletal system The bony framework of the body.

skin debris Skin cells that have been shed.

skip wave A hairstyle that combines pin curls and finger waving.

slip The soft, slippery feeling talc imparts to face powder.

slithering Cutting hair with shears or scissors by sliding up and down the hair strand in order to remove lengths at various intervals.

small intestine The region of the digestive system where absorption of nutrients takes place.

smooth muscle *See* **involuntary muscle**.

soap cap A type of glamour shampoo.

sodium hydroxide (heye DROK syd) Caustic in chemical used in hair straightening.

sodium hypochlorite (heye poh KLOR ite) An inexpensive disinfectant used to cleanse implements; household bleach.

sodium perborate (per BOH rayt) Ingredient in hair lighteners; forms peroxide when mixed with water.

softening Applying a chemical to the hair to make it more receptive to waving, straightening, and coloring.

soft press A hairpressing treatment that removes 60 to 70 percent of the curl.

soft water Water that is low in minerals and that lathers easily with soap.

solution A mixture of two or more substances, one of which is dissolved in the other.

solvent A compound that will dissolve another substance.

space Movements, directions, and shapes within a form.

spectrum The name for the whole set of wavelengths present in electromagnetic radiation; specifically, the band of colored light that results when light passes through a prism.

sphenoid (SFEE noid) Bone that forms the front base of the skull behind the eyes and the nose.

spinal A division of the 11th cranial nerve; acts on the sternocleidomastoid and trapezium muscles. **spinal cord** The portion of the central nervous system contained in the spine.

spiral curl A curl formed by feeding hair into a curling iron so that it "spirals" toward the tip of the iron.

spiraled rollers Rollers that are placed on a flat base, with the ends of the hair rolled up completely to create volume or fullness.

spirilla (spy RIL ah) Corkscrew- or comma-shaped bacteria.

spirillum (spy RIL um) Singular of spirilla.

spleen An organ serving as a storage place for red blood cells.

spore An inactive bacterium that forms a hard shell-like outer covering.

square Describing a face with a fairly even width from forehead to jaws.

square parting A box-shaped section as the base for a sculpture or pin curl.

stand-up curl A coiled curl that stands up from the scalp.

staphylococci (staf lo KOK seye) Cocci that divide and grow in clusters or bunches; found in pustules, boils, abscesses.

steamer A device that provides moist heat for conditioning the scalp or face.

steatoma (stee ah TOH mah) A tumor of the sebaceous glands that forms under the skin.

stemmed base A curl foundation that consists of sectioned hair directed away from the scalp.

sterilization The process of killing all microorganisms. **sternocleidomastoid** (ster noh kly do MAS toid) Muscle that runs from the collarbone and chest bones to

behind the ear; draws head forward, back, and sideways.

sternum The breastbone.

straightener A product used to break hair bonds in order to relax curly or kinky hair.

straightening comb Comb used for straightening curly hair.

strong irritants See **secondary irritants**.

strand test Application of a chemical-waving straightening, or coloring product to an individual strand of hair to determine its effect before continuing with the service.

stratum corneum (STRAT um KOHR nee um) The tough, nearly waterproof surface layer of the skin. **stratum germinativum** (jur mi noh TIV um) The innermost or deepest layer of the epidermis in which new skin cells are formed.

stratum granulosum (gran yoo LOH sum) The layer of the epidermis that contains nearly dead cells that move toward the surface of the skin to replace cells in the cornified layer that have worn away.

stratum lucidum (LOO si dum) The clear layer of the epidermis through which light can pass.

streaking The process by which strips of hair are sectioned out and lightened.

streptococci (strep to KOK seye) Cocci that grow in chains; cause sore throat and blood poisoning.

stretch base A wig cap made of elastic that stretches to fit most heads.

stretch wig Wig made of reinforced elastic to permit a greater variation of fit.

striated muscle (STRY ayt ed) See **voluntary muscle**.

stripping Lightening or removing color from the hair.

style comb A comb with a numbered scale that can be used to measure lengths of hair; it has both coarse and fine teeth so that it can be used on any texture of hair.

styling aid A product used in wet or thermal styling to prevent hair damage.

styling chair The chair in which the patron sits while his or her hair is being styled.

styling station The work area that is allotted to each operator in the salon.

subcutaneous (sub kyoo TAY nee us) Located beneath the surface of the skin.

subjective symptom A symptom of a disorder that is felt by the person but is not visible to others. See **objective symptom**.

subsection To part off sections within a section.

sudoriferous glands (soo dohr IF er us) The glands that excrete sweat.

sulfur A nonmetallic element; two sulfur atoms form crosslinks that give hair its shape.

sulphonated oil (SUL fuh nay ted) An oil mixed or treated with sulfuric acid; used in hair lighteners and soapless shampoos.

sun protection factor A measurement of the degree of protection from the sun's harmful rays found in suntanning products; abbreviated SPF.

superficial temporal The main artery that supplies blood to the skin and muscles at the front, sides, and top of the head; the muscles of chewing.

superfluous Unwanted; excessive.

superior auricularis Muscle located above the ar; draws ear upward.

superior vena cava (VEE na KAY va) The large vein that carries blood from the head, chest, and arms to the heart.

supinator (SOO pi nay tohr) Muscle located in the forearm, turns hand so that the palm faces forward.

surfactant (sir FACT ant) A surface active agent that reduces surface tension when it is dissolved in water.

swab A stick wrapped with

absorbent cotton used for the application of solutions.

sweat pore A tiny opening on the surface of the skin through which sweat reaches the surface.

switch A woven length of hair with one, two, or three strands; can be used to create a number of hairstyles, including the French twist, chignon, and ponytail.

swivel clamp A clamp used to attach the wig block to a work table.

synovial fluid (si NOH vee al) A white fluid surrounding the joints that keeps them lubricated.

synthetic bristle brush A brush made of artificial bristles, usually nylon.

synthetic hair Artificial fibers used in the construction of wigs and hairpieces; not as manageable as human hair.

tactile corpuscles Nerve endings responsible for the sense of touch.

tapering shears Shears used to thin hair where there is too much bulk; may also be used to blend and shape stubby and blunt ends.

tapotement (ta POHT mahnt) A massage movement that involves taping the surface of the skin with the hand or flexed fingers.

teasing See **lacing**.

telogen phase The period during which the hair rests and does not grow.

temporal A division of the 7th cranial nerve; acts on muscles above and in front of the ears, eyelids, eyebrows, and upper cheeks.

temporal bones Two bones that form the sides of the skill below the parietals.

temporalis (tem poh RAY lis) Muscle located beneath the superior auricular; opens and closes jaw during chewing.

temporary color A tint that coats the hair shaft and affects only the cuticle layer.

tendon A membrane that attaches muscles to bones, cartilage, and ligaments.

tensile strength (TEN sill) The resistance any material offers to forces trying to pull it apart.

tepid Moderately warm.

testes (TES teez) Small reproductive glands.

testosterone (tes TAHS teh rohn) A male hormone.

tetanus A disease that causes spasms of the voluntary muscles; known as lockjaw when confined to the muscles of the lower jaw.

texture The general quality and feel of the hair; coarseness or fineness.

thermal Relating to heat.

thermal cap A heating cap used with corrective hair preparations such as oils, proteins, and moisturizers.

thermal hair straightening The process of temporarily rearranging the basic structure of overly curly hair into a form by pressing with a hop pressing comb.

thermal styling Dressing the hair by means of electrical equipment or heat.

thinning shears See **tapering shears**.

thioglycolate (THEYE oh GLEYE kol ayt) See **ammonium. thioglycolate**.

thioglycollic acid (theye oh GLEYE kol ik) A reducing agent typically combined with ammonia or another amine.

thoracic duct (tho RAS ik DUKT) A major lymph channel that helps to drain the body.

thorax The portion of the body between the neck and the abdomen; the cavity in which the heart and lungs lie.

three-color effect A high-fashion effect in which the hair is prelightened to one shade, while two shades of toner are used in various other sections.

three-dimensional shading An effect in which the hair is prelightened and then two shades of toner and one shade of tint are used.

three-wire system A system that used a ground wire in addition to the usual feed and return wires of an electric plug.

thrombocytes (THROM boh syts) Blood platelets.

thyroid A large ductless gland in the neck.

thyroxine (thy ROX zeen) A hormone secreted by the thyroid gland that regulates the body metabolism and controls weight.

tincture of iodine A solution used to cleanse cuts and small wounds.

tinea (TIN ee ah) Ringworm.

tinea capitis (KAP i tis) Ringworm of the scalp.

tinea corporis (KOR por is) Ringworm of the hands.

tinea pedis (PED is) Ringworm of the feet; athlete's foot.

tinea unguium (UN gwee um) Ringworm of the fingernail.

tint To color the hair; a product used to color the hair.

tint back A technique to return lightened hair to its natural hair color or to go to a darker shade.

tipping Lightening the hair ends, especially at the front of the head.

tissue A collection of cells, usually of a similar kind, that form one of the structural materials of a plant or animal.

tonality The warmness or coolness of a color.

toner An aniline derivative of very delicate, light shades that is used on previously lightened hair.

top coat A liquid applied over colored nail polish to prevent chipping; gives a hard, glossy finish and strengthens the nail.

toupee (too PAY) A small wig or hairpiece used to cover the top or crown of the head.

toxin (TOX in) Poison produced by chemical substances that enter the bloodstream and tissues.

T-pins Pins used for holding a hairpiece on a block while it is being styled.

trachea (TRAY kee ah) The air passageway to the lungs; the windpipe.

traction baldness (TRAC shun BALD nes) Hair loss caused by stress from pulling. Tight braids often cause this type of baldness.

transverse capular (TRANZ vurs SKAP yoo lar) The main artery that supplies blood to the front and back of the shoulder and the shoulder joint.

trapezius (tra PEE zee us) Muscle located at the back of the neck and upper part of the back; raises and lowers shoulders.

triangle Describing a face with a narrow forehead and wide jaw.

triangularis (treye ang yoo LAY ris) Muscle from the side of the chin to the corner of the mouth; draws mouth down.

triceps (TREYE seps) Muscle located at the back of the upper arm; extends forearm.

trichology (treye KOHL oh jee) The study of hair.

trichoptilosis (TRIK op ti LOH sis) Split hair ends, a disease of the hair shaft.

trichorrhexis nodosa (TRIK oh rek sis no DOH sah) Knotted hair, a disease of the hair shaft.

tricolor blonding (TREYE KUL ohr BLAHND ing) A technique in which various shades of color graduate from the darkest to the lightest according to the structure of the head.

trigeminal (treye GEM i nal) The 55th cranial nerve.

tuck A folded-over flat seam used in altering a wig cap.

turbinates (TUR bi nayts) Two bones located at the side walls of the nasal cavity.

tweezing Removal of excess hair in the eyebrow area by means of tweezers.

tyrosine (TIE ro seen) An amino acid essential for the creation of natural melanin.

T-zone (TEE ZOHN) An area of the face that cuts across the forehead and down the nose.

ulna (UL nah) The smaller bone of the forearm, located on the little finger side.

ulnar (UL nar) The main artery that supplied blood to the back of the forearm and hand.

ultraviolet A portion of the spectrum lying outside the visible range and above the violet band; abbreviated UV.

underprocessed hair Hair that had little or no change in structure because of insufficient exposure to the chemical action of waving lotion.**ureter** (yoo REE ter) A duct that carries urine away from a kidney to the bladder.

urine Liquid that passes from the kidneys to the bladder, containing waste materials that the kidneys have filtered from the blood.

USP Abbreviation for United States Pharmacopoeia, the official United States book of standard drugs; on a label, USP means that the product meets the standards of the United States Pharmacopoeia.

UV *See* **ultraviolet**.

vaccination Administration of a vaccine, usually by injection.

vaccine Any substance used for preventive inoculation that is designed to produce or increase immunity to a particular disease.

valence (VAY lens) The combining capicity of an atom.

value The lightness or darkness of a color. Also known as *level* or *depth*.

vector *See* **disease vector**.

vegetable dye A coating tint made from a plant; henna is an example.

veins Tubelike vessels that transport blood to the heart.

ventricle The chamber of the heart that receives the blood from the auricle.

vertical Running or moving from top to bottom.

vibrate To shake.

vibrator An electrical device used for massage purposes; causes a shaking motion that stimulates circulation.

villi (VIL ee) Minute projections in the intestine that aid in absorbing nutriments into the blood.

virgin hair Normal hair which has had no previous bleaching or tinting treatments.

virus Microscopic pathogenic particles of unknown origin.

visible light Light that can be seen.

vitamin An organic substance essential to good health and proper nutrition.

vitamin A A vitamin essential to the health of the skin, hair, and nails; main sources are butter, carrots, leafy vegetables, sweet potatoes.

vitamin B A group of vitamins important to the nervous system and the skin; main sources are breads, cereals, milk, green leafy vegetables, fresh meat.

vitamin C A vitamin essential for healthy teeth and gums; main sources are citrus fruits, tomatoes, melons, strawberries.

vitamin D A vitamin important for strong bones and teeth; main sources are milk, egg yolks, liver.

vitiligo (vit ih LEYE goh) White blotches, usually on the arms, and neck, caused by the absence of pigment.

volt The unit used to measure voltage.

voltage The pressure or push that moves the current in an electric circuit.

volume Term used to describe the amount of oxygen a particular amount of hydrogen peroxide can produce; for example, 20-volume hydrogen peroxide can produce an amount of oxygen equal to 20 times its own volume; also, height or lift in a hairstyle.

voluntary muscle A muscle whose activity is controlled by the will.

vomer (VOH mer) Bone located at the back of the nasal cavity.

washing soda Sodium carbonate; a water softener.

water-wrapped perm A permanent wave that is wrapped with water; the waving lotion is applied after the entire head is wrapped for greater control in timing.

watt The unit used to measure electrical power.

wax A special kind of organic compound that is often used to remove excessive hair growth.

weak irritants *See* **primary irritants**.

weaving Used to camouflage thining or balding hair, this technique involves the sewing or gluing of wefts of artificial hair in tracks of the client's own hair.

weft A machine-stitched or hand-woven strip of hair.

wedged parting A triangular section used as the base for a stand-up curl.

wen *See* **steatoma**.

wet sanitizer A container that is filled with enough germicidal solution to cover tools and implements completely.

wetting agent A substance, such as a detergent, that helps tint to penetrate into the hair.

whitehead *See* **milia**.

wig An artificial head covering made of human hair or a synthetic fiber.

wig block A leather, wood canvas, or styrofoam form to which a wig is attached during styling, cleaning, and so forth.

wig cap The mesh foundation to which hair is attached in the manufacture of a wig.

wiglet A hairpiece with a flat base that is used to create special styles; smaller than a wig.

wiry hair Hair that has a smooth, hard, glossy surface that makes it resistant to waving.

wrinkles Lines that occur as skin loses its elasticity.

yak A type of long-haired ox whose hair is used in making wigs; matches the lightest white human hair.

yeast A one-celled fungus.

zinc oxide A chemical used in some face packs to neutralize excess acid or alkali on the skin.

zygomatic (zeye goh MAT ik) A division of the 7th cranial nerve; acts on muscles of the upper cheeks, upper lips, and sides of the nose.

zygomatic bones Two bones located in the upper cheeks; form the floor of the eye cavity.

zygomaticus (zeye goh MAT i kus) Muscle from the corner of the mouth to the zygomatic bone; draws mouth up and back.

INDEX